DISEASE IN EVOLUTION

GLOBAL CHANGES AND EMERGENCE
OF INFECTIOUS DISEASES

ANNALS OF THE NEW YORK ACADEMY OF SCIENCES
Volume 740

DISEASE IN EVOLUTION

GLOBAL CHANGES AND EMERGENCE
OF INFECTIOUS DISEASES

Edited by Mary E. Wilson, Richard Levins, and Andrew Spielman

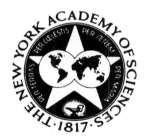

The New York Academy of Sciences
New York, New York
1994

COVER: The art on the printed cover is taken from the paper in this volume by Tamara Awerbuch and appears on p. 233.

Library of Congress Cataloging-in-Publication Data

Disease in evolution : global changes and emergence of infectious
   diseases / edited by Mary E. Wilson, Richard Levins, and Andrew
   Spielman.
       p.   cm. — (Annals of the New York Academy of Sciences, ISSN
   0077-8923 ; v. 740)
       Includes bibliographical references and indexes.
       ISBN 0-89766-876-6 (cloth : alk. paper). — ISBN 0-89766-877-4
   (paper : alk. paper)
       1. Epidemiology—Congresses.   2. Medical geography—Congresses.
   I. Wilson, Mary E.   II. Levins, Richard.   III. Spielman A. (Andrew)
   IV. Series.
       [DNLM: 1. Communicable Diseases—transmission—congresses.
   2. Communicable Disease Control—congresses. 3. Environmental
   Health—congresses. 4. Evolution—congresses. W1 AN626YL v. 740
   1994 / WA 110 D612 1995]
   Q11.N5 vol. 740
   [RA648.6]
   500 s—dc20
   [614.4′9]
   DNLM/DLC
   for Library of Congress   94-34169
                                                                        CIP

BiComp/PCP
Printed in the United States of America
ISBN 0-89766-876-6 (cloth)
ISBN 0-89766-877-4 (paper)
ISSN 0077-8923

ANNALS OF THE NEW YORK ACADEMY OF SCIENCES
Volume 740
December 15, 1994

DISEASE IN EVOLUTION

GLOBAL CHANGES AND EMERGENCE OF INFECTIOUS DISEASES[a]

Editors

MARY E. WILSON, RICHARD LEVINS, AND ANDREW SPIELMAN

Conference Coordinator

IRINA ECKARDT

Conference Organizers

TAMARA AWERBUCH, UWE BRINKMANN, PAUL R. EPSTEIN, LAURIE GARRETT, RICHARD LEVINS, CRISTINA DE A. POSSAS, CHARLES PUCCIA, ANDREW SPIELMAN, AND MARY E. WILSON

CONTENTS

[a] This volume is the result of a conference entitled **Emerging Diseases Workshop** held November 7–10, 1993 in Woods Hole, Massachusetts.

Part II. Remote Sensing Images

Part III. Vector-borne/Terrestrial Diseases
Edited by Mary E. Wilson and Andrew Spielman

Part IV. Mathematical Modeling
Edited by Richard Levins

Part V. Theoretical and Social Approaches
Edited by Irina Eckardt

Part VI. Surveillance
Edited by Irina Eckardt

Part VII. Conceptual Framework
Edited by Irina Eckardt

Part VIII. Research Agenda

Financial assistance was received from:

- **The John D. and Catherine T. MacArthur Foundation—a grant made to Harvard University in support of the Human Security Program of the Common Security Forum**
- **The Rockefeller Foundation**

Preface

This volume emerges from ideas shaped during a workshop held at Woods Hole, Massachusetts in November 1993. The intellectual groundwork for the workshop was built over many years. In the fall of 1991 two professors at the Harvard School of Public Health, Richard Levins and Uwe Brinkmann, invited a handful of colleagues and acquaintances to join in a series of discussions about new diseases. Those who participated in those early discussions brought experience and training from a range of disciplines—ecology, entomology, epidemiology, infectious diseases, population biology, mathematical modeling, international health, evolutionary biology, climate, environmental analysis, and marine ecology, among others. We threw ideas into a crucible for testing and remolding. We marveled at concepts and ideas that were at the fringe of our understanding. We strained to look at data and events simultaneously through the prism of other disciplines and across a range of approaches. We tried to bridge the gulfs that separated us by language, paradigms, scientific tools, and priorities. We discussed causality, conceptual frameworks, evolution, epistemology, vulnerability, as well as specific diseases—cholera, tuberculosis, malaria and others.

We invited outside speakers to share with us their ideas and intellectual energy. The exchanges were often unruly, escaping any conventional format or structure. The process, while always challenging and sometimes exhilarating, exposed each of us to the gaps in our own knowledge and experience.

We decided to organize a workshop with invited experts to expand the disciplines represented and to catalyze our thinking. We wanted to capture our ideas in a book to reach a wider audience so that others could critically evaluate, learn from and move beyond our experiences.

In June 1993 Uwe Brinkmann, one of the founding members of our group, died suddenly and unexpectedly while on a field trip to Brazil. His death left a void we felt personally and intellectually. We had lost a friend and someone who facilitated our work through his leadership, broad experience, capacity to think creatively across disciplines, and his love of intellectual exploration. After discussion and reorganization, we decided to continue with plans for the meeting and book and to dedicate both to him. This book would have been enriched by his participation in the meeting, though his thinking certainly shaped our content and approach. We hope it is worthy of his high standards.

Many participants prepared papers that were distributed to all participants the month before the meeting. The primary goal of our workshop was to advance the intellectual understanding of disease emergence. We brought together participants from diverse disciplines in hopes of uncovering creative, new ways to approach the field. We included persons whose work focused on plants and animals, as important lessons can come from kingdoms biologically remote from the human species. We aimed to devise a transdisciplinary conceptual framework for approaching the problem of emerging diseases, to identify research priorities, and to create a research agenda as a policy guide for individuals and institutions trying to predict and interdict emerging diseases. We took a broad view and sought a comprehensive understanding of disease emergence, drawing on the biological and ecological context and looking beyond surveillance to identify ways to anticipate disease emergence.

The format of the meeting shaped both our discussions and organization of the book. We conducted small group working sessions as well as plenary sessions, intended to allow exchange across disciplines along with integration and conceptualization. Sections of this book include papers prepared for the meeting as well as concept papers and summaries of discussions held by the working groups prepared during the workshop. The edited versions of exchanges during the plenary sessions are also included.

The diseases used in case studies reflect research activities of the participants. Although we did not specifically devote sessions to AIDS and tuberculosis, two diseases that are arguably among the most important infectious diseases confronting us, the process of thinking and the approach we want to foster are relevant to all diseases. The specific examples chosen are of secondary importance. Even though early in our discussions we decided to focus on infectious diseases, the need exists for broad transdisciplinary approaches to other emerging diseases and problems, such as asthma, certain types of malignancies, environmental toxins, violence, and others.

We see this volume as work in progress. It reflects our attempt to capture dialogue across disciplines while trying to think creatively about approaches to infectious disease threats of today and tomorrow. The Woods Hole workshop was one stage in a process we hope will continue.

Acknowledgments

We owe thanks to many. Lincoln Chen, the Chair of Population and International Health offered steadfast support for our work. We received early financial support from the John D. and Catherine T. MacArthur Foundation through a grant made to Harvard University in support of the Human Security Program of the Common Security Forum. We also received generous support from The Rockefeller Foundation. The book could not have been completed without this assistance.

We thank the New York Academy of Sciences for their assistance in recording and transcribing the meeting and in the preparation of the book.

Several members of the New Disease group who did not prepare formal papers for this volume were actively involved throughout our discussions and seminar series and influenced our thinking and approaches to problems. Richard Cash, Agnes Brinkmann, Najwa Makhoul, and Paul Wise were among those who gave energy and ideas to the group through many seasons.

Irina Eckardt and Paul Epstein deserve special thanks for their contributions before, during and after the meeting. As section editors they helped to shape the book. Through the seminars they have been instrumental in helping to educate participants and to reach out to other disciplines.

MARY E. WILSON
Harvard University
Cambridge, Massachusetts

New Disease Workshop: Dedication to Uwe Brinkmann

The members of the Harvard Working Group on New and Resurgent Disease want to dedicate this conference and the resulting publication to the memory of our colleague and friend Uwe Brinkmann, who worked with us from the start of our project more than a year ago and who died suddenly in June while this conference was being planned.

Uwe arrived at Harvard in a whirlwind of activity three years ago, full of energy, ideas and enthusiasm. He was a happy man, doing the work he loved. He had multiple rewards: the joy of discovering solutions to difficult problems, the awareness of helping to meet urgent human needs, the exhuberance of play on encountering a new toy such as some software package that allowed more colorful displays of data in exotic juxtapositions. He twinkled with the special pleasure of recounting how he thwarted or evaded a particularly stubborn obstruction or with the wry irony as he reported on frustrations still in place. He glowed with the satisfaction of sharing his insights and experiences with students and colleagues.

He was a physician, the first to treat a patient with Lassa Fever in Europe although this meant living in total quarantine for weeks while the press denounced him for threatening the survival of Germany. He was also a critic of medical narrowness. He was completely without the defensiveness with which that profession often responds to external criticism and added the rich detail of his own knowledge to developing that criticism. He worked mostly at the levels of field epidemiology and epidemiological policy and from there reached out to engage with excitement the frontier issues of molecular biology, climatology, and economic development.

He was a political person, a social democrat in the best tradition of German social democracy, and saw clearly that disease was as much a matter of poverty and injustice as of vectorial capacity and mutation, that the explosions of AIDS and Malaria in southeast Asia are as much matters of the political economy of prostitution or of deforestation as of immunosuppression and drug resistance. Indeed, his contribution to this conference is not a paper on the ecology of malaria resurgence or any of his other current projects but is on the ambiguous and even harmful effects of economic development as it is most widely conceived and promoted, both curing and spreading disease, generating at the same time affluence and misery, modern health services and the habitats and social relations that make those services necessary, with population displacements and relations of debt that almost guarantee that those services are inadequate.

Uwe had a special interest in the dynamics of working together across disciplinary boundaries. He was generous in sharing his ideas without worrying about putting his name tag on them, open to receiving and using immediately the ideas of others, always exploring ways to assure that everybody was heard and that half-formed ideas were not crushed by criticism before they can show their possibilities. He wanted very much for this conference to produce something that goes beyond what each of us brings with us, and that our discussions be rooted in the strength of disciplinary rigor but also recombine in unexpected ways. The unfamiliar and experimental way in which the sessions have been organized reflect those concerns.

Thus our dedication of this conference to Uwe Brinkmann is more than our remembering a tragic loss. It is also acknowledging an active presence.

RICHARD LEVINS
Harvard University
Cambridge, Massachusetts

The Challenge of New Diseases

RICHARD LEVINS

Department of Population and International Health
Harvard School of Public Health
665 Huntington Avenue
Cambridge, Massachusetts 02115

What brings us here to this workshop is the shared recognition that Public Health as a whole was caught by surprise. The expectation that infectious disease was in decline and that we would continue to see a unidirectional decline toward complete elimination, held on tenaciously even in the face of well known and dramatic exceptions. It was widely assumed that if not the particular means at least the major approaches at our disposal—pesticides, antibiotics, and vaccines—made that decline unproblematic in principle even if difficult in detail.

But finally, this could be asserted no longer. The accumulation of "exceptions" and the frustration of our efforts forced a new awareness that diseases rise and fall, evolve and spread and retreat and spread again, and that we have to prepare for a more complex tomorrow than naive progressivism and simple extrapolation would have us anticipate.

But how do we prepare for tomorrow? One way is to predict tomorrow. Science knows only one way to predict, and that is to imagine tomorrow will be like today. But like what about today?

Vibrios will spread cholera toxin in Bangladesh tomorrow because they do so today. Anopheline mosquitoes will spread malaria as they do today. *Ixodes damini* will continue to transmit Lyme disease in northeast North America as it does today. The aphid *Toxoptera citri* will continue its propagation of tristeza disease of citrus in Panama as it does today. Therefore we have to know better what is happening today in order to know tomorrow.

But tomorrow may be different from today: the vibrio may be transported to new suitable locations and infect new populations or climate change may allow the cyanobacteria and marine invertebrates the vibrio associates with to increase. Anopheles may spread as forests are cleared, Ixodes as forests return, Toxoptera because they feel like it.

So tomorrow will be like today after all: the vibrio will continue to associate with cyanobacteria or copepods tomorrow as it does today, Anopheles will continue in semiopen country and the deer tick will continue to follow the deer. The clandestine trade in citrus budwood will spread tristeza, ocean commerce will continue and even expand, deforestation proceeds apace and global warming will continue as it has. Therefore if we know, not the present locations, but the environmental requirements and mobilities of *Anopheles gambiae,* of *Vibrio cholerae, Ixodes damini* and *Toxoptera citri* today we will know where to look for them tomorrow.

But tomorrow may be different from today: as fishing, climate change and eutrophication continue, the species composition of the plankton community may change, and the vibrio may associate with new species of plankton. Other species of Anopheles, perhaps more tolerant of cold, may pick up Plasmodium from infected animals so that the distribution of *A. gambiae* will no longer be a sufficient guide to the malarial region. Tristeza may spread to other aphids even more expansive and effective as vectors than *Toxoptera citri*.

But then tomorrow will be like today after all: species will continue to expand and contract and adapt as climate and habitat change; species will continue to meet as competitors, mutualists, and comensals, vectors will exchange pathogens through shared hosts. If we know how species interact today we will know about tomorrow.

But tomorrow may be different from today: the mosquitoes will not only expand to the boundaries of their tolerance but that tolerance itself may change. The virulent tristeza virus may be replaced by more benign genotypes, Borelia may adapt from mice to other rodents and allow their ticks to vector Lyme disease.

Then tomorrow will be like today after all: mutation, recombination and natural selection will continue to operate as they do today, and if we understand the microevolutionary processes that operate today we will understand tomorrow.

But tomorrow may be different from today: From among the millions of unknown or rare microorganisms, which of them, like Legionella, will succeed in escaping from the control of their competitors and predators and prosper in the new environments we are creating for them? Which free-living bacteria will adopt the parasitic way of life? Which benign symbiont of our gut will invent a new toxin that gives it access to intracellular nutrients? Among the hundreds of thousands or millions of insects, which will newly come into intimate contact with us and offer its own viruses new opportunities? How will bacteria like the Clavibacteria of tomatoes change their virulence for tomatoes as they pass through potatoes or onions or grasses?

But even that tomorrow will be like today: evolution proceeds as before in every new context, groups with evolutionary plasticity spin off new taxa and invade new niches. And if we know the patterns of macroevolution we are better prepared for that tomorrow as well.

At each step in this narrative we find that the more different tomorrow may be, the more broadly we have to root our theory in order to find the more encompassing similarities that remain. We are already able to prepare for those tomorrows that are most like today, but we remain helplessly exposed to the surprises in those tomorrows that are the most different.

Each expansion of our theoretical breadth transforms more of the different into the similar within the new perspective. Our task in a coherent strategy to face the new is to develop nested theoretical structures, some more general and long range, some more precise, specific and immediate, that together allow us to expect the previously unexpected.

This is not easy to do. It means reaching out beyond the common sense that not only informs our particular disciplines but that many of us helped to create. It means resisting the temptation, so common in interdisciplinary projects, to passively accept each others' expertise and biases in one package and assign chapters for a book that merely summarizes what we already brought in with us. It means looking skeptically at the almost automatic recipes that have guided us in the past so that we inquire of a method, before it breaks down, what are its limitations, what do we do next, what are the alternatives to it, and what do we do if we're wrong?

We hope that both the composition of this workshop and the unfamiliar way in which we have structured the next three days, will bring us closer to these goals. We attempted to achieve many kinds of combinations: detailed intimate knowledge of cases, but drawn from different habitats and taxonomic groups of pathogens; a focus both on human and plant disease; the perspectives from medicine, ecology, evolutionary genetics, social science and philosophy; methodologies of the laboratory, field and blackboard; different approaches to mathematical modeling; occupations that direct us toward immediate as well as long-range results; veteran researchers and new innovators; people whose interests center on the subject matter of this workshop and those whose peripheral interest can bring quite different kinds of insight.

What we are hoping for as a final product from this conference is not recommendations for specific measures to combat particular diseases but rather the beginning of an over all strategy for facing the new and unexpected.

Disease in Evolution

Introduction

MARY E. WILSON

Mount Auburn Hospital
330 Mount Auburn Street
Cambridge, Massachusetts 02238
and
Department of Population and International Health
Harvard School of Public Health
665 Huntington Avenue
Boston, Massachusetts 02115

New diseases are not new. Throughout recorded history previously unknown diseases have appeared or resurfaced in new populations. Until well into the twentieth century, infections were an expected part of the human condition. Then the triumphs of modern science and technology led the public—and many experts—to expect instead nearly complete freedom from infectious diseases. Today, the pendulum of expectation is swinging back. Arguably, the process of emerging disease may be accelerating. Profound changes in the world increase the likelihood that some of the known infectious diseases will increase and that additional, currently unknown infections will be recognized.[1] This new reality challenges our confidence in the power of science and technology to control nature.

Western medicine tends to see the human at the center of an environment that contains microbes with the capacity to invade the human host and cause disease. Microbes are described as invasive, pathogenic, virulent, as hostile enemies. Medicine has sought to eradicate these microbial foes, or at least to eliminate disease caused by them. The imagery is that of a battlefield. And humans have often prevailed. Interventions such as provision of clean water and adequate housing, antimicrobials, vaccines, and vector control, have been remarkably effective. We live in an era that was conditioned by the experience with smallpox, polio, and other public health successes. Even tuberculosis, so much in the news recently, is a minor problem in the United States today relative to the toll it exacted at the turn of this century. (It remains an enormous and growing problem in many parts of the world.) We adopted a way of thinking about infectious diseases predicated on a sequence of identification, intervention, and control or eradication of the pathogen. The declines for tetanus, smallpox, measles, and polio shown in FIGURE 1 set our pattern of expectation—a linear progression from high to low.

An alternative view envisions the human as one of many species eating, assisting and competing with each other in a world where many processes are cyclical or waxing and waning and evolving. Our anthropomorphic view of the serial eradication or control of microbial species to help assure infection-free human survival is shortsighted and probably impossible. Microbes, like

1

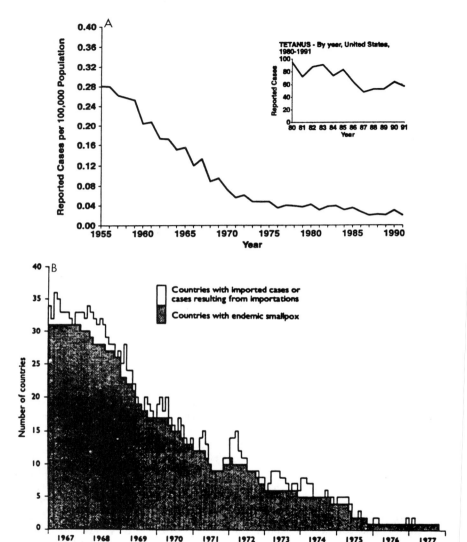

FIGURE 1. Declines in tetanus, smallpox, measles and polio in recent decades. **A**: Tetanus, by year, United States, 1955–1991. **B**: Number of countries experiencing smallpox each year from 1967 to 1978. **C**: Measles (rubeola), by year, United States, 1950–1991. **D**: Poliomyelitis (paralytic), by year, United States, 1951–1991. (**A, C, D** are from the Centers for Disease Control. Summary of notifiable diseases, United States, 1991. *Morbidity and Mortality Weekly Report* **40** [53]. **B** is from F. Fenner, D. A. Henderson, I. Arita, *et al.* 1988. WHO, Geneva.)

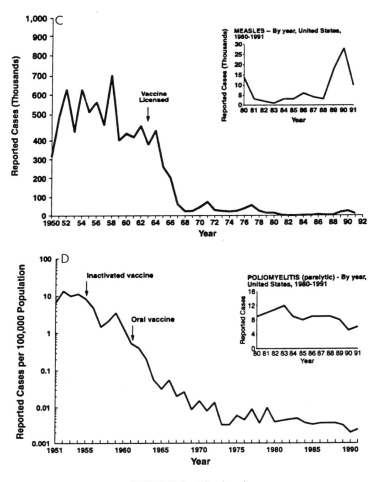

FIGURE 1. (*Continued*)

all life forms, have been selected for survival. Many are essential for life on earth, participating in the growth of plants and animals, the recycling of materials, the synthesis of chemicals, the production of food and antimicrobials. Those that multiply in or on a human host and whose presence causes tissue damage we term pathogens. In the process of multiplying and surviving, some coincidentally kill the human host. Microbes whose survival depends on the human host adapt to the biologic and social environment created by the host. Microbes undergo mutation, recombination, genetic drift and shift; variants escape from vaccine-induced immunity.[2]

Ironically, many of the forces that contribute to the appearance of new diseases and emergence of old ones are created by human activity—in many instances by what we consider extraordinary achievements. We have underestimated the complexity of our environment and the capacity of other species to adapt and evolve. We have overestimated the power of tools, such as antimicrobials, pesticides, and vaccines to free us of disease. We have failed to recognize that events in plants and animals can teach us and affect our health. We have paid little attention to the geoclimatic influences on health. We have too often ignored the social, economic, and political contributions to disease. This book and the conference on which it is based attempt to begin to remedy these shortcomings in knowledge, attention, and expectation.

Several general concepts can help focus the discussions that follow and summarize themes that will run through this volume.

- Disease emergence is complex; often several factors must change sequentially or simultaneously to allow a disease to emerge.
- Infectious diseases are dynamic. New infections will continue to appear, possibly at increasing rates.
- Known infectious diseases will change in distribution, severity and frequency.
- Most new infections are not caused by novel pathogens.
- Human activities are the most potent factors leading to the appearance of new infectious diseases and the change in known infectious diseases.
- Social, economic, climatic, and political forces shape disease patterns and influence emergence.
- Interventions to control infections can paradoxically increase the burden of disease.
- Understanding disease emergence requires looking beyond the organism to the milieu, the ecosystem, and society. A global perspective is essential.

These concepts inform our discussion both of familiar epidemiological issues and of matters previously assumed to lie outside public health practice, including disease recognition, pathogen evolution, the vulnerability of populations, environmental and demographic change, and the role of technology in both the creation and amelioration of health problems. Although many of the illustrative examples that follow come from human disease, examples from plants and animals are also relevant.

RECOGNITION

The pathogens identified in most of the newly named diseases, such as Legionnaires' disease, toxic shock syndrome, Lyme disease, and AIDS are not novel pathogens that appeared *de novo* just prior to the recognition of disease. In most instances of new diseases, the pathogens have been present for centuries or longer. The process that leads to the recognition and naming of a disease often involves social and economic, as well as scientific events. Factors that favor recognition of a disease as new are several: clustering of cases in time or space; increase in prevalence; distinctive signs, symptoms or laboratory findings; short incubation; rapid progression; high mortality or serious sequelae; appearance in a new geographic area or a new population; presence in a highly visible or affluent population.[3] New infectious diseases are most readily identified in a population with good medical resources and low rates of endemic infectious diseases. A new disease associated with high fever, for example, is more likely to be overlooked in an area with high background rates of malaria and other infectious diseases causing fevers. The background noise from other diseases that are common in many tropical and developing countries may camouflage a new disease and delay its recognition. Diseases with very long incubation periods might become evident only with increasing life spans of humans. Technologic advances that allow the identification of microbes or the pathologic or immunologic changes they induce, may be essential not only in naming a disease but in characterizing its clinical range and epidemiology. Cat scratch disease was long assumed to be caused by a microbe carried by cats; only with the development of newer diagnostic technologies has it become possible to identify the agent in humans and cats and to learn that the same microbe is also associated with a totally different pathologic process, bacillary angiomatosis, in AIDS patients.[4]

VULNERABILITY

Many factors affect the vulnerability of populations, whether plants or animals, to disease and death. The current vulnerability of the human population derives from many factors: aging of the population, immunosuppression from AIDS or from medical treatment (such as chemotherapy), medical devices (such as prosthetic valves and joints), and treatments (such as dialysis) that have prolonged the lives of many with disease and disability, crowding, pollution, social upheaval, and movement into new habitats where populations have not yet adapted. One consequence of increased vulnerability is that organisms living in and around us and previously considered harmless commensals are now causing death and disability. Medical journals regularly report the first cases of infection with organisms either never previously identified or not previously recognized as pathogenic. As host defenses fall, a wider range of organisms can enter and survive in the human and, if they can successfully transfer to other humans, may adapt to the human body as a new habitat. An improving standard of living and freedom from exposure to some infections early in life can shift upward the age at which initial infection tends to occur, and for some microbes, paradoxically produce an increase in disease severity when infection does occur. If vaccine-induced immunity wanes more rapidly than immunity after natural infection or if viruses change so that they can escape antibodies induced by a vaccine, we could see diseases in unexpected populations and with unanticipated clinical manifestations. The tenuous nature of control of vaccine-preventable diseases was highlighted by the appearance of outbreaks of diphtheria and polio in 1993 and 1994 in parts of the former Soviet Union at a time of socioeconomic and political instability.

MIGRATION

Natural phenomena—the winds, migrating birds, ocean currents, mobile animals—can carry microbes, seeds, insects, and other biota over great distances. Superimposed on the natural currents of wind, water and migration, are people and their conveyances. The world is crisscrossed by transport mechanisms that carry people as well as animals, plants, and other goods to distant destinations. The rapidity and frequency of travel and extent of migration have profound implications for the introduction and exchange of plant and animal life. Humans may carry a pathogen or vector or both into an area where conditions allow spread to other humans and persistence in the new environment. Genetic differences in a new population may make them unusually vulnerable to introduced infections. One hypothesis for the excess mortality in the New World from infections introduced by Europeans is the lesser genetic diversity in persons in the New World.[5] Humans also carry customs and behavioral patterns which, if introduced and adopted, may lead to disease in a new environment. Human activity has not only increased the rate of spread of organisms but also changed the meaning of distance. Previously, most spread of organisms had been to adjacent areas, a gradual expansion of range. But preferred routes or destinations may make Miami "closer" to New York than to Montgomery, San Salvador closer to San Francisco than to Guatemala City, Sarajevo closer to Vienna than to Belgrade.

In addition to transporting people and goods to new locations, ships convey marine organisms (flora and fauna) on their hulls and in their ballast water, which is taken on at one site and discharged at another. In one survey, 367 different species were identified in ballast water of ships traveling between Japan and Coos Bay, Oregon.[6] Some may be harmless though many introductions have been detrimental to their new ecosystem. In Australia, an estimated 60 million tons of ballast water are discharged each year to 40 ports.[7] Introduced species, such as jelly-fish like, tentacled creatures called ctenophores (*Mnemiopsis leidyi*), have devastated local fishing in the Black and Azov Seas.[8] Ships may have been the vehicle for the recent introduction of *Vibrio cholerae* into South America and the subsequent massive and ongoing epidemic of human disease. Vibrio O139 has spread along waterways, though the human traffic along these routes may be critical elements in its spread.

Many events contribute to migration of humans—war, political unrest, economic crisis, natural disasters such as earthquakes, climatic change, work, and exploration. Movement into remote or previously unexplored geographic areas, whether for adventure or land development, is frequently accompanied by the appearance of new diseases. Pathogens are often ones not previously known. These microbes often live in or on animals or in the soil. Arthropod vectors and animals may be involved in maintenance and spread.

Movement from rural to urban areas often leads to different kinds of diseases. In many countries migration from the countryside to urban areas has led to the development of an historically new habitat, the huge periurban slum areas that provide an environment permissive for the spread of infections not typically seen in urban areas. New construction sites, poor garbage disposal, inadequate piped water leading to water storage in open containers, and unscreened dwellings permit breeding grounds for arthropod vectors and rodents and ready access to humans. Traffic between periurban slums and rural areas provides ongoing exchange of microbes in both directions. Poor access to medical care means that treatment may be delayed and diseases may go unrecognized and spread of infection facilitated. Slum dwellers are often more vulnerable to infection due to malnutrition, exposure to pollutants, crowding, and loss of their rural support networks.

TECHNOLOGIC PROGRESS

Technologic advances have expanded the spectrum of possible diseases and the capacity for transmission. Medical advances allowing survival of persons vulnerable to a broader range of pathogens have already been mentioned. Antimicrobials have doubtlessly saved millions of lives—but for a price. The selective pressure exerted by the wide use of antimicrobials in humans and animals has fostered the emergence and spread of resistant organisms. Use of antimicrobials has set the stage for outbreaks of *Clostridium difficile* colitis and nosocomial infections with organisms resistant to all known antimicrobials.

Tissue and organ transplantation offers a new route for disease transmission. Use of animals as a source of organs expands the possible range of organisms that may be introduced and makes it critical to understand better the transfer of microbes from one species to another.[9] At the same time, immunosuppression in transplantation patients makes it easier for new pathogens to invade the body successfully. With respect to species barriers, the outbreak of bovine spongiform encephalopathy in the United Kingdom has put a spotlight on the issue and is an instructive case. Scrapie, a disease of sheep, has long been recognized in the United Kingdom. Sheep unfit for human consumption are sent to rendering plants where ruminant meat and bone meal are prepared as a cheap source of animal protein, fed to weaned calves. Economic pressures brought on by the oil crisis in the early 1980s apparently led renderers to adopt energy efficient methods to prepare animal tissues. The altered technique was less likely to destroy the highly heat-resistant scrapie agent. In late 1986 a dairy farmer in Kent, noting strange behavior in his cows, sent brain tissue to a special laboratory where the neuropathologist noted a pathologic appearance consistent with scrapie. The disease in cows was named bovine spongiform encephalopathy (BSE) and became known colloquially as mad cow disease. Although use of ruminant-derived protein in food for cattle or sheep was banned in the United Kingdom in 1987, in 1990 there were still reported roughly 600 new cases of BSE per month in cows.

We have insufficient understanding of species differences in the factors that permit microbes to infect and cause disease. When can we expect species-to-species spread? The hantavirus, seemingly a harmless commensal in rodents, can produce fulminant disease in humans. A recent outbreak of a yet-to-be-identified virus that caused encephalitis-like symptoms in a colony of baboons used for human organ transplants underscores the urgent need for research in species differences in susceptibility to various microbes.

Modern technology has done much to protect public facilities, such as municipal water supplies, recycled air masses in buildings and subways, central-ized meat packing and hospital wards, from contamination. But the low probability of disaster is partially offset by a growing number of opportunities and the much greater impact when something goes wrong. Large municipal systems supply large populations with water. When a break in the system or contamination occurs, the magnitude of the resulting epidemic can be massive, as was seen in the Milwaukee outbreak of cryptosporidiosis in the spring of 1993, estimated to have caused illness in 403,000 persons.[10] More than 4000 persons required hospitalization. Mass processing and wide distribution networks have expanded the size of outbreaks from salmonella traced to milk, chicken and other foods.

> Land development often alters the environment in ways that reduce biodiversity; agricultural practices increasingly rely on a few species of plants, chosen for market potential. Biodiversity in many spheres may lend resiliency and stability to populations. For example, studies in grasslands show that primary productivity in a more diverse plant com-munity is more resistant to and recovers more fully from a major drought.[11]

The history of tuberculosis illustrates the many forces that affect disease frequency, and expression, and spread. Urbanization and crowding in the 19th century facilitated the spread of tuberculosis, which remained the most common cause of death in many parts of Europe and North America into the early 20th century. At the turn of the century, annual mortality rates from tuberculosis exceeded 200 per 100,000 population in New York, Boston, and Philadelphia. For comparison, annual mortality rates from tuberculosis in the United States in the early 1990s were less than 1 per 100,000; reported cases of tuberculosis are approximately 10 per 100,000 population. In the United States and Europe, morbidity and mortality from tuberculosis declined long before there was any effective chemotherapy or vaccine (FIG. 2). Addition of these modalities had a modest influence on the overall rates in the United States. The influence of socioeconomic and political factors on rates of disease are strikingly evident in the rise in tuberculosis during WW I and WW II that occurred even in unoccupied countries (FIG. 3). Genetic changes in populations may also have influenced the impact of tuberculosis over a long time frame. Tuberculosis often killed before reproductive, age so it could have had a selective influence over several generations. The upsurge of tuberculo-sis in many parts of the world in the last decade has been pushed by many factors: expansion of the HIV-infected population, lack of access to

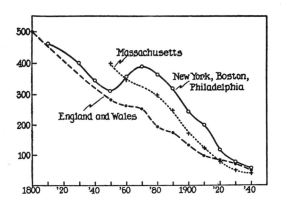

FIGURE 2. Deaths from tuberculosis. The figures at the bottom indicate the years, those at the left the number of deaths per year, per 100,000 population. (Modified from *The White Plague: Tuberculosis, Man, Society.* René Dubos and Jean Dubos. New Brunswick, NJ & London: Rutgers University Press. Used with permission.)

therapy, increasing resistance of *M. tuberculosis* to commonly used drugs, communal living conditions that favor spread. At the same time disease has increased, the spectrum of clinical findings has expanded to include rare and previously unreported syndromes, so that recognition may be delayed. In the United States today we see the convergence of changes in the host, changes in the microbe, and changes in the social milieu, which favor exposure and decrease the likelihood of early recognition and effective treatment. In many parts of the world, the drugs that can effectively cure drug-susceptible disease have been unavailable for economic reasons.

Infections with nontuberculous mycobacteria (especially *Mycobacterium avium* complex or MAC) have increased dramatically in recent years. A contributing factor is the substrate provided by the enlarging population of persons made vulnerable because of HIV, increasing age, underlying diseases, and chemotherapy. Studies in progress suggest exposure may also be increasing.[12] In the United States piped water systems used to deliver water to institutions and homes may also distribute nontuberculous mycobacteria, organisms found widely in soil and in natural water sources. MAC can survive in chlorinated water. The usual temperatures used for water in institutions, such as hospitals, do not kill MAC. In fact, the warm temperatures in hospital water supplies encourage the proliferation of MAC.[13] Holding tanks and continuous recirculation of hot water, common to many institutions, may allow these mycobacteria to persist and even multiply. Composition of water pipes may also affect growth. For example, presence of higher concentrations of zinc in natural waters is associated with increased rates of recovery of MAC. Yet unknown is whether pipes made from zinc alloys affect bacterial composition of water. Recent work suggests that water distribution systems in hospitals may be an important source of nontuberculous mycobacteria that infect HIV-infected persons.[14]

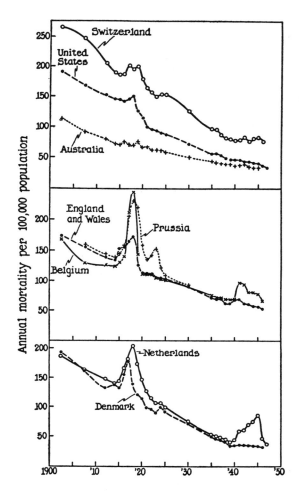

FIGURE 3. Deaths from tuberculosis. The figures at the bottom indicate the years, those at the left the number of deaths per year, per 100,000 population. (Modified from *The White Plague: Tuberculosis, Man, Society*. René Dubos and Jean Dubos. New Brunswick, NJ & London: Rutgers University Press. Used with permission.)

PERSPECTIVE

In confronting the prospect of new and emerging diseases we must avoid both complacency and panic. Recent newspaper articles proclaim that deaths from infections such as meningococcus and streptococcus herald a new wave of death and destruction. Deaths from these usually treatable infections have never been eliminated. We need a better organized approach that allows us to monitor, anticipate, and respond to threats. Baseline data are essential in helping to identify when a change has occurred. The extent of migration and movement makes it evident that any approach to new diseases must be global in scope.

More attention should be given to massive die-offs in other species that may hold important lessons. Recent reports detail an epizootic disease sweeping through the lions of Serengeti National Park in Tanzania and killing a third or more of them. Studies have identified canine distemper virus as the cause. Of concern is that the canine distemper virus, as suggested by its name, is primarily a pathogen of dogs and wolves (not felines) though it has also caused disease in skunks, raccoons, and ferrets. Outbreaks of canine distemper virus occurred in wild animal parks in California in 1993, killing lions, leopards, and tigers. Why the virus is now appearing in felines is being investigated. Critically important will be the studies to determine if the virus has mutated, allowing it to infect a new species, whether the virus has been present in felines in the past but has gone unrecognized, and whether other factors have increased the vulnerability of this population of lions.[15]

Tungro virus of rice is spread by the brown leaf hopper and devastated Indonesian rice after heavy pesticide use and the reduced diversity of rice varieties that accompanied the Green Revolution allowed the vector population to explode. The spread of a new species of whitefly, *Bemisia argentifolia*, has carried with it the bean golden mosaic virus and the tomato gemini virus in tropical America. Tristeza of citrus is spreading in part due to the widespread use of sour orange rootstocks that offered protection against blight. In the United States, the use of a cytoplasmic genotype for male sterility, convenient in production of hybrid corn, made it possible for the fungus of southern cornleaf blight to sweep through the Midwest in 1971–72. R. Levins

---

The traditional biomedical model tends to focus narrowly on the human host and pathogen. The papers and discussions recorded in this volume enlarge the frame of reference to the ecosystems and the earth and begin to try to integrate social sciences, human behavior, climate change, and evolutionary ecology in a framework that will help foster new ways of thinking about new diseases.

Many questions posed for the workshop remain unanswered at its conclusion. Is the process of emergence related to the process of adaptation of one species to the presence of another, *e.g.,* stable cohabitation or conversely a consequence of the removal of previous competitors or predators? Is emergence of diseases just the visible end of the spectrum of the ongoing process of adaptation and evolution? Are there fundamental limitations in the concepts of causality, which hamper efforts to detect and monitor new diseases? How do we comprehend the complexity of the systems that influence the presence, abundance, and distribution of species?

While we may occasionally eradicate a particular pathogen (such as smallpox), infectious diseases as a class will not disappear. Although we will not eliminate most species that cause disease in humans, we may limit transmission and prevent disease. The microbial life of earth is diverse, versatile, and huge, and new interactions with humans are inevitable. Some organisms may disappear, and new ones will appear.[16] Known microbes may mutate, undergo recombination, and change in resistance patterns. They may cause new disease syndromes in persons with different genetic make-up or interact with other microbes or environmental forces to create new patterns of disease. What is certain is that an evolving nature and ever changing activity will produce the unexpected. The magnitude and diversity of the sea of microbes we live in must instill a sense of wonder and humility as we strive to assure the health and survival of the human species in a continually evolving world.

REFERENCES

1. LEVINS, R., T. AWERBUCH, U. BRINKMANN, et al. 1994. The emergence of new diseases. Am. Scientist **82:** 52–60.
2. FORTUIN, M., V. KARTHIGESU, L. ALLISON, C. HOWARD, S. HOARE, M. MENDY & H. C. WHITTLE. 1994. Breakthrough infections and identification of a viral variant in Gambian children immunized with hepatitis B vaccine. J. Infect. Dis. **169:** 1374–1376.
3. WILSON, M. E. 1991. A World Guide to Infections: Diseases, Distribution, Diagnosis. New York: Oxford University Press.
4. ADAL, K. A., C. J. COCKERELL & W. A. PETRI, JR. 1994. Cat scratch disease, bacillary angiomatosis, and other infections due to Rochalimaea. New Engl J. Med. **330:** 1509–1515.
5. BLACK, F. L. 1992. Why did they die? Science **258:** 1739–1740.
6. CARLTON, J. T. & J. B. GELLER. 1993. Ecological roulette: The global transport of non-indigenous marine organisms. Science **261:** 78–82.
7. LOCKWOOD, A. P. M. 1993. Aliens and interlopers at sea. Lancet **342:** 942–943.
8. TRAVIS, J. 1993. Invader threatens Black, Azov Seas. Science **262:** 1366–1367.
9. FISHMAN, J. A. 1994. Miniature swine as organ donors for man: Strategies for prevention of xenotransplant-associated infections. Xenotransplantation **1**(1).
10. MACKENZIE, W. R., H. M. HOXIE, M. E. PROCTOR, et al. 1994. A massive outbreak in Milwaukee of cryptosporidium infection transmitted through the public water supply. N. Engl. J. Med. **331:** 161–167.
11. TILLMAN, D. & J. A. DOWNING. 1994. Biodiversity and stability in grasslands. Nature **367:** 363–365.
12. VON REYN, C. F., R. D. BADDELL, T. EATON, et al. 1993. Isolation of *Mycobacterium avium* complex from water in the United States, Finland, Zaire, and Kenya. J. Clin. Microbiol. **31:** 3227–3230.
13. DU MOULIN, G. C., K. D. STOTTMEIER, P. A. PELLETIER, A. Y. TSANG & J. HEDLEY-WHYTE. 1988. Concentration of *Mycobacterium avium* by hospital hot water systems. JAMA **260:** 1599–1601.
14. VON REYN, C. F., J. N. MASLOW, T. W. BARBER, J. O. FALKINHAM & R. D. ARBEIT. 1994. Persistent colonization of potable water as a source of *Mycobacterium avium* infection in AIDS. Lancet **343:** 1137–1141.
15. MORELL, V. 1994. Serengeti's big cats going to the dogs. Science **264:** 1664.
16. WALDOR, M. K. & J. J. MEKALANOS. 1994. *Vibrio cholerae* O139 specific gene sequences. Lancet **343:** 1466.

Marine Ecosystem Health
Implications for Public Health

PAUL R. EPSTEIN

Harvard Medical School
The Cambridge Hospital
1493 Cambridge Street
Cambridge, Massachusetts 02139

TIMOTHY E. FORD, CHARLES PUCCIA,
AND CRISTINA DE A. POSSAS

Harvard School of Public Health
665 Huntington Avenue
Boston, Massachusetts 02115

AGENDA FOR THE WATERBORNE DISEASE DISCUSSION

A recurrent theme across disciplines of health, ecology, and medicine suggests that alterations to the aquatic environment directly and indirectly result in increases in waterborne disease outbreaks. A new research agenda to address the effect of environmental change on human health must be comprehensive and result in implementation plans for mitigation and prevention. The ability to understand the connection between ecosystem structure and function, and the epidemiology of disease can result in informed policy decisions in such diverse areas as resource management, water and waste treatment, agricultural and industrial practice, education, and in disease treatment options.

There are at least four subtopics for this workshop:

1. We need to improve our understanding of the environmental factors involved in the emergence, uncontrolled growth, persistence and transmission of pathogens and pests.

2. While we cannot forecast an organism's response to habitat alterations, we can identify stressed ecosystems and critical regions where pathogen/pest emergence becomes more probable. We need to identify the potential risks associated with specific environmental vulnerabilities and perturbations.

3. We need to develop surveillance to detect habitat changes and shifts in bioclimatic conditions relevant to natural biota. Total surveillance, beyond being impractical, may be unnecessary: Key species and elements may serve as biological indicators of ecosystem stress and vulnerability. We need to set goals for surveillance and explore the appropriate use of new technologies while emphasizing simple, inexpensive, easily transferrable information systems and methodologies. And we need to integrate health surveillance with

13

other programs to monitor environmental and ecological health (diversity, resilience, dynamic stability, productivity and vigor—see Epstein, this volume).

4. Lastly, we need to discuss the nature of public health measures to control, prevent, or ameliorate new and recurrent disease. Part of disease recognition derives from the social implications of a disease and the perception of risk. Interventions involve assessment of effectiveness and feasibility of application, and of how best to surmount the social and economic barriers that invariably present major obstacles to implementing successful public health policies.

This introductory paper will briefly review our current understanding of the interrelationships between the health of aquatic environments and waterborne disease.

WATERBORNE DISEASES

Eighty percent of reported disease outbreaks are caused by waterborne organisms (*e.g.,* cryptosporidiosis and cholera) or can be traced to a waterborne source (*e.g.,* legionellosis). Environmental conditions, stresses and perturbations contribute directly to all these diseases. Between the 1960s and 1990, the average annual number of documented waterborne disease outbreaks (WBDOs) in the United States increased almost fourfold. *Giardia* was the most commonly identifiable WBDO, but improved techniques implicate *Cryptosporidium* in an increasing number of episodes.[1] (Note the thousands infected in Milwaukee in March, 1993.) In addition, the majority of cases of acute gastroenteritis caused by waterborne organisms, although of unknown etiology, are most likely of viral origin.[2] Although many of the WBDOs in developed countries can be traced to failure of treatment systems, or leakage within distribution networks, an alarming number of outbreaks are caused by resistance to commonly used concentrations of disinfectants. The obvious example are the cysts that enable protozoa such as *Giardia* and *Cryptosporidia* to survive in treated water systems. In addition, algae in freshwater systems absorb chlorine (forming hazardous chlorinated hydrocarbons) and reduce effective free chlorine. Increasing evidence suggests that even in developed countries there is a public health issue not addressed by current water quality criteria, many of which themselves are rarely met.

Cholera

In marine systems, the story of cholera highlights how environmental change (or anthropogenic influence) affects disease transmission. In the 1990s, following a decade of relative stability, cholera invaded the American continent and resurged in Africa, and a new strain has now emerged in Asia. This raises a variety of public health issues concerning food and water safety (the "internal" environment of affected nations). However, the major focus of this workshop is on environmental factors influencing the "inoculum," penetration, and persistence of organisms, including this ancient pathogen.

In 1961 cholera left Asia, arriving in southeastern Europe and Africa in the 1970s, tracking coastlines and inland waterways. During the 1980s the sum of cases worldwide declined but the number of affected nations grew threefold.[3] In 1991 cholera struck Peru, penetrating its poor populations from multiple epicenters along the Atlantic coast.[4] The pandemic spread rapidly to Ecuador (February), Colombia (March), and Chile (April), in seaports up to 1700 km from the initial assault. Cholera later entered Brazil, Venezuela, and Bolivia, again following rivers and streams. Over 15 months, more than 0.5 million persons fell ill and close to 5,000 died in nineteen Latin American nations;[5] the toll in Africa was greater, with case-fatality rates over 9%. From March to August, 1991, *Vibrio cholerae* O1, biotype El Tor, serotype Inaba was isolated from marine plankton near Lima.[6] *V. cholerae* O1 has been recovered from the bilge of Latin American vessels docked in US Caribbean ports[7] and it presumably crossed the Pacific as a stow-away,[8] as DNA probing demonstrates "genetic identity" with the strain in Bangladesh.[9]

Since 1960 researchers in Bangladesh have related the seasonality of cholera to coastal algal blooms,[10,11] but the reservoir remained a mystery. In seeking to understand the survival strategy, Colwell and colleagues used fluorescent antibody and polymerase chain reaction techniques, and identified a viable but non-culturable, "quiescent," form of *V. cholerae* (see Colwell and Huq, this volume), associated with a wide range of surface marine life.[12] Under adverse conditions, organisms contract 15- to 300-fold and reduce their metabolic rates, in effect "hibernating," in order to tolerate shifts in pH, temperature, salinity, and nutrients. With favorable conditions (*e.g.*, sufficient nitrogen and phosphorus and proper water temperature) conducive to algal blooms, *Vibrio cholerae* revert to a culturable and infectious state. Chitinases[13] and mucinases[14] facilitate attachment to aquatic organisms, while algal-derived surface films and slimes enhance growth by creating turbulence-free micro-environments.[15] Prolonged survival of *Vibrio cholerae* O1 and non-O1 strains is associated with cyanobacteria (*Anabaena variabilis*), silicate diatoms and drifting dinoflagellates, seaweeds and macroalgae (*Ascophyllum nodosum*), duckweed (*Lemna minor*) and water hyacinths (*Eichhornia crassipes*). Up to 10^6 bacteria have been detected on the egg sacs of the zooplankton copepods. Near Lima, *Vibrio cholerae* O1 was isolated from mollusks, and from the skin and intestines of fish.[6]

In Asia multiple-drug resistant strains of *V. cholerae* O1, biotype El Tor are increasingly widespread. In 1992, chlorine-resistant forms of El Tor *V. cholerae* were isolated in sewage lagoons near Lima, and several variants of an entirely new strain, *V. cholerae* non-O1 CT+ (non-agglutinating with cholera enterotoxin) are now spreading in India, Bangladesh and Thailand. Tendering a new antigen (O139) and bearing a pilus colonization factor, *V. cholerae* non-O1 CT+(O139 Bengal) appears to be exceptionally hardy in terms of environmental adaptation (R. B. Sack, personal communication). Extensive monsoon flooding in July 1993 enhanced its dissemination. The genetic shifts in *V. cholerae* are especially disruptive as recombinant vaccine trials for El Tor are beginning, and, with the potential of spread to immunologically naive populations in Africa and Latin America, O139 Bengal could become the agent of an eighth pandemic of cholera.

Marine Viruses

Massive North Sea seal kills (18,000) in 1988, and dolphin die-offs in the western (1990) and eastern Mediterranean (1992) have been associated with several strains of morbilli (phocine distemper) viruses.[16] While pollutants (*e.g.*, PCBs) may increase sea mammal susceptibility to infection, it is now clear that vast numbers of viruses exist in marine waters (see below). The role of environmental changes in increasing the pathogenicity of marine viruses, or creating conditions for the survival of known pathogenic viruses may become a crucial question for the health of aquatic ecosystems.

Work of Paul and others,[17] suggests that viruses are extremely abundant in marine systems though we are uncertain of their role. However, there is increasing evidence through improved enumeration techniques and electron microscopy of high viral "infection" rates in bacteria—estimated to possibly be as high as 70 percent of heterotrophic bacteria—contributing to 10–100 percent of bacterial mortality.[18] If this is the case, viruses may play a crucial role in regulating productivity within the marine ecosystem, completely changing our understanding of trophic dynamics.

We are beginning to see strong correlations between drinking water and gastrointestinal disease outbreaks,[19] suspected to be caused by viruses that have survived treatment systems and that are substantially more abundant in drinking water than previously suspected.[20] This is not limited to coastal waters polluted by human sewage, where hepatitis A and Norwalk viruses in shellfish often cause epidemics.[21] We should therefore not be surprised at the magnitude of the potential roles for viruses in marine ecosystem health.

For example, at the November, 1993 meeting of the Environmental Management of Enclosed Coastal Seas (EMEX) it was reported that the Long Island brown tide, causing anoxic damage to scallops for several years, is now producing a toxin, and a virus may be involved.

Advances in Technology

Improvements in nucleic acid technology throughout the 1980s have enabled us to characterize the community DNA of natural bacterial and viral populations. Further purification of the DNA (or RNA) can enable molecular probing for target gene sequences representing specific bacterial metabolic potential.[22] Polymerase chain reaction technology (PCR) now enables detection of specific gene sequences from microorganisms that are present in environmental samples at very low concentrations. For example, PCR has been used successfully to detect viable but non-culturable *Legionella pneumoph-*

ila in water samples.[23] In addition, PCR is now routinely used to detect presence of the cholera toxin gene in *Vibrio cholerae* samples.[24]

Our perception of the potential significance and risks of gene transfer in the environment is dramatically changed by these new measurements of viral and bacterial abundance. Anthropogenic activities may have created conditions for increased gene transfer through discharge of heated, nutrient- and pathogen-enriched waters. Although there are a number of mechanisms of gene transfer,[25] the apparent abundance of viruses, and the high viral infection rates of bacteria, suggest that transduction (whereby DNA is packaged into viral capsids and subsequently transferred to a recipient bacterial cell) could be a significant route for dissemination of genes coding for antibiotic resistance and virulence factors. Genetic alteration by mutation has been shown to increase under environmental stress,[25] and as with infection of higher organisms, viral infection of bacteria may also increase under environmental stress. What this could mean in terms of "newly created pathogens" is a hotly debated topic. It would certainly seem that the potential for an eighth cholera pandemic discussed previously, could have been caused by the non-O1 strain of *V. cholerae* either obtaining the cholera toxin gene by mutation or gene transfer.

HARMFUL ALGAL BLOOMS

Survival and proliferation of pathogens in algal blooms are not the only concern. Toxic phytoplankton blooms are associated with paralytic (PSP), diarrheic (DSP), neurotoxic (NSP), and amnesic (ASP) shellfish poisoning as well as with histamine (scromboid), and ciguatera (CFP) fish poisoning. Phytoplanktonologists describe a global increase of red, green, golden, bioluminescent, and brown algal blooms in marine, estuarine, and inland waters, from points as diverse as California, North Carolina, Guatemala, Iceland, Japan, Thailand, and the Tasman Sea.[26,27]

Harmful algal blooms (HABs) affect tourism, aquaculture, and human health. The following is a sample of reports: in 1973 and 1974 blooms of brevetoxin-producing (NSP-related) *Gymnodinium breve* blanketed Florida beaches; in 1976 saxitoxin-producing *G. catenatum* bloomed off the Spanish coast causing hundreds of cases of mussel poisoning; *Pyrodinium* blooms have spread from New Guinea (1972) to Brunei and Sabah (1976), to the Philippines in 1983 and 1987 (1,127 cases and 34 deaths), and to the Pacific coast of Costa Rica and Guatemala (1987) (26 deaths). In 1988, immense toxic green gelatinous blooms caused by *Chrysochromulina polyepsis* devastated 200 salmon farms in Norway and Sweden (an estimated $200 million loss) [pollution from rivers of eastern Germany was blamed]; and during the 1980s, DSP from dinoflagellates spread from Japan, North and South America to previously uncontaminated areas of Ireland, Portugal, Italy, India, Thailand[28] (see Todd and Tester, this volume).

The new appearances of HABs coincide with El Niño years (see p. 19);

is this "global epidemic"[26,27] of HABs one of the first biological signals of global change (T. Smayda, personal communication)?

ENVIRONMENTAL FACTORS

While sunlight, pH, upwelling currents, winds, and river runoff plumes govern the precise location and timing of plankton blooms, the major anthropogenic influences are as discussed below.

Pollution

Excess nutrients from sewage and fertilizer effluents are the primary cause of marine eutrophication; eroding soil and acid rain (from fossil fuel and forestry combustion) add additional nitrogen and phosphorus. Small freshwater bodies lack dissolved carbonates, thus increased atmospheric CO_2 can also "fertilize" algal growth on ponds and sewage lagoons. Toxins, such as lipophilic organic compounds (PCBs, PAHs), heavy metals, and pesticides bioaccumulate in the food chain, causing histopathological changes (e.g., hepatic tumors in fish), physiological, and genetic damage in marine organisms; additionally they alter immune function, algal growth, and thus ecosystem dynamics. Increased ultraviolet-B waves pose a similar threat to individuals, populations and the community structure of species within ecosystems. Oil slicks and solid plastics have had major impacts on marine mammals and seabirds, altering predation pressures.

Over-Harvesting

The over-harvesting of fin and shellfish (beyond levels to sustain long-term potential yields), reinforces algal growth by reducing algivorous grazing. According to the UN, nine of the world's seventeen major fisheries are in serious decline, four are depleted, and the remainder "fully-" or "over-exploited."[29] During the 1970s over-fishing in the Northeast U.S. Shelf system replaced cod and haddock with benthic species (e.g., skates); but the system rebounded in the 1980s under international agreement to limit coastal fishing.[30] The ability of a marine ecosystem to recover from one stress (its resilience) depends on the stability of other ecosystem elements.

Habitat Loss

Wetlands bridge terrestrial and marine systems with grasses tolerant of both. These coastal habitats have multiple functions: as "nature's kidneys," they filter nitrogen and phosphorus, store carbon, remove toxins, and support fish and seabird communities. Salt marshes are suffering from coastal development; each year the United States loses 300,000 acres of wetlands. Mangroves are removed for mariculture. Coral reefs (the "oceans' rainforests"), which cradle diverse marine flora and fauna and buffer coasts from storms, are being widely mined to supply material for road and housing construction in poor nations.[29] In addition, warming and other stresses unsettle the algal symbiont, bleaching coral by expelling swarms of dinoflagellates;[31] additionally, algal mats block light and deoxygenate the shoals. Most of the east African and Indian reefs are severely disfigured, while marine reserves have begun to protect some of the Caribbean and Pacific reefs.[29]

Warming and Algal Growth

Ship recordings ("sea truth") since 1850 demonstrate ocean as well as terrestrial warming.[32] Warming reduces dissolved oxygen, and, within ranges, stimulates algal photosynthesis and metabolism. Warming also favors cyanobacteria and dinoflagellates, many toxic to rival species and less palatable to zooplankton and fish grazers (a positive feedback on algal growth). During the 1980s, the warmest decade of the century, several large-scale natural experiments occurred. In 1982/83 a strong El Niño (the strongest known climate signal, with the broadest, reproducible impacts on regional weather patterns throughout the world) warmed North Atlantic seas, altering zooplankton, finfish, seal, and seabird communities throughout the decade. In the Pacific, elevated sea surface temperatures overwhelmed cool upwelling water, altering Peruvian sardine and anchovy yields for years.[33] In 1987 (an El Niño year) there was extensive coral bleaching in the Caribbean and large die-offs of sea-grass in the Florida Keys. In 1987 the first recorded *G. breve* red tide was observed off Cape Hatteras, North Carolina. The Gulf Stream, in which *G. breve* were always present at low levels (<10 cells/l), probably transported this phytoplankton. Blooms were apparently fostered by favorable environmental conditions, including the presence of a semi-stable gulf stream eddy serving as a "chemostat" for *G. breve*[34] (see Tester, this volume).

Further up the Atlantic coast in 1987 a new phenomenon occurred. Following heavy rains subsequent to drought (increasing runoff), and accompanying warm eddies of the gulf stream which swept unusually close to Canada's Prince Edward Island, the pennate diatom (*Nitzschia pungens*) bloomed. The diatom produced domoic acid causing 156 cases of amnesia (some permanent) and five deaths in Canadian mussel consumers[35] (see Todd, this volume). During the same period, hundreds of dead bottlenose dolphins and humpback whales appeared on Northeast coasts, with PCBs, biotoxins and "viruses" implicated.[36] Since 1987, outbreaks of domoic acid poisoning have spread: in 1991/92 (also an El Niño year), in Monterey Bay, California (now a marine reserve), hundreds of pelicans and cormorants were poisoned from ingestion of fish contaminated with domoic acid; then, in the summer of 1992, massive blooms of a close relative, *Pseudonitzschia pseudodelicatissima,* occurred in Scandinavian waters.[37] 1991/1992 also saw the first appearance of PSP saxitoxins as far south as the Straits of Magellan,[38] concurrent with the penetration of *V. cholerae* into the Americas.

LARGE MARINE ECOSYSTEMS

Just as the major pandemics cross regional, national and international boundaries, the underlying ecosystem functions that permit biological communities to exist and persist depend on energy and material flow plus organismic migrations across large regions. Some 49 large marine ecosystems (LMEs) have been identified,[33] with each area representing at least 200,000 km². Global temperature changes, alterations in hydrography, and massive human interventions such as overfishing, pollution or diversion of major watershed areas disrupt LMEs, as dominant species migrate away, become restricted, or are forced to change behavior patterns (see Sherman, this volume).

Remote Sensing and Algal Blooms

Remote sensing provides a potentially important tool for monitoring the health of LMEs. The global distribution of coastal blooms can be visualized on images from the Coastal Zone Color Scanner (CZCS), a satellite that collected data from 1978 to 1985. Detecting visible red and near infrared emissions, CZCS images provided estimates of the amount of chlorophyll ā, thus generating values for primary production and the biomass of phytoplankton (see FIGS. 2–5 in Remote Sensing section). These values are used to evaluate the role of marine life in the global carbon cycle. As algae are a reservoir for enteric pathogens and a source of toxins, such images can also be used for public health purposes. The Advanced Very High Resolution Radiometer (AVHRR), detecting far infrared (heat), on satellites of the National Oceanic and Atmospheric Administration (NOAA), is now used to monitor phytoplankton blooms (see FIGS. 6–9 in Remote Sensing section). AVHRR generates images revealing river plumes, often associated with blooms, which can indicate where sampling should be done for monitoring toxic species (D. Anderson, WHOI, personal communication). The next generation of satellites, Sea-Viewing Wide Field Sensor (Sea-WiFS), is scheduled for launching in 1994.

CONCLUSIONS

The public health crises of new and resurgent diseases can in large part be traced to a failure in understanding the interactions between the human population and the environment. Anthropogenic influence on the marine environment, for example, enables development of conditions for pathogen survival through eutrophication and heated waters. Genetic transfer can also be affected/accelerated by these conditions, resulting in enhanced development of antibiotic resistance, exposure to virulence factors and to environmental stresses that help to select for virulence. Public health may be affected indirectly through the food chain; we are only beginning to understand that community health is closely tied to the health of the ecosystem.

Several research questions follow, moving from the specific to the more general.

1. How extensive are viable but non-culturable stages of human pathogens (refuge strategies) and can we identify the environmental factors that result in the return to virulent (and transmissible) states?

2. Can we quantify risks of genetic transfer/mutation within a specific polluted aquatic environment?

3. How do we prioritize ecological questions in order to model and assess degrees of risk, and respond to the potential as well as actual outbreaks of waterborne disease?

4. How might harsh environments and changes in predator/prey dynamics, competitors and insurance species, contribute to the emergence, resurgence and/or redistribution of pathogens and pests?

5. Can we measure the direct and indirect cascading effects of localized pollution events at the large marine ecosystem or even global level?

6. How do global signals and changes within LMEs integrate to create new habitats that permit the proliferation of new disease?

7. How can environmental monitoring be enhanced to include indicators of potential disease (*e.g.*, algal toxins and bacterial symbionts) and the surveillance of health outcomes?

8. How will environmental management to improve ecosystem health effect disease emergence and resurgence?

Our advances in detection technology raise the question as to how extensively our surveillance of environmental samples for pathogens or toxins should become? In theory the applications and numbers of pathogens or potentials to become pathogens are vast. Resources are, however, limited and must be directed towards the major health crises that currently exist (*e.g.*, cholera) and the most informed estimates of where, and what emerging epidemics might occur. Of immediate concern is O139 Bengal. Development of an early warning system for O139 Bengal, monitoring plankton and ballast water for vibrios (speciated) could constitute this system. This will involve monitoring the basic parameters of LMEs with the participation of the International Maritime Organization, the WHO and CDC. An interdisciplinary approach is required to begin to understand and close the gaps between environmental and human health.

REFERENCES

1. ROSE, J. B., GERBA, C. P. & W. JAKUBOWSKI. 1991. Survey of potable water supplies for *Cryptosporidium* and *Giardia*. Environ. Sci. Technol. **25**: 1393–1400.
2. GERBA, C. P. & J. B. ROSE, 1990. Viruses in source and drinking water. *In* Drinking Water Microbiology. G. A. McFeters, Ed.: 380–396. New York: Springer.
3. WHO, 13 March 1991. Cholera: The epidemic in Peru—Part I. Weekly Epidemiological Record No.9. **66**: 61–63.
4. WHO, 17 May 1991. Cholera in Peru—Update. Weekly Epidemiological Record No. 20. **66**: 141–145.

5. SWERDLOW, D. L., E. D. MINTZ, M. RODRIQUEZ, *et al.* 1992. Waterborne transmission of epidemic cholera in Trujillo, Peru: Lessons for a continent at risk. Lancet **340**: 28–33.
6. TAMPLIN, N. L. & C. C. PARODI. 1991. Environmental spread of *Vibrio cholerae* in Peru. Lancet **338**: 1216–1217.
7. DEPAOLA, A., G. M. CAPERS, M. L. MOTES, *et al.* 1992. Isolation of Latin American epidemic strain of *Vibrio cholerae* O1 from US Gulf Coast. Lancet **339**: 624.
8. CARLTON, J. T. & J. B. GELLER. 1993. Ecological roulette: The global transport of nonindigenous marine organisms. Science **261**: 78–82.
9. FARUQUE, S. M. & J. ALBERT. 1992. Genetic relation between *Vibrio cholerae* O1 strains in Ecuador and Bangladesh. Lancet **339**: 740–741.
10. COCKBURN, T. A. & J. G. CASSANOS. 1960. Epidemiology of epidemic cholera. Public Health Reports **75**: 791.
11. SAMADI, A. R., N. K. CHOWDHURY, M. I. HUQ & M. U. KHAN. 1983. Seasonality of classical and El Tor cholera in Dhaka, Bangladesh: 17 year trends. Trans. R. Soc. Trop. Med. Hyg. **77**: 853.
12. BYRD, J. J., X. U. HUAI-SHU & R. R. COLWELL. 1991. Viable but non-culturable bacteria in drinking water. Appl. Environ. Microbiol. **57**: 875–878.
13. NALIN, D. R., V. DAYA, A. REID, M. M. LEVINE & L. CISNAROS. 1979. Adsorption and growth of *Vibrio cholerae* on chitin. Infect. Immun. **25**: 768–770.
14. SCHNEIDER, D. R. & C. D. PARKER. 1982. Purification and characterization of the mucinase of *Vibrio cholerae*. J. Infect. Dis. **145**: 474–482.
15. JENKINSON, I. 1992. New—A seawater rheology group. Harmful Algae News. Suppl to International Marine Science (UNESCO) **62**: 5.
16. HEIDE-JORGENSEN, M.-P., T. HARKONEN, R. DIETZ & P. M. THOMPSON. 1992. Retrospective of the 1988 European seal epizootic. Dis. Aquat. Org. **13**: 37–62.
17. PAUL, J. H. 1993. The advances and limitations of methodology. *In* Aquatic Microbiology: An Ecological Approach. T. E. Ford, Ed.: 483–511. Boston: Blackwell.
18. PROCTOR, L. M. & J. A. FUHRMAN. 1990. Viral mortality of marine bacteria and cyanobacteria. Nature **343**: 60–62.
19. PAYMENT, P., L. RICHARDSON, J. SIEMIATYCKI, R. DEWAR, M. EDWARDES & E. FRANCO. 1991. A randomized trial to evaluate the risk of gastrointestinal disease due to consumption of drinking water meeting current microbiological standards. Am. J. Pub. Health **81**: 703–708.
20. BITTON, G., S. R. FARRAH, C. L. MONTAGUE & E. W. AKIN. 1986. Viruses in drinking water. Environ. Sci. Technol. **20**: 216–222.
21. EASTAUGH, J. 1989. Infectious and toxic syndromes from fish and shellfish consumption. Arch. Intern. Med. **149**: 1735–1740.
22. HAZEN, T. C. & L. JIMENEZ. 1988. Enumeration and identification of bacteria from environmental samples using nucleic acid probes. Microbiol. Sci. **5**: 340–343.
23. BEJ, A. K., M. H. MAHUBANI & R. M. ATLAS. 1991. Detection of viable legionella pneumophila in water by polymerase chain reaction and gene probe methods. Appl. Environ. Microbiol. **57**: 597–600.
24. SHIRAI, H., M. NISHIBUCHI, T. RAMAMURTHY, *et al.* 1991. Polymerase chain reaction for detection of cholera enterotoxin operon of *Vibrio cholerae*. J. Clin. Microbiol. **29**: 1517–2521.
25. MILLER, R. V. 1993. Genetic stability of genetically engineered microorganisms in the aquatic environment. *In* Aquatic Microbiology: An Ecological Approach. T. E. Ford, Ed.: 483–511. Boston: Blackwell.
26. SMAYDA, T. J. & Y. SHIMIZU. 1993. Toxic Phytoplankton Blooms in the Sea. UK: Elsevier.
27. ANDERSON, D. M. 1992. The fifth international conference on toxic marine phytoplankton: A personal perspective. Harmful Algae News, Suppl. to International Marine Science (UNESCO) **62**: 6–7.
28. LASSUS, P. 1993. Prospectus: Sixth International Conference on Toxic Marine phytoplankton. Nantes Cedex O1, France. (Contains multiple citations.)
29. SIMONS, M. 6 Aug 1993. Mining is ravaging the Indian Ocean's coral reefs. New York Times, p. 3.

30. VALIELA, I. 1984. Marine Ecological Processes. New York: Springer-Verlag.
31. HAYES, L. & T. J. GOREAU. 1991. The tropical coral reef ecosystem as a harbinger of global warming. World Resource Rev. **3:** 306–322.
32. HOUGHTON, J. T., G. L. JENKINS & J. J. EPHRAUMIS, Eds. 1990. Climate Change: The IPCC Scientific Assessment. New York: Cambridge University Press.
33. SHERMAN, L., L. M. ALEXANDER & B. D. GOLD, Eds. 1993. Large Marine Ecosystems: Stress, Mitigation, and Sustainability.: 301–319. AAAS Press.
34. TESTER, P. A., R. P. STUMPF, F. M. VUKOVICH, P. K. FOWLER & J. T. TURNER. 1991. An expatriate red tide bloom, transport, distribution, and persistence. Limnol. Oceanogr. **36**(5): 1053–1061.
35. TODD, E. C. D. 1993. Domoic acid and amnesic shellfish poisoning—a review. J. Food Protection **56:** 69–83.
36. MACKENZIE, D. 1988. Mystery of mussel poisoning deepens in Canada as the chain of death spreads to whales. New Scientist **30** (28 Jan.).
37. LUDLOHM, N. & J. SKOV. 1993. *Pseudonitzchia pseudodelicatissima* in Scandinavian waters. Harmful Algae News. Suppl to International Marine Science (UNESCO) **62:** 4.
38. CARRETO, J. I. & H. R. BENEVIDES. 1993. World record of PSP in southern Argentina. Harmful Algae News. Suppl to International Marine Science (UNESCO) **62:** 7.

Coastal Ecosystem Health

A Global Perspective

KENNETH SHERMAN

National Oceanic and Atmospheric Administration
National Marine Fisheries Service
Northeast Fisheries Science Center
28 Tarzwell Drive
Narragansett, Rhode Island 02882-1199

INTRODUCTION

A significant milestone in marine resource development was achieved in July 1992 with the adoption by a majority of coastal countries of follow-on actions to the United Nations' Conference on Environment and Development (UNCED). The UNCED declarations on the ocean explicitly recommended that nations of the globe: 1) prevent, reduce, and control degradation of the marine environment so as to maintain and improve its life-support and productive capacities; 2) develop and increase the potential of marine living resources to meet human nutritional needs, as well as social, economic, and development goals; and 3) promote the integrated management and sustainable development of coastal areas and the marine environment. UNCED also recognized the general importance of capacity building, as well as the important linkage between monitoring and the achievement of marine resource development goals. The UNCED recommendations should lead to programs that will enhance the health of coastal ecosystems.

Achievement of UNCED recommendations and the improvement in the health of coastal ecosystems will require the implementation of a new paradigm in ocean monitoring and management that can overcome traditional geopolitical and interdisciplinary sectorization. Such an approach should be based on principles of ecology and sustainable development. The large marine ecosystem (LME) concept provides the framework for achievement of UNCED commitments. LMEs are areas which are being subjected to increasing stress from growing exploitation of fish and other renewable resources, coastal zone damage, river basin runoff, dumping of urban wastes, and fallout from aerosol contaminants. The LMEs are regions of ocean space encompassing near-coastal areas from river basins and estuaries on out to the seaward boundary of continental shelves and the seaward margins of pelagic current systems adjacent to the continents. They are relatively large regions on the order of 200,000 km² or larger, characterized by distinct bathymetry, hydrography, productivity, and trophically dependent populations.[1] The theory, measurement, and modeling relevant to monitoring the changing states of LMEs are embedded in reports on multistable ecosystems, and on the pattern formation and spatial diffusion within ecosystems.[2,3] Because LMEs usually subsume the coastal waters of more than one state, coordination between those states in monitoring and resource management is desirable. The utility of a regional approach for implementation of ecological research, monitoring, and stress mitigation has been recognized.[4-6] In the application of the LME concept to management, coastal states would maintain ultimate responsibility for their territorial sea and exclusive economic zone resources. Although recognition of the LME concept engenders no legal commitment by coastal states to share their resources, it would be in their enlightened self-interest to do so.

It is within the nearshore coastal domains of the LMEs that the human-induced stress on ecosystems requires mitigating actions to ensure the continued productivity and economic viability and health of marine resources. Although the management of LMEs is an evolving scientific and geopolitical process, sufficient progress has been made to allow for useful comparisons among the primary, secondary, and tertiary driving forces influencing large-scale changes in the biomass yields and long-term sustainability of LMEs. Results from a series of LME studies are presented in this report. The information provided is intended to encourage dialogue and debate on strategies for linking scientific and societal interests. It is aimed at promoting the health of coastal ecosystems and assisting in the short-term and long-term development and sustainability of coastal ocean ecosystems in the post-UNCED decade of the 1990s, bearing in mind the need to meet the objectives of Agenda 21 aimed at reducing the degradation of marine ecosystems and promoting their integrated management and sustainable development. Mitigating actions to reduce stress on marine ecosystems are required to ensure the long-term sustainability of marine resources. The principles adopted by coastal states under the terms of the United Nations Convention for the Law of the Sea (UNCLOS) have been interpreted as supportive of the management of living marine resources and coastal habitats from an ecosystems perspective.[7,8] However, at present no single international institution has been empowered to monitor the changing ecological states or health of marine ecosystems and to reconcile the needs of individual nations with those of the community of nations in taking appropriate mitigation actions.[9] In this regard, the need for a regional approach to implement research, monitoring, and stress mitigation in support of marine resources development and sustainability at less than the global level has been recognized from a strategic perspective.[10,11]

LARGE MARINE ECOSYSTEM CHARACTERISTICS

From the ecological perspective, the concept that critical processes controlling the structure and function of biological communities can best be addressed on a regional basis has been applied to ocean space in the utilization of marine ecosystems as distinct global units for marine research, monitoring, and management. The concept of monitoring and managing renewable resources from a regional ecosystem perspective has been the topic of a series of symposia and workshops initiated in 1984 and continuing through 1992, wherein the geographic extent of each region is defined on the basis of ecological criteria (TABLE 1). As the regional units under consideration are large, the term LME is used to characterize them. Several occupy semi-enclosed seas, such as the Black Sea, the Mediterranean Sea, and the Caribbean Sea. Some of these can be divided into domains, or subsystems—for example the Adriatic Sea, a subsystem of the Mediterranean Sea LME. In other LMEs geographic limits are defined by the scope of continental margins. Among these are the U.S. Northeast Continental Shelf, the East Greenland Sea, the Northwestern Australian Shelf. The seaward limit of the LMEs extends beyond the physical outer limits of the shelves, themselves, to include all or a portion of the continental slopes. Care was taken to limit the seaward boundaries to the areas affected by ocean currents around the margins of the continents, rather than relying simply on the 200-mile Exclusive Economic Zone (EEZ) or fisheries zone limits. Among the ocean current LMEs are the Humboldt Current, Canary Current, and Kuroshio Current ecosystems.

CHANGING ECOSYSTEM STATES (HEALTH)

The topic of change and persistence in marine communities and the need for multispecies and ecosystem perspectives in the management of marine resources in general and fishery resources in particular relate to the reports of changing states of marine ecosystems.[12] Collapses of the Pacific sardine in the California Current Ecosystem, the pilchard in the Benguela Current Ecosystem, and the anchovy in the Humboldt Current Ecosystem, are but a few examples of cascading effects on other ecosystem components including marine birds.[13-16] The removal of millions of metric tons of fish from LMEs can affect the changing states or health of LMEs. Recent observations suggested that excessive nutrient loadings and other pollutants can generate changes in the state of health of LMEs.[17-19] Ecosystem "health" is a concept of wide interest for which a single precise scientific definition is problematical. Ecosystem health is used herein to describe the resilience, stability, and productivity of the ecosystem in relation to the changing states of ecosystems. In present practice, assessing the health of LMEs relies on a series of indicators and indices.[20-23] The overriding objective is to monitor changes in health from an ecosystem perspective as a measure of the overall performance of a complex system.[20] The health paradigm is based on the multiple-state comparisons of ecosystem resilience and stability[20,24,25] and is an evolving concept. Definitions of several variables important to the changing states and health of marine ecosystems are given in TABLE 2. Following the definition of Costanza[20] (1992), to be healthy and sustainable, an ecosystem must maintain its metabolic activity level, its internal structure and organization, and must be resistant to external stress over time and space frames relative to the ecosystem (TABLE 3). These concepts were discussed at a workshop convened by the National Oceanic and Atmospheric/National Marine Fisheries Service (NOAA/NMFS) at the Northeast Fisheries Science Center's Narragansett

TABLE 1. List of 29 Large Marine Ecosystems and Sub-systems for Which Syntheses Relating to Principal, Secondary, or Tertiary Driving Forces Controlling Variability in Biomass Yields Have Been Completed by February 1993 [a]

Large Marine Ecosystem	Volume No.[b]	Authors
U.S. Northeast Continental Shelf	1	M. Sissenwine
	4	P. Falkowski
U.S. Southeast Continental Shelf	4	J. Yoder
Gulf of Mexico	2	W. J. Richards and M. F. McGowan
	4	B. E. Brown et al.
California Current	1	A. MacCall
	4	M. Mullin
	5	D. Bottom et al.
Eastern Bering Shelf	1	L. Incze and J. D. Schumacher
West Greenland Shelf	3	H. Hovgaard and E. Buch
Norwegian Sea	3	B. Ellertsen et al.
Barents Sea	2	H. R. Skjoldal and F. Rey
	4	V. Borisov
North Sea	1	N. Daan
Baltic Sea	1	G. Kullenberg
Iberian Coastal	2	T. Wyatt and G. Perez-Gandaras
Mediterranean-Adriatic Sea	5	G. Bombace
Canary Current	5	C. Bas
Gulf of Guinea	5	D. Binet and E. Marchal
Benguela Current	2	R. J. M. Crawford et al.
Patagonian Shelf	5	A. Bakun
Caribbean Sea	3	W. J. Richards & J. A. Bohnsack
South China Sea-Gulf of Thailand	2	T. Piyakarnchana
Yellow Sea	2	Q. Tang
Sea of Okhotsk	5	V. V. Kusnetsov
Humboldt Current	5	J. Alheit and P. Bernal
Indonesia Seas-Banda Sea	3	J. J. Zijlstra and M. A. Baars
Bay of Bengal	5	S. N. Dwivedi
Antarctic Marine	1 & 5	R. T. Scully et al.
Weddell Sea	3	G. Hempel
Kuroshio Current	2	M. Terazaki
Oyashio Current	2	T. Minoda
Great Barrier Reef	2	R. H. Bradbury and C. N. Mundy
	5	G. Kelleher
South China Sea	5	D. Pauly and V. Christensen

[a] The ecological criteria for designation of the distinct LMEs includes information on bathymetry, hydrography, productivity, and trophodynamics.

[b] Vol. 1, Variability and Management of Large Marine Ecosystems, edited by K. Sherman & L. M. Alexander, AAAS Selected Symposium 99, Westview Press, Boulder, CO, 1986. Vol. 2, Biomass Yields and Geography of Large Marine Ecosystems, edited by K. Sherman & L. M. Alexander, AAAS Selected Symposium 111, Westview Press, Boulder, CO, 1989. Vol. 3, Large Marine Ecosystems: Patterns, Processes, and Yields, edited by K. Sherman, L. M. Alexander, & B. D. Gold, AAAS Symposium, AAAS Press, Washington, DC, 1990. Vol. 4, Food Chains, Yields, Models, and Management of Large Marine Ecosystems, edited by K. Sherman, L. M. Alexander, & B. D. Gold, AAAS Symposium, Westview Press, Boulder, CO. 1991. Vol. 5, Large Marine Ecosystems: Stress, Mitigation, and Sustainability, edited by K. Sherman, L. M. Alexander, & B. D. Gold, AAAS Press, Washington, DC, 1993.

TABLE 2. Definitions of Some Important Variables for Use in the Indexing of Changing Ecosystem States (Health)[a]

Variable	Definition	Units
Stability		
Homeostasis	Maintenance of a steady state in living organisms by the use of feedback control processes.	
Stable	A system is stable if, and only if, the variables all return to the initial equilibrium following their being perturbed from it. A system is locally stable if this return applies to small perturbations, and globally stable if it applies to all possible perturbations.	Binary
Sustainable	A system that can maintain its structure and function indefinitely. All non-successional (i.e., climax) ecosystems are sustainable, but they may not be stable (see resilience below). Sustainability is a policy goal for economic systems.	Binary
Resilience	1. How fast the variables return towards their equilibrium following a perturbation. Not defined for unstable systems (Pimm, 1984). 2. The ability of a system to maintain its structure and patterns of behavior in the face of disturbance (Holling, 1986).	Time
Resistance	The degree to which a variable is changed, following a perturbation.	Nondimensional and continuous
Variability	The variance of population densities over time, or allied measures such as the standard deviation or coefficient of variation (sd/mean).	
Complexity		
Species richness	The number of species in a system.	Integer
Connectance	The number of actual interspecific interactions divided by the possible interspecific interactions.	Dimensionless
Interaction strength	The mean magnitude of interspecific interaction: the size of the effect of one species' density on the growth rate of another species.	
Evenness	The variance of the species abundance distribution.	
Diversity indices	Measures that combine evenness and richness with a particular weighting for each. One important member of this family is the information theoretic index, H.	Bits
Ascendency	An information theoretic measure that combines the average mutual information (a measure of connectedness) and the total throughput of the system as a scaling factor (see Ulanowicz, 1992).	
Other Variables		
Perturbation	A change to a system's inputs or environment beyond the normal range of variation.	Varies
Stress	A perturbation with a negative effect on a system.	
Subsidy	A perturbation with a positive effect on a system.	

[a] Adapted and expanded from Costanza.[20]

TABLE 3. Indices of Vigor, Organization, and Resilience in Various Fields[20]

Component of Health	Related Concepts	Existing Related Measures	Fields of Origin	Probable Method of Solution
Vigor	Function Productivity System Throughput	GPP, NPP, GEP → GNP → Metabolism →	Ecology Economics Biology	Measurement
Organization	Structure Biodiversity	Diversity index Average mutual information Predictability →	Ecology	Network analysis
Resilience		Scope for growth →	Ecology	Simulation modeling
Combinations		Ascendancy →	Ecology	

Laboratory in April 1992. Among the indices discussed by the participants were five that are being considered as experimental measures of changing ecosystem states and health—1) diversity, 2) stability, 3) yields, 4) production, and 5) resilience.[26]

The data from which to derive the experimental indices are obtained from time-series monitoring of key ecosystem parameters. A prototype effort to validate the utility of the indices is under development by NOAA at the Northeast Fisheries Science Center. The ecosystem sampling strategy is focused on parameters relating to the resources at risk from overexploitation, species protected by legislative authority (marine mammals), and other key biological and physical components at the lower end of the food chain (plankton, nutrients, hydrography).[27] The parameters of interest depicted in FIGURE 1 include zooplankton composition, zooplankton biomass, water column structure, photosynthetically active radiation (PAR), transparency, chlorophyll-a, NO_2, NO_3, primary production, pollution, marine mammal biomass, marine mammal composition, runoff, wind stress, seabird community structure, seabird counts, finfish composition, finfish biomass, domoic acid, saxitoxin, and paralytic shellfish poisoning (PSP). The experimental parameters selected incorporate the behavior of individuals, the resultant responses of populations and communities, as well as their interactions with the physical and chemical environment. The selected parameters, if measured in all LMEs, will permit comparison of relative changing states and health status among ecosystems. The interrelations between the datasets and the selected parameters are indicated by the arrows leading from column 1 to column 2 in the figure. The measured ecosystem components are depicted in relation to ecosystem structure in a diagrammatic conceptualization of patterns and activities within the LME at different levels of complexity (FIG. 2).

Initial efforts to examine changing ecosystem states and relative health within a single ecosystem are underway for four subareas of the U.S. Northeast Continental Shelf Ecosystem—Gulf of Maine, Georges Bank, Southern New

England, and Mid-Atlantic Bight. Initial studies of the structure, function, and productivity of the system have been reported.[28] It appears that the principal driving force in relation to sustainable ecosystem yield is fishing mortality expressed as predation on the fish stocks of the system, and that long-term sustainability of high economic yield species will be dependent on the application of adaptive management strategies.[29,30]

Several alternative management strategies for the fish stocks of the U.S. Northeast Continental Shelf Ecosystem are under consideration by the New England Fishery Management Council and the Atlantic States Marine Fisheries Commission. In addition to fisheries management issues and significant biomass flips among dominant species, the Northeast Continental Shelf Eco-

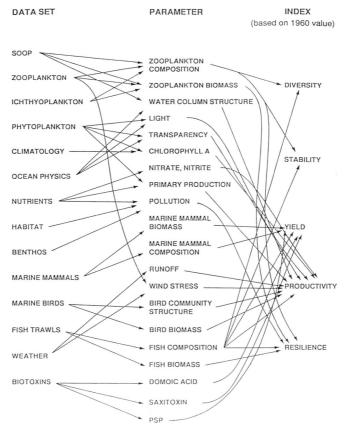

FIGURE 1. A schematic representation of the data bases and experimental parameters for indexing the changing states of large marine ecosystems. The data base represents time-series measurements of key ecosystem components from the U.S. Northeast Continental Shelf Ecosystem. Indices will be based on changes compared with the ecosystem state in 1960.[68]

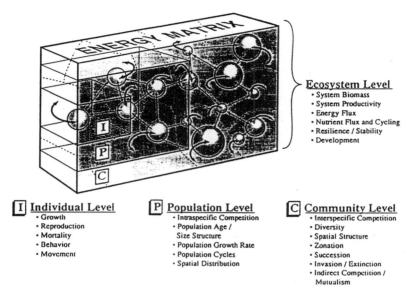

Ecosystem Level
- System Biomass
- System Productivity
- Energy Flux
- Nutrient Flux and Cycling
- Resilience / Stability
- Development

[I] Individual Level
- Growth
- Reproduction
- Mortality
- Behavior
- Movement

[P] Population Level
- Intraspecific Competition
- Population Age / Size Structure
- Population Growth Rate
- Population Cycles
- Spatial Distribution

[C] Community Level
- Interspecific Competition
- Diversity
- Spatial Structure
- Zonation
- Succession
- Invasion / Extinction
- Indirect Competition / Mutualism

FIGURE 2. Diagrammatic conceptualization of patterns and activities at different levels of complexity. Each sphere represents an individual abiotic or biotic entity. Abiotic is defined as nonliving matter. Broad, double-headed arrows indicate feedback between entities and the energy matrix for the system. The thin arrows represent direct interactions between individual entities. Much of ecology is devoted to studying interactions between biotic and abiotic entities with a focus on the effects of such interactions on individuals (I), populations (P), or communities (C) of organisms. Ecosystem ecology studies these interactions from the viewpoint of their effect on both the biotic and abiotic entities and within the context of the system. The boundaries of the system must be established to conduct quantitative studies of flux.

system is also under stress from the increasing frequency of unusual plankton blooms, and eutrophication within the nearshore coastal zone resulting from high levels of phosphate and nitrate discharges into drainage basins. Whether the increases in the frequency and extent of nearshore plankton blooms are responsible for the rise in incidence of biotoxin-related shellfish closures and marine mammal mortalities, remains an important open question that is the subject of considerable concern to state and federal management agencies.[31,32]

LARGE MARINE ECOSYSTEM STRESS

It is the coastal ecosystems adjacent to the land masses that are being stressed from habitat degradation, pollution, and overexploitation of marine resources. Nearly 95% of the usable annual global biomass yield of fish and other living marine resources is produced in 49 LMEs within, and adjacent to, the boundaries of the EEZs of coastal nations located around the margins of the ocean basins, where levels of primary production are persistently higher than for the open-ocean pelagic areas of the globe (FIG. 3).

Pollution at the continental margins of marine ecosystems can impact on natural productivity cycles, including eutrophication from high nitrogen and phosphorus effluent from estuaries. The presence of toxins in poorly treated sewage discharge, and loss of wetland nursery areas to coastal development are also ecosystem-level problems that need to be addressed.[33] Overfishing has caused biomass flips among the dominant pelagic components of fish communities resulting in multimillion metric ton losses in potential biomass yield.[34] The biomass flip, wherein a dominant species rapidly drops to a low level to be succeeded by another species, can generate cascading effects among other important components of the ecosystem, including marine birds,[35] marine mammals, and zooplankton.[36,37] Recent studies implicate

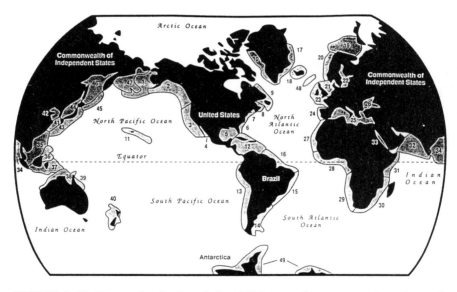

FIGURE 3. World map showing boundaries of 49 large marine ecosystems located around the margins of the ocean basins, where the influence of overexploitation, pollution and habitat degradation, and climate change are affecting the structure and function of the ecosystems.[69] **1.** Eastern Bering Sea; **2.** Gulf of Alaska; **3.** California Current; **4.** Gulf of California; **5.** Gulf of Mexico; **6.** Southeast U.S. Continental Shelf; **7.** Northeast U.S. Continental Shelf; **8.** Scotian Shelf; **9.** Newfoundland Shelf; **10.** West Greenland Shelf; **11.** Insular Pacific-Hawaiian; **12.** Caribbean Sea; **13.** Humboldt Current; **14.** Patagonian Shelf; **15.** Brazil Current; **16.** Northeast Brazil Shelf; **17.** East Greenland Shelf; **18.** Iceland Shelf; **19.** Barents Sea; **20.** Norwegian Shelf; **21.** North Sea; **22.** Baltic Sea; **23.** Celtic-Biscay Shelf; **24.** Iberian Coastal; **25.** Mediterranean Sea; **26.** Black Sea; **27.** Canary Current; **28.** Guinea Current; **29.** Benguela Current; **30.** Agulhas Current; **31.** Somali Coastal Current; **32.** Arabian Sea; **33.** Red Sea; **34.** Bay of Bengal; **35.** South China Sea; **36.** Sulu-Celebes Seas; **37.** Indonesian Seas; **38.** Northern Australian Shelf; **39.** Great Barrier Reef; **40.** New Zealand Shelf; **41.** East China Sea; **42.** Yellow Sea; **43.** Kuroshio Current; **44.** Sea of Japan; **45.** Oyashio Current; **46.** Sea of Okhotsk; **47.** West Bering Sea; **48.** Faroe Plateau; and **49.** Antarctic.

climate and natural environmental changes as prime driving forces of variability in fish population levels.[38-40] The growing awareness that biomass yields are being influenced by multiple driving forces in marine ecosystems around the globe has accelerated efforts to broaden research strategies to encompass food chain dynamics and the effects of environmental perturbations and pollution on living marine resources from an ecosystem perspective.

MONITORING STRATEGY

A monitoring strategy for measuring the changing states of the biological, physical, and chemical states of LMEs was recommended by a panel of international experts that met at Cornell University in July 1991 (TABLE 4).[27] Monitoring methods included were: 1) regular trawling using a stratified random sampling design, and 2) plankton surveys. The large-scale changes in the fisheries of the North Sea and the Northeast Continental Shelf of the United States have been successfully detected using trawling techniques for

TABLE 4. Core Marine Ecosystem Monitoring Program

Candidate parameters for the Core Program include:		
Chlorophyll fluorescence[b]	Salinity structure[b]	Temperature structure[b]
Primary production[c]	Nutrients[b]	
Diatom/flagellate ratio[b]	NO$_2$	Stratification index[b]
Zooplankton composition and biomass	NO$_3$	Transparency[b]
Copepod diversity[b]	Pollution index (e.g., hydrocarbons, sewage)	PAR[b]
Fisheries survey		Rainfall or runoff, wind strength and direction
Assessment		
Changes in abundance and distribution		
Biology		
Length		
Age and growth		
Predator-prey		
Pathology		
Acoustics for pelagics		
Nets for demersals		
Physical measurements		
Temperature		
Salinity		
Chemical measurements		
Water samples (nutrients, productivity, pollutants)		

[a] The Core Program is based on transects sampled by UOR or instrumented CPR, supplemented by satellite oceanography and systematic trawl and acoustic surveys.[27]

[b] Measurements derived from instrumented CPR/UOR sensors.

[c] Based on inclusion of double-flash pump and probe system.

several decades.[41] The surveys have been conducted by relatively large research vessels. However, standardized sampling procedures, when deployed from small calibrated trawlers, can provide important information on fish stocks. The fish catch provides biological samples, demography, biodiversity, and community analyses for stomach analyses, age and growth, fecundity, and size comparisons,[42] and data for clarifying and quantifying multispecies trophic relationships. Samples of trawl-caught fish can also be used to monitor pathological conditions that may be associated with coastal pollution.

An important component of the core monitoring program will be the definition of routes of exposure to toxic contaminants of selected finfish and shellfish and the assessment of exposure to toxic chemicals by several life history stages. In addition, the routes of bioaccumulation and trophic transfer of contaminants are assessed and critical life history stages and selected food-chain organisms will be examined for a variety of parameters that indicate exposure to, and effects of, contaminants. Contaminant-related effects that will be measured include certain diseases, impaired reproductive capacity, and impaired growth. Many of these effects can be caused by direct exposure to contaminants, or by indirect effects, such as those resulting from alterations in prey organisms. The core program for assessing chemical contaminant exposure and effects in fishing resources and food-chain organisms will consist of a suite of parameters, including biochemical responses that are clearly linked to contaminant exposure coupled with measurements of organ disease and reproductive status that have been used in previous studies to establish links between exposure and effects. The specific suite of parameters measured will cover the same general responses and thus allow comparable assessment of the physiological status of each species sampled as it relates to chemical contaminant exposure and effects.

Physical measurements can be made from small trawlers or ships-of-opportunity, using readily available and relatively cost-effective systems for measuring physical characteristics of the water column. Standard logs for weather observations, important in detecting global change, are an important component of the data-collecting effort. The monitoring of changes in fish stocks is ongoing in LMEs across the North Atlantic basin, including the Northeast U.S. Shelf, the Canadian Scotian Shelf, and Newfoundland Shelf, and on the Greenland Shelf, Icelandic Shelf, Norwegian Shelf, Barents Sea Shelf, and the North Sea. The plankton, nutrient loadings, and selected potentially harmful constituents (*e.g.*, petrogenic hydrocarbons, toxic phytoplankton) of LMEs can be measured in a cost-effective manner by deploying CPR systems from commercial vessels of opportunity.[43] The advanced plankton recorders can be fitted with sensors for temperature, salinity, chlorophyll, nitrate/nitrite, light, bioluminescence, zooplankton, and ichthyoplankton,[44,45] providing the means to monitor changes in phytoplankton, zooplankton, primary productivity, species composition and dominance, and long-term changes in the physical and nutrient characteristics of the LME, as well as longer term changes relating to the biofeedback of the plankton to the stress of climate change.[46–49] Plankton monitoring using the CPR (Continuous Plankton Recorder) system is at present expanding in the North Atlantic.

NORTHEAST SHELF LME STUDIES

A critical feature of the LME monitoring strategy is the development of a consistent long-term data base for understanding interannual changes and multi-year trends in biomass yields for each of the LMEs. An ecosystem monitoring strategy similar to the proposed core program has been operable in the waters of the Northeast Shelf Ecosystem by NOAA's National Marine Fisheries Service since the 1960s. During the late 1960s and early 1970s, when there was intense foreign fishing within the Northeast U.S. Continental Shelf Ecosystem, marked alterations in fish abundances were recorded. Significant shifts among species abundances were observed. The finfish biomass of important species (*e.g.*, cod, haddock, flounders, herring, and mackerel) declined by approximately 50% (FIG. 4). This was followed by increases in the biomass of sand lance (FIG. 5) and elasmobranchs (dogfish and skates) (FIG. 6) and led to the conclusion that the overall carrying capacity of the ecosystem for finfish did not change. The excessive fishing effort on highly valued species allowed for low-valued species to increase in abundance. Analyses of catch-per-unit-effort and fishery-independent bottom trawling survey data were critical sources of information used to implicate overfishing as the cause of the shifts in relative abundance among the species of the fish community within the shelf ecosystem. It is important to note, however, that the lower-end of the food chain in the offshore waters of the ecosystem remained unchanged, largely as described by Bigelow[50] and Riley *et al.*[51] during the earlier studies of the 1900s through the 1950s, suggesting that ecosystem productivity remained high during a period of species dominance shifts among the fish community caused by human interventions through fishing.[52] The natural "resilience" of the ecosystem in relation to recovery from stress can be documented in the recovery of mackerel to former (pre-1960) levels of abundance and the apparent recovery of herring to 1960s level of abun-

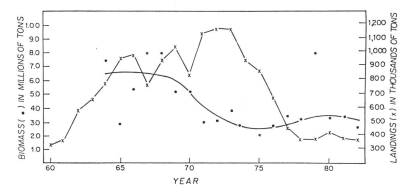

FIGURE 4. Annual catch trends, excluding menhaden and large pelagic species (*e.g.*, large sharks and tuna) and estimated biomass of "exploitable" fish and squid of the Northeastern Continental Shelf Ecosystem, 1960 to 1982.[70]

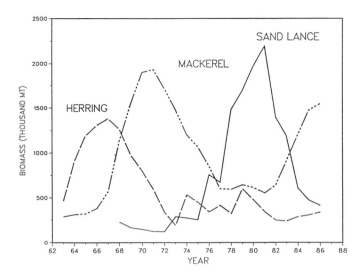

FIGURE 5. Trends in biomass of mackerel (age 1+) and herring (age 3+) derived from virtual population analysis (VPAs) and trends in relative abundance (stratified mean catch per tow [kg]) of sand lance (age 2+) based on research vessel surveys.[34]

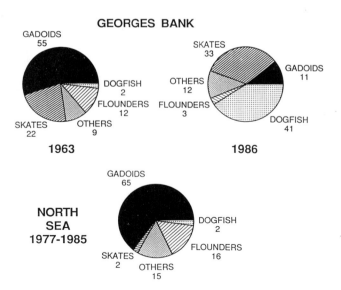

FIGURE 6. Species shift and abundance of small elasmobranchs (dogfish and skates) on Georges Bank within the Northeast Continental Shelf Ecosystem of the United States compared with the North Sea Ecosystem.[49]

dance on Georges Bank.[30,53] The gyre systems of the Gulf of Maine and Georges Bank subsystems and the nutrient enrichment of the estuaries in the southern half of the Northeast Shelf Ecosystem contribute to the maintenance on the shelf of relatively high levels of phytoplankton and zooplankton prey fields for planktivores including fish larvae, menhaden, herring, mackerel, sand lance, butterfish, and marine birds and mammals.

GLOBAL PERSPECTIVE

The topics of change and persistence in marine communities, and the need for multispecies and ecosystem perspectives in the management of marine resources were reviewed at the Dahlem Conference on Exploitation of Marine Communities in 1984.[54] The designation and management of LMEs is, at present, an evolving scientific and geopolitical process.[55,56] Sufficient progress has been made to allow for useful comparisons among different processes influencing large-scale changes in the biomass yields of LMEs.[57]

Among the ecosystems being managed from a more holistic perspective are: the Yellow Sea Ecosystem, where the principal effort is underway by the Peoples Republic of China;[58] the multispecies fisheries of the Benguela Current Ecosystem under the management of the government of South Africa;[16] the Great Barrier Reef Ecosystem;[59] and the Northwest Australian Continental Shelf Ecosystem[60] under management by the state and federal governments of Australia; the Antarctic Marine Ecosystem under the Commission for the Conservation of Antarctic Marine Living Resources (CCAMLR) and its 21-nation membership.[61,62] Within the EEZ of the United States, the state governments of Washington and Oregon have developed a comprehensive plan for the management of marine resources within the Northern California Current Ecosystem.[63]

The broad-spectrum approach to LME research and monitoring provides a conceptual framework for collaboration in process-oriented studies conducted by the National Science Foundation (NSF)-NOAA sponsored GLOBal ocean ECosystems dynamics (GLOBEC) program on the Northeast Continental Shelf[64] and proposed for other LMEs (e.g., California Current, Antarctic Marine Ecosystem) and the proposed Indian Ocean-Somalia Current Ecosystem study planned as part of the Joint Global Ocean Flux Studies (JGOFS).

With a minimum of expense and effort, ongoing FAO and UNEP marine programs can be strengthened by refocusing them around the natural boundaries of regional LMEs. The United Nations Environment Program (UNEP) Regional Seas programs can be enhanced by taking a more holistic ecosystems approach to pollution issues as part of an overall effort to improve the health of the oceans. The LME research and monitoring strategies are compatible with the Global Ocean Observing System (GOOS) proposed by the Intergovernmental Oceanographic Commission (IOC), and will, in fact, strengthen GOOS by adding an ecosystem module to the existing physical and meteorological modules.[65] The LME approach will complement the GLOBEC studies and provide useful data inputs to JGOFS. The concept has been discussed at meetings of ICES, International Council for the Scientific Exploration of the Mediterranean Sea (ICSEM), FAO, IOC, International Union for Conservation of Nature and Natural Resources (IUCN), and United Nations Environment Program (UNEP) with generally favorable responses for developing the concept more fully and implementing it more widely within the United Nations framework of ongoing programs. The concept is wholly compatible with the FAO interest in studying "catchment basins" and quantifying their impact on enclosed and semi-enclosed seas (*e.g.*, LMEs). The observations presently underway under the IOC/OSLR (Ocean Studies Related to Living Resources) program now operating within the California Current, Humboldt Current, and Iberian Coastal ecosystems provide an important framework for expanded LME studies of these systems in relation to not only fisheries issues, but also problems of pollution and coastal zone management.

FOCUS OF LME HEALTH STUDIES IN THE 1990s

Future effort directed at an improved definition of ecosystem health that will consider both natural environmental perturbation as well as the effects of human intervention on the changing states of ecosystems will focus on:

1) The development of ecosystem change and health indices and indicators for LMEs.

2) The development of component models of LMEs incorporating measurements of changing states and health indicators rather than single, large models that generally have limited prediction capability.

3) The development and evaluation of models using health indicators that are directly applicable to management decisions. They should be simple in construction, allow for interaction with resource managers, and provide sufficient flexibility for testing hypotheses for a range of scenarios.

Efforts are underway to link scientific and societal needs to support long-term, broad-area coastal ocean assessment and monitoring studies. If the proposition for time-series monitoring of changing ecosystem states is to be realized in this period of shrinking budgets, it would be in the best interests of science and society to be tightly linked in the endeavor. The basis for the linkage can be found in a series of recent developments revolving around: 1) recent interest in global climate change; 2) legal precedent for international cooperation implicit in the Law of the Sea; 3) a growing interest in marine ecosystems as regional units for marine research, monitoring, and management; and 4) the effort of the IOC to encourage the implementation of a GOOS. Global climate change has become a factor in the sustainability of biomass production in LMEs. The rather large-scale fluctuations in marine biomass yields of LMEs over the past several decades, when considered in the light of the growing concerns over coastal pollution and habitat loss, are serving to accelerate movement toward the development and implementation of a coastal component for GOOS. The core monitoring strategy for large marine ecosystems proposed for the coastal GOOS is designed to provide biological, physical, and chemical data pertinent to the development of indices to monitor changing states of LMEs. The indices are the basis for improving the dialogue between scientists and resource managers, for implementing mitigation strategies where appropriate, and for reinforcing the need for the long-term (multidecadal) ecosystem-wide monitoring programs.

The more holistic, ecosystem-wide approach to broad-area coastal and ocean marine resource assessment through monitoring studies is a means for fostering international cooperation and support in regions where the resources of the ecosystem are shared by several countries. The 49 large marine ecosystems that have been identified are located around the margins of the ocean basins and extend over the coastlines of several countries. They are in regions of the world's oceans most affected by overexploitation, pollution, and habitat degradation, and collectively represent target areas for mitigation effort. The Global Environment Facility (GEF) of the World Bank, in collaboration with NOAA, IOC, UNEP, FAO, Natural Environment Research Council (NERC), the Sir Alister Hardy Foundation for Ocean Science, and scientists from national marine resource agencies of several countries (*e.g.,* Belgium, Cameroon, China, Denmark, Estonia, Germany, Ivory Coast, Japan, Kenya, Korea, the Netherlands, Nigeria, Norway, Philippines, Poland, Thailand) are prepared to support LME assessment, mitigation, and coastal monitoring activities of the kind proposed recently in a commentary by Duarte *et al.*[66] These efforts will include a comparative approach to long-term monitoring of the environment which allows for examination of data sets from various areas, and is supported by "robust international management and funding systems." It appears that resource managers and scientists are being responsive in reversing the cancellation of monitoring programs described by Duarte *et al.,*[66] and that monitoring initiatives related to the long-term sustainability of marine resources are underway in Europe and elsewhere.[67]

REFERENCES

1. SHERMAN, K. & L. M. ALEXANDER, Eds. 1986. Variability and Management of Large Marine Ecosystems. American Association for the Advancement of Science (AAAS) Selected Symposium 99. Boulder, CO: Westview Press, Inc.
2. LEVIN, S. 1993. Approaches to forecasting biomass yields in large marine ecosystems. *In* Large Marine Ecosystems: Stress, Mitigation, and Sustainability. K. Sherman, L. M. Alexander & B. D. Gold, Eds.: 36–39. Washington, DC: AAAS Press.
3. MANGEL, M. 1991. Empirical and theoretical aspects of fisheries yield models for large marine ecosystems. *In* Food Chains, Yields, Models, and Management of Large Marine Ecosystems. K. Sherman, L. M. Alexander & B. D. Gold, Eds.: 243–261. Boulder, CO: Westview Press.
4. RICKLEFS, R. E. 1987. Community diversity: Relative roles of local and regional processes. Science 235(4785): 167–171.
5. LEVIN, S. A. 1990. Physical and biological scales, and modelling of predator-prey interactions in large marine ecosystems. *In* Large Marine Ecosystems: Patterns, Processes, and Yields. K. Sherman, L. M. Alexander & B. D. Gold, Eds.: 179–187. Washington, DC: AAAS Press.
6. GRAHAM, R. L., C. T. HUNSAKER, R. V. O'NEILL & B. L. JACKSON. 1991. Ecological risk assessment at the regional scale. Ecol. Applications 1: 196–206.

7. BELSKY, M. H. 1986. Legal constraints and options for total ecosystem management of
    large marine ecosystems. *In* Variability and Management of Large Marine Ecosystems.
    K. Sherman & L. M. Alexander, Eds. AAAS Selected Symposium 99: 241–261. Boulder,
    CO: Westview Press, Inc.

8. BELSKY, M. H. 1989. The ecosystem model mandate for a comprehensive United States
    ocean policy and Law of the Sea. San Diego L. Rev. **26**(3): 417–495.

9. MYERS, N. 1990. Working towards one world. Book review. Nature **344**(6266): 499–500.

10. TAYLOR, P. & A. J. R. GROOM, Eds. 1989. Global Issues in the United Nation's Frame-
    work. London: Macmillan.

11. MALONE, T. C. 1991. River flow, phytoplankton production and oxygen depletion in
    Chesapeake Bay. *In* Modern and Ancient Continental Shelf Anoxia. R. V. Tyson &
    T. H. Pearson, Eds. Geological Society Spec. Publ. No. 58: 83–93.

12. SUGIHARA, G., S. GARCIA, J. A. GULLAND, J. H. LAWTON, H. MASKE, R. T. PAINE,
    T. PLATT, E. RACHOR, B. J. ROTHSCHILD, E. A. URSIN & B. F. K. ZEITZSCHEL.
    1984. Ecosystem dynamics: Group report. *In* Exploitation of Marine Communities.
    R. M. May, Ed.: 130–153. Berlin: Springer-Verlag.

13. MACCALL, A. D. 1986. Changes in the biomass of the California Current system. *In*
    Variability and Management of Large Marine Ecosystems. K. Sherman & L. M. Alexan-
    der, Eds. AAAS Selected Symposium 99: 33–54. Boulder, CO: Westview Press, Inc.

14. CROXALL, J. P., Ed. 1987. Seabirds: Feeding Ecology and Role in Marine Ecosystems.
    London: Cambridge University Press.

15. BURGER, J. 1988. Interactions of marine birds with other marine vertebrates in marine
    environments. *In* Seabirds and Other Marine Vertebrates. J. Burger, Ed.: 3–28. New
    York: Columbia University Press.

16. CRAWFORD, R. J. M., L. V. SHANNON & P. A. SHELTON. 1989. Characteristics and
    management of the Benguela as a large marine ecosystem. *In* Biomass Yields and Geogra-
    phy of Large Marine Ecosystems. K. Sherman & L. M. Alexander, Eds. AAAS Selected
    Symposium 111: 169–219. Boulder, CO: Westview Press, Inc.

17. KULLENBERG, G. 1986. Long-term changes in the Baltic Ecosystem. *In* Variability and
    Management of Large Marine Ecosystems. K. Sherman & L. M. Alexander, Eds. AAAS
    Selected Symposium 99: 19–32. Boulder, CO: Westview Press, Inc.

18. ZAITSEV, YU. P. 1992. Recent changes in the trophic structure of the Black Sea. Fish.
    Oceanogr. **1**(2): 180–189.

19. CADDY, J. 1993. Contrast between recent fishery trends and evidence for nutrient enrich-
    ment in two large marine ecosystems: The Mediterranean and the Black Seas. *In* Large
    Marine Ecosystems: Stress, Mitigation, and Sustainability. K. Sherman, L. M. Alexander
    & B. D. Gold, Eds.: 137–147. Washington, DC: AAAS Press.

20. COSTANZA, R. 1992. Toward an operational definition of ecosystem health. *In* Ecosystem
    Health: New Goals for Environmental Management. R. Costanza, B. G. Norton &
    B. D. Haskell, Eds.: 239–256. Washington, DC: Island Press.

21. RAPPORT, D. J. 1992. What is Clinical Ecology? *In* Ecosystem Health: New Goals for
    Environmental Management. R. Costanza, B. G. Norton & B. D. Haskell, Eds.:
    144–156. Washington, DC: Island Press.

22. NORTON, B. G. & R. E. ULANOWICZ. 1992. Scale and biodiversity policy: A hierarchical
    approach. AMBIO **21**(3).

23. KARR, J. 1992. Ecological integrity: Protecting earth's life support systems. *In* Ecosystem
    Health: New Goals for Environmental Management. R. Costanza, B. G. Norton &
    B. D. Haskell, Eds.: 223–238. Washington, DC: Island Press.

24. PIMM, S. L. 1984. The complexity and stability of ecosystems. Nature **307**: 321–326.

25. HOLLING, C. S. 1986. The resilience of terrestrial ecosystems local surprise and global
    change. *In* Sustainable Development of the Biosphere. W. C. Clark & R. E. Munn,
    Eds.: 292–317. London: Cambridge University Press.

26. SHERMAN, K. 1993. Emerging Theoretical Basis for Monitoring Changing States (Health)
    of Large Marine Ecosystems. U.S. Department of Commerce, NOAA Tech. Mem.
    NMFS-F/NEC-100.

27. SHERMAN, K. & T. LAUGHLIN, Eds. 1992. Large marine ecosystems monitoring workshop
    report. U.S. Department of Commerce, NOAA Tech. Mem. NMFS-F/NEC-93.

28. SHERMAN, K., M. GROSSLEIN, D. MOUNTAIN, D. BUSCH, J. O'REILLY & R. THEROUX. 1988. The continental shelf ecosystem off the northeast coast of the United States. *In* Ecosystems of the World 27: Continental Shelves. H. Postma & J. J. Zilstra, Eds.: 279–337. Amsterdam, the Netherlands: Elsevier

29. SISSENWINE, M. P. & E. B. COHEN. 1991. Resource productivity and fisheries management of the northeast shelf ecosystem. *In* Food Chains, Yields, Models, and Management of Large Marine Ecosystems. K. Sherman, L. M. Alexander & B. D. Gold, Eds.: 107–123. Boulder, CO: Westview Press, Inc.

30. MURAWSKI, S. A. 1991. Can we manage our multispecies fisheries? Fisheries. 16(5): 5–13.

31. SHERMAN, K., N. JAWORSKI & T. SMAYDA. 1992a. The Northeast Shelf Ecosystem: Stress, Mitigation, and Sustainability, 12–15 August 1991 Symposium Summary. U.S. Department of Commerce, NOAA Tech. Mem. NMFS-F/NEC-94.

32. SMAYDA, T. 1991. Global epidemic of noxious phytoplankton blooms and food chain consequences in large ecosystems. *In* Food Chains, Yields, Models, and Management of Large Marine Ecosystems. K. Sherman, L. M. Alexander & B. D. Gold, Eds.: 275–308. Boulder, CO: Westview Press, Inc.

33. GESAMP [GROUP OF EXPERTS ON THE SCIENTIFIC ASPECTS OF MARINE POLLUTION]. 1990. The state of the marine environment. UNEP Regional Seas Reports and Studies No. 115. Nairobi.

34. FOGARTY, M., E. B. COHEN, W. L. MICHAELS & W. W. MORSE. 1991. Predation and the Regulation of Sand Lance Populations: An Exploratory Analysis. ICES Marine Sci. Symp. 193: 120–124.

35. POWERS, K. D., & R. G. B. BROWN. 1987. Seabirds. *In* Georges Bank. R. H. Backus, Ed. Chapter 34: 359–371. Cambridge, MA: MIT Press.

36. OVERHOLTZ, W. J. & J. R. NICOLAS. 1979. Apparent feeding by the fin whale *Balaenoptera physalus*, and humpback whale, *Megoptera novaeangliae*, on the American sand lance, *Ammodytes americanus*, in the Northwest Atlantic. Fish. Bull. U.S. 77: 285–287.

37. PAYNE, P. M., D. N. WILEY, S. B. YOUNG, S. PITTMAN, P. J. CLAPHAM & J. W. JOSSI. 1990. Recent fluctuations in the abundance of baleen whales in the southern Gulf of Maine in relation to changes in selected prey. Fish. Bull. U.S. 88: 687–696.

38. KAWASAKI, T., S. TANAKA, Y. TOBA & A. TANIGUCHI, Eds. 1991. Long-term Variability of Pelagic Fish Populations and Their Environment. Proceedings of the International Symposium, Sendai, Japan, 14–18 November 1989. Pergamon Press, Tokyo, Japan.

39. BAKUN, A. 1993. The California Current, Benguela Current, and Southwestern Atlantic Shelf ecosystems: A comparative approach to identifying factors regulating biomass yields. *In* Large Marine Ecosystems: Stress, Mitigation, and Sustainability. K. Sherman, L. M. Alexander & B. D. Gold, Eds.: 99–221. Washington, DC: AAAS Press.

40. ALHEIT, J. & P. BERNAL. 1993. Effects of physical and biological changes on the biomass yield of the Humboldt Current ecosystem. *In* Large Marine Ecosystems: Stress, Mitigation, and Sustainability. K. Sherman, L. M. Alexander & B. D. Gold, Eds.: 53–68. Washington, DC: AAAS Press.

41. AZAROVITZ, T. R. & M. D. GROSSLEIN. 1987. Fishes and squids. *In* Georges Bank. R. H. Backus, Ed.: 315–346. Cambridge, MA: MIT Press.

42. ICES [INTERNATIONAL COUNCIL FOR THE EXPLORATION OF THE SEA]. 1991. Report of the Multispecies Working Group. ICES C.M. 1991/Assess:7.

43. GLOVER, R. S. 1967. The Continuous Plankton Recorder survey of the North Atlantic. Symp. Zool. Soc. Lon. 19: 189–210.

44. AIKEN, J. 1981. The Undulating Oceanographic Recorder Mark 2. J. Plankton Res. 3: 551–560.

45. UNESCO [UNITED NATIONS EDUCATIONAL, SCIENTIFIC AND CULTURAL ORGANIZATION]. 1992. Monitoring the health of the oceans: Defining the role of the Continuous Plankton Recorder in global ecosystems studies. The Intergovernmental Oceanographic Commission and The Sir Alister Hardy Foundation for Ocean Science. IOC/INF-869, SC-92/WS-8.

46. COLEBROOK, J. M. 1986. Environmental influences on long-term variability in marine plankton. Hydrobiologia 142: 309–325.

47. DICKSON, R. R., P. M. KELLY, J. M. COLEBROOK, W. S. WOOSTER & D. H. CUSHING.

         1988. North winds and production in the eastern North Atlantic. J. Plankton Res.
         10: 151–169.
48. Jossi, J. W. & D. E. Smith. 1990. Continuous plankton records: Massachusetts to
         Cape Sable, N.S., and New York to the Gulf Stream, 1989. NAFO Ser. Doc. **90/
         66:** 1–11.
49. Sherman, K., E. B. Cohen & R. W. Langton. 1990. The Northeast Continental
         Shelf: An Ecosystem at Risk. *In* Gulf of Maine: Sustaining our Common Heritage. V.
         Konrad, S. Ballard, R. Erb & A. Morin, Eds.: 120–167. Proceedings of an International
         Conference held at Portland, Maine, December 10–12, 1989. Published by Maine State
         Planning Office and the Canadian-American Center of the University of Maine.
50. Bigelow, H. B. 1926. Plankton of the offshore waters of the Gulf of Maine. Bull. of the
         Bureau of Fish. XL Part 2. Washington DC: Government Printing Office.
51. Riley, G. A., H. Stommel & D. F. Bumpus. 1949. Quantitative ecology of the plankton
         of the western North Atlantic. Bull. Bingham Oceanogr. Coll. **XII**(3): 169 pages.
52. Sherman, K., J. R. Green, J. R. Goulet & L. Ejsymont. 1983. Coherence in
         zooplankton of a large Northwest Atlantic Ecosystem. Fish. Bull. U.S. **81:** 855–862.
53. Smith, W. G. & W. W. Morse. 1993. Larval distribution patterns: Early signals for
         the collapse/recovery of Atlantic herring *Clupea harengus* in the Georges Bank area. Fish.
         Bull. U.S. **91:** 338–347.
54. May, R. M., Ed. 1984. Exploitation of Marine Communities. Berlin: Springer-Verlag.
55. Morgan, J. R. 1988. Large marine ecosystems: An emerging concept of regional manage-
         ment. Environment **29**(10): 4–9 & 26–34.
56. Alexander, L. M. 1989. Large marine ecosystems as global management units. *In* Biomass
         Yields and Geography of Large Marine Ecosystems. K. Sherman & L. M. Alexander,
         Eds.: AAAS Selected Symposium 111: 339–344. Boulder, CO: Westview Press, Inc.
57. Bax, N. J. & T. Laevastu. 1990. Biomass potential of large marine ecosystems: a systems
         approach. *In* Large Marine Ecosystems: Patterns, Processes and Yields. K. Sherman,
         L. M. Alexander & B. D. Gold, Eds.: 188–205. Washington, DC: AAAS Press.
58. Tang, Q. 1989. Changes in the biomass of the Yellow Sea ecosystems. *In* Biomass Yields
         and Geography of Large Marine Ecosystems. K. Sherman & L. M. Alexander, Eds.
         AAAS Selected Symposium 111: 7–35. Boulder, CO: Westview Press, Inc.
59. Bradbury, R. H. & C. N. Mundy. 1989. Large-scale shifts in biomass of the Great
         Barrier Reef ecosystem. *In* Biomass Yields and Geography of Large Marine Ecosystems.
         K. Sherman & L. M. Alexander, Eds. AAAS Selected Symposium 111: 143–167.
         Boulder, CO: Westview Press, Inc.
60. Sainsbury, K. J. 1988. The ecological basis of multispecies fisheries, and management
         of a dermersal fishery in tropical Australia. *In* Fish Population Dynamics, 2nd edit.
         J. A. Gulland, Ed.: 349–382. New York: John Wiley & Sons.
61. Scully, R. T., W. Y. Brown & B. S. Manheim. 1986. The Convention for the
         Conservation of Antarctic Marine Living Resources: A model for large marine ecosystem
         management. *In* Variability and Management of Large Marine Ecosystems. K. Sherman
         & L. M. Alexander, Eds. AAAS Selected Symposium 99: 281–286. Boulder, CO:
         Westview Press, Inc.
62. Sherman, K. & A. F. Ryan. 1988. Antarctic marine living resources. Oceanus
         31(2): 59–63.
63. Bottom, D. L., K. K. Jones, J. D. Rodgers & R. F. Brown. 1989. Management
         of living resources: A research plan for the Washington and Oregon continental margin.
         National Coastal Resources Research and Development Institute, Newport, OR. NCRI-
         T-89-004, 80 pp.
64. Global Ocean ECosystems Dynamics [GLOBEC]. 1991. Report Number 1. Initial
         science plan. February 1991. Washington, DC: Joint Oceanographic Institutions Inc.
65. IOC [International Oceanographic Commission of UNESCO]. 1992. GOOS.
         Global Ocean Observing System, An initiative of the Intergovernmental Oceanographic
         Commission (of UNESCO). Paris, France: IOC, UNESCO.
66. Duarte, C. M., J. Cebrian & N. Marba. 1992. Uncertainty of detecting sea change.
         Nature **356:** 190.

67. SHERMAN, K., H. SKJOLDAL & R. WILLIAMS. 1992b. Global ocean monitoring. Nature 359: 769.
68. SHERMAN, K. & A. SOLOW. 1992. The changing states and health of a large marine ecosystem. ICES C.M. 1992/L:38, Session V.
69. LIKENS, G. E. 1992. The Ecosystem Approach: Its Use and Abuse. Excellence in Ecology. Vol. 3. O. Kinne, Ed. W-2124 Oldendorf/Luhe, Germany: Ecology Institute.
70. SISSENWINE, M. P. 1986. Perturbation of a predator-controlled continental shelf ecosystem. *In* Variability and Management of Large Marine Ecosystems. K. Sherman & L. M. Alexander, Eds. AAAS Selected Symposium 99: 55–85. Boulder, CO: Westview Press, Inc.

Environmental Reservoir of *Vibrio cholerae*

The Causative Agent of Cholera[a]

RITA R. COLWELL[b,c,d] AND ANWARUL HUQ[c]

bUniversity of Maryland Biotechnology Institute
4321 Hartwick Building,
College Park, Maryland 20740

cDepartment of Microbiology
College Park, Maryland 20742

BACKGROUND

Until the late 1970s and early 1980s, *Vibrio cholerae* was believed to be highly host-adapted and incapable of surviving longer than a few hours or days outside the human intestine. This view, enunciated by Felsenfeld,[1] was that "some authors claimed that cholera vibrios may survive in water, particularly seawater, for as long as 2 months. This is, however, scarcely possible under natural conditions, if reinfection of the water does not take place." This perspective of cholera ecology dominated the literature since the organism was first identified by Robert Koch in 1884.[2]

For *V. cholerae* the term "survival" had been viewed to reflect a high degree of host-adaptation, *e.g.*, "cholera vibrios" being able to exist for only very short periods of time outside the human intestine. But Koch's speculation that multiplication takes place in river water, without any assistance, has proven to be prescient, since the most recent data show that toxigenic *V. cholerae* O1 exist for long periods in laboratory microcosm water.[3] In fact, the evidence accumulated over the past decade shows that *V. cholerae* is an autochthonous inhabitant of brackish water and estuarine systems.[4] The autochthonous nature of *V. cholerae* O1 is an important factor in the epidemiology of cholera, significantly so in endemic areas. Thus, the very early studies of *V. cholerae*, prior to 1970, were aimed at identifying environmental conditions associated with unusual delays in the inevitable "death" of the "cholera vibrios," in order to establish the length of time after which an environment could be considered cholera-free, unless recontaminated with infected stool.

The remarkable discoveries of the past decade have revealed the existence of the dormant or somnabulant (*i.e.*, viable but non-culturable) state into which *V. cholerae* O1 and *V. cholerae* non-O1 enter in response to nutrient

[a] The work reported here was supported, in part, by NOAA Grant No. NA16RU0264-02, National Science Foundation Grant No. BSR-9020268, and Environmental Protection Agency Cooperative Agreement No. CR817791-01.

[d] Address correspondence to: Rita R. Colwell at the University of Maryland Biotechnology Institute; Tel: 301-403-0105; Fax: 301-454-8123.

deprivation and other environmental conditions.[5] This phenomenon represents a new perspective and imparts a dynamic meaning to the term "survival," suggesting that *V. cholerae* cells do not necessarily die when discharged into aquatic environments, but instead remain viable, and capable of transforming into a "culturable state," if environmental conditions again become favorable.[6] The implications of dormancy of *V. cholerae* O1 are both significant and relevant, considering that dormant (viable but non-culturable) forms are not recoverable on conventional bacteriological media routinely used to isolate and maintain cells of *V. cholerae* in culture. However, non-culturable forms of *V. cholerae* O1, when inoculated in rabbit ileal loops and tested in human volunteers, caused large amounts of fluid accumulation and diarrhea, respectively.[5,7]

EVIDENCE FOR A VIABLE, NON-CULTURABLE STATE

The evidence, primarily based on physiological studies of *V. cholerae* in aquatic environments, is such that the dormant or viable but non-culturable state transcends mere survival and addresses the more fundamental questions of adaptation and response of microorganisms to environmental conditions.[8] Studies, based on observations using microcosms simulating saline, estuarine, brackish and fresh-water environments, have provided new and important information on *V. cholerae* physiology in relation to temperature and salinity, adherence, and colonization of chitinaceous and mucilaginous macrobiota.

Studies prior to 1970 were all based on methods for isolation and characterization of *V. cholerae* originally developed for diagnosis of cholera in hospital laboratories.[9] The many difficulties associated with isolation of *V. cholerae* O1 from the aquatic environment can be related to the simple fact that methods for isolating *V. cholerae* were developed for clinical specimens containing large numbers of actively growing cells. Such methods do not work for environmental samples that are likely to contain cells exposed to and, thereby, adapted to a variety of environmental conditions including, most commonly, low nutrient concentration, pH in the range of 7–8 (seawater), fluctuating temperatures and pH, variations in oxygen tension, exposure to UV via sunlight, *etc.*[10] The findings of Colwell *et al.*[5] that *V. cholerae* O1 in environmental samples may not grow on laboratory media routinely used for isolation was a pivotal point in the debate concerning the ecology of *V. cholerae*, namely, that viable but "non-culturable" cells may go undetected unless appropriate methods for detection, *e.g.,* molecular, immunological, or direct microscopy, are employed. With modern molecular biology techniques, combined with immunological direct detection methods, it can be convincingly demonstrated that viable but non-culturable *V. cholerae* O1 occur, even in clinical specimens from patients with the disease.[5,7,11]

It has traditionally been known that cholera can be transmitted via water, wastewater, and food.[12] However, a consistent theme of the reports on this subject in the literature on *V. cholerae* O1 is that, when cells of *V. cholerae* are suspended in fresh or saline water, they show a steady decrease in number of cells enumerable over time by plate counts. To address this issue, the conversion of *V. cholerae* from the culturable to the viable but non-culturable state was demonstrated in laboratory microcosms.[13,14] Subsequent studies showed that survival is enhanced in saline waters but that the organism maintains itself less well in potable water. In any case, there is an absolute requirement of Na^+ for growth of *V. cholerae* in water.[15] The traditional argument in support of the view that *V. cholerae* O1 does not survive in environmental waters has been the failure to isolate the organism from environmental water sources unless existing cases of cholera were in close proximity. For example, epidemiologic surveillance in the intensively monitored Matlab area in Bangladesh in 1969, failed to isolate *V. cholerae* O1 from water sources between cholera seasons or from water not subject to contamination by active cholera cases.[16] In contrast, Huq *et al.*[6] showed that *V. cholerae* O1 could be detected throughout the year by direct immunofluorescent microscopy in these waters even at times when the organism could not be isolated (*i.e.,* cultured) from water.

Huq *et al.*[6] for the first time, reported the presence of *V. cholerae* O1 throughout the year by detecting the organism in > 63% of plankton specimens, using a fluorescent antibody detection method. Results for water samples collected in Matlab, Bangladesh, were FA positive for *V. cholerae* O1 when < 1% of the same specimens collected were positive for culturable *V. cholerae* O1. Earlier, Tamplin *et al.*[17] reported attachment of *V. cholerae* O1 to zooplankton and phytoplankton from natural waters. By using the direct detection technique, Islam *et al.*[3] have demonstrated the persistence of *V. cholerae* O1 under laboratory conditions for over 15 months in association with blue green bacteria. Thus, the most recent findings show the existence of a viable but non-culturable state for *V. cholerae* O1. Clearly, the microorganism is able to adapt and maintains itself in the aquatic environment in a form that will be missed by surveillance methodologies other than direct detection by fluorescent antibody or gene probes.

Probably the most profound challenge to prior dogma concerning *V. cholerae* O1 ecology derives from studies by Colwell *et al.*[5] suggesting that *V. cholerae* O1 possesses the ability to enter a state of (or one approximating to) dormancy in response to nutrient deprivation, elevated salinity, and/or reduced temperature. Exposure to low nutrient conditions has recently been recognized as one important stimulus to enter the viable but non-culturable state, and represents a common strategy for survival among bacteria in nutrient-poor environments.[8] Novitsky and Morita[18–20] demonstrated that cultures of the marine psychrophilic *Vibrio* sp. ANT-300 responded to starvation in either natural or artificial seawater by increasing the number of cells producing progeny cells with decreased volume. Morphology also was altered from the typical bacillus—rod-shape—to coccoid cells. The coccoid cells exhibited an endogenous respiration less than 1% of the original, as well as a 40% decrease in cellular DNA, but remained culturable. Novitsky and Morita[20] did not postulate a viable but non-culturable state, but, rather, presented excellent evidence of adaptation of cells to a low nutrient environment, since they studied only those cells remaining culturable, not recognizing cells that were viable but non-culturable.

Colwell et al.,[5] Huq et al.,[6] Roszak et al.,[8] Xu et al.,[14] and Brayton et al.,[13] demonstrated, by both field and laboratory studies, that *V. cholerae*, indeed, undergoes conversion to a viable but non-culturable state, whereby the cells are reduced in size, become ovoid, but, in contrast to starved cells, do not grow at all on standard laboratory media, but remain responsive to nalidixic acid and continue to assimilate radiolabeled substrate.[8,21] In other experiments, cells of *V. cholerae* O1 (strain CA401) were inoculated into microcosms of chemically defined sea-salts solution adjusted to 0.5% salinity and incubated at 10°C or 25°C for 24 or 96 hours. The direct viable count (DVC) represented, in all cases, *ca.* 98% of the acridine orange direct count (AODC), while the percentage of culturable cells, compared with AODC counts, ranged from 13% (10 C, 2.5% salinity) to 87% (25 C, 0.5% salinity).

ESTUARINE SURVIVAL

Hood and Ness[22] reported results similar to those obtained by Xu et al.[14] but used a non-toxigenic *V. cholerae* O1 strain isolated from oysters and five non-toxigenic *V. cholerae* non-O1 environmental isolates, as well as a clinical isolate of *V. cholerae* O1. Survival was monitored in sterile and non-sterile estuarine waters and sediments at 20°C by AODC and plate count on Trypticase Soy-1.5% NaCl agar. All of the strains showed similar patterns, in sterile estuarine water, where the culturable counts remained relatively constant for the duration of monitoring (up to 15 days) and were consistently 0.5 to 1 $\log_{10}$ less than the AODC counts.

Later, Baker et al.[23] provided evidence for the formation of small coccoid cells by both an environmental strain (WF110) from shellfish and a clinical strain of *V. cholerae* CA401 exposed to nutrient-free artificial seawater and filter-sterilized natural seawater microcosms. Total counts (TC) were determined by direct epifluorescence microscopy on preparations stained with 4', 6-diamino-2-phenylinodole (DAPI). Viability was determined by DVC and plate counts on a seawater-based, complete medium incubated for 72 hours at 30°C. Microcosms were maintained at 21°C for up to 330 days following inoculation, yielding approximately 5×10^3 cells by culturable count. The results showed no significant difference between the two seawater solutions or between the two strains of *V. cholerae*, with respect to starvation-survival. Upon exposure to starvation conditions, the clinical as well as the environmental isolate underwent reductive cell division, increased cell numbers, and formed coccoid cells, while greatly reducing individual cell volume. By two days after inoculation, the culturable counts increased approximately 2.5 $\log_{10}$. From that peak, all counts decreased steadily and gradually (< 0.5 $\log_{10}$ overall) until the experiment was terminated at 55 or 75 days. At the time of inoculation, the total (AODC) count was approximately 0.5 $\log_{10}$ greater than the DVC and 1 $\log_{10}$ greater than the culturable count. By 20 days and, thereafter, this difference increased to 1 $\log_{10}$ and 2 $\log_{10}$, respectively. The relationship between the slopes for TC, DVC, and culturable counts remained essentially constant throughout; there was no sudden or rapid decrease in viability or increase in viable but non-recoverable cells in any of the time periods monitored. Since incubation was at 21°C, in contrast to the much lower temperature employed by Xu et al.,[14] these data indicate the importance of temperature in inducing the viable but non-culturable state in V. cholerae. The morphological response to starvation, monitored by electron microscopy, appeared to be uniform for the two strains studied.

SEASONALITY AND ENVIRONMENTAL CONDITIONS

The annual distribution of V. cholerae detected by fluorescent antibody method has been reported by Huq et al.[6] However, the seasonality of this organism, coupled with the starvation response and non-culturable phenomenon was earlier reported by Colwell et al.,[5] and reflects the origin of V. cholerae as an autochthonous estuary-dweller. The capacity of V. cholerae to undergo starvation response, as well as enter the viable but non-culturable state makes it clear that long-term survival of this organism in the environment, perhaps for years, must be considered a source of the organism in cholera epidemics. When the cells are subjected to nutrient depletion or addition, reduction, or elevation in salinity and temperature, the cells rapidly go non-culturable, but remain viable and potentially pathogenic, as demonstrated by Colwell et al.[5] who employed rabbit loop assays to recover viable but not culturable cells of V. cholerae from cold, full strength seawater. Furthermore, non-culturable cells of a vaccine strain of V. cholerae (i.e., with the CT gene removed) when ingested by volunteers in feeding experiment produced diarrhea.[7]

Isolation of V. cholerae from the natural aquatic environment has been patchy and the concentration of cells varies, depending upon the culture methods used for detection. More frequent isolation occurring in the summer months may be a result of higher temperatures and increased concentrations of available nutrient. A linear correlation with salinity was observed, with greater frequency of isolations at sites of salinities between 0.2–2.0‰. The effect of temperature was more strongly correlated with the frequency of isolation; that is, there was more frequent isolation when the water temperature was greater than 17°C. From these data, Colwell et al.[24] concluded that V. cholerae is autochthonous in brackish water and estuarine environments, a finding supported by Hood and co-workers,[25,26] who reported strong linear correlations between V. cholerae non-O1 and temperature and salinity in two estuaries in Florida. The constantly changing conditions in tidal estuaries suggests an association of the ability of V. cholerae to adapt to a wide range of salinity and temperature conditions, with its natural ecological habitat being brackish, riverine, and estuarine waters.

To obtain an understanding of salinity and temperature relationships for V. cholerae, laboratory microcosms were prepared, simulating environmental conditions, which can be controlled and replicated as required. This approach provided an advantage of being able to measure quantitatively those environmental effects on *V. cholerae* O1, as well as effects of environmental parameters on pathogenic properties during exposure to water of varying salinities, temperatures, *etc.* Cells of *V. cholerae* O1 in natural waters are not consistently detectable by culture methods, as discussed above. In fact, detection, enumeration, and monitoring *V. cholerae* in the environment are not yet feasible unless a method is used that allows detection of non-culturable organisms. The fluorescent antibody direct staining approach has proven to be very effective for samples collected from the natural environment.[6]

The first extensive studies of salinity and temperature relationships using microcosms was reported by Singleton *et al.*[15,27] using *V. cholerae* O1 strain LA4808 isolated during the 1978 El Tor cholera outbreak in Louisiana, and nine other clinical or environmental strains, including both O1 and non-O1 *V. cholerae.* The number of bacterial cells in the microcosms, over time, were calculated from viable plate and AODC microscopic counts, using samples taken from microcosms prepared with a chemically defined sea salts solution in which the salinity, organic nutrient concentration, or temperature was varied. Following initial studies by Singleton *et al.*,[15] survival and growth of *V. cholerae* under various conditions of salinity, pH, temperature, and presence of cations was reported by Miller *et al.*[28] A total of 59 strains, representing a variety of biovars, were examined, using viable plate counts on Trypticase Soy Agar. Six *V. cholerae* O1 isolates were extensively studied. Results from these studies showed that strains of *V. cholerae* varied greatly in survival in the culturable state under conditions of low salinity (0.05%) and this response was unrelated to serotype, *i.e.*, O1 or non-O1, source (clinical or environmental), or country of origin (*e.g.*, Tanzania or Bangladesh). At 25°C, 18 of the 20 strains tested remained viable, with less variation at optimal salinity.

VIBRIO CHOLERAE AND PLANKTON

It has been demonstrated from *in situ* studies that vibrios make up a significant portion of the normal flora in many aquatic environments, with presence of *V. cholerae* strongly influenced by salinity and temperature, as discussed above. Parallel laboratory microcosm studies showed that the strict requirement for Na^+ is not limiting in natural waters, but that salinity, as the key determinant of osmolarity, normally would restrict the distribution of *V. cholerae* to water of more than potable salinity. By studying the influence of water temperature, salinity, and pH on survival and growth of toxigenic *V. cholerae* O1 associated with live copepods,[29] it was concluded that 15‰ salinity, 30°C water temperature, and 8.5 pH supported increased attachment and multiplication of *V. cholerae* on copepods. Results provided by Colwell *et al.*[4,24] and Kaper *et al.*[30] also suggest that growth of *V. cholerae* in the environment is limited to waters with temperatures above 10°C. Survival through cold seasons, however, depends upon the capacity of the organism to enter the dormant state, as discussed earlier.

Tamplin and Colwell[31] demonstrated that toxin production in microcosm cultures was related to salinity, demonstrating a salinity optimum between 2.0%–2.5% for toxin production, that was independent of cell concentration and toxin stability. A study reported by Miller et al.[32] showed that cells do not lose enterotoxigenicity after long-term exposure (64 days) in microcosms under a variety of conditions, nor did a selection for either hyper- or hypo-toxigenic mutants occur. However, increased toxin production by toxigenic V. cholerae O1 has been reported when the organism is associated with Rhizoclonium fontanum, a green alga commonly found in natural water.[33] Clearly, cholera toxin-positive strains of V. cholerae O1 do not dramatically alter their toxigenic character, even after entering into the non-culturable state in the aquatic environment.

The phenomenon of the non-culturable stage of V. cholerae and its association with phyto- and zooplankton and survival in the aquatic environment are very important in the ecology of this organism. Huq et al.[34] demonstrated that V. cholerae, when associated with planktonic live copepods, survived longer in laboratory microcosms, compared to exposure to dead copepods, or in the presence of Pseudoisochrysis sp., a blue-green alga used to feed live copepods. In this study, cells of V. cholerae were enumerated by plate count and it was found that the organisms could be cultured on plates up to 336 hours. However, no attempts were made to detect the presence of viable cells of V. cholerae that entered into the non-culturable state, as the fluorescent antibody method had not yet been developed nor was an established method for detection of toxigenic V. cholerae, such as PCR, available at that time. In a subsequent study, Huq et al.[6] were able to detect cells of V. cholerae O1 in 63% of plankton samples collected in Bangladesh during a 3-year study. In this same study, they were able to culture V. cholerae O1 on plates from < 1% of the water samples and none from plankton samples. These findings suggested that cells of V. cholerae, when attached to plankton, enter into the non-culturable stage as a part of their mechanism for survival in the environment. Further evidence showing the natural habitat of this organism to be in the environment will be reported elsewhere (R. R. Colwell et al. 1994, unpublished data).

Most recently, toxigenic V. cholerae O1 were detected in a non-epidemic area.[35] The study was carried out on divers diving in the Chesapeake Bay region of the United States and the Black Sea off the coasts of Russia and the Ukraine. V. cholerae O1 were isolated using culture methods and also were detected in seawater and from swabs of the ears, nose, and throat of divers, using the fluorescent antibody method, when culture was unsuccessful. Blood samples drawn from the divers before and two weeks after the dives demonstrated clinically significant rise in vibriocidal antibody titer, even when the divers did not manifest clinical symptoms. It is interesting to note that in June, 1991, V. cholerae O1 was detected in water and plankton specimens collected in the Black Sea, using direct detection kits and fluorescent antibody direct staining. These same samples, however, were not culture positive, except in a few instances. Approximately four weeks after this field work was completed, in the same coastal area where swimming and bathing beaches are located, an outbreak of cholera was reported in a local newspaper, *Recher-nya Odessa,* on September 11, 1991.

A few examples of adherence to non-chitinaceous surfaces described for *V. cholerae* include attachment to roots of water hyacinth by *V. cholerae* O1[36] in fresh water of cholera endemic areas and to green algae.[37,38]

CONCLUSION

In summary, in Bangladesh, thousands of water samples can be analyzed without a single isolation of *V. cholerae* O1 in culture. At the same time, millions of people, several times daily, ingest water directly from these water sources, creating a much greater "sampling" intensity that leads to a finite number of primary cases, *i.e.*, cases arising from ingestion of autochthonous *V. cholerae* O1. Thus, the conclusion is that *V. cholerae* O1 resides in the environment and enters into a stage whereby it cannot be cultured but, at the same time, conversion of the organism to the culturable state occurs, either in the environment or via human or animal passage. A possible hypothetical cycle has been suggested[39] (FIG. 1). What the actual sequence of events

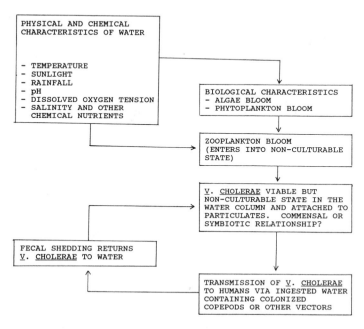

FIGURE 1. Hypothetical model for the transmission of *Vibrio cholerae* in nature. (Modified from the original published in *Biological Monitoring of Environmental Pollution,* 1988 Tokai University Press, Japan.)

is in the "life cycle" of *V. cholerae* remains to be eludicated fully, but the hypothesis which we have described in this paper offers the most workable explanation to date.

REFERENCES

1. FELSENFELD, O. 1974. The survival of cholera vibrios. *In* Cholera. D. Barua & W. Burrows, Eds.: 359–366. Philadelphia: W.B. Saunders.
2. KOCH, R. 1884. An address on cholera and its bacillus. Br. Med. J. **2**: 403–407, 453–459.
3. ISLAM, M. S., B. S. DRASER & D. J. BRADLEY. 1990. Survival of toxigenic *Vibrio cholerae* O1 with common duckweed, *Lema minor* in artificial aquatic ecosystem. Trans. Royal Soc. Trop. Med. Hyg. **84**: 422–424.
4. COLWELL, R. R., J. KAPER & S. W. JOSEPH. 1977. *Vibrio cholerae, Vibrio parahaemolyticus* and other vibrios: Occurrence and distribution in Chesapeake Bay. Science **198**: 394–396.
5. COLWELL, R. R., P. R. BRAYTON, D. J. GRIMES, D. R. ROSZAK, S. A. HUQ & L. M. PALMER. 1985. Viable, but non-culturable *Vibrio cholerae* and related pathogens in the environment: Implication for release of genetically engineered microorganisms. Biotechnology **3**: 817–820.
6. HUQ, A., R. R. COLWELL, R. RAHMAN, A. ALI, M. A. R. CHOWDHURY, S. PARVEEN, D. A. SACK & E. RUSSEK-COHEN. 1990. Detection of *Vibrio cholerae* O1 in the aquatic environment by fluorescent-monoclonal antibody and culture methods. Appl. Environ. Microbiol. **56**: 2370–2373.
7. COLWELL, R. R., M. L. TAMPLIN, P. R. BRAYTON, A. L. GAUZENS, B. D. TALL, D. HARRINGTON, M. M. LEVINE, S. HALL, A. HUQ & D. A. SACK. 1990. Environmental aspects of *V. cholerae* in transmission of cholera. *In* Advances in Research on Cholera and Related Diarrhoeas. R. B. Sack & Y. Zinnaka, Eds., 7th edit.: 327–343. Tokyo: K. T. K. Scientific Publishers.
8. ROSZAK, D. B., D. J. GRIMES & R. R. COLWELL. 1984. Viable but non-recoverable stage of *Salmonella enteritidis* in aquatic systems. Can. J. Microbiol. **30**: 334–338.
9. FINKELSTEIN, R. A. 1973. Cholera. CRC Crit. Rev. Microbiol. **2**: 553–623.
10. LITSKY, W. 1979. Gut critters are stressed in the environment, more stressed by isolation procedures. *In* Aquatic Microbial Ecology. R. R. Colwell & J. Foster, Eds.: 345–347. Proceedings of the conference sponsored by the American Society for Microbiology. Maryland Sea Grant Publication UM-SG-TS-80-03. University of Maryland, College Park, MD.
11. COLWELL, R. R., J. A. K. HASAN, A. HUQ, L. LOOMIS, R. J. SIEBLING, M. TORRES, S. GALVEZ, S. ISLAM & D. BERNSTEIN 1992. Development and evaluation of a rapid, simple sensitive monoclonal antibody-based co-agglutination test for direct detection of *V. cholerae* O1. FEMS Microbiol. Lett. **97**: 215–220.
12. GLASS, R. I. & R. BLACK. 1992. The epidemiology of cholera. *In* Cholera. D. Barua & W. B. Greenough, Eds.: 129–154. New York: Plenum Book Co.
13. BRAYTON, P. R. & R. R. COLWELL. 1987. Fluorescent antibody staining method for enumeration of viable environmental *Vibrio cholerae* O1. J. Microbial. Methods **6**: 309–314.
14. XU, H.-S., N. ROBERTS, F. L. SINGLETON, R. W. ATWELL, D. J. GRIMES & R. R. COLWELL. 1982. Survival and viability of non-culturable *Escherichia coli* and *Vibrio cholerae* in the estuarine and marine environment. Microb. Ecol. **8**: 313–323.
15. SINGLETON, F. L., R. W. ATTWELL, M. S. JANGI & R. R. COLWELL. 1982. Influence of salinity and nutrient concentration on survival and growth of *Vibrio cholerae* in aquatic microcosms. Appl. Environ. Microbiol. **43**: 1080–1085.
16. McCORMACK, W. M., M. S. ISLAM, M. FAHIMUDDIN & W. H. MOSLEY. 1969. Endemic cholera in rural East Pakistan. Am. J. Epid. **89**: 393–404.

17. TAMPLIN, M. L., A. L. GAUZENS, A. HUQ, D. A. SACK & R. R. COLWELL. 1990. Attachment of *V. cholerae* serogroup O1 to zooplankton and phytoplankton of Bangladesh waters. Appl. Environ. Microbiol. **56:** 1977–1990.

18. NOVITSKY, J. S. & R. Y. MORITA. 1976. Morphological characterization of small cells resulting from nutrient starvation of a psychrophilic marine vibrio. Appl. Environ. Microbiol. **32:** 617–622.

19. NOVITSKY, J. S. & R. Y. MORITA. 1977. Survival of a psychrophilic marine vibrio under long-term nutrient starvation. Appl. Environ. Microbiol. **33:** 635–641.

20. NOVITSKY, J. S. & R. Y. MORITA. 1978. Possible strategy for the survival of marine bacteria under starvation conditions. Mar. Biol. **48:** 289–295.

21. STEVENSON, L. H. 1978. A case for bacterial dormancy in aquatic systems. Microb. Ecol. **4:** 127–133.

22. HOOD, M. A. & G. E. NESS. 1982. Survival of *Vibrio cholerae* and *Escherichia coli* in estuarine waters and sediments. Appl. Environ. Microbiol. **43:** 578–584.

23. BAKER, R. M., F. L. SINGLETON & M. A. HOOD. 1983. Effects of nutrient deprivation on *Vibrio cholerae*. Appl. Environ. Microbiol. **46:** 930–940.

24. COLWELL, R. R., P. A. WEST, D. MANEVAL, E. F. REMMERS, E. L. ELLIOT & N. E. CARLSON. 1984. Ecology of pathogenic vibrios in Chesapeake Bay. *In* Vibrios in the Environment. R. R. Colwell, Ed.: 367–387. New York: John Wiley and Sons.

25. HOOD, M. A., G. E. NESS, G. E. RODRICK & N. J. BLAKE. 1983. Distribution of *Vibrio cholerae* in two Florida estuaries. Microb. Ecol. **9:** 65–75.

26. HOOD, M. A., G. E. NESS, G. E. RODRICK & N. J. BLAKE. 1984. The ecology of *Vibrio cholerae* in two Florida estuaries. *In* Vibrios in the Environment. R. R. Colwell, Ed. Chapter 23: 399–409. New York: John Wiley and Sons.

27. SINGLETON, F. L., R. W. ATWELL, M. S. JANGI & R. R. COLWELL. 1984. Effects of temperature and salinity on *Vibrio cholerae* growth. Appl. Environ. Microbiol. **44:** 1047–1058.

28. MILLER, C. J., B. S. DRASAR & R. G. FEACHEM. 1984. Response to toxigenic *Vibrio cholerae* O1 to physico-chemical stresses in aquatic environments. J. Hyg. **93:** 475–495.

29. HUQ, A., P. A. WEST, E. B. SMALL, M. I. HUQ & R. R. COLWELL. 1984. Influence of water temperature, salinity, and pH on survival and growth of toxigenic *Vibrio cholerae* serovar O1 associated with live copepods in laboratory microcosms. Appl. Environ. Microbiol. **48:** 420–424.

30. KAPER, J. B., H. LOCKMAN, R. R. COLWELL & S. W. JOSEPH. 1979. Ecology, serology, and enterotoxin production of *Vibrio cholerae* O1 in Chesapeake Bay. Appl. Environ. Microbiol. **37:** 91–103.

31. TAMPLIN, M. L. & R. R. COLWELL. 1986. Effect of microcosm salinity and organic substrate concentration on production of *Vibrio cholerae* enterotoxin. Appl. Environ. Microbiol. **52:** 297–301.

32. MILLER, C. J., B. S. DRASAR, R. G FEACHAM & R. J. HAYES. 1986. The impact of physico-chemical stress on the toxigenicity of *Vibrio cholerae*. J. Hyg. Camb. **96:** 49–57.

33. ISLAM, M. S. 1990. Increased toxin production by *V. cholerae* O1 during survival with a green algae, *Rhizoclonium fontanam*, in an artificial aquatic environment. Microbiol. Immun. **34:** 557–563.

34. HUQ, A., E. B. SMALL, P. A. WEST, M. I. HUQ, R. RAHMAN & R. R. COLWELL. 1983. Ecology of *Vibrio cholerae* O1 with special reference to planktonic crustacean copepods. Appl. Environ. Microbial. **45:** 275–283.

35. HUQ, A., J. A. K. HASAN, G. LOSONSKY & R. R. COLWELL. 1994. Occurrence of toxigenic *V. cholerae* O1 and *V. cholerae* non-O1 in professional divers and dive sites in the United States, Ukraine and Russia. FEMS Microbiol Letters **120:** 137–142.

36. SPIRA, W. M., A. HUQ, Q. S. AHMAD & Y. A. SAYEED. 1981. Uptake of *V. cholerae* biotype El Tor from contaminated water by water hyacinth (*Eichornia crassipis*). Appl. Environ. Microbiol. **42:** 550–553.

37. ISLAM, M. S., B. S. DRASAR & D. J. BRADLEY. 1989. Attachment of toxigenic *V. cholerae* O1 to various fresh water plants and survival with a filamentous green algae, *Rhizoclonium fontanam* J. Trop. Med. Hyg. **92:** 396–401.

38. ISLAM, M. S. 1992. Seasonality and toxigenicity of *Vibrio cholerae* non-O1 isolated from

different components of ponds ecosystem of Dhaka City, Bangladesh. World J. Microbio-
tech. **8:** 160–163.

39. HUQ, A., M. A. R. CHOWDHURY, A. FELSENSTEIN, R. R. COLWELL, R. RAHMAN &
K. M. B. HOSSAIN, 1988. Detection of *V. cholerae* from aquatic environments in Bangla-
desh. *In* Biological Monitoring of Environment Pollution. M. Yasuno & B. A. Whitton,
Eds.: 259–264. Tokyo: Tokai University Press.

Cholera El Tor in Latin America, 1991–1993 [a]

LEONARDO MATA

Section of Infection-Nutrition,
Institute of Investigations in Health (INISA)
University of Costa Rica,
Ciudad "Rodrigo Facio," Costa Rica

NATIONAL EPIDEMICS

Cholera El Tor appeared in Peru in 1991 and spread rapidly to nearly all neighboring countries (TABLE 1; FIG. 1).[1] The disease evolved more explosively than anything recorded since the beginning of the 7th pandemic in Sulawesi (the Celebes) in 1961. National epidemics varied in magnitude according to prevailing levels of poverty, health education, sanitation, risk factors and response from the community at large.

Spread in South America

In Peru cholera appeared in January 1991 in late summer, striking in Chancay, Chimbote, Piura, Lima, Trujillo and other localities in succession or simultaneously, along 1200 km of coast.[1–3] Toxigenic *Vibrio cholerae* O1, biotype El Tor, serovar Inaba was recovered from cases and carriers and from all kinds of untreated drinking water; it was occasionally found in poorly prepared or insufficiently cooked foods. In three weeks the epidemic covered the Pacific coast, with 30,000 cases and 114 deaths. Within one month it reached all highland Departments but Cusco, and in six weeks, the forested region where fatalities were greatest.[1] The epidemic waned at the end of April, with the lowest levels in the colder period of May–August (FIG. 2). Cholera hit again in the summer of 1992, but with less intensity; in the third year it became endemic, a pattern observed in most countries affected by significant morbidity (TABLE 1; FIG. 2).

The epidemic reached Ecuador six weeks later, apparently carried by fishermen who had drunk water from a well in Túmbez, a neighboring Peruvian village.[1,2,4] After two months, it had spread in the entire country, but with less intensity than in Peru (TABLE 1). The epidemic was milder in 1992 and even less in 1993. Colombia followed with smaller outbreaks than in Peru and Ecuador. In Brazil, cholera began in the Amazon basin, at the

[a] This work was supported, in part, by the University of Costa Rica, the Association for Investigation in Health (ASINSA), the Rockefeller Foundation, the Swedish Agency for Research and Cooperation (SAREC) and the Harvard School of Public Health.

TABLE 1. Cholera Epidemics and Total Cases, 1991–1993[a]

Country	Onset	1991	1992	1993	Total
Peru	Jan 23	322,562	212,642	70,671	605,875
Ecuador	Mar 01	46,320	31,870	5,391	83,585
Colombia	Mar 10	11,979	15,129	230	27,338
Brazil	Apr 08	2,101	30,054	37,300	69,455
USA	Apr 09	26	102	13	141
Chile	Apr 12	41	73	28	142
Mexico	Jun 13	2,690	8,162	7,586	18,438
Guatemala	Jul 24	3,674	15,395	18,845	37,914
El Salvador	Aug 19	947	8,106	4,139	13,192
Bolivia	Aug 26	206	22,260	8,510	30,976
Panama	Sep 10	1,178	2,416	42	3,636
Honduras	Oct 13	11	384	486	881
Nicaragua	Nov 12	1	3,067	2,776	5,844
Venezuela	Nov 29	13	2,842	380	3,235
French Guiana	Dec 14	1	16	2	19
Costa Rica	Jan 03		12	11	23
Belize	Jan 09		159	24	183
Argentina	Feb 05		553	1,523	2,076
Suriname	Mar 06		12	0	12
Guyana	Nov 05		556	58	614
Paraguay	Jan 25			3	3
TOTAL		391,750	351,810	158,018	901,578

[a] Number of cases reported to Ministries of Health and PAHO as of 2 October 1993.

junction with Colombia and Peru, rising tenfold from July to September.[4] While the outbreak was unexpectedly moderate, there were cases in slums of São Paulo, Rio de Janeiro and other cities. The epidemic took eight months to reach Bolivia, favored by illicit trade at the border with Peru, which usually increases after mid-year.[2] Argentina and Paraguay had cases one year later (TABLE 1; FIG. 1).

Spread in Middle America

The epidemic did not continue towards Central America (FIG. 1). Instead, it broke out in Mexico on June 13 with two dozen cases in San Miguel Totolmaloya, an isolated highland village presumed to be engaged in illicit activities with South America.[2] Rapidly, most Mexican states reported the disease and one month later it had reached Guatemalan communities along the border. Here it followed the path of rivers and dirt roads used by migrant workers, mimicking the great epidemic of Shiga dysentery of 1969–1971 in the Central American Isthmus[5] (FIG. 1, TABLE 1). From the southern Mexican border, cholera advanced to the Guatemalan west coast, the highlands and the lowlands to the north and east. The disease appeared in El Salvador one month later and evolved in the entire country as in Guatemala. A few weeks later it was in Honduras with much less intensity than in Guatemala and El Salvador, among people settled along the border who had drunk untreated

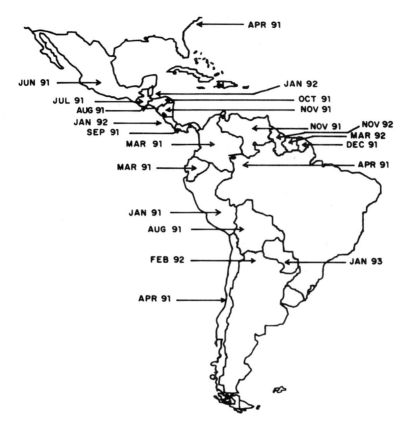

FIGURE 1. Spread of cholera in the Americas, 1991–1993.

water from the Goascarán River. Cholera began in Nicaragua early in 1992, but the greatest epidemic was in 1993, with less intensity than in El Salvador and Guatemala.

Countries without Epidemics

Uruguay and the Caribbean had not reported cholera as of October 2, 1993.[4] Canada, the United States, Paraguay, and Costa Rica have had sporadic cases. Chile, Suriname, and Argentina had limited outbreaks, and all these nations have better socioeconomic conditions than those countries experiencing large epidemics.

Forty cholera cases were diagnosed in Santiago, Chile, 1700 km south of Peru, in April 1991, but no epidemic occurred due to the adequate hygiene and sanitation of its population as well as the preventive measures effected

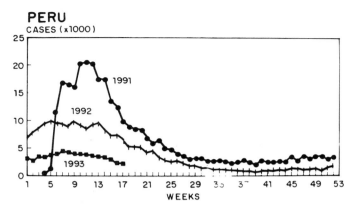

FIGURE 2. Epidemics of cholera in Peru, 1991–1993.

during the emergency. Only ninety additional cases were reported in 1992 and 1993.

In January 1992 the first imported case was recognized in Costa Rica; eleven additional cases were diagnosed in 1992, six acquired in neighboring countries to the north.[2] There was one isolated case and six symptomless carriers associated with a toxigenic *V. cholerae* O1, more related to strains of the 7th Asian pandemic than to those of Latin America (Dr. Joy Wells, Centers for Disease Control, unpublished). Through November 1993, Costa Rica had 23 cholera cases, mostly imported from Nicaragua.

Morbidity

Rates were estimated from cases admitted to hospitals, clinics and health centers (TABLE 2, FIG. 3). The figures probably include many non-cholera diarrheas, but most investigators agree that the figures are underestimates. The wide range in rates of infection and death reflect varying socioeconomic differences across nations. Peru had the highest morbidity rate, 1437 cases per 100,000 population. It was estimated that 1.5 per cent of the population became infected with *V. cholerae* O1 within the first three epidemic months.[1–4] Ecuador, Bolivia, Guatemala and El Salvador followed with relatively high rates, but significantly lower than those of Peru. Mexico and Honduras had unexpectedly low rates (less than 0.6 cases per 100,000), while the disease was negligible in Chile, Costa Rica, and Paraguay.

Risk Factors

In Peru, Ecuador, Bolivia, and Guatemala, the largest outbreaks affected the Amerindians who are known to have predominantly blood O group, and

TABLE 2. Cholera Morbidity per 100,000, 1991–1993[a]

	Population (millions)	1991	1992	1993
Peru	21.9	1,436.7	947.1	260.5
Ecuador	10.8	416.6	286.7	8.9
Bolivia	7.3	2.7	287.8	86.5
Guatemala	9.5	37.7	158.0	8.6
El Salvador	5.3	17.2	147.1	28.9
Panama	2.5	46.8	96.1	1.7
Belize	1.0		85.5	7.5
Nicaragua	3.8	<0.05	74.2	12.4
Guyana	1.0	35.0	69.1	3.0
Colombia	32.8	1.3	44.2	0.5
Brazil	151.4	0.9	19.2	2.8
French Guiana	0.1	0.1	14.5	1.8
Venezuela	19.8	2.9	13.7	0.3
Mexico	83.3	0.2	8.8	0.2
Honduras	5.3		7.0	0.2
Argentina	32.7		1.7	3.5
Suriname	0.4		2.7	0
Chile	13.4	0.3	0.5	0.2
Costa Rica	3.1		0.4	0.3
Paraguay	4.4		0.07	0.1
USA	262.7	<0.05	<0.05	<0.05

[a] Rates from figures in TABLE 1.
[b] World Bank, WHO, and Encyclopedia Britannica, 1991.

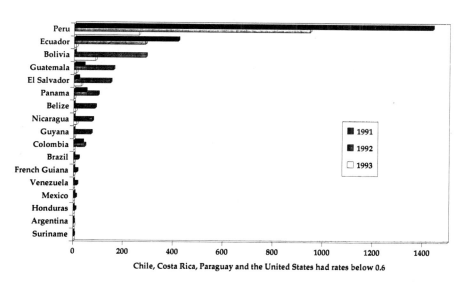

FIGURE 3. Cholera morbidity per 100,000 population, 1991–1993.

who live in increasingly vulnerable ecosystems. In countries experiencing smaller epidemics, such as in El Salvador, the northwest of Argentina and the Indian territories of Panama, most cases were seen among Amerindians. Explosive epidemics in slums and rural areas were characteristically found in populations living in deprived and impoverished neighborhoods.

Detailed case-control studies in Peru[3,6-8] revealed several risk factors, including drinking untreated water and consumption of the following foods: raw sea molluscs and crustaceans, unheated food leftovers (mainly rice), "juanes" ("tamales" of corn dough stuffed with meats and potatoes), foods sold by street vendors, and ice prepared with untreated water (TABLE 3).

Protective Factors

Washing hands, health education, and drinking "toronjada" (home-made grapefruit beverage) were protective against developing cholera.[7] Consumption of cooked fish and "ceviche" (raw fish marinated for several hours in lemon juice) were found not to be associated with cholera in Peru and other Latin American nations. At the beginning of the epidemic, fish and ceviche were blamed for the spread of cholera without scientific proof.[2] Such unfounded assertions had three negative effects: an immediate reduction in fish consumption, an attrition of fish exports and a delayed identification of contaminated water as the source of contagion.

Regarding ceviche, *in vitro* experiments revealed a strong vibriocidal capacity of the juice and pulp of all citrus and other acidic fruits found in the tropics.[2,9] Millions of toxigenic *V. cholerae* O1 are killed within 5–10 minutes

TABLE 3. Risk Factors for Cholera in Peru, 1991

Location	Risk Factors
Larco-Herrera	• unboiled water • home water, hand-contaminated • water from shallow wells • food and drink at parties • cabbage sprayed with sewage
Piura	• food/beverages of street vendors • unboiled water • leftover rice (>3 hr), unheated • home water, hand-contaminated • ice from street vendors
Ventanilla/Callao	• unboiled water • deficient/lack of knowledge on contagion
Iquitos	• unboiled water • unwashed fruits and vegetables • leftover poorly heated rice • eating "juanes"

Source: references 3, 6–8.

TABLE 4. Number of *Vibrio cholerae* O1 Killed by the Juice of Acidic Fruits of Tropical America

Substrate	Number Killed (millions)	Killing Time (min)
1. Expressed lemon juice	100	5
2. Home beverages made of sour orange, lemon, sour guava, tamarind, naranjilla, maracuja, carambola, blackberry, pineapple, orange	100	10
3. Cabbage salad dressed with lemon juice	100	5
4. Lettuce salad dressed with lemon juice	100	5
5. Raw fish marinated with lemon juice (commercial ceviche)	100–1000	5
6. Contaminated raw fish marinated with lemon juice (laboratory ceviche)	10–1000	30

Source: Mata and Vives.[9]

when exposed to the juice or pulp of acidic fruits (TABLE 4).[2,9] The effect is mediated by the high concentration of hydrogen ions (pH ranging from 1.9 to 3.5). Traditional home refreshments made from these fruits also have a strong vibriocidal capacity. Indigenous populations intuitively believe that lemon juice protects against intestinal disease.

Toxigenic *V. cholerae* O1 could be isolated, but infrequently, from intestines and skin of fish and in molluscs during the epidemics in Latin America.[10] Meantime, the vibrio was readily found in all types of drinking water during epidemics, in sites separated by large distances from each other, and from coastal regions. (Dr. Óscar Grados, National Institute of Health, Lima, Perú, unpublished data).[2] The situation in the aquatic reservoir will be described later.[11–14]

ORIGIN OF CHOLERA IN LATIN AMERICA

Pathogenic Cultivars

Most strains of *V. cholerae* O1 El Tor isolated from cases, carriers and drinking water during the Latin American epidemics belong to serovar Inaba. Several Ogawa strains appeared later in humans and water sources. Inaba strains share similar molecular characteristics,[15] but depart from those strains found in the 1970s in cases in the coasts of the United States and in the Gulf of Mexico. Prior to the current epidemic, sporadic cholera infections in the U.S. were acquired from the aquatic reservoir;[16,17] recently there have been importations from Latin America, with limited secondary spread resulting from the good environmental sanitation and personal hygiene in the U.S. An indigenous presence of the novel serogroup O139, but cholera-toxin negative, *V. cholerae* was reported from Argentina in 1993.[18]

Aquatic Reservoir

The brackish water in an estuary or lagoon (atoll) serves as the aquatic reservoir and harbors epidemic and non-epidemic *V. cholerae* O1 among its plankton.[15] In the reservoir, bacteria, algae, protozoa, copepods, plants, and organic sediment harbor dormant stages while salinity, temperature, and pH determine seasonal blooming of algae and growth of attached vibrios. In the reservoir, strains of *V. cholerae* O1 may be non-culturable. Some strains of *V. cholerae* non-O1 apparently become toxigenic.[16] In estuaries and lagoons, fish may harbor pathogenic vibrios. These fish, if salted, stored and eaten raw may induce outbreaks traced to lagoons (such as those in Guam and Kiribati[11,12]) or epidemics related to estuaries (like those in the Indian sub-continent[13,14]).

It could not be determined if the epidemic organism in Peru was introduced by vessels emptying sewage or ballast water in coastal waters, or if it was present in plankton long before the epidemic. During the current outbreak, *V. cholerae* non-O1 was isolated from all types of non-acid untreated drinking water. Furthermore, in Costa Rica, with only a few cases, 7,000 strains of *V. cholerae* non-O1 were isolated (with Moore swabs) from 11,000 water samples from sewers, rivers, creeks, and ponds throughout the country (Dr. Darner Mora, Aqueducts and Sewers Institute, San José, Costa Rica, unpublished data). This finding suggests that the epidemic strain—or a precursor—was present in pre-epidemic times in brackish, non-acidic, and slow moving water. Yet, it is difficult to explain the absence of cholera before 1991, when sanitary conditions were more deficient than they are now.

Algal Blooms and Amplification of Vibrios

It can be hypothesized that the epidemic strain lived in brackish water in Peru, and proliferated when promoting factors became optimal for its growth.[15] After introduction, the vibrio moved upstream along with an expanding reservoir, offering new opportunities for *V. cholerae* amplification and introduction into human populations. The main factor in transmission remains the contamination of drinking water and food.[2,3,6–8]

Sporadic Disease

Cholera was not recognized in Latin America before the current pandemic, for at least two reasons: 1) the lack of recognition of the existence of an aquatic reservoir in Latin America, and 2) the lack of routine investigation of O1 and non-O1 cholera vibrios. The appreciation of the reservoir in the United States assisted in the identification of sporadic disease since the 1970s.[16] The minuscule outbreak of indigenous cholera in the Costa Rican highland village already mentioned would have remained unrecognized if the threat of cholera had not existed.[19]

CHOLERA CONTROL

Mortality

Since January 1991, more than 8,000 deaths attributable to cholera have been recorded in the Americas (TABLE 5). Deaths were more numerous in those countries with the highest morbidity.

Case Fatality

Before the advent of oral rehydration therapy (ORT) and rapid intravenous rehydration therapy (RIT), as many as 50 per cent of untreated or poorly treated cholera cases died of dehydration or its sequelae. ORT and RIT were rendered practical in the last two decades,[20-22] and they are responsible for the very low case fatality ratio (CFR) during the current epidemic. Even so, wide and paradoxical differences in CFRs were noted across nations (TABLE 6, FIG. 4). Peru showed an excellent record in handling dehydrated patients[4] while relatively more advanced nations were less successful, experiencing CFRs greater than 2.5. El Tor is considerably less severe than classic cholera. On the other hand, most cases admitted to clinics are dehydrated. Thus, low CFRs in Peru and other impoverished nations speak highly for the application of ORT and RIT.

TABLE 5. Cholera Deaths in the Americas, 1991–1993[a]

Country	1991	1992	1993	Total
Peru	2,909	727	497	4,133
Ecuador	697	208	43	948
Brazil	26	359	397	782
Bolivia	12	383	211	606
Guatemala	50	207	207	464
Colombia	207	158	4	369
Mexico	34	99	148	281
Nicaragua	0	46	111	157
El Salvador	34	45	9	88
Panama	29	49	4	82
Venezuela	2	68	9	79
Argentina		15	24	39
Honduras	0	17	12	29
Guyana		8	2	10
Belize		4	0	4
Chile	2	1	0	3
USA	0	1	0	1
Suriname		1	0	1
French Guiana	0	0	0	0
Costa Rica		0	0	0
Paraguay			0	0
TOTAL	4,002	2,396	1,678	8,076

[a] Ministries of Health and PAHO as of 2 October, 1993.

TABLE 6. Cholera Case Fatality Ratio, 1991–1993[a]

Country	1991	1992	1993
Venezuela	15.38	2.39	2.37
Panama	2.46	2.03	9.52
Suriname		8.33	
Bolivia	5.82	1.72	2.47
Chile	4.87	1.37	0
Honduras	—[b]	4.42	2.50
Guyana		1.44	3.45
El Salvador	3.59	0.55	0.22
Argentina		2.71	1.57
Belize		2.51	—
Mexico	1.26	1.21	1.95
Nicaragua	—	1.50	1.90
Colombia	1.72	1.04	1.73
Ecuador	1.50	0.65	0.80
Guatemala	1.36	1.34	1.10
Brazil	1.23	1.19	1.06
Peru	0.90	0.34	0.70
USA	0	0.25	0

[a] As of October 2, 1993, PAHO, revised. No deaths reported for Costa Rica, French Guiana, and Paraguay. Ratio of number of deaths to number of cases of cholera, expressed as %. As an example, for Venezuela in 1991, there were 2 deaths among the 13 reported cases for a ratio of 2/13 or 15.38%.

[b] — Indicates insufficient data.

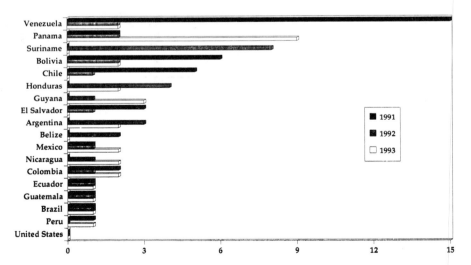

FIGURE 4. Percent case fatality for cholera, 1991–1993.

The main factor accounting for this success has been the emphasis during the past decade on these therapies by governments, the Pan American Health Organization (PAHO), and the International Children's Fund (UNICEF). The prompt response of PAHO and other international bodies with financial assistance and technical support were fundamental for local action. The role of local and international news media was also crucial. The obvious result was improved awareness of the need for prompt ORT in all patients, including those seriously dehydrated requiring transport to a health facility for RIT. The high CFRs in Venezuela, Panama, Chile, and Mexico may reflect superior reporting systems. Alternatively they may be due to incomplete or timid adoption of ORT and RIT, limited availability of ORT in rural, sparsely populated communities, or to inadequate primary health care systems. In fact, CFR rose to 10% in rural areas of the Amazon, regardless of availability of oral rehydration salt solution at home or homemade sugar salt solution.[23] A case-control study showed that death was related to "multiple barriers to health care."[24]

PREVENTION OF CHOLERA

Successful Programs

Chile's program included appropriate waste control in buses, trains and airplanes arriving from Peru; national health education (radio, television, and posters), to improve hand-washing and provide instruction on treating raw water and the proper preparation of food. Raw vegetables in restaurants and food sold by street vendors were banned. Vegetable crops shown to be irrigated with sewage-contaminated water were destroyed. There was emphasis on chlorination and bacteriologic monitoring of drinking water, and investigation and follow up of cholera cases.[2,4]

Costa Rica implemented a similar program of education and prevention using the mass media, primary health care, schools, nongovernmental organizations, and churches. The emphasis was on hand washing, breastfeeding infants, proper reheating of food, and treatment of drinking water and waste.[2,4] Costa Rica set the target of universally available safe water and fecal waste control. The program emphasized prompt rehydration of cases and antibiotic treatment of cases and contacts; wide distribution of sachets for ORT and training for modern rehydration therapy in hospitals, clinics and health centers. It also included food surveillance and control; development of a national network of laboratories for routine culture of cases and investigation of carriers; and treatment of municipal water supplies. In Chile and Costa Rica, such measures contributed to a significant decline in overall diarrhea morbidity and mortality, and prevented cholera epidemics in these nations.

Treatment of Cases

Confinement and treatment of moderate and severe cholera cases (known to excrete the largest number of vibrios) limited dissemination of infection in the family and in the community. In Chile, Venezuela, and other relatively more developed nations, there was routine treatment of cases and family contacts with effective antibiotics that shorten the period of communicability of epidemic vibrios. This practice was carried out in rural areas of Costa Rica as well.

COMMENT

Cholera in Latin America is transmitted primarily through water and secondarily by food contaminated with toxigenic *V. cholerae* O1. The magnitude and intensity of the national epidemics reflected individual differences in socioeconomic conditions. Decades of slow but steady upgrading of sanitation and water supply systems around the world during the first half of this century have reduced the overall risk of diarrhea morbidity and mortality. However, *V. cholerae* has adapted to a contemporary human with better health and nutrition, living in an improved sanitary environment, but one still plagued by crowding and urban deprivation.

Contrasting with the classic biotype, the adapted El Tor survives better outside the human organism in the aquatic reservoir. It causes a milder disease with considerably more asymptomatic carriers than the classic biotype. Current epidemics may have resulted from the amplification of one virulent variety in algal blooms in an aquatic reservoir.

The emergence of the novel variant *V. cholerae* O139, now epidemic in the Indian subcontinent,[24-26] illustrates the endless interaction of humans and microbes, and the unquestionable potential of the latter to adapt to new sanitary and behavioral strategies aimed to control and prevent their spread. In this regard, the theories of developmental biologists[27] and pragmatic epidemiologists[28] are relevant. The lower magnitude of the 1993 El Tor epidemic and the amelioration of the pandemic throughout Latin America in the second and third years, suggests that protection is being attained through acquisition of immunity and improvements in water supplies and in sanitation, and with health education.

REFERENCES

1. SEMINARIO L., A. LÓPEZ, E. VÁSQUEZ & M. RODRÍGUEZ. 1991. Epidemia de cólera en el Perú. Vigilancia epidemiológica. Rev. Per. Epidemiol. (Perú) **4:** 8–41.
2. MATA, L. 1992. El Cólera. Historia, Prevención y Control. UNED and UCR, La Paulina, Costa Rica, pp. XV + 366 pp.
3. RIES, A. A., D. J. VUGLIA, A. M. P. BEINGOLEA, E. VÁSQUEZ, J. G. WELLS, N. GARCÍA-BACA, N. SWERDLOW, M. POLLACK, N. H. BEAN, L. SEMINARIO & R. V. TAUXE. 1992. Cholera in Piura, Peru: A modern urban epidemic. J. Infect. Dis. **166:** 1429–1433.

4. PAN AMERICAN HEALTH ORGANIZATION. 1994. Health conditions in the Americas. Pan American Health Organization, Washington, D.C. In press.

5. MATA, L. J., E. J. GANGAROSA, A. CÁCERES, D. PERERA & M. L. MEJICANOS. 1970. Epidemic Shiga bacillus dysentery in Central America. I. Etiologic investigations in Guatemala, 1969. J. Infect. Dis. **122:** 170–180.

6. RODRÍGUEZ, M., E. TEJADA, L. SEMINARIO, D. L. SWERDLOW, E. D. MINTZ, P. A. BLAKE, J. G. WELLS, C. OCAMPO, W. SALDAÑA, M. POLLACK & R. V. TAUXE. 1991. Epidemia de cólera en el Distrito de Víctor Larco Herrera, Trujillo, La Libertad, Perú. Rev. Per. Epidemiol. (Perú) **4:** 42–46.

7. MUJICA, O., R. QUICK, A. PALACIOS, L. BEINGOLEA, R. VARGAS, D. MORENO & L. SEMINARIO. 1991. Cólera en la selva peruana: Factores de riesgo y protección. Rev. Per. Epidemiol. (Perú) **4:** 62–69.

8. VÁSQUEZ E., A. PALACIOS, L. BEINGOLEA, L. SEMINARIO, A. A. RIES, D. VUGLIA, J. G. WELLS, L. M. POLLACK & R. V. TAUXE. 1991. Epidemia de cólera en Perú: Estudio de caso-control de Piura, febrero-marzo, 1991. Rev. Per. Epidemiol. (Perú) **4:** 47–50.

9. MATA, L. & M. VIVES. 1992. Efecto del jugo y de la pulpa de frutas ácidas sobre el *Vibrio cholerae*. *In* El Cólera. Historia, Prevención y Control, Chapter 10: 275–310. UNED/UCR, La Paulina, Costa Rica.

10. TAMPLIN, M. L. & C. C. PARODI. 1991. Environmental spread of *Vibrio cholerae* in Peru. Lancet **338:** 1216–1217.

11. MERSON, M. H., W. T. MARTIN, J. P. CRAIG, G. K. MORRIS, P. A. BLAKE, G. F. CRAUN, J. C. FEELEY, J. C. CAMACHO & E. J. GANGAROSA. 1977. Cholera on Guam. 1974. Am. J. Epidemiol. **105:** 349–361.

12. MCINTYRE, R. C., T. TIRA, T. FLOOD & P. A. BLAKE. 1979. Modes of transmission of cholera in a newly infected population on an atoll: Implications for control measures. Lancet **i:** 311–314.

13. MILLER, C. J., B. S. DRASAR & R. G. FAECHEM. 1982. Cholera and estuarine salinity in Calcutta and London. Lancet **i:** 1216–1218.

14. GLASS, R. I. & R. E. BLACK. 1992. The epidemiology of cholera. *In* Cholera. D. Barua & W. B. Greenough, III, Eds.: 129–154. New York: Plenum Medical Books.

15. WACHSMUTH, I. K., C. A. BOPP, P. FIELDS & C. CARRILLO. 1991. Difference between toxigenic *Vibrio cholerae* O1 from South America and US gulf coast. Lancet **1:** 1097–1098.

16. COLWELL, R. R. & W. M. SPIRA. 1992. The ecology of *Vibrio cholerae*. *In* Cholera. D. Barua & W. B. Greenough, III, Eds.: 107–127. New York: Plenum Medical Books.

17. SHANDERA, W. X., B. HAFKIN, D. L. MARTIN, J. P. TAYLOR, D. L. MASERANG, J. G. WELLS, M. KELLY, K. GHANDI, J. B. KAPER, J. V. LEE & P. A. BLAKE. 1983. Persistence of cholera in the United States. Am. J. Trop. Med. Hyg. **32:** 812–817.

18. RIVAS M., C. TOMA, E. MILIWEBSKY, M. CAFFER, M. GALAS, P. VARELA, M. TOUS, A. M. BRU & N. BINSZTEIN. 1993. Letter to the *Lancet*. Lancet **342:** 926–927.

19. MATA, L. 1992. Cholera en Costa Rica, 1992. *In* El Cólera. Historia, Prevención y Control, Chapter 11: 311–328. UNED/UCR, La Paulina, Costa Rica.

20. NALIN, D. R., M. M. LEVINE, L. MATA, C. DE CÉSPEDES, W. VARGAS, C. LIZANO, A. R. LORÍA, A. SIMHON & E. MOHS. 1978. Comparison of sucrose with glucose in oral therapy of infant diarrhoea. Lancet **ii:** 277–279.

21. POSADA, G. & D. PIZARRO. 1986. Rehidratación por vía endovenosa rápida con una solución similar a la recomendada por la OMS para rehidratación oral. Bol. Méd. Hosp. Inf. México **43:** 463–469.

22. MOLLA, A. M., R. A. SARKER, M. HOSSAIN, A. MOLLA & W. B. GREENOUGH, III. 1982. Rice-powder electrolyte solution as oral therapy in diarrhoea due to *Vibrio cholerae* and *Escherichia coli*. Lancet **i:** 1317–1319.

23. QUICK, R. E., R. F. VARGAS, D. MORENO, O. MUJICA, L. BEINGOLEA, A. M. PALACIOS, L. SEMINARIO & R. V. TAUXE. 1993. Epidemic cholera in the Amazon: The challenge of preventing death. Am. J. Trop. Med. Hyg. **48:** 597–602.

24. ALBERT, M. J., A. K. SIDDIQUE, M. S. ISLAM, A. S. G. FARUQUE, M. AUSARUZZAMAN,

         S. M. FARUQUE & R. B. SACK. 1993. Large outbreak of clinical cholera due to *Vibrio cholerae* non-O1 in Bangladesh. Lancet **341:** 704.

25.   RAMMAMURTHY, T., S. GARG, R. SHARMA, S. BHATTACHARYAM, G. B. NAIR, T. SHIMADA, T. TAKEDA, T. KARSAWA, H. KURAZANO, A. PAL & Y. TAKEDA. 1993. Emergence of novel strains of *Vibrio cholerae* with epidemic potential in southern and eastern India. Lancet **341:** 703–704.

26.   SHIMADA, T., G. B. NAIR, B. C. DEB, M. J. ALBERT, R. B. SACK & Y. TAKEDA. 1993. Outbreak of *Vibrio cholerae* non-O1 in India and Bangladesh. Lancet **341:** 1347.

27.   EWALD, P. W. 1993. The evolution of virulence. 1993. Scientific American, April: 86–93.

28.   GLASS, R. I., M. CLAESON, P. S. BLAKE, R. J. WALDMAN & N. F. PIERCE. 1992. Cholera in Africa: Lessons on transmission and control for Latin America. Lancet **338:** 791–795.

Harmful Marine Phytoplankton and Shellfish Toxicity

Potential Consequences of Climate Change[a]

PATRICIA A. TESTER

National Oceanic and Atmospheric Administration
National Marine Fisheries Service
Southeast Fisheries Science Center, Beaufort Laboratory
101 Pivers Island Road
Beaufort, North Carolina 28516

INTRODUCTION

Concern about global warming has increased as the concentrations of greenhouse gases have risen since the start of the industrial revolution. Currently, global climate change models predict a non-uniform warming of 0.5°C to 2.5°C during the next decade, including a disproportionate warming[1] with minimum temperatures expected to increase more than the maximum temperatures. A consequence of a more uniform temperature gradient between tropical and polar regions will be reduced atmospheric circulation and oceanic mixing. Modified wind and rain patterns will influence upwelling intensity, amount of runoff and subsequently nutrient availability.

Climate changes affect the physics and chemistry of the world's oceans and will alter every functional relationship in the marine food web either directly or indirectly. These effects will be noticed first in the lower trophic levels and portend significant changes in phytoplankton biomass and shifts in species dominance. Phytoplankton blooms and red tides have been known since biblical times and are associated with shellfish toxicity and fish kills.

> . . . . all the waters in the river turned to blood. And the fish that were in the river died; and the river stank and the Egyptians could not drink of the water of the river.
>
> Exodus 7:20–21

Yet, phytoplankton researchers[2-5] have noted an increasing frequency of harmful phytoplankton blooms worldwide. Of the ~5,000+ phytoplankton species fewer than 50 are known to be toxic. Once established these toxic or nuisance blooms persist because they deplete the available nutrients, or their toxins may inhibit the growth of other phytoplankton or reduce grazing pressure by zooplankton.[6] The ramifications of harmful/toxic phytoplankton blooms are extensive. The loss of human life and health are of primary concern.

---

[a] The U.S. Government has the right to retain a nonexclusive royalty-free license *in* and *to* any copyright covering this paper.

Regional economies are disproportionally impacted when shellfish resources are toxic and cannot be harvested because the market for all seafood suffers; mass mortality of finfish and loss of environmental quality result in further economic losses. Marine mammal deaths are linked to the concentration of phycotoxins within marine food chains,[7] and the impact of toxic phytoplankton on non-commercial species can only be conjectured. Because the subject area is extensive, the focus of this working paper will be on toxic marine phytoplankton, their effects on humans, and the potential for climate change to exacerbate these effects. Unfortunately, it is not possible to review the blue-green algae or cyanobacteria. While represented by only a few marine genera, these organisms in freshwater systems pose significant threats worldwide to human health.

PHYCOTOXINS

Phycotoxins are either water or lipid soluble, nonproteinaceous, low molecular weight ($\sim 1,000$) compounds that are relatively stable to heat and cold. Numerous forms of the toxins are present within the same phytoplankton cell and the toxin content can vary owing to genetic differences and environmental factors. While only a small proportion of the phytoplankton species are toxic, or produce hemolytic agents, there are few similarities among them. In her review Steidinger[8] provides no definitive answers to why some phytoplankton species are toxic, but the possibilities range from a specific adaptation to produce a toxic metabolic by-product that conveys an inter-specific advantage, to events involving infestations and resultant viral or bacterial recombinant DNA.

Filter-feeding bivalves accumulate and concentrate phycotoxins and these toxins can be bioconcentrated as they move through the food chain to top carnivores. Human intoxication follows ingestion of tainted shellfish or finfish. Severity of symptoms is dependent on amount of toxin ingested, weight and general health of the individuals, and their susceptibility to the toxin. General clinical symptoms of fish and shellfish poisoning include nausea, vomiting, abdominal pain, and diarrhea. Phycotoxins have a high affinity for specific receptor sites leading to critical changes in intracellular ion concentrations of sodium, calcium or potassium. Consequently action potential and nerve transmission impulses are affected.

Generally there is a satisfactory control and/or monitoring in regions where shellfish poisoning presents a threat to human safety and fishery economics in developed countries, but the situation is vastly different in developing countries, and therein lies a major health problem. Worldwide, the International Council for the Exploration of the Sea gathers and exchanges information on "exceptional plankton blooms." In the United States the Food and Drug Administration is responsible for food safety and conducting methodological research, though the duty of routine inspections of shellfish growing areas and shellfish safety falls to state agencies through participation in the National Shellfish Sanitation Program. Currently testing for shellfish toxins in U.S. waters is based on a mouse bioassay. Toxicity is expressed in mouse units; one mouse unit is that amount of crude toxin contained in 100 g shellfish tissue after extraction with diethyl ether that, on average, will kill 50% of the test mice (20 g weight) in 15.5 hours after intraperitoneal injection.[9] This bioassay procedure is slow, cumbersome, costly, non-specific and the subject of continuing debate. Development of alternatives to the mouse bioassay has gained increasing support. Receptor binding assays are favored because they are specific and provide a true measure of potency.[8] The only exception to the mouse bioassay method is HPLC detection of domoic acid, a toxin produced by certain diatoms.

CIGUATERA FISH POISONING

Ciguatera fish poisoning (CFP) was first recognized in the 1550s in the Caribbean[10] but the causative agent was not identified until the last decade. CFP has a pantropical distribution between 34°S and 35°N and is known from the Caribbean basin, Florida, the Hawaiian Islands, French Polynesia and Australia.[11] It is caused by a suite of at least 6 toxins produced by a multispecies assemblage of benthic (sessile, epiphytic) dinoflagellates including *Gambierdiscus toxicus* which is responsible for ciguatoxin production. These toxins are bioconcentrated by higher carnivores, especially reef fish, which may remain toxic for more than 2 years after becoming contaminated.[12]

Worldwide 50,000 victims are stricken annually[13] with CFP, and cases per thousand residents per year vary between 3–9 in the Caribbean to 5–13 in French Polynesia. It is estimated that only 20–40% of the cases are reported. In the acute phase of CFP, gastrointestinal distress is followed by neurological and cardiovascular symptoms which may be, but rarely are, fatal. A chronic phase can persist for weeks, months or years.[14] There is no antidote for CFP and supportive therapy is the rule. In extreme cases of CFP, death through respiratory paralysis may occur within 2–24 hours of ingesting tainted fish. Repeated exposure to ciguatoxins exacerbates the symptoms. CFP is considered a major health and economic problem in many tropical islands where fish is a large part of the diet. CFP is one of the most important constraints to fisheries resources development in these regions.[15] It also poses a threat to uninformed tourists.[14]

NEUROTOXIC SHELLFISH POISONING

Neurotoxic shellfish (NSP) produces gastrointestinal and neurological symptoms, less severe but, nearly identical to those of CFP. Blooms of *Gymnodinium breve*, the dinoflagellate responsible for NSP, are usually marked by large patches of discolored water and massive fish kills. In addition, this unarmored dinoflagellate can be ruptured easily by wave action, whereupon its toxins become aerosolized and cause asthma-like symptoms. Consequently,

G. breve red tides were documented early (1844), and their correlation with shellfish toxicity was recognized by 1880. However the identification and characterization of the first of 10 brevetoxins was not completed until 1981 when toxin purification techniques became available.[16]

Historically the distribution of *G. breve* blooms was centered in the Caribbean Sea and Gulf of Mexico with isolated occurrences recorded in Trinidad, northern Venezuela, and Florida's east coast. During the fall and winter of 1987–88 there was a large, persistent *G. breve* bloom in the coastal waters of North Carolina, a range extension of 800–900 km for this species.[17] Forty-eight cases of NSP were documented and more than $24 million dollars was lost to the local economy when many shellfish harvesting areas were closed for the entire season.[18] Subsequently, this dinoflagellate was found in low but consistent numbers in the Gulf Stream and the transport mechanism for the 1987–88 expatriate bloom was elucidated.[19]

PARALYTIC SHELLFISH POISONING

Paralytic shellfish poisoning (PSP) was recognized by Native Americans before the arrival of European explorers. Several members of Captain George Vancouver's crew succumbed to PSP while they explored the Pacific Northwest in 1798. PSP is caused by saxitoxin, which was first characterized in 1957[20] and now includes 21 recognized forms. Saxitoxins contaminate shellfish, and marine mammal deaths have resulted from food chain concentration in mackerel.[7] These toxins are water soluble and act on the peripheral nervous system and secondarily on the central nervous system. The mode of action is as a sodium channel block, binding to receptor sites and inhibiting nerve transmission to muscles. The onset of symptoms is rapid; gastrointestinal distress, tingling, numbness and ataxia are typical. Death, if it occurs, is by respiratory failure.

Examples of cells containing saxitoxins are *Alexandrium catenella, A. tamarense, Gymnodinium catenatum, Pyrodinium bahamense* var. *compressum.* These may be found from the sub-Arctic to the tropics. Most of these species produce cysts or resting stages, and excystment is, in some cases, associated with temperature change.[21] Until 1970 PSP was known only from temperate waters of North America, Europe, and Japan; by 1990 PSP was documented in South Africa, South America, the Philippines, Australia, and India.[5] At present, one dinoflagellate species responsible for PSP, *P. bahamense*, is confined to tropical coastal waters of the Atlantic and Indo-Pacific but a survey of its fossil cysts indicate a much wider geographic range in the past.[5]

DIARRHETIC SHELLFISH POISONING

Diarrhetic shellfish poisoning (DSP) was first reported from Japan in 1976.[22] Okadaic acid produced by several species of the dinoflagellate *Dinophy-*

sis was found to be its cause. DSP is not fatal and recovery is within three days, with or without medical treatment. Its symptoms are easily mistaken for bacterial gastroenteritis. Over a five year period (1976–1982) 1,300 DSP cases were reported in Japan; in 1981 5,000+ cases were reported in Spain; in 1983 3,300± cases were reported in France.[5] DSP has been documented in Japan, Europe, Chile, Thailand, and New Zealand, but prior to 1990 DSP was not known to occur in North America. In 1990 there was a DSP incident along the southern coast of Nova Scotia, followed by another in 1992.[23] Some consider DSP to be the most serious and globally widespread phyco-toxin-caused seafood illness, and while DSP-producing species of phytoplankton occur throughout all temperate coastal waters of the United States, no outbreaks of DSP have been confirmed there.

AMNESIC SHELLFISH POISONING

Amnesic shellfish poisoning (ASP) was recognized for the first time in 1987 on Prince Edward Island when over 100 acute cases and 4 deaths resulted after the victims consumed blue mussels.[24] The neurotoxin domoic acid produced by a diatom, *Nitzschia pungens* f. *multiseries,* was found responsible for the ASP. Symptoms of gastroenteritis followed by dizziness, headache, seizures, disorientation, short-term memory loss, and respiratory difficulty are typical of severe cases.

In the Bay of Fundy there are generally two blooms of *Nitzschia* each year. One occurs when the water temperature warms to ~10°C and the later bloom follows the highest water temperatures of the year in late August.[25] Despite the annual blooms of the diatoms that cause ASP in Canadian waters, contaminated shellfish have been kept off the market by vigilant management practices. Public confidence in the local mussel industry is high; mussel harvests there now exceed the 1987 levels.[26]

In the fall of 1991 domoic acid was detected in dead sea birds in Monterey Bay. They had been feeding on anchovies that had ingested *Pseudonitzschia australis*, the source of the domoic acid. Further tests found domoic acid present in razor clams and crabs from Oregon and Washington where both recreational and commercial fisheries were closed.[26] Although no human intoxication resulted from this incident, it was a clear warning that domoic acid can accumulate in marine food chains. The several diatom species responsible for ASP are widely distributed in coastal waters of Europe, the United States, the Mediterranean, North Africa, Australia, New Zealand, South America, and Japan.

DISCUSSION

There are two types of factors important to phytoplankton biology in relation to climate change; the first concerns large-scale environmental changes and the second focuses on the physiological species-specific responses of individual taxa. There is general appreciation today that the circulation of the world ocean is driven from sinking surface water in the North Atlantic. This circulation is intimately linked to the large-scale hydrological cycle. One of the most disturbing predictions of the effects of climate warming is slowing of the worldwide "conveyor belt" of currents that flushes the deep ocean with oxygenated surface water and returns nutrient-rich deep water to the surface. Further climate disruption would result when the atmospheric carbon dioxide could no longer be transported to the deep-ocean "carbon sinks" and thus intensify the Greenhouse Effect. Reduced oceanic mixing would lead to greater stratification/stability of the water column, a condition known to be important in dinoflagellate blooms.[2] As a more specific example of the effects of an imbalance in atmospheric pressure and sea surface temperature, the El Niño-Southern-Oscillation in the Pacific basin has been implicated in *Pyrodinium bahamense* blooms in the tropical Indo-Pacific.[27] Atypical weather and circulation/ meander patterns of the Gulf Stream were considered important factors in unusual toxic phytoplankton blooms from Prince Edward Island and North Carolina.[19] Such instabilities are not unlikely if the steady state ocean is challenged by climate disruptions.

In the scenario of global warming, the toxic phytoplankton species with tropical and sub-tropical distributions would be the most likely to experience significant changes in bloom dynamics or range extensions to higher latitudes. Such possibilities have been explored for *Gymnodinium catenatum* blooms along the coast of Spain (rias)[28] and for *Gymnodinium breve*.[29] Ciguatera, paralytic, and neurotoxic shellfish poisoning could become increasingly common health threats in higher latitudes where there are large human population centers. Eutrophication could increase the possibility of some blooms by providing a source of nutrients. The distribution of fossil cysts of toxic species indicate a wider range of some species during different climate regimes and may be viewed as "latent" distributional maps. We should also consider the possibility that undescribed or "shadow" species[30] of toxic phytoplankton or accidental introductions of toxic species[31] could be favored by climate change. Too, we need to set aside the dogma that a species has to be present in large numbers (bloom concentrations) or dominate the phytoplankton assemblage before we will consider it a causative factor in shellfish toxicity.

Despite the international efforts of researchers who meet periodically to share their findings on toxic marine phytoplankton, a recently completed national (U.S.) plan on marine biotoxins and harmful algae,[23] computerized data bases,[32] and workshops on specific areas of interest,[26] our research, monitoring, and regulatory infrastructure is not adequately prepared to meet an expanding global threat. This is especially true when we consider the greatest impact of climate change on toxic marine phytoplankton may be in underdeveloped nations or in island groups where isolation prevents rapid detection and assistance.

REFERENCES

1. WHITE, R. M. 1990. Sci. Am. **262**: 36–43.
2. STEIDINGER, K. A. & D. G. BADEN. 1984. *In* Dinoflagellates. D. L. Spector, Ed. **1**: 201–261. Orlando, FL: Academic Press.
3. ANDERSON, D. M. 1989. *In* Red Tides: Biology, Environmental Science and Toxicology. T. Okaichi, D. M. Anderson & T. Nemoto, Eds. **1**: 11–16. New York: Elsevier Sci. Publ.
4. SMAYDA, T. J. 1990. *In* Toxic Marine Phytoplankton. E. Graneli, B. Sundstron, L. Edler & D. M. Anderson, Eds. **1**: 29–40. New York: Elsevier Sci. Publ.
5. HALLEGRAEFF, G. M. 1993. Phycologia **32**: 79–99.
6. TURNER, J. T. & P. A. TESTER. 1989. *In* Novel Phytoplankton Blooms. Causes and Impacts of Recurrent Brown Tides and Other Unusual Blooms. E. M. Cosper, V. M. Bricelj & E. J. Carpenter, Eds. **1**: 359–374. New York: Springer Verlag
7. GERACI, J. R., D. M. ANDERSON, R. J. TIMPERI, D. J. ST. AUBIN, G. A. EARLY, J. H. PERSCOTT & C. A. MAYO. 1989. Can. J. Fish. Aquat. Sci. **46**: 1895–1898.
8. STEIDINGER, K. A. 1983. Prog. Phycol. Res. **2**: 147–188.
9. DELANEY, J. E. 1985. *In* Laboratory Procedures for the Examination of Seawater & Shellfish, A. E. Greenbery & D. A. Hunt, Eds. **1**: 64–80. Washington DC: Am. Publ. Health Assoc.
10. MARTYR, P. 1912. De Orbo Novo, the Eight Decades of Peter Martyr. F. A. MacNutt, Translator, Vol. 2. New York: G. A. Putnam Sons.
11. ANDERSON, D. M. & P. S. LOBEL. 1987. Biol. Bull. **172**: 89–107.
12. HELFRICH, P. & A. H. BANNER. 1968. Bernice P. Bishop Mus. Occas. Pap. **23**: 371–382.
13. BOMBER, J. W. & K. E. AIKMAN. 1988/89. Biol. Oceanogr. **6**: 291–311.
14. FREUDENTHAL, A. R. 1990. *In* Toxic Marine Phytoplankton. E. Graneli, B. Sundstron, L. Edler & D. M. Anderson, Eds. **1**: 463–468. New York: Elsevier Sci. Publ.
15. OLSEN, D. A., D. A. NELLIS & R. S. WOOD. 1984. Marine Fish. Rev. **46**: 13–18.
16. LIN, Y. Y., M. A. RISK, S. M. RAY, D. VANENGEN, J. CLARDY, J. GOLICK, J. C. JAMES & K. NAKANISHI. 1981. J. Am. Chem. Soc. **103**: 6773–6775.
17. TESTER, P. A., P. K. FOWLER & J. T. TURNER. 1989. *In* Novel Phytoplankton Blooms. Causes and Impacts of Recurrent Brown Tides and Other Unusual Blooms. E. M. Cosper, V. M. Bricelj & E. J. Carpenter, Eds. **1**: 349–358. New York: Springer Verlag.
18. TESTER, P. A. & P. K. FOWLER. 1990. *In* Toxic Marine Phytoplankton. E. Graneli, B. Sundstron, L. Edler & D. M. Anderson, Eds. **1**: 499–503. New York: Elsevier Sci. Publ.
19. TESTER, P. A., R. P. STUMPF, F. M. VUKOVICH, P. K. FOWLER & J. T. TURNER. 1991. Limnol. Oceanogr. **36**: 1051–1061.
20. SCHANTZ, E. I., J. D. MOLD, D. W. STRANGER, J. SHAVEL, F. J. REIL, J. P. BOWDEN, J. M. LYNCH, R. S. WYLER, B. RIEGEL & H. SOMMER. 1957. J. Am. Chem. Soc. **79**: 5230–5235.
21. ANDERSON, D. M., S. W. SHISHOLM & C. J. WATRAS. 1983. Marine Biol. **76**: 179–189.
22. YASUMOTO, T., Y. OSHIMA & W. SUGAWARA. 1978. Bull. Jap. Soc. Sci. Fish. **46**: 1405–1411.
23. ANDERSON, D. M., S. B. GALLOWAY & J. D. JOSEPH, Eds. 1993. Marine Biotoxins and Harmful Algae: A National Plan. **1**: 1–44. Woods Hole Oceanogr. Inst. Tech. Rept., WHOI 93-02. Woods Hole, MA.
24. BATES, S. S., C. J. BIRD, A. S. W. DEFREITAS, R. FOXALL, M. GILGAN, L. A. HANIC, G. A. JOHNSON, A. W. MCCULLOUGH, P. ODENSE, R. POCKLINGTON, M. A. QUILLIAM, P. G. SIM, J. C. SMITH, D. V. SUBBAO, E. C. D. TODD, J. A. WALTER & J. L. C. WRIGHT. 1989. Can. J. Fish. Aquat. Sci. **46**: 1203–1215.
25. MARTIN, J. L., K. HAYA & D. J. WILDISH. 1993. *In* Toxic Phytoplankton Blooms in the Sea, T. J. Smayda & Y. Shimizu, Eds. **1**: 613–618. Amsterdam: Elsevier Sci. Publ. B.V.
26. WOOD, A. M. & L. M. SHIPIRO, Eds. 1993. Domoic Acid Final Report of the Workshop. **1**: 1–12. Oregon State Univ. Sea Grant, Corvallis, OR.
27. MCMINN, A. 1989. Micropaleontology **35**: 1–9.

28. FRAGA, S. & A. BAKUM. 1993. *In* Toxic Phytoplankton Blooms in the Sea, T. J. Smayda & Y. Shimizu, Eds. **1:** 59–65. Amsterdam: Elsevier Sci. Publ. B.V.
29. TESTER, P. A., M. E. GEESEY & F. M. VUKOVICH. *In* Toxic Phytoplankton Blooms in the Sea, T. J. Smayda & Y. Shimizu, Eds. **1:** 67–71. Amsterdam: Elsevier Sci. Publ. B.V.
30. BURKHOLDER, J. M., E. J. NOGA, C. H. HOBBS & H. B. GLASGOW, JR. 1992. Nature **358:** 407–410.
31. CARLTON, J. T. & J. B. GELLER. 1993. Science **261:** 78–82.
32. WHITE, A. J. 1990. *In* Toxic Marine Phytoplankton. E. Graneli, B. Sundstron, L. Edler & D. M. Anderson, Eds. **1:** 509–511. New York: Elsevier Sci. Publ.

Emerging Diseases Associated with Seafood Toxins and Other Water-borne Agents

EWEN C. D. TODD

Bureau of Microbial Hazards, Food Directorate
Health Protection Branch, Health Canada
Sir Frederick G. Banting Research Centre
Ottawa, Ontario, Canada, K1A 0L2

NEW TOXIC EVENTS

Although paralytic shellfish poisoning (PSP) has been well documented over the years, recent observations indicate that the associated dinoflagellates or their toxins are occurring in new areas. *Alexandrium excavatum* was first observed in the Argentinian Sea in 1980, and since then blooms have increased in frequency and range along the coasts.[1] An exceptionally large bloom of *Alexandrium catenella* was documented from southern Argentina in 1991/92; this caused mortalities in fish and birds, as well as many human intoxications.[2] The intensity of the bloom was sufficient to produce discoloration of the water and luminescence. Off the south Brazilian coast in March 1993 the normal diatom community was replaced by toxic dinoflagellates *Gyrodinium, Prorocentrum* and *Dinophysis,* and another unknown species that caused shellfish mortality; the weather was unusually warm and calm.[3] Another indicator of spread is the fact that *A. tamarense* was first detected in Long Island Sound in 1985, the most southerly location of its appearance in the eastern United States.[4] A similar new occurrence was reported from Newfoundland.[5] The first PSP incident occurred there in late summer of 1982 after a long warm calm period which presumably allowed a local *Alexandrium* bloom to develop. Although no further illnesses have been documented, PSP toxins have been found in many more sites around Newfoundland since 1982, indicating that spreading by natural or human-induced means is taking place. PSP toxins have also been more frequently detected in the Gulf of St. Lawrence.[6] *Alexandrium minutum* has expanded its range in France since its first detection in 1988 in Brittany.[7] In addition, the mouse bioassay has detected toxins of unknown origin from cultured mussels in France[8] and in Norway.[9] PSP toxins are now found in a variety of molluscan and non-molluscan shellfish. For instance, in the United Kingdom toxins were present not only in shellfish for the first time in many northern areas in 1990,[10] but crabs were found to be sufficiently toxic that their sale was banned, and, following complaints of illness in 1990, the hepatopancreases of some lobsters on the Atlantic coast of Canada, mainly in the Gaspé area of Quebec, were examined and found to contain up to 722 μg PSP toxins/100 g.[11,12]

PSP originating from a different species, *Pyrodinium bahamense* var. *compressa,* has also been reported from tropical countries. Cases were first documented in Papua New Guinea in 1972, Brunei and Malaysia in 1976, the Philippines in 1983 and Guatemala in 1987.[13] Since aquaculture is becoming established in tropical countries, the risks for PSP and other intoxications will increase. An example of this occurred in the Philippines in 1992 when 141 persons were poisoned (8 died) following consumption of molluscan shellfish including cultured green mussels, sardines, cuttlefish and crabs.[14]

In 1983 about 3,000 diarrhetic shellfish poisoning (DSP) intoxications from okadaic acid occurred in southern Brittany after cultured mussels were ingested. Since then *Dinophysis* spp have been monitored regularly,[7] and there is evidence of a gradual spread of these dinoflagellates along French coasts and northwest Spain. Each year *Dinophysis* cells originate in the open sea without the requirement of nutrients from land run-off, and they then migrate to the shore[15] in the summer through currents driven by the predominantly south to southwest winds.[16] The first DSP episode in North America arose from consumption of cultured mussels containing dinophysis toxin 1 (DTX1) in Nova Scotia in 1990. *Dinophysis norvegica* was found in the digestive glands of the mussels, but *Prorocentrum lima* may have been the toxin source.[17] Episodes of gastroenteritis have been reported every year following consumption of shellfish since then, but insufficient dinophysis toxin 1 or okadaic acid has been found in leftover shellfish to verify them as DSP. DSP has been suspected in the United States but no episode has yet been confirmed.[18]

Only one confirmed outbreak of amnesic shellfish poisoning (ASP) has been reported worldwide. This occurred in Canada in November and December, 1987, due to consumption of cultured mussels harvested in Prince Edward Island (PEI).[19] The domoic acid originated from a diatom *Pseudonitzschia pungens* f. *multiseries*, which was blooming in the area where the mussels were harvested. These blooms seem to be dependent on available nitrate which increases in the fall after rain and strong winds. Local conditions in the inner estuaries are important and agricultural runoff, rather than upwelling of nutrients, is the probable source of the nitrate. Water turbulence is more important for offshore blooms. Domoic acid production depends not only on availablity of nitrate, but also on cessation of diatom cell division and presence of light. Cells in the stationary phase remain viable for weeks and continue to release domoic acid into the water, even at sea temperatures of 0°C.[20] Blooms occurred but were less extensive in subsequent years when the domoic acid concentration in the fall was sufficient to close harvesting only for a short period of time. In October 1991 a small bloom was recorded from northern PEI for the first time. In addition, toxin-producing blooms have been documented from Maine and Texas coasts.[19] Also, low levels of domoic acid produced by *Pseudonitzschia pseudodelicatissima* were found in the Bay of Fundy and Danish and Norwegian waters.[21-23] *P. australis* caused deaths of pelicans and cormorants eating anchovies off Monterey Bay in California in September 1991.[19] Domoic acid has also been recovered from shellfish and crabs harvested on the west coast of the United States, and may have caused 24 illnesses in Washington State.[19]

Neurotoxic shellfish poisoning (NSP) has only been regularly reported from the Gulf of Mexico and once from North Carolina in 1987,[24] but was identified as the cause of over 180 shellfish-related illnesses in New Zealand in January 1993.[25] Other persons seemed to suffer from DSP-like symptoms and symptoms unrelated to any of the known shellfish toxins. *Gymnodinium* cf *breve, Dinophysis,* and *Alexandrium* were all found in coastal waters. The main shellfish eaten were cultured mussels, oysters and scallops. Unusual weather patterns associated with the El Niño-Southern Oscillation phenomenon allowed the development of the blooms through southerly winds and cooler water temperatures; there had been no previous record of shellfish toxicity in New Zealand.[26] The unusual wind patterns coupled with the cooler waters created new environments for phytoplankton and appeared favorable for the *Gymnodinium*.

A newly identified form of fish toxicity was recently identified in Pimlico Sound estuaries, North Carolina,[27] where a new dinoflagellate *Pfiesteria piscimorte* disorients and kills fish with toxin(s). The organism then feeds on the dying fish before encysting. The toxin(s) produced were sufficent to cause respiratory distress and disorientation in one of the laboratory workers (Burkholder, personal communication, 1993). This may indicate the existence of a whole new class of toxic compounds that could have implications for human acute and chronic illness.

NATURAL ENVIRONMENTAL CHANGES

Changes in the environment because of local or global effects appear to be major factors determining the range of phytoplankton blooms and increasing the risk of toxin being present in seafood. At present, there is limited understanding of the dynamics of bloom formation and dissolution, but many separate observations and experiments show that there are multiple forces effecting change. Sunlight, wind velocities and tidal fronts are important, but also local hydrography and preceding blooms of other phytoplankton.[28,29] In the British Isles PSP has been documented since 1968; local conditions favorable for blooms include neap tides, periods of weak winds, and runoff.[10] However, increase in toxic events may also coincide with other long-term phenomena, *e.g.,* decreasing populations of herring, cod, sprat and kittiwakes, which are dependent on adequate sources of plankton. The presence of nitrogen, medium sunlight intensities, and cool water temperatures were important for toxic *A. catenella* blooms in Hong Kong bays in 1988 and 1989.[30] In southern Chile and southern Argentina in 1991 and 1992 particularly large blooms of *A. catenella* with very high toxin levels in shellfish (127,200 μg saxitoxin eq/100 g mussels), caused many illnesses and some deaths. The intensity of these blooms may be related to the increased radiation resulting from the Antarctic ozone hole.[31] Some phytoplankton, *e.g., Phaeocystis* and *Alexandrium* can withstand an increase in UV radiation much better than zooplankton including copepods. It has also been postulated that PSP toxin levels, at least in the Bay of Fundy which has the highest tides in the world, are related to the 18.5 year lunar tidal cycle.[32] An unusual red tide from a bloom of *Cochlodinium* in 1990 off the Chinese coast killed fish, including one-ton of devilfish, and shellfish, causing an economic loss of 2.6 million yuan (RMB).[33] Heavy rainfall preceded the outbreak and warm water temperatures in calm weather assisted in the development of the bloom.

An outbreak of neurologic shellfish poisoning was first documented in North Carolina in 1987/88,[24] and since then *Gymnodinium breve*, its causative dinoflagellate, has continued to be present in the South Atlantic Bight north of Florida (see also Tester, this volume). Increased water temperatures giving rise to shoreward eddies may have been important, and predicted global warming will probably give rise to more such incidents.[24] Global warming and associated changes in ocean currents may also contribute to the observed increased upwelling of cold nutrient-rich water into the warmer surface water off the Spanish coast where mussels are cultured.[34] This, possibly combined with mussel fecal matter, allows rapid growth of *G. catenatum* and may explain the recent blooms of this organism. *Gyrodinium aureolum* blooms off the Norwegian coast have followed heavy precipitation and land runoff,[35] and the very large bloom of *Chrysochromulina polylepis* in Scandinavian waters in 1988 was probably due to exceptional hydrographic conditions, rather than long-term change in the environment such as eutrophication.[36] Increase in cobalt and a decrease in phosphorus may have been more significant factors. Unfortunately, prediction of large *Chrysochromulina* blooms is not currently possible. The 1988 bloom caused $US 200 million in losses to salmon farms.[37]

HISTORIC AND PREHISTORIC DATA

All these data are based on observations over a short time scale. At present, there are limited data on the distribution of toxic phytoplankton over historic or prehistoric times and their relationship with environmental changes. However, the fossil record of other lifeforms may be useful for suggesting possible relationships. Extinction of animal and plant species is caused by habitat reduction and global cooling.[38] These two effects can be connected, *e.g.*, the loss of the continental shelf habitat to marine species during glaciation and associated lowering of the sea level. Habitat reduction has much more of an impact in tropical than boreal and temperate regions, because of the far greater diversity of life in the former. Species may occupy very small areas in tropical forests and to a lesser extent on coral reefs compared with the large areas occupied by species in higher latitudes. Cooling also affects tropical species more than others because the latter are used to seasonal temperature changes and can retreat to more hospitable habitats if cooling persists. Several times in geologic history extinction has been high, most notably at the end of the Permian age, when 80–95% of all species, particularly marine types, disappeared. The cause of this extinction is not known but may be linked to recession of the sea level and decreased oxygen content.[39] However, new varieties replaced them rapidly on the geologic time scale, and these were more vigorous, predatory and able to adapt to environmental change.

The message from this is that species tend to remain in stable communities with little change until a habitat becomes vacated. In this respect disease-causing agents may have a chance of migrating to new areas if changing conditions favor them. The only data on fossil dinoflagellate cysts are from Europe. The historical record of PSP-associated *Gymnodinium catenatum* has been traced in southern Scandinavian waters from 6,000 years BP (before present) to 300 years BP when it became locally extinct. [40,41] Warm temperatures appear to have been a major factor in encouraging blooms, and conversely, cold temperatures in causing their extinction. Reintroduction of cysts by human means could allow development of modern blooms, since the temperatures of these waters have since moderated. This may have happened in northern Spain. The organism was first detected there in 1976, but core samples revealed no cysts in sediments dating back 9,000 years. Therefore, toxic phytoplankton can be transferred into a new habitat and quickly spread, or possibly be present in low numbers until conditions are favorable for their rapid growth. The expected effect of global warming would be to extend the range of tropical and subtropical toxic phytoplankton into higher latitudes. [42]

THE EFFECT OF BACTERIA ON PHYTOPLANKTON BLOOMS

There is evidence that interactions between microorganisms and plankton may increase or decrease toxicity. Tetrodotoxin (TTX) is produced in puffer fish possibly through the metabolism of *Vibrio* spp in or on the fish. TTX has been reported along with PSP toxins in Japanese scallops through ingestion of *Alexandrium tamarense,* which may contain intracellular bacteria, such as *Moraxella.* [43] Bacteria have also been found in *A. tamarense,* [44] *A. lusitanicum* [45] and *Ostreopsis lenticularis.* [46] In addition, a range of bacteria have been found to produce sodium channel–blocking agents in Scottish seawater. [47] Non-axenic cultures [a] of *Pseudonitzschia pungens* f. *multiseries* produce 20 times as much domoic acid as axenic cultures, indicating that production is enhanced by specific bacteria. [48] In addition, destruction of phytoplankton blooms by parasitizing or toxigenic microorganisms is a possibility which may may affect the types and intensities of succeeding blooms of toxic species. For instance, it is claimed that a *Flavobacterium* sp. kills the dinoflagellate *Gymnodinium nagasakiense.* [49] *Vibrio cholerae* has been found in a non-culturable state but still capable of infection in a variety of habitats around the world. [50] The *Vibrio* attaches to copepods and can be transported to new areas by these means; since the cells are concentrated on the copepods, they can cause infections if these are ingested.

---

[a] Axenic culture—the growth of organisms of a single species in the absence of cells or living organisms of another species. For phytoplankton this is normally considered to be culturing of a species in the absence of bacteria.

HUMAN INFLUENCES ON THE ENVIRONMENT

Enriching sea water with large amounts of nutrient from agricultural run-off, human sewage and industial waste increases nitrogen and phosphorus levels relative to silicon. This favors growth of non-siliceous phytoplanktonic groups, *e.g.*, bluegreen algae and *Phaeocystis*, at the expense of dinoflagellates.[51] Several genera of bluegreen algae such as *Anabaena, Aphanizomenon, Microcystis, Nodularia, Oscillatoria*, produce neurotoxins, hepatotoxins, cytotoxins, and dermatotoxins.[51] Economically damaging blooms, deaths of animals, and human gastroenteritis and dermatitis have been linked to drinking and recreational water contaminated with these algae in North and South America, Europe, Israel, Australia, New Zealand, South Africa, Zimbabwe, Thailand, China, and other parts of the world.[53] A new toxin causing hepatoenteritis is cylindrospermin from *Cylindrospermopsis raciborskii* which caused illnesses in Queensland residents using a local reservoir; attempts to remove the dense algal bloom with copper sulfate resulted in the release of the toxin which affected 148 persons drinking the water.[54] Because of eutrophication, bluegreen algae blooms are occurring more frequently in the Baltic Sea,[55-57] and as more lakes and reservoirs receive organic runoff from fertilizers, new species of toxic bluegreen algae will be discovered. The existence of new classes of toxins from the genera *Coelosphaerium, Gloetrichia, Lyngbya, Nostoc*, and *Trichodesmium* is already suspected.[54] Pollution may be a factor in the Northern Adriatic Sea which has been prone to algal blooms since 1975.[58] These have intensified since the development of large gelatinous aggregates composed of microalgae, bacteria and protozoa in the summer months after 1988.[59] Toxicity by *Alexandrium tamarense* (PSP), *Dinophysis* (DSP) and *A. minutum* (PSP) were first detected in 1982, 1988, and 1989, respectively. DSP was first reported in 1989, but levels of *Dinophysis* spp did not seem to change substantially; the dinoflagellate was found frequently but not in high numbers.[58] Toxicity may be related to the choice of plankton available to the mussels. A limited supply of other species could mean more *Dinophysis* would be ingested. The Black Sea is one of the most polluted in the world, with increasing numbers of phytoplankton blooms occurring.[60-62]

Human activity is not restricted to eutrophication. In Australia there is good evidence that ballast water from visiting cargo ships released in harbors has allowed toxic *Alexandrium* and *Gymnodinium* species to become established in local waters, causing PSP and preventing shellfish harvesting for lengthy periods.[63] *Vibrio cholerae*, seaweeds, and the zebra mussel have similarly been spread by ballast water.[36] In the 1980s jellyfish-like ctenophores of the genus *Mnemiopis* were transported in ballast water from a coast on the Americas and released into the Black Sea, where because of lack of a controlling predator, they multiplied to pest proportions.[64] They also spread to the nearby Sea of Azov. Their consumption of zooplankton and fish eggs is not only devastating the fishing industy in these seas, but may change the phytoplankton compostion to allow more toxic species to grow. *Mnemiopis* has now reached the eastern Mediterrean Sea where it is being monitored for harmful effects. Another concern for the Mediterranean Sea is the tropical water seaweed *Caulerpa taxifolia* since it contains toxins that could enter the food chain through grazing by herbivores.[65] It was first seen in 1984 and appears to have escaped from a museum tropical aquarium; it has now adapted to the colder water temperatures in winter and has increased its extent. This may indicate that a new genetic variety able to colonize the colder water of the Mediterranean Sea and out-compete the existing flora has developed. Spread has been most likely from drifting of fronds in currents, transfer through fishing nets, and attachment to anchors. It is expected to colonize the whole Mediterranean Sea in about 20 years and affect inshore fishing.[65] Many eukaryotic species have been transported throughout the oceans not only through ballast discharge and attachment to ship hulls and equipment, but also through relaying of shellfish in new areas.[66] Toxic phytoplankton could similarly be transferred inadvertently in these shellfish to extend the range of these toxic species.

Since historically most fishing and eutrophication has occurred in temperate waters, our awareness for the potential for emergence of new diseases or spread of known diseases in new areas is greatest in these regions. However, as more human activity is pursued in tropical waters through more intensive fishing, aquaculture, industrial development and pollution, it may be that this environment is more likely to be affected by change than temperate waters, and the possibility of emerging diseases is greater. Unlike viruses with close host associations which tend to favor rapid coevolution,[67] there is little evolutionary pressure other than environmental changes for new toxic species of phytoplankton to occur. Evidence from fossilized cysts indicates that little morphological change has taken place, but global warming and eutrophication may change the biota sufficient to stimulate new toxic forms.

HARVESTING OF NEW SEAFOOD PRODUCTS AND DEVELOPMENT OF NEW FISHERIES

Aquaculture is a relatively new venture that interacts with toxic phytoplankton. Fish deaths are substantial from some of these blooms, but also there is increased risk of human intoxication through consumption of higher volumes of contaminated products. This can result from naturally occurring blooms in the area coming in contact with actively feeding cultured fish or shellfish, but there is also the possibility that increased nutrients from aquaculture, *e.g.,* salmon farming and mussel growing, may stimulate the formation of local phytoplankton blooms. Although problems with aquaculture in the United States are rare, this has not always been the experience of other countries. DSP has been reported from Japan, France, Spain, the Netherlands, Scandinavia, New Zealand, Chile and Canada; PSP from Morocco and the Philippines; and ASP from Canada as a result of consumption of contaminated cultured mussels. When a massive *Dinophysis* bloom shut down the mussel industry in southern Chile at a cost of $100,000, sea urchins were harvested instead.[68] This type of action could lead to new problems from unidentified toxins if the seafood has not previously been tested for acceptability. Toxic dinoflagellates can also affect fish and crustacean farming in brackish water. *Gymnodinium mikimotoi* has killed tilapia and other fish and also shrimps in India.[69,70] Other blooms may introduce toxins into the product without destroying the fish or crustaceans, and possibly be a hazard to consumers.

A potential new seafood—the northern moonshell—in the southern part of the Gulf of St. Lawrence has, since 1989, been shown to contain PSP toxins.[6] The source of these is not known but *A. excavatum* is present in significant numbers under the ice ($< -1°C$) and could explain why shellfish may be toxic in early spring. Moonshells, along with *Buccinum undatum*, another carnivorous mollusk, on the Georges Bank between Nova Scotia and Massachusetts have also been found to be toxic.[71] The source of this toxicity can only be speculated—perhaps movement of inshore blooms to the Bank region or undetected local blooms—but it was unknown before 1988. However, these, and other predatory snails such as whelks and dog winkles, can concentrate the toxin to unsafe levels even though the prey has non-detectable levels of PSP toxins (< 40 μg saxitoxin equivalents/100 g shellfish tissue), and have caused illnesses and deaths in many parts of the world.[72] This may also be related to the source of PSP toxins being found in hepatopancreases of lobsters found in the canyons on the Georges Bank in 1990. These lobsters have been harvested relatively recently. In the United Kingdom, because of declines in lobster stock, there has been an increase in crab fishing in the last decade. Subsequent findings of PSP toxins in the crab body (although not the meat) has led to seasonal bans on their harvesting.

Also, in the 1990s PSP toxins were found in the adductor muscles of scallops, as well as in other organs, in Scotland (queen scallops) and British Columbia (rock scallops).[73] Up till now work done in North America on the east coast giant scallop has indicated that adductor muscles are free of PSP toxins. There is also an increasing demand for whole scallops through aquaculture in both North America and Europe. Since scallops retain PSP toxins in their organs for long periods, these cultured scallops have to be carefully monitored. These findings may affect the future marketability of these shellfish.

Swordfish was the cause of illness in a small outbreak in Quebec in 1991, but the specific agent could not be determined. High levels of the decomposition products putrescine and cadaverine were found in leftover swordfish at levels indicative of bacterial spoilage. Since these amines are potentiators of histamine poisoning, they could have contributed to the illness, but negligible amounts of histamine were found in the fish.[74] From this it would appear that amines, apart from histamine, or other spoilage compounds could be responsible for fish poisonings.

SOCIAL CHANGE AFFECTING EATING HABITS

Residents of temperate countries are affected by ciguatera through consumption of tropical fish when they visit Caribbean and Pacific island communities, or through the importation of the fish. Intoxications are frequently misdiagnosed by physicians because of their lack of knowledge of ciguatera. Generally, no fish samples are available for analysis, and so, diagnosis is based on symptomatic data. For instance, a large outbreak occurred in 1987 when 57 of 61 Canadians, who ate a fish casserole in Cuba hours before they returned to Montreal, developed symptoms on the flight or shortly after landing.[75] The species of fish was not determined.

The second group of persons exposed to ciguatoxins are those who buy imported tropical fish from the fish market or eat such fish at restaurants. Incidents have been documented in the 1980s from Canada, northern United States, and the United Kingdom. One example of these incidents occurred in 1984 involving 9 individuals of oriental origin in Toronto who ingested different parts of a grouper purchased separately.[76] The reason that ciguatera poisoning in temperate regions has been recognized only in the last decade is threefold: 1) the increase in emigrants from tropical countries who are familiar with these fish; 2) the purchase of tropical fish by restaurants and fish markets to answer an increasing demand by consumers who have eaten such fish abroad or those who wish to try more exotic foods; and 3) the greater likelihood that today's investigators of fish poisonings will consider ciguatera as a possible cause of illness.

Whelks are not eaten frequently in most countries, but the Japanese obtain them from domestic and imported sources, and have documented poisoning resulting from tetramine present in the salivary glands of certain species. Similar illnesses have also been recorded in Scotland,[77] where some of the whelks destined for Japan were sold locally without extraction of the glands. In Nova Scotia several episodes have been described in the past, but only in 1991 were whelks examined for tetramine.[77] The source of the tetramine was *Neptunea decemcostata* whelks, which were a byproduct of scallop trawling. In two concurrent episodes blurred vision, lightheadedness, staggering, flushing, and weakness were experienced by 7 persons shortly after they ate the whelks. Two factors contributed to these incidents: only a small Acadian population in southwest Nova Scotia eats these regularly, and although *N. decemcostata* has a wide distribution in eastern Canada, it is only in the Bay of Fundy that these contain tetramine. The commercial harvesting of whelks in this area is now banned. Presumably some environmental factors are important for tetramine production by the salivary gland, but these are not known. For the whelk, the tetramine may be a defensive or predatory mechanism.

In some countries mackerel are frequently eaten ungutted and they are exported in this form from the United States and Canada. Recent examinations of mackerel from the east coast of North America show that mackerel livers contain PSP toxins.[19,71] Consumption of these by humpback whales may have contributed to their deaths in 1987. Therefore, there are potential risks to consumers of ungutted mackerel.

When the herring stock had decreased to non-harvestable levels in the United Kingdom in the 1950s and 1960s, the fishing industry turned to mackerel as a substitute. This resulted in a dramatic increase in scombroid fish poisonings because mackerel spoil more easily than herring with production of histamine in the flesh.[78] Marlin is currently being promoted as a fish to export from tropical countries. Unlike other fish, its quality deteriorates on freezing. Therefore, marlin are being kept refrigerated for long periods of time between capture and sale. In the 1990s spoilage in these fish was sufficient to allow development of histamine and cause two outbreaks in both the United States and Canada.[79]

Today's demand for sushi and other raw seafood products increases the risk of parasitic infections. Cases of anisakiasis are occasionally documented. Illnesses from freshwater fish parasites are probably more frequent because of the number of species infecting freshwater fish in many different parts of the world, especially tropical areas. When raw or incompletely cooked fish are eaten, sooner or later parasitic infections will result. As an example, a new fish-associated parasitic disease occurred in May 1993 when several Koreans ate uncooked white suckers taken from a local Quebec river.[80] They were infected by *Metorchis conjunctis* present in the fish. This was the first time that illnesses have been proven to be caused by this parasite, even though the eggs have occasionally been reported in stools of Canadian native people from eastern Canada, and some parts of the United States for 50 years. The opportunity for infection, therefore, had always been there but required a group of persons who were culturally accepting of eating raw sucker flesh to achieve this.

MORE AWARENESS OF PUBLIC HEALTH AGENCIES OF TOXIC PHYTOPLANKTON AS CAUSES OF ILLNESS

Local awareness of toxic phytoplankton blooms is important to determine potential health hazards. For instance, the November 1991 Washington/Oregon closures for domoic acid in shellfish were based on mouse deaths that were similar to those noted in the investigation of the Californian pelican deaths two months earlier. These were caused by their anchovy food source being contaminated with domoic acid originating from *P. australis* growing in Monterey Bay.[19] This environmental observation would probably have gone unsolved without the awareness of the PEI episode and the assistance of the Canadian researchers involved. So, one ASP outbreak triggered analyses of many samples in Canada and the United States (and also in many other countries) which indicated that low levels of domoic acid, perhaps from a variety of sources, may not be uncommon in the marine environment but only reach amounts sufficient to cause human illness under unusual circumstances.

Similarly, increased testing for domoic acid and other possible shellfish toxins in eastern Canada in 1987/88, led to the identification of low levels of PSP toxins present in some of the extracts (on average $< 50 \ \mu g/100$ g). The conclusion drawn was that small numbers of toxic *Alexandrium* had been in the Magdalen Islands' waters, but not enough to cause human illness.[19] While it is probable that the *Alexandrium* had been there for years but was not recognized, there is also the possiblity that cysts were brought into these areas by artificial means. Low numbers of *Alexandrium* and *Dinophysis* species have been found in the ballast water of ships discharging into harbors in the Magdalen Islands.[81]

Since the 1990 DSP episode in Nova Scotia, fisheries and health officials are more likely to investigate sporadic episodes of DSP-like illnesses. With rapid follow-up of consumer complaints it may be possible to identify the toxic components, and whether or not they originate from *Dinophysis* spp or from other sources. In the fall of 1993 a second confirmed DSP outbreak was reported from eastern Newfoundland.

Along with increased awareness have come the availability of more analytical methods for detecting PSP, DSP, and ASP toxins and the sharing of scientific data at the international level. More sophisticated methods for identifying ciguatoxin and parasites are currently being developed and evaluated. Methods are also becoming more capable of detecting low levels of toxins. These advances should help public health officials take appropriate action for control.

THE ECONOMIC IMPACT OF SEAFOOD TOXIN ILLNESSES

Few attempts have been made to estimate the number of food-borne or water-borne cases in a country or their costs. Even though these estimates may be limited in accuracy, they do give a measure for the effectiveness of existing control programs and whether the benefit-cost ratio justifies the need for new programs. There are three types of costs associated with seafood toxins: 1) costs associated with human illness; 2) costs of monitoring potentially toxic areas and inspection and analysis of finished products; and 3) loss of product sales because of closure of harvest areas (short- or long-term), embargo of imported product, or less demand through decrease in purchasers through adverse publicity and loss of tourism. Illness costs include those to society for health care and investigation of the cause of illness, to the individual who loses both the opportunity for work and leisure (lost productivity), and to the fishing, processing and foodservice industries for lost business. In Canada, costs have been calculated for seafood toxins.[82] Those with most impact are PSP, ASP, scombroid poisoning, and ciguatera. The medical and lost productivity costs for the estimated 150 PSP cases is probably over $225,000 each year. In 1988, the PSP monitoring program cost $3,300,000. Only one episode of ASP caused by ingestion of domoic acid has been documented in Canada with illness-related costs and lost business of $8.4 million. In 1988, the cost for implementing a domoic acid monitoring program was $1,390,000. Because of the effectiveness of the monitoring program no further illnesses or public concern for ASP has occurred. There may be about 300 scombroid poisonings costing over $150,000 each year. The expense of analyzing suspect lots of fish for spoilage amines is $27,000. For a possible 325 ciguatera poisoning cases each year the total annual cost would be $350,000. Costs for DSP and tetramine poisoning account for about $95,000 annually. The total annual costs associated with the estimated 845 illnesses caused by seafood toxins, therefore, is about $820,000, and the

TABLE 1. Human Interventions in the Aquatic Environment Leading to
Human Illness

Action	Consequence	Diseases That Have Occurred
Aquaculture	New harvest areas in possible polluted water or water with risk of harmful algal blooms	Norwalk-type viral diseases ASP, DSP, PSP Salmonellosis from anti- biotic resistant strains?
	Products distributed more widely with increased sales volume	Cholera
	Use of human and animal fe- ces as nutrient	
	Use of antibiotics to prevent fish and shellfish diseases	
Relaying of shellfish	Introduction of new toxic spe- cies and pathogens	Salmonellosis? cholera? PSP?
Eutrophication of water	Increased phytoplankton blooms	Probable DSP and PSP
Construction of harbors, ship wrecks, destruction of coral	Exposure of inanimate surfaces to allow growth of benthic dinoflagellates	Ciguatera poisoning
	Dumping of contaminated ballast water in new loca- tions	Cholera, PSP
	Transport of shellfish in fecally contaminated barges	Hepatitis A
	International transport of con- taminated foodstuffs (egg powder, cocoa beans, cocoa- nut, spices, *etc.*)	Salmonellosis from serovars rare in the importing countries
Cruise ships	Passenger consumption of con- taminated food and water	Shigellosis, *E. coli* infect- ions, salmonellosis, cigua- tera poisoning

product monitoring and analytical costs are $4.7 million. In the United States the losses for the estimated 58,200 cases of illnesses from PSP, scombroid and ciguatera poisoning was $125 million, and for 42,000 vibrio infections was $50 million.[83] Losses because of shellfish or fish kills, or temporary bans on harvesting, are often in the millions of dollars, *e.g.,* $US 2 million in the Philippines in 1988, 1.5 billion yen in the Seto Inland Sea, Japan, in 1991.[84] Other examples are cited in the IOC 1992 report on harmful algal blooms[84] and in this text. Even if these figures are limited in number and accuracy, it is clear that diseases associated with seafood can have a severe economic impact which can be expected to increase if these types of disease continue to spread or new ones emerge.

CONCLUSIONS

Phytoplankton blooms are increasingly being reported in many parts of the world, with more varieties being documented and their geographic ranges extended. Changes in climate and more extensive human influences appear to be major factors on the growth of phytoplankton. These factors are not easily controlled in the short term, and it can be assumed that problems with harmful algal blooms will continue to worsen. Human interventions in the aquatic environment have also increased the risk of human disease, both from bacterial food-borne agents and seafood toxins (TABLE 1). A more focused approach to assess the potential health hazards of new fisheries ventures, including aquaculture, and evaluating the quality of new seafood products, will help determine the risks before the products are marketed. Educating people, *e.g.*, sport fishermen and recreational shellfish harvesters, of the hazards of eating seafood from closed areas or consuming raw or undercooked fish and shellfish, is an ongoing process with predictably limited success, especially for emigrants from other countries. The only mechanism of reducing risk is to monitor fish and shellfish for increasing amounts of known toxins and infectious agents, and to halt harvesting or sale when a threshold limit is reached. Predicting the potential for toxicity can also be achieved though early detection of blooms, using techniques such as remote sensing[22,85] and identification of specific toxic phytoplankton,[7,23] or warning the public of imminent potential hazards.[86-88] With this kind of information it may be possible to minimize the effect of the bloom, for example, by moving cultured fish or shellfish to non-toxic areas, or adopt other actions and management policies.

REFERENCES

1. CARRETO, J. I., C. EL BUSTO, H. SANCHO, M. CARIGNAN, D.C. COLLEONI, S. DE MARCO & A. FERNANDEZ. 1993. An exploratory analysis of the Mar del Plata shellfish toxicity area (1980–1990). *In* Toxic Phytoplankton Blooms in the Sea. T. J. Smayda & Y. Shimizu, Eds.: 377–382. Amsterdam: Elsevier Science Publishers B.V.
2. BENAVIDES, H. R., L. PRADO & J. I. CARRETO. 1993. Exceptional bloom of *Alexandrium catenella* in the Beagle Channel (Southern Argentine). Abstract 6th International Conference on Toxic Marine Phytoplankton, Nantes, France, Oct. 18–22, 1993, 32.
3. ODEBRECHT, C., L. RORIG, V. GARCIA, J. S. YUNES & P. C. ABREU. 1993. Shellfish mortality and a red tide event in Southern Brazil. Abstract 6th International Conference on Toxic Marine Phytoplankton, Nantes, France, Oct. 18–22, 1993, 150.
4. NUZZI, R. & R. M. WATERS. 1993. The occurrence of PSP toxin in Long Island, New York, USA. *In* Toxic Phytoplankton Blooms in the Sea. T. J. Smayda & Y. Shimizu, Eds.: 305–310. Amsterdam: Elsevier Science Publishers B.V.
5. HOCKIN, J., D. WHITE, K. SPENCER, G. POWER & J. REID. 1983. Paralytic shellfish poisoning first cases in Newfoundland. Can. Dis. Weekly Rep. 9(7): 25.
6. WORMS, J., N. BOUCHARD, R. CORMIER, K. E. PAULEY & J. SMITH. 1993. New occurrences of paralytic shellfish poisoning toxins in the southern Gulf of St. Lawrence, Canada. *In* Toxic Phytoplankton Blooms in the Sea. T. J. Smayda & Y. Shimizu, Eds.: 353–358. Amsterdam: Elsevier Science Publishers B.V.
7. BELIN, C. 1993. Distribution of *Dinophysis* spp. and *Alexandrium minutum* along French coasts since 1984 and their DSP and PSP toxicity levels. *In* Toxic Phytoplankton Blooms in the Sea. T. J. Smayda & Y. Shimizu, Eds.: 469–474. Amsterdam: Elsevier Science Publishers B.V.
8. MARCAILLOU-LE BAUT, C. 1993. Toxicity episodes along the French coasts apparently different from PSP or DSP. Abstract 6th International Conference on Toxic Marine Phytoplankton, Nantes, France, Oct. 18–22, 1993, 129.

9. TANGEN, K. & E. DAHL. 1993. Harmful phytoplankton in Norwegian waters—an overview. Abstract 6th International Conference on Toxic Marine Phytoplankton, Nantes, France, Oct. 18–22, 1993, 195.

10. WYATT, T. & F. SABORIDO-REY. 1993. Biography and time-series analysis of British PSP records, 1968 to 1990. In Toxic Phytoplankton Blooms in the Sea. T. J. Smayda & Y. Shimizu, Eds.: 73–78. Amsterdam: Elsevier Science Publishers B.V.

11. TODD, E. 1993. Seafood-associated diseases in Canada. J. Assoc. Food and Drug Officials. 56(4): 45–52.

12. DESBIENS, M. & A. CEMBELLA. 1993. Occurrence and elimination kinetics of PSP toxins in the American lobster (Homarus americanus). Abstract 6th International Conference on Toxic Marine Phytoplankton, Nantes, France, Oct. 18–22, 1993, 61.

13. AZANZA-CORRALES, R. & S. HALL. 1993. Isolation and culture of Pyrodinium bahamense var compressum from the Philippines. In Toxic Phytoplankton Blooms in the Sea. T. J. Smayda & Y. Shimizu, Eds.: 725–730. Amsterdam: Elsevier Science Publishers B.V.

14. GONZALES, C.L. 1993. Pyrodinium bloom in Central Philippines. Harmful Algae News, IOC, UNESCO, Paris. No. 5: 1, 3.

15. DELMAS, D., A. HERBERLAND & S. MAESTRINI. 1993. Do Dinophysis spp. come from the open sea along the French Atlantic coast? In Toxic Phytoplankton Blooms in the Sea. T. J. Smayda & Y. Shimizu, Eds.: 489–494. Amsterdam: Elsevier Science Publishers B.V.

16. LASSUS, P., F. PRONIEWSKI, P. MAGGI, P. TRUQUET & M. BARDOUIL. 1993. Wind-induced looms of Dinophysis cf acuminata in the Antifer area (France). In Toxic Phytoplankton Blooms in the Sea. T. J. Smayda & Y. Shimizu, Eds.: 519–523. Amsterdam: Elsevier Science Publishers B.V.

17. QUILLIAM, M. A., M. W. GILGAN, S. PLEASANCE, A. S. W. DEFREITAS, D. DOUGLAS, L. FRITZ, T. HU, C. SMYTH & J. L. C. WRIGHT. 1993. Confirmation of an incident of diarrhetic shellfish poisoning in Eastern Canada. In Toxic Phytoplankton Blooms in the Sea. T. J. Smayda & Y. Shimizu, Eds.: 547–552. Amsterdam: Elsevier Science Publishers B.V.

18. FREUDENTHAL, A. & J. JIJINA. 1985. Shellfish episodes involving or coincidental with dinoflagellates. In Toxic Dinoflagellates. D. M. Anderson, A. W. White & D. G. Baden, Eds.: 461–466. New York: Elsevier Science Publishing Co. Inc.

19. TODD, E. 1993. Domoic acid and amnesic shellfish poisoning—a review. J. Food Protect. 56(1): 69–83.

20. SMITH, J. C., J. L. MCLACHLAN, P. G. CORMIER, K. E. PAULEY & N. BOUCHARD. 1993. Growth and domoic acid production and retention by Nitzschia pungens forma multiseries at low temperatures. In Toxic Phytoplankton Blooms in the Sea. T. J. Smayda & Y. Shimizu, Eds.: 631–636. Amsterdam: Elsevier Science Publishers B.V.

21. MARTIN, J. L., K. HAYA & D. WILDISH. 1993. Distribution and domoic acid content of Nitzschia pseudodelicatissima in the Bay of Fundy. In Toxic Phytoplankton Blooms in the Sea. T. J. Smayda & Y. Shimizu, Eds.: 613–618. Amsterdam: Elsevier Science Publishers B.V.

22. ANDERSEN, P., H. EMSHOLM, J. JOHANNESEN & B. HALD. 1993. Report on the Danish monitoring programme on toxic algae and algal toxins 1991–1992. Abstract 6th International Conference on Toxic Marine Phytoplankton, Nantes, France, Oct. 18–22, 1993, 22.

23. AUNE, T., E. DAHL, & K. TANGEN. 1993. Algal monitoring, a useful tool in early warning of shellfish toxicity? Abstract 6th International Conference on Toxic Marine Phytoplankton, Nantes, France, Oct. 18–22, 1993, 22.

24. TESTER, P. A., M. E. GEESEY & F. M. VUKOVICH. 1993. Gymnodinium breve and global warming: What are the possibilities? In Toxic Phytoplankton Blooms in the Sea. T. J. Smayda & Y. Shimizu, Eds.: 67–72. Amsterdam: Elsevier Science Publishers B.V.

25. MACKENZIE, L., L. RHODES, D. TILL, F. H. CHANG, B. WALKER, J. KAPA & A. HAYWOOD. 1993. Spatial and temporal relationships between Gymnodinium sp. abundance and the contamination of shellfish with lipid soluble toxins in New Zealand. Abstract 6th International Conference on Toxic Marine Phytoplankton, Nantes, France, Oct. 18–22, 1993, 126.

26. CHANG, F. H., L. MACKENZIE, D. TILL, D. HANNAH & L. RHODES. 1993. The first

toxic shellfish outbreaks and the associated phytoplankton blooms in early 1993 in New Zealand. Abstract 6th International Conference on Toxic Marine Phytoplankton, Nantes, France, Oct. 18–22, 1993, 50.

27. BURKHOLDER, J. M., H. B. GLASGOW & K. A. STEIDINGER. 1993. Unraveling environmental and trophic controls on stage transformations in the complex life cycle of an ichthyotoxic "ambush predator" dinoflagellate. Abstract 6th International Conference on Toxic Marine Phytoplankton, Nantes, France, Oct. 18–22, 1993, 43.

28. EL BUSTO, C., J. I. CARRETO, H. R. BENAVIDES, H. SANCHO, D. C. COLLEONI, M. O. CARIGNAN & A. FERNANDEZ. 1993. Paralytic shellfish toxicity in the Argentinian Sea, 1990: An extraordinary year. In Toxic Phytoplankton Blooms in the Sea. T. J. Smayda & Y. Shimizu, Eds.: 229–233. Amsterdam: Elsevier Science Publishers B.V.

29. BORKMAN, D. G., R. W. PIERCE & J. T. TURNER. 1993. Dinoflagellate blooms in Buzzards Bay, Massachusetts. In Toxic Phytoplankton Blooms in the Sea. T. J. Smayda & Y. Shimizu, Eds.: 211–216. Amsterdam: Elsevier Science Publishers B.V.

30. HO, K.-C. & I. J. HODGKISS. 1993. Characteristics of red tides caused by *Alexandrium catenella* (Whedon & Kofoid) Balech in Hong Kong. In Toxic Phytoplankton Blooms in the Sea. T. J. Smayda & Y. Shimizu, Eds.: 263–268. Amsterdam: Elsevier Science Publishers B.V.

31. CARRITO, J. I. & H. R. BENAVIDES. 1993. World record of PSP in Southern Argentina. Harmful Algae News, IOC, UNESCO, Paris. No. **5:** 2.

32. MORGAN, S. 1993. Bay of Fundy lunar tide cycles may increase PSP. Sou'wester, Aug 15. **25**(22):10.

33. QI, D., Y. HUANG & X. WANG. 1993. Toxic dinoflagellate red tide by a *Cochlodinium* sp. along the coast of Fujian, China. In Toxic Phytoplankton Blooms in the Sea. T. J. Smayda & Y. Shimizu, Eds.: 235–238. Amsterdam: Elsevier Science Publishers B.V.

34. FRAGA, S. & A. BAKUN. 1993. Global climate change and harmful algal blooms: The example of *Gymnodinium catenatum* on the Galician coast. In Toxic Phytoplankton Blooms in the Sea. T. J. Smayda & Y. Shimizu, Eds.: 59–65. Amsterdam: Elsevier Science Publishers B.V.

35. DAHL, E. & K. TANGEN. 1993. 25 years of experience with *Gymnodinium aureolum* in Norwegian waters. In Toxic Phytoplankton Blooms in the Sea. T. J. Smayda & Y. Shimizu, Eds.: 15–20. Amsterdam: Elsevier Science Publishers B.V.

36. GRANELI, E., E. PAASCHE & S. MAESTRINI. 1993. Three years after the *Chysochromulina polylepis* bloom in Scandinavian waters in 1988: Some conclusions of recent research and monitoring. In Toxic Phytoplankton Blooms in the Sea. T. J. Smayda & Y. Shimizu, Eds.: 23–32. Amsterdam: Elsevier Science Publishers B.V.

37. EPSTEIN, P. R., T. E. FORD, C. PUCCIA & C. DE A. POSSAS. 1994. Marine ecosystem health: Implications for public health. Ann. N.Y. Acad. Sci. **740:** 13–23. This volume.

38. ELDREDGE, N. 1991. The Miner's Canary. New York: Prentice Hall Press.

39. KERR, R. A. 1993. The greatest extinction gets greater. Science **262:** 1370–1371.

40. DALE, B., A. MADSEN, K. NORDBERG & T. A. THORSEN. 1993. Evidence for prehistoric and historic " blooms" of the toxic dinoflagellate *Gymnodinium catenatum* in the Kattegat-Skagerrak region of Scandinavia. In Toxic Phytoplankton Blooms in the Sea. T. J. Smayda & Y. Shimizu, Eds.: 47–52. Amsterdam: Elsevier Science Publishers B.V.

41. DALE, B. & K. NORDBERG. 1993. Possible environmental factors regulating prehistoric and historic "blooms" of the toxic dinoflagellate *Gymnodinium catenatum* in the Kattegat-Skagerrak region of Scandinavia. In Toxic Phytoplankton Blooms in the Sea. T. J. Smayda & Y. Shimizu, Eds.: 53–57. Amsterdam: Elsevier Science Publishers B.V.

42. TESTER, P. A. 1994. Harmful algal phytoplankton and shellfish toxicity: Potential consequences of climate change. Ann. N.Y. Acad. Sci. **740:** 69–76. This volume.

43. KODAMA, M., H. SHIMIZU, S. SATO, T. OGATA & K. TERAO. 1993. Infection of bacteria in the liver cells of toxic puffer: A possible cause for organisms to be made toxic by tetrodotoxin in association with bacteria. Abstract 6th International Conference on Toxic Marine Phytoplankton, Nantes, France, Oct. 18–22, 1993, 112.

44. DOUCETTE, G. J. & C. G. TRICK. 1993. Characterization of bacteria associated with

different isolates of *Alexandrium tamarense*. Abstract 6th International Conference on Toxic Marine Phytoplankton, Nantes, France, Oct. 18–22, 1993, 65.

45. FRANCA, S., S. VIEGAS, V. MASCARENHAS, L. PINTO & G. J. DOUCETTE. 1993. Prokaryotes in association with a toxic *Alexandrium lusitanicum* in culture. Abstract 6th International Conference on Toxic Marine Phytoplankton, Nantes, France, Oct. 18–22, 1993, 80.

46. GONZALES, I., C. G. TOSTESON, V. HENSLEY & T. R. TOSTESON. 1993. Associated bacteria and toxicity development in cultured *Ostreopsis lenticularis*. Abstract 6th International Conference on Toxic Marine Phytoplankton, Nantes, France, Oct. 18–22, 1993, 89.

47. GALLACHER, S. & T. H. BIRKBECK. 1993. Seasonal changes in the incidence of marine bacteria which produce sodium channel blocking toxins in Scottish waters. Abstract 6th International Conference on Toxic Marine Phytoplankton, Nantes, France, Oct. 18–22, 1993, 84.

48. BATES, S. S., D. J. DOUGLAS, G. J. DOUCETTE & C. LEGER. 1993. Effect on domoic acid production of reintroducing bacteria to axenic cultures of the diatom *Pseudonitzschia pungens* f. *multiseries*. Abstract 6th International Conference on Toxic Marine Phytoplankton, Nantes, France, Oct. 18–22, 1993, 84.

49. ISHIDA, Y., I. YOSHINAGA & T. KAWAI. 1993. Lysis of *Gymnodinium nagasakiense* by marine bacteria. Abstract 6th International Conference on Toxic Marine Phytoplankton, Nantes, France, Oct. 18–22, 1993, 104.

50. COLWELL, R. R. & A. HUQ. 1994. The environmental reservoir of *Vibrio cholerae*: The causative agent of cholera. Ann. N.Y. Acad. Sci. **740:** 44–54. This volume.

51. SMAYDA, T. J. 1990. Novel and nuisance phytoplankton blooms in the sea: Evidence for a global epidemic. *In* Toxic Marine Phytoplankton. E. Graneli, B. Sundstrom, L. Edler & D. M. Anderson, Eds.: 29–40. New York: Elsevier Science Publishing Co. Inc.

52. CARMICHAEL, W. W., N. A. MAHMOOD & E. G. HYDE. 1990. Cellular mechanisms of action for freshwater cyanobacteria (blue-green algae) toxins. *In* Microbial Toxins in Foods and Feeds. A. E. Pohland, V. R. Dowell, Jr. & J. L. Richard, Eds.: 553–573. New York: Plenum Press.

53. CARMICHAEL, W. W. & I. R. FALCONER. Diseases related to freshwater blue-green algal toxins and control measures. *In* Algal Toxins in Seafood and Drinking Water. I. R. Falconer, Ed.: 187–209. London: Academic Press Ltd.

54. MOORE, R. E., I. OHTANI, B. S. MOORE, C. B. DE KONIG, W. Y. YOSHIDA, M. T. C. RUNNEGAR & W. W. CARMICHAEL. 1993. Cyanobacterial toxins. Gazzetta Chimica Italiana **123:** 329–336.

55. BALODE, M. 1993. Bloom dynamics of toxic blue-green algae in the Baltic Sea, Gulf of Riga. Abstract 6th International Conference on Toxic Marine Phytoplankton, Nantes, France, Oct. 18–22, 1993, 27.

56. KONONEN, K., K. SIVONEN & J. LEHTIMAKI. 1993. Toxicity of phytoplankton blooms in the Gulf of Finland and the Gulf of Bothnia, Baltic Sea. *In* Toxic Phytoplankton Blooms in the Sea. T. J. Smayda & Y. Shimizu, Eds.: 269–273. Amsterdam: Elsevier Science Publishers B.V.

57. ZERNOVA, V. V. & M. M. DOMANOV. 1993. Effects of increasing eutrophication on the phytoplankton community of Baltic Sea. Abstract 6th International Conference on Toxic Marine Phytoplankton, Nantes, France, Oct. 18–22, 1993, 229.

58. BONI, L., A. MILANDRI, R. POLETTI & M. POMPEI. 1993. DSP cases along the coast of Emilia-Romagna (northwestern Adriatic Sea). *In* Toxic Phytoplankton Blooms in the Sea. T. J. Smayda & Y. Shimizu, Eds.: 475–481. Amsterdam: Elsevier Science Publishers B.V.

59. HONSELL, G. 1993. First report of *Alexandrium minutum* in Northern Adriatic waters (Mediterranean Sea). *In* Toxic Phytoplankton Blooms in the Sea. T. J. Smayda & Y. Shimizu, Eds.: 127–132. Amsterdam: Elsevier Science Publishers B.V.

60. BODEANU, N. 1993. Red tides in Mamaia Bay (Romanian coast of Black Sea). Abstract 6th International Conference on Toxic Marine Phytoplankton, Nantes, France, Oct. 18–22, 1993.

61. GEORGIEVA, L. V. 1993. Distribution of potentially toxic phytoplankton species in the

Black Sea. Abstract 6th International Conference on Toxic Marine Phytoplankton, Nantes, France, Oct. 18–22, 1993, 85.

62. MONCHEVA, S. P. 1993. Harmful algal blooms along the Bulgarian Black Sea coast and possible patterns of fish and zoobenthic mortalities. Abstract 6th International Conference on Toxic Marine Phytoplankton, Nantes, France, Oct. 18–22, 1993, 143.

63. RIGBY, G. R., I. G. STEVERSON, C. J. BOLCH & G. M. HALLEGRAEFF. 1993. The transfer and treatment of shipping ballast waters to reduce the dispersal of toxic marine dinoflagellates. In Toxic Phytoplankton Blooms in the Sea. T. J. Smayda & Y. Shimizu, Eds.: 169–176. Amsterdam: Elsevier Science Publishers B.V.

64. TRAVIS, J. 1993. Invader threatens Black, Azov Seas. Science. 262: 1366–1367.

65. JENKINSON, I. 1993. Mediterranean invasion by the toxic seaweed Caulerpa taxifolia. Harmful Algae News, IOC, UNESCO, Paris. No. 5: 7.

66. LOCKWOOD, A. P. M. 1993. Aliens and interlopers at sea. Lancet. 342: 942–944.

67. MORSE, S. S. 1994. Hantaviruses and the hantavirus outbreak in the United States: A case study in disease emergence. Ann. N.Y. Acad. Sci. 740: 199–207. This volume.

68. LEMBEYE, G., T. YASUMOTO, J. ZHAO & R. FERNANDEZ. 1993. DSP outbreak in Chilean fiords. In Toxic Phytoplankton Blooms in the Sea. T. J. Smayda & Y. Shimizu, Eds.: 525–529. Amsterdam: Elsevier Science Publishers B.V.

69. KARUNASAGAR, IN., B. B. NAYAK & ID. KARUNASAGAR. 1993. Mortality in shrimp farm associated with Gymnodinium mikimotoi bloom. Abstract 6th International Conference on Toxic Marine Phytoplankton, Nantes, France, Oct. 18–22, 1993, 108.

70. KARUNASAGAR, ID. & IN. KARUNASAGAR. 1993. Fish kills due to Gymnodinium mikimotoi red tide in brackish water fish farm in India. Abstract 6th International Conference on Toxic Marine Phytoplankton, Nantes, France, Oct. 18–22, 1993, 108.

71. WHITE, A. W., J. NASSIF, S. E. SHUMWAY & D. K. WHITTAKER. 1993. Recent occurrence of paralytic shellfish toxins in offshore shellfish in the Northeastern United States. In Toxic Phytoplankton Blooms in the Sea. T. J. Smayda & Y. Shimizu, Eds.: 441–446. Amsterdam: Elsevier Science Publishers B.V.

72. MATTER, A. 1993. Paralytic shellfish poisoning: Toxin accumulation in the marine foodweb, with emphasis on carnivorous gastropods and human exposure. Abstract 6th International Conference on Toxic Marine Phytoplankton, Nantes, France, Oct. 18–22, 1993, 136.

73. IOC. 1992. Programme on Harmful Algal Blooms. IOC-SCOR Workshop, Newport, RI, USA, 2–3 November 1991. Workshop Report No. 80(SC-92/WS-26), Annex VI. Intergovernmental Oceanographic Commission—UNESCO, Paris, France.

74. TODD, E. C. D. & C. F. B. HOLMES. 1993. Recent illnesses from seafood toxins in Canada: Doses relating to fish poisonings. In Toxic Phytoplankton Blooms in the Sea. T. J. Smayda & Y. Shimizu, Eds.: 341–346. Amsterdam: Elsevier Science Publishers B.V.

75. FRENETTE, C., J. D. MACLEAN & T. W. GYORKOS. 1988. A large common-source outbreak of ciguatera fish poisoning. J. Infect. Dis. 158: 1128–1130.

76. HO, A. M. H., I. M. FRASER & E. C. D. TODD. 1986. Ciguatera poisoning: A report of three cases. Ann. Emerg. Med. 15: 1225–1228.

77. WATSON-WRIGHT, W. M., G. G. SIMS, C. SMYTH, M. GILLIS, M. MAHER, T. VANTROTTIER, D. E. SINCLAIR & M. GILGAN. 1992. Identification of tetramine as toxin causing food poisoning in Atlantic Canada following consumption of whelks (Neptunea decemcostata). In Emerging Food Safety Problems Resulting from Microbial Contamination. M. Katsutoshi & J. L. Richard. Eds.: 555–561. Proceedings 7th International Symposium on Toxic Microorganisms, Nov. 12–14, 1991, Tokyo.

78. BARTHOLOMEW, B. A., P. R. BERRY, J. C. RODHOUSE & R. J. GILBERT. 1986. Scombrotoxic fish poisoning in Britain; Features of over 250 suspected incidents from 1976 to 1986. Epidemiol. Infect. 99: 775–782.

79. TODD, E. C. D., D. J. BROWN, A. GROLLA, H. SAARKOPPEL, A. CHAN, J. MCGREGOR, S. REFFLE, S. RYAN & N. JERRETT. 1992. Scombroid poisoning—an outbreak in two Ontario communities. Can. Comm. Dis. Report 18(3): 17–19.

80. MACLEAN, J. D., R. J. ARTHUR, B. WARD, M. A. CURTIS, T. W. GYORKOS & E. KOKOSKIN. 1993. Common source outbreaks of acute metorchiasis due to the Canadian liver fluke, Metorchis conjunctus. Abstract Joint Annual Meeting of the American Society

of Tropical Medicine and Hygiene and The American Society of Parasitology, Atlanta, Ga., USA, Oct. 31–Nov. 4, 1993.

81. GOSSELIN, S., M. LAVASSEUR & D. GAUTHIER. 1993. Transport and introduction of toxic dinoflagellates via ballast water on the eastern Atlantic coast of North America. Abstract 6th International Conference on Toxic Marine Phytoplankton, Nantes, France, Oct. 18–22, 1993, 90.

82. TODD, E. C. D. 1993. Costs of diseases associated with seafood toxins in Canada. Abstract 6th International Conference on Toxic Marine Phytoplankton, Nantes, France, Oct. 18–22, 1993, 202.

83. TODD, E. C. D. 1989. Preliminary estimates of costs of foodborne disease in the United States. J. Food Protect. **52:** 595–601.

84. IOC. 1993. IOC-FAO Intergovernmental Panel on Harmful Algal Blooms, First Session, Paris, France, June 23–25, 1992 (IOC-FAO/PHAB-I/3), Annex V. Intergovernmental Oceanographic Commission—UNESCO, Paris, France.

85. KEAFER, B. A. & D. M. ANDERSON. 1993. Use of remotely-sensed sea surface temperatures in studies of *Alexandrium tamarense* bloom dynamics. *In* Toxic Phytoplankton Blooms in the Sea. T. J. Smayda & Y. Shimizu, Eds.: 763–768. Amsterdam: Elsevier Science Publishers B.V.

86. FYLLINGEN, I. & I. MARTINUSSEN. 1993. Norwegian monitoring and forecasting of algal occurrence. Abstract 6th International Conference on Toxic Marine Phytoplankton, Nantes, France, Oct. 18–22, 1993, 83.

87. PETTERSSON, K. 1993. Information service regarding acute threats, including toxic algal blooms, to the marine environment in Sweden, emphasized on the Swedish west-coast. Abstract 6th International Conference on Toxic Marine Phytoplankton, Nantes, France, Oct. 18–22, 1993, 160.

88. SOTTO, F. B., J. YOUNG & J. RODRIGUEZ. 1993. A red tide management scheme in the Philippines at the regional level. Abstract 6th International Conference on Toxic Marine Phytoplankton, Nantes, France, Oct. 18–22, 1993, 160.

Marine Ecosystems: Discussion

Part A: Sustainability, Stresses, and Contamination

KENNETH SHERMAN: A number of us have been studying marine resource sustainability for several decades and we can report to you that the marine environment is under significant stress. In the political realm there is great sensitivity to this stress and an interest in generating mitigating action; so this is where science and policy meet. On the one hand the political process has helped focus on ecosystems in the marine and fresh water aquatic environments; unfortunately the science to support this kind of political interest is way behind the curve. We're not fully up to the task, but clearly there are people who would like to see us move ahead much more rapidly in the next 10 years than we have in the past 10 years.

We have attempted to develop a framework in which multidisciplinary groups like this one might find a place to bring their talents to bear on some rather significant problems. Now what are the significant problems? One is toxins, algal toxins, that have direct human consequences with regard to biotoxins in shellfish. Another is coliform bacteria that have been responsible for closing down significant components of the U.S. shellfish industry from time to time over many years. We have problems of contaminant loading in relation to coastal pollutants. We have trends in pollution and in primary productivity (production of primary nutrients through photosynthesis) that seem to be exacerbating the situation. So given that we have a significant problem with regard to stress, we need to prioritize our efforts. We would argue that the highest priority are those areas adjacent to the continental land masses for several reasons: high biological productivity, most of the population pressures that are generating contaminant loading are there, and 95% of the world's fishery resources are extracted in near coastal regions.

We also have the background of global change and a fairly significant high probability of a warming in process now that has impacts in different regions of the global ocean.

In terms of the primary productivity of phytoplankton, we are looking at a scale of a few days to less than a day for turnover rates and very short spatial distances, generally less than 10 kilometers. Here new technology is available which allows us to make that kind of high frequency observation (*i.e.,* undulating collectors and instruments). The most difficult component in any of these marine systems is the 300 plankton whose turnover rates in terms of population is around 30 days.

There are very high levels of eutrophication, of increases in primary productivity from nitrate and phosphate over-loading, in places like the Baltic, the Adriatic, and the Black Sea. In these three areas biomass yields and the structure of the system have changed significantly. One case study for the Black Sea would, in my opinion, classify that area as the most stressed marine ecosystem on the globe. Over the last 10 years the levels of productivity from nitrate and phosphate loadings from the rivers of Eastern Europe have resulted in high levels of primary productivity and a stress on the system with significant O_2 depletions (hypoxia from algal mats) around the periphery of that system. Most recently the introduction of jelly fish, in the millions of metric tons, is very likely to crowd out any fish in that system. So there's very significant structural change associated with excessive primary productivity and algal abundance.

PATRICIA TESTER: The contribution of river systems to nutrient input is certainly of concern to us in terms of phytoplankton blooms. In the Adriatic, there is a large phytoplankton bloom in this Landsat image that is simply downstream of the Po River System (see FIG. 11 in Remote Sensing section). We have taken an eye of God, hand of man approach with satellite images to look at the environmental system and the contributions that fresh water and nutrient effluents can make to marine systems.

I think Ken Sherman's thoughts are well considered and I think that the probability of things happening today are simply much greater in estuarine systems. Rivers, simply put, are collecting mechanisms for the waste of large cities. The demographics of the United States is such that in many areas people are moving into coastal regions, at least on the eastern seaboard from Chesapeake South, Chesapeake being the largest estuary in the country. The two largest estuaries are very shallow, perhaps very poorly drained most times, and are regions capable of collecting a great deal of material and holding on to it. That material then can be resuspended by wind mixing and such. I think that we are perhaps developing cesspools at the end of our major rivers. That may be a bit of an overstatement but these are perhaps environmental changes loaded and waiting to happen; and that is environmental, not in terms of climate, but environmental spaces that are being taxed very heavily.

And we're asking more and more of these systems as we begin to develop aquaculture. Where our natural systems are not providing us with the amount and kinds of seafood that we choose, aquaculture systems then begin to be a self-fulfilling prophecy in terms of input of nutrients and things that simply feed both phytoplankton and perhaps pathogenic agents as well.

In terms of absolute global change I'm not sure that we need to advocate that as such. It's one of those things where it will be very difficult to provide enough information to convince everyone that this is indeed happening. But if we take it upon ourselves to say that we don't need to be convinced that this is happening, if we're not looking for a level of—let us say—scientific proof that is undisputable, we simply understand that there are people working in these systems who have a good deal of intuition and a long track record of knowing what are normal perturbations in these systems; and as those begin to fall further and further outside the norm these people are probably then the ones that need to draw up red flags and say the system is in danger. I can't prove it perhaps point by point in every system down the line, but this system is in danger and these are some key points. If there are trends going in that direction it would perhaps be amiss for us to miss those and go on with life as usual.

SHERMAN: In the United States there are seven large marine ecosystems (LMEs) under investigation. The Northeast Shelf, about 260,000 square kilometers, the Southeast Shelf, Gulf of Mexico, California Current, Gulf of Alaska, East Bering Sea, and Insular Pacific. Activities are being supported at a level of about $250 million from the National Marine Fishery Service and approximately another $100 million from other federal agencies. So we have an infrastructure for monitoring that's ongoing.

In each of these systems subsystems can be identified. Just off the Gulf of Maine and offshore bank there is an area under the influence of major estuaries. Here we have a very stressed system where the biomass produced here naturally has been reduced over the past 20 years by about 50%, mostly by excessive fishing. However, we understand that and we have proposals for reducing the amount of fishing effort in the system by 50–70%. Now from a socioeconomic point of view that's drastic.

With regard to the present U.S. administration, the executive is going to move forward plans for reducing fishing efforts to that degree. There's a lot of resiliency at the lower end of the food chain so we would expect that the fish populations may recover the structure that existed in that region in the 1960s before a major perturbation of over-fishing occurred. However, in the course of our studies over the shelf we discovered something we hadn't anticipated and that was elevated levels of primary productivity in the near shore area. And that's related to an intense influx of nitrates and phosphates coming into the system. One of the most degraded environments in the U.S. is Boston Harbor.

Of interest to this group, however, is that disease from pollution and the stress on the system are not directly associated with commercial fisheries, and this is an area we need to address. We suspect that these diseases (from biotoxins) are related to elevated levels of primary productivity, but we don't have that link yet sorted out.

TESTER: In terms of the drainage basins of the Mississippi River, what's occurring in the northern Gulf of Mexico is also beginning to, or also has the potential to, affect regions in other parts of our ecosystem. We're tied together much more closely than many of us would have ever believed. This is a satellite image showing sea surface temperature (see FIG. 10 in Remote Sensing section). We have found that other items or products, biological sometimes, move from the Gulf of Mexico in this very fast moving high temperature river known as the Gulf Stream. It is a western boundary current and its contents are moving off of this region at about 4 to 5 knots, after which they depart from the land mass at about Cape Hattaras. The shelf is very narrow in this area and then meanders of the Gulf Stream go shoreward. Near shore water (that shows up as a lighter color) is where cooler temperature water has been captured by the Gulf Stream and will probably be retained in it. The alternative to that situation is when the Gulf Stream makes a very strong meander onto the continental shelf near the coastal region and actually deposits material from the Gulf Stream in those regions.

In 1987 *Gymnodinium breve*, a toxic dinoflagellate, was part of the product of the Gulf of Mexico that was deposited on our shelf. The ensuing bloom of about 6 million cells per liter caused about 6 months of shellfish bed closures, 48 cases of neurotoxic shellfish poisoning, and we estimate about $25 million loss to the local fishing economy. This example demonstrates how remote sensing may be used in tracking river flows and fresh water entries into a marine system.

EWEN TODD: In 1987 we had several events that occurred all at one time. We had PSP outbreaks in India for the first time, we had the domoic acid story in Canada for the first time. We had humpback whales die not far from the Massachusetts coast apparently with shellfish poisoning and found it subsequently isolated in mackerel they had eaten. We had *Chrysochromulina* bloom in Sweden which was a few months later in 1988. And then there were the dolphins that died just north of Florida, and there were seals that died in the Mediterranean from viruses. However a lot of these did not repeat themselves as far as I know and they diminished. So were these coincidences? Was there a warming trend? The Prince Edward Island story of domoic acid was as far as we know a local issue not related to global warming. The whale die-off may have occurred before and we just didn't notice it. The dolphin story may be related to neurotoxic shellfish poisoning and warming, that's possible. So we can go back and look at these but we've got to be careful not to lock them all together and say that it's an event.

Part B: Cholera Emergence

RITA COLWELL: The first critical concept is that epidemiology has neglected basic principles of microecology. Physicians who practice epidemiology have little knowledge of interactions of microorganisms through the environment and with each other, particularly with their survival strategies in the natural ecosystems.

In 1991 there was an explosive outbreak of cholera that occurred in Peru with 285,000 cases. (And remember that the 108,000 hospitalized represented something like 2–10% of the actual number of cases.) So this was a fairly dramatic infection, if you will, of the population. There were 2,700 deaths; but that's because public health authorities just did not know what they were dealing with initially, given such a sudden onset and massive epidemic. It was better understood when it spread to Ecuador and Colombia and those nations were better able to contain it and reduce the death rate.

One of the features of cholera is the rapidity of onset of the disease. One can be fairly normal one day, have a meal, and the next day literally be dead, if you have cholera gravis form of the disease. John Snow, 100 years ago, was able, through some elegant epidemiology (simply plotting cases), to track cholera to the water source in central London. Tracking cholera over the last 30 years one finds that it is first related to coastal areas.

In the Latin American outbreak it is very interesting that the spread followed the El Niño and the Humboldt current. In fact, sea surface temperatures off the coast of Chile, Ecuador and Peru, according to oceanographers, have increased detectably; while the increase is only fractions of a degree, in seawater *that* is highly significant. And the initial data suggest that there have been changes in the plankton population compositions. As far as I can deduce (and I was in Chile a couple of weeks ago working at the Fisheries Institute) there is an indication that there has been an abundance of copepods; however, we don't have enough data as yet to determine the statistical significance. In any case, anecdotally there seems to have been an increase in copepod abundance over the last few years, and the pattern of the epidemic seems to follow the current.

THOMAS MONATH: But again where is the vehicle; is it in the water or in the plankton, copepods, *etc.?*

COLWELL: Pathogens, including viruses, that we are dumping into the oceans persist. Many go into a dormant stage and persist. In the Galapagos (unpublished data) there were at least 25 cases of cholera that preceded the outbreaks in Peru. In the Galapagos the only water supply is rain water and it's collected in the system in the volcanic rock. Plankton were examined with monoclonal antibodies using a slide illumination technique, and they were positive for *V. cholerae*. Furthermore, collected rain water in houses was also positive.

Now with respect to transmission via contact with water, that's not really understood. Capelli did a very interesting study interviewing bathers on beaches in New Jersey and New York. However, that was prior to understanding that culturing potentially pathogenic bacteria and viruses doesn't give a true measure of what's present. So his experiments essentially have to be done all over again using gene probes, monoclonal antibodies, and other direct detection techniques in order to get greater precision of the numbers of organisms that are present in the water. We've found that divers in polluted waters, even though they don't have overt disease, will seroconvert forming antibodies to *V. cholerae*. These studies have been done in the water in which Navy divers trained near Washington, D.C., and in polluted sites in Russia (particularly the Black Sea). One can easily culture *Pseudomonas* species from these waters (a good indicator of pollution) and demonstrate the presence of many other pathogens.

Yes, I think it's instructive that all of the vibrio species are pathogenic and transmission is by ingestion, particularly of shellfish and crabs that are probably either inappropriately cooked or stored, then "reinfection" of the water source. We've done a lot of work on the effects of ocean dumping and we found that in the pile six dumpsite, for example, (where it was assumed that the dumping of certain spores didn't reach the sediment) that you can detect *Clostridium perfringens*, which is easier to culture than other pathogens. We're now going to be using some gene probes for *Salmonella* to confirm that there are other pathogens.

The point is that the pathogens that we are dumping into the oceans persist. They go into dormant stage and viruses in particular can be detected and persist. We are essentially providing not only a reservoir but kind of a trough of human pathogens.

Part C: Climate Signals, Ecosystems, and Complexity

PATRICIA TESTER: Currently our global climate change models predict a non-uniform warming of about ½ to 2½°C during the next decades, possibly to include a disproportionate warming in the higher latitudes of the northern hemisphere. As a consequence of this more uniform temperature gradient between the middle latitudes and the poles we expect that there will be reduced atmospheric circulation, and thus, possibly, reduced ocean circulation and oceanic mixing.

Modified wind and rain patterns will influence the amount of river runoff and subsequently the nutrient availability in near shore regions. We expect to see a significant sea level rise in the low lands of the Gulf of Mexico and possibly up along the Southeast U.S. coast. Climate change affects the physics and the chemistry of the world's oceans and thus has the potential to alter every functional relationship in the marine food web. We expect that these will first occur in the lower trophic (planktonic) levels.

I believe that 1987 was a peculiar year. Not only did the new event that Ewen Todd mentioned take place (domoic acid-induced amnesic shellfish poisoning), but there was a large first time ever *Gymnodinium breve* bloom along the North Carolina coast, and that might have been implicated in some of the dolphin die-offs further up the east coast (through contamination of migrating mackerel).

From a local perspective in North Carolina, I will say that it was a unique climate period. During the entire fall there had been very little wind, so very little mixing of the upper ocean layer. It was also an unusually warm fall and our temperature records will bear that out. There was no rainfall during the entire fall period, until about a week before a major bloom was recognized. There had been a bloom of *G. breve* in Florida and we were able, by timing the speed of the Gulf Stream (which was pretty steady and pretty well known in terms of its transport capabilities) to say that, from the time the bloom initiated off the Florida coast to when the cells were supposedly delivered off of our near coastal region, these calculations were consistent with the timing of the outbreak in North Carolina. The satellite imagery track was also consistent with this means of transport.

Our coast is bathed almost periodically on about a five- or seven-day time scale with meanders of the Gulf Stream. One particular meander stalled and we were able to place it in roughly the same position on the shelf for up to 19 days. That's a highly unusual situation. In fact it really hadn't been recognized by physical oceanographers until we had a biological reason to start asking questions about the longevity of this particular feature on the coast.

Now I don't know whether 1987 was one of those years that is simply going to go off the scale in terms of unusual events; possibly there were other regional climate differences that haven't been appreciated or published at this point. From discussions with people in a coastal community that had been settled for roughly 250 years by subsistence level fishermen, there was nothing in the corporate memory of these small communities that indicated that there had ever been a red tide bloom before. So I don't know whether 1987 represents what happens if we are changing climate regimes; but indeed 1987 was a unique year in our coastal environment between the Gulf of Mexico and the eastern seaboard of the United States.

HARVEY FINEBERG: Could I pursue this Pat? You've essentially said it was a unique year, but what would you say are imaginable ways that we could develop a system of surveillance observation based on accumulated knowledge that would help to distinguish these aberrant (I think Dr. Epstein said "anomalous") conditions from the beginnings of a more secular change in the status of, in this case, coastal ecology?

TESTER: We are at early stages in understanding the global connections among climate signals and distant events, and I do not believe the link between El Niño and Gulf Stream warming has been determined.

PAUL EPSTEIN: One way of relating distant signals and local events is to better understand how stressed ecosystems are vulnerable to climatic factors, whatever the climate regime is. Increased variability in climate (predicted by coupled atmospheric-oceanic global circulation models) will have large impacts. If the climate regime (the means in temperatures and precipitation) is also changing, climatic factors are going to have an even greater impact on marine ecosystems in the future. For the record, 1987 was an El Niño year.

STEPHEN MORSE: Would it be safe to say that the increasing eutrophication and degradation of some of these ecosystems would make the effect of a temporary anomaly in the Gulf Stream climate more severe; that is, would it increase the consequence of such an anomaly, and is there some modeling on the increased consequences that might ensue?

TESTER: Forgive this rather crude vernacular, but if you take a cesspool and warm it up a lot it's a very potent situation.

FINEBERG: When one thinks about systems that are of the scale that we are considering in both size and temporal dimensions, the actual account of an observation, or what counts as an observation, can take a very long time to acquire. And so the capacity to be able to describe a phenomenon may take a very substantial amount of time because the system we're observing undergoes change which is orders of magnitude slower than the *E. coli*.

LEONARDO MATA: Many things are happening concurrently in Central America. You know we had hurricane Joanna, after which we had a dengue epidemic in Nicaragua; then the outbreaks of cholera in Peru that spread so rapidly—in 3 months—throughout the coast and to Mexico and all through Central America. And now we have dengue in Costa Rica at altitudes higher than have been previously reported. How a country like Costa Rica, 55,000 square kilometers, can be covered with *Aedes aegypti* in 3 or 4 months—when we have mountains that are huge—the minimum is 2,000 meters and the highest is 3,800 meters—between the Pacific and the Atlantic, altitudes which mosquitos don't normally reach, raises new questions. These phenomena call on the expertise in this gathering in the fields of entomology, virology, and social science; something bigger is happening. Alterations of the environment and also climatic changes occur at frequent intervals, as Dr. Epstein has mentioned. I wonder if we could go back to records and see what happened in the 1940s because in the 1940s there were huge epidemics of dengue in Central America and 20 years later we had the epidemics of shigella dysentery. So these phenomena have now to be examined in a holistic way and also as far back as possible retrospectively to see if we are witnessing another episode of multiple diseases appearing, similar to former periods.

EPSTEIN: I think it's not a question of predicting one place with certainty but that one can talk about patterns and about places, critical regions, which are particularly vulnerable: Those regions are important to monitor.

I would like to return to the question of surveillance for a moment and whether we should be considering monitoring vulnerable or critical regions. Steve, I remember in the *New York Times* article back in July you talked about the ecological conditions related to the hantavirus emergence—the 6 years of drought followed by one year of rain, increasing the food for deer mice. Also an Indian Chief from the Navajo nation was quoted as saying *we've lost our balance with nature*. Now he may have been overstating his own role in creating that imbalance, but I think it's telling in terms of what that region has become. And that region has been identified as critical by researchers at Clark University who are looking at critical regions where diseases may emerge.

MORSE: It would be helpful perhaps if we set up criteria for identifying critical regions. One obvious one is areas of high biodiversity that are also undergoing ecological change. What other criteria could we establish that would enable us to target the right areas?

EPSTEIN: A book in manuscript coming out of Clark University looks at nine critical or threatened regions, looking at basic life support systems such as water (availability and quality), soil fertility and forest cover.

Additionally, global forces may be superimposed on local environmental susceptibilities. We can't say an outbreak of brown tide is going to occur on Long Island or that domoic acid poisoning will occur on Prince Edward Island, but we may say that because of the changes in the sea temperature this year we can expect some events along the East coast.

We have direct and indirect effects of the climate system on ecosystems. Direct effects of warming may be increased cardiovascular disease in heat waves, while there may be indirect effects in terms of disease vectors.

We can analyze the climate system in two ways: We may have a change in means of temperatures and precipitation, thus a change in regimes, meaning that the system has "jumped" states and climate parameters are oscillating around new means. That is what happened 9,500 years ago at the end of the ice age; the state jumped for reasons we don't understand and went into the current regime known as the holocene era. Whether the means are going to jump again—whether the climate system will change or not—is a crucial issue today.

We must also examine more than the means because there is evidence that minimum (nighttime and winter) temperatures may go up disproportionately more than maximum temperatures—and this may affect vectors and parasite cycles much more than a change in means would affect them.

Then we have the variations about the means known as anomalies, *i.e.,* deviations from the means. Here we must consider the frequency, amplitude, duration and onset of anomalies, all which may vary in an unstable climate system and may begin to vary before the means shift.

Anomalous events such as storms, floods and drought—more perturbations, more chaotic factors—which is what seems to be occurring—may overwhelm direct effects (of sea level rise, for example). The coupled global circulation models predict more El Niño events, more warming events, with increased carbon dioxide. El Niño events happen about 2 every decades; but since 1983 we have had four El Niño events. In fact climatologists are reporting that we are locked into a prolonged El Niño, a period of stagnating ocean warmth. (The warming is reflected in lower atmospheric pressures between Tahiti and Darwin, Australia—the Southern Oscillation—in a negative mode for four years.) How this will affect weather patterns this winter is very uncertain now, more so than in recent years. But the Western Pacific Warming Pool is a chief climate signal and determines patterns of weather, rain, floods worldwide, and that may obviously cause problems with vectors in ways that are different than just indicated by calculation of the means.

RITA COLWELL: I think I would rather use the analogy of our being in the descriptive stage of let's say ecological epidemiology rather than synoptic or actually dealing with quantification in cause and effect. I think that what we're really trying to do is seek out correlations and patterns from which we may be able to derive the causations. We're still in the very earliest stage. This is not in any way a negative statement; I simply wish to redefine it and step back. I think first of all the finding that the flood body of Mississippi water moved into the Atlantic is pretty dramatic. Now that gives credence to the kinds of things we're trying to do, but I think if we leap to the conclusion that there is a direct cause and effect, we open ourselves up to ridicule and I wouldn't want to do that. I think it would be sufficient right now to seek out, which has never been done before, a global approach to epidemiology, one taking into account ecological perspectives and parameters that give a kaleidoscopic view instead of a unidimensional view. I think that if we can achieve that, we would be making a major step.

IRINA ECKARDT: If dolphins are dying in one place and whales are dying in another, the question arises how these scattered events are related. If we would assume that these events are related and that we are dealing with a complex ecosystem, we should be aware that such complex and changing systems can collapse. A collapse of a system might be described with a phase in which the necessary feedback- and repair-mechanisms for reproduction of the systems and its sub-systems are not functioning anymore. Seemingly isolated incidents may be correlated even if we don't see the correlations now, and we need an overall perspective to view these events and try to put them together.

Complex systems may be very sensitive to initial boundary conditions, and slight changes in boundary conditions can have large impacts on the evolution of a system. Thus slight changes in a complex system can produce large impacts. We are doing a lot of environmental destruction; thus it is important not only to install a global surveillance system, but to work to prevent the stresses we are introducing into ecosystems.

RICHARD LEVINS: If you have a complex system, with a lot of simultaneous equations representing it, and ask what is its sensitivity to a unit change from some external force, the answer will be the ratio of two determinants. The numerator will depend on the particular variable that you're looking at and the denominator is a system property that depends on the interactions of all the variables. So if the denominator gets closer to zero (which means that there's a relative increase of the positive feedback with respect to the negative feedback) then every perturbation will produce a greater response than previously. But the model doesn't determine what those perturbations will be; that will depend on extrinsic factors. Therefore, we can be talking about unique events but yet have something which has simultaneously caused vulnerability at the general level.

FINEBERG: I do think, we were all impressed by the simplicity and beauty of the bifurcation between "macrobial" and microbial phenomena and we'll look forward to hearing more about that.

Part D: Report on Water-borne Diseases Workshop
(*Report prepared by Rudi Slooff*)

Problems: The phenomenon of "new disease" needs to be broken down into cases where rather stable species are causing problems in "new" environments (such as toxic algae) and those where rapidly differentiating, evolving species are causing problems in "old" and "new" environments alike (such as *V. cholerae*).

Some discussion was devoted to the potential role of biofilms in harboring pathogens and bringing them in contact with vectors, such as copepods. Biofilms may play a role in places such as sewage systems, water pipes, canal linings, where there is a chance for interaction with humans (*e.g.*, role in *Legionella*).

When discussing environmental factors related to marine-derived diseases, the "internal environment" of host nation elements facilitating the movement of infectious agents from the marine or freshwater environment into the human population, also requires attention, as do the stress factors determining (sub)population vulnerability. A better understanding of all these issues is needed for setting up effective monitoring and surveillance systems.

Modeling: There is a need for predictive epidemiological models that enable the use of monitoring systems for improved forecasting and early warning. Such models may not be able to predict "new" diseases in "new" environments; therefore, efforts should be focused on models to predict the appearance of known diseases, such as cholera, in new areas. One complication, however, is presented by the appearance of new strains of known diseases (such as *Vibrio* "O139 Bengal"). Additionally, there is the need to identify and monitor areas, regions and ecosystems most vulnerable to invasions and/ or emergence of pathogens.

Model components need to include: 1) estimates of reservoirs and vectors, 2) the presence and distribution of dormant (non-culturable) strains of pathogens, 3) factors determining reservoir size (such as surface area for adhesion, or proxy parameters for this, such as suspended particles), 4) factors affecting infectivity, and 5) factors facilitating human-to-human transmission.

There is also a need for the development of life-cycle laboratory models for testing hypotheses on host-pathogen and vector-pathogen relationships. These need to be based on suitable laboratory species and standardized studies to allow results to be extrapolated to natural situations without losing predictive power.

Interventions: Most of our discussion on interventions dwelt on surveillance systems. It is estimated that current surveillance systems for seafood poisoning fail to pick up the majority of cases (*e.g.*, > 90%), and need to be improved. In this context, it was suggested to distinguish between *late*, *intermediate* and *early* surveillance. Late surveillance is instituted once cases have occurred, so as to improve intervention methodology to curb subsequent cases. Intermediate surveillance covers areas near or similar to areas where cases occur, while early surveillance would cover areas where cases are likely to occur. Such a grading would enable stratified expenditure in accordance with need.

An early surveillance system could be modeled on the International Mussel Watch program of UNEP/UNESCO, financed by the Global Environment Facility (GEF) fund of the World Bank. In this program, coastal bivalves are used as biomarkers for contaminants. The program can be expanded to include observations on plankton species, nutrients, temperatures, primary production, and fish pathology. An extension of the Mussel Watch program into the Gulf of Guinea is being prepared and one also for the Yellow Sea (see under research proposals in the Research Agenda section at the end of this volume).

These programs can be complemented by UNEP/WHO recordings on human exposures (GEMS/HEALS) and WHO monitoring for Food Safety, by identifying existing or new collaborating centers with trained staff, or recruitment and training of suitable persons. This proposal needs further development on close coordination with WHO (PEP/CWS/PEP), at both global and regional levels.

REMOTE SENSING IMAGES

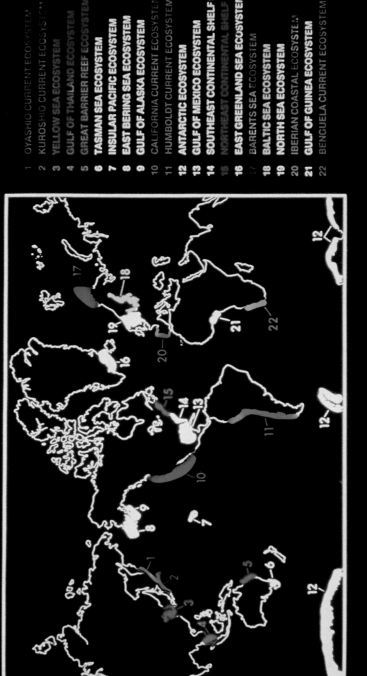

PREDOMINANT VARIABLE   PREDATION   ENVIRONMENT   POLLUTION   INSUFFICIENT INFORMATION

1 OYASHIO CURRENT ECOSYSTEM
2 KUROSHIO CURRENT ECOSYSTEM**
3 YELLOW SEA ECOSYSTEM
4 GULF OF THAILAND ECOSYSTEM
5 GREAT BARRIER REEF ECOSYSTEM
6 TASMAN SEA ECOSYSTEM
7 INSULAR PACIFIC ECOSYSTEM
8 EAST BERING SEA ECOSYSTEM
9 GULF OF ALASKA ECOSYSTEM
10 CALIFORNIA CURRENT ECOSYSTEM
11 HUMBOLDT CURRENT ECOSYSTEM
12 ANTARCTIC ECOSYSTEM
13 GULF OF MEXICO ECOSYSTEM
14 SOUTHEAST CONTINENTAL SHELF ECOSYSTEM
15 NORTHEAST CONTINENTAL SHELF ECOSYSTEM
16 EAST GREENLAND SEA ECOSYSTEM
17 BARENTS SEA ECOSYSTEM
18 BALTIC SEA ECOSYSTEM
19 NORTH SEA ECOSYSTEM
20 IBERIAN COASTAL ECOSYSTEM
21 GULF OF GUINEA ECOSYSTEM
22 BENGUELA CURRENT ECOSYSTEM

FIGURE 1. World map depicting 22 of the world's 49 large marine ecosystems (LMEs); colors indicate predominant driving forces influencing the health and integrity of these systems.

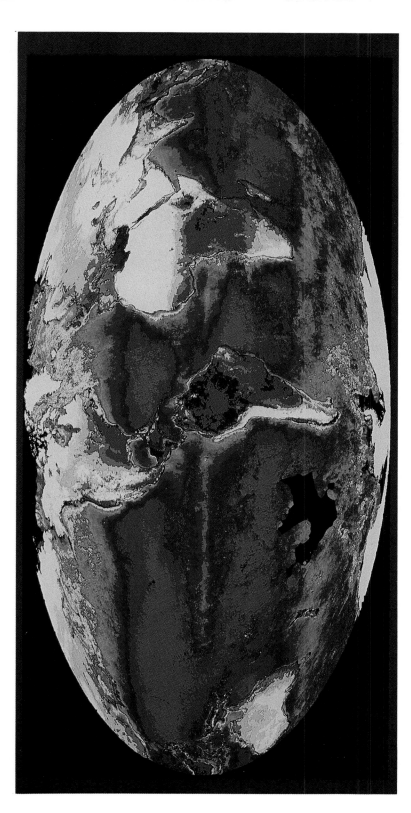

FIGURE 2. The first truly global view of the Earth's biosphere is seen here. The composite image of the ocean chlorophyll concentration was produced from 31,352, 4-km resolution Coastal Zone Color Scanner (CZCS) scenes from November 1978 through June 1981, each of which corresponds to approximately 2 million square kilometers of ocean surface. Nearly 400 billion bytes of raw CZCS data located on more than 12,000 9-track computer tapes were used to make this image. Land vegetation patterns are derived from three years of daily images from NOAA-7's visible and near infrared sensors (credit: C. J. Tucker, NASA/GSFC). **Note:** In Figures 2 through 5, the ocean color indicates phytoplankton biomass. CZCS detects chlorophyll, which is an indicator of phytoplankton biomass.

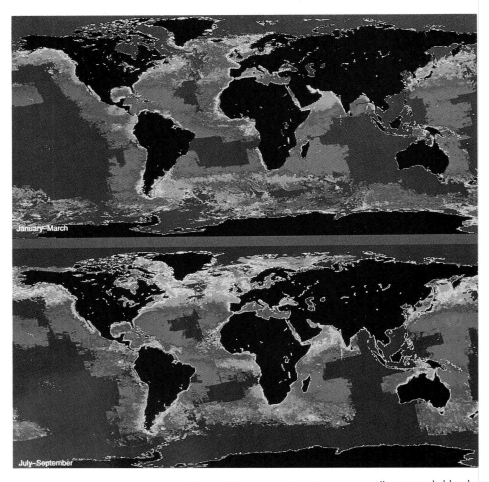

FIGURE 3. Global phytoplankton (chlorophyll) concentrations change seasonally, as revealed by these three-month composites for 1979: January–March (*upper left*), April–June (*upper right*), July–September (*lower left*), and October–December (*lower right*). Note the "blooming" of phytoplankton over the entire North Atlantic with advent of northern hemisphere spring and seasonal increases in equatorial phytoplankton concentrations in both Atlantic and Pacific Oceans and off the western coasts of Africa and Peru. (NASA)

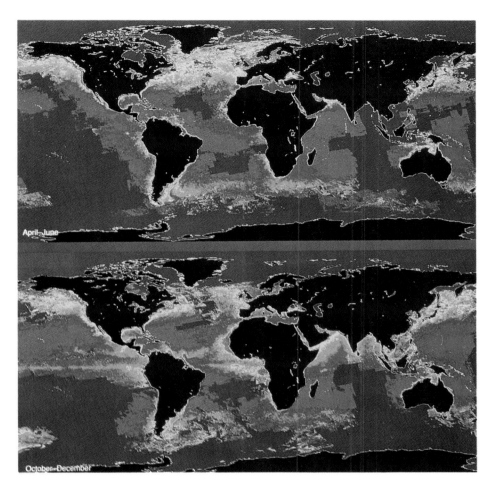

FIGURE 3. (*Continued*).

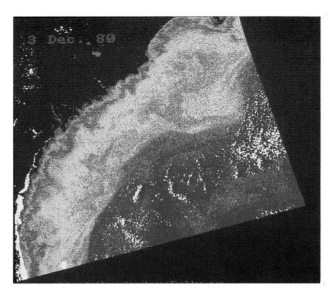

FIGURE 4. Chlorophyll concentration, southeast coast of the United States (parts of North Carolina, South Carolina, Georgia and Florida) on 3 December 1980. The chlorophyll concentrations are comparatively low. Note the Gulf Stream deflection (to the right) at the topographic feature called the "Charleston Bump" (dark blue water = low biomass). (CZCS processed by Martin and Tester)

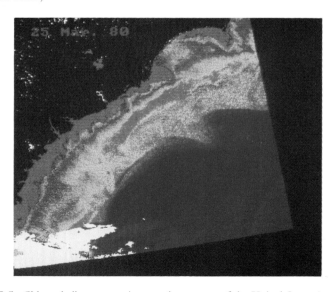

FIGURE 5. Chlorophyll concentration, southeast coast of the United States (parts of North Carolina, South Carolina, Georgia and Florida) on 25 March 1980. Note the high chlorophyll concentration at the mouth of the Cape Fear River (very top of slide). Note that deflection (to the right) of the Gulf Stream (dark blue water = low biomass) at the "Charleston Bump" is less pronounced than on 3 December 1980 (FIG. 4). Evidence of upwelling at the continental shelf edge characterized by the pattern of high biomass at the coast line, low biomass at the mid-shelf and higher biomass parallel to the shelf edge where the Gulf Stream meanders over the shelf and causes upwelling. (CZCS processed by Martin and Tester)

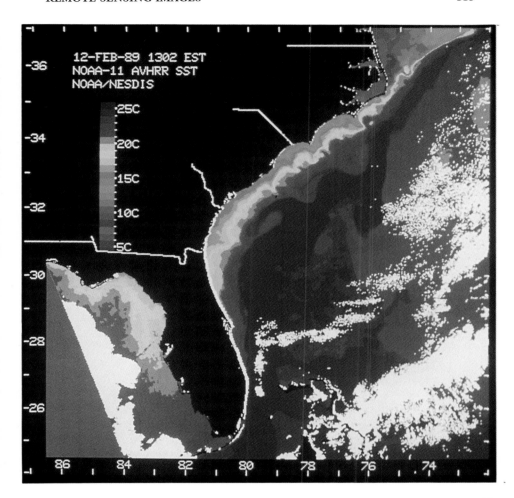

FIGURE 6. Note: Images in Figures 6 through 9 indicate Sea Surface Temperature (SST) measured by the Advanced Very High Resolution Radiometer (AVHRR) sensor flown on NOAA polar-orbiting weather satellites. This image is from NOAA-11 and shows the southeastern coast of the United States on 12 February 1989. It illustrates the meander pattern of the Gulf Stream, and there is a cold core ring off the North Carolina coast (yellow = cooler water enclosed by warmer, Gulf Stream water). Note that the Gulf Stream departs from its coast parallel flow at Cape Hatteras, North Carolina. (NOAA)

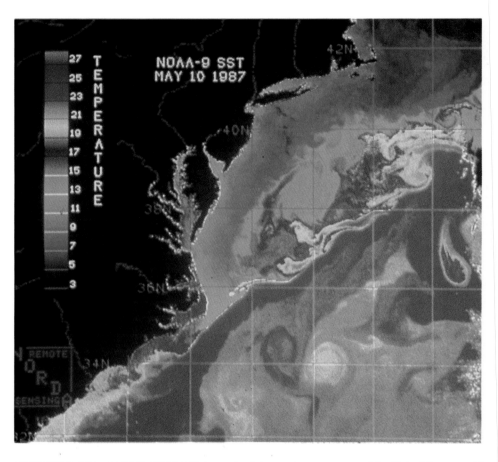

FIGURE 7. This AVHRR (NOAA-9) image is of the northeastern coast of the United States on 10 May 1987. It illustrates the meander pattern of the Gulf Stream and its departure from the coast as it flows toward the center of the North Atlantic. Note the cold core ring (green) at the right margin (midway down the image). (NOAA/NESDIS)

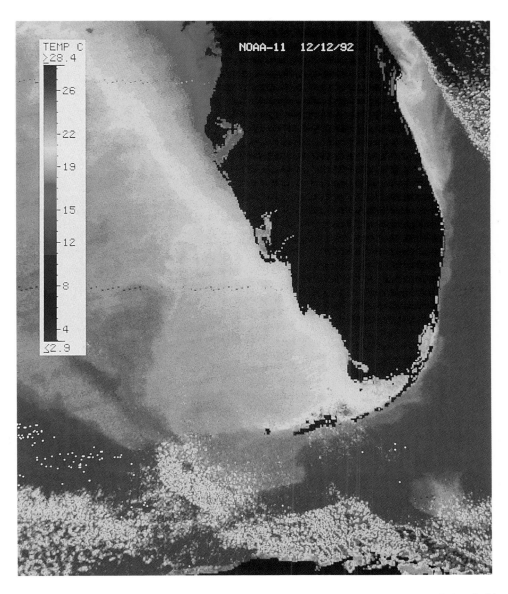

FIGURE 8. This AVHRR (NOAA-11) image shows southern Florida, Florida Bay, and the Florida Current on 12 December 1992. (NOAA/COASTWATCH, Tester)

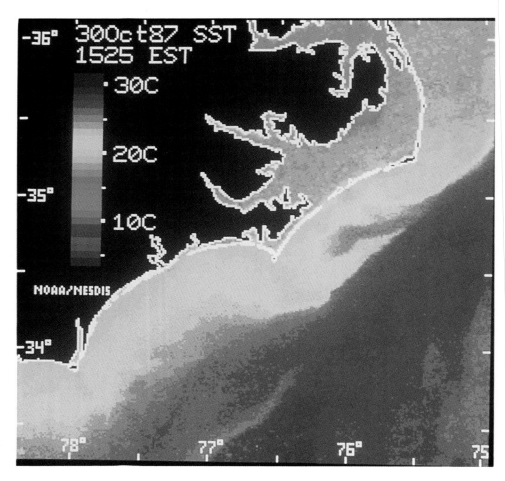

FIGURE 9. This AVHRR (NOAA-9) image of the North Carolina coast was made on 30 October 1987. The meander of the Gulf Stream is seen to override the continental shelf, and it was responsible for the transport of the toxic dinoflagellate red tide organism *Gymnodinium breve* into nearshore waters. The ensuing red tide bloom resulted in 48 cases of neurotoxic shellfish poisoning and a $25 million loss to the local economy over the next 4 to 6 months. (NOAA/NESDIS, Stumpf)

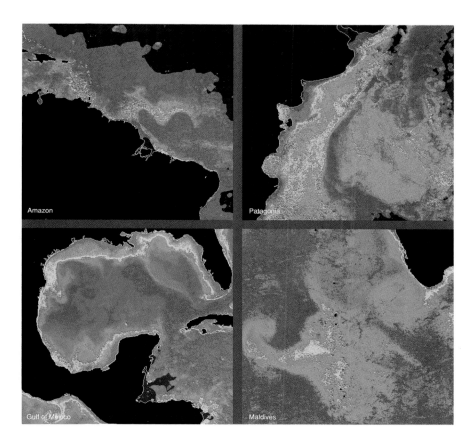

FIGURE 10. Coastal Features: Pigment distributions off the northeast coast of South America (*upper left*, Oct 1979) are dominated by the influence of two great rivers—the Amazon and the Orinoco—which together contribute 20% of the global river discharge to the ocean. The Orinoco plume extends into the Caribbean, while the Amazon plume flows north along the Brazilian coast and then meanders eastward across the Atlantic, influenced by the North Equatorial Countercurrent. The tongue of cold, nutrient-rich water of the Malvinas/Falkland Current borders on the productive waters at the edge of the Argentinian continental shelf (*upper right*, April 1979). The shallow coastal waters bordering the Gulf of Mexico (*lower left*, Oct 1979) support rich fisheries. Ocean currents flowing past the Maldive Islands off the southern coast of India (*lower right*, Dec 1979) stimulate plumes of plankton-rich water.

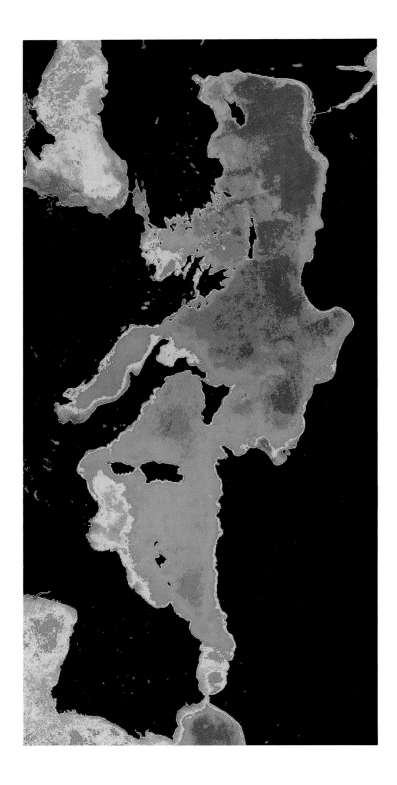

FIGURE 11. Mediterranean: The relatively clear, pigment-poor waters of the Mediterranean contrast sharply with the plankton-rich Atlantic waters off northwest Spain (*upper left*). Clearly evident in this view of the Mediterranean is the well-known pigment front along southern France and Spain. This image is produced from 30 scenes acquired during May 1980. The gyre in the Alboran Sea near the Straits of Gibraltar is caused by complex circulation patterns resulting from water exchange between the Mediterranean and Atlantic Ocean. In some cases, localized areas of high production are due to pollution from human activities.

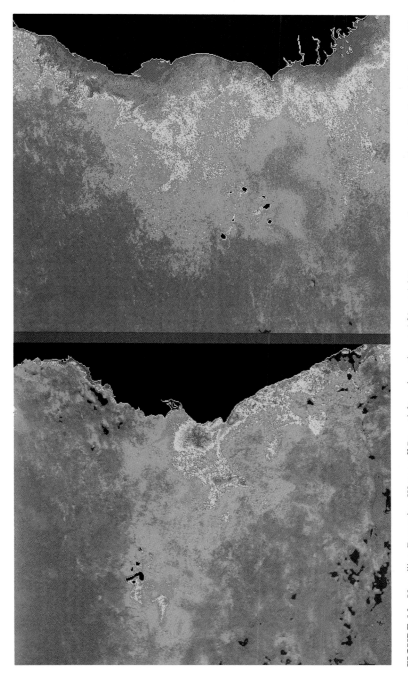

FIGURE 12. Upwelling Dynamics: Waters off Peru (*left*) and northwest Africa (*right*) are among the most productive in the global ocean. The Peru/Pacific composite covers 16–26 January 1980 and the Africa/Atlantic composite 16 and 22 December 1979. Nutrients injected by wind-driven coastal upwelling result in high phytoplankton biomass and productivity, which supports some of the world's richest fisheries. The upwellings are reflected here as 100-km-wide chlorophyll-rich bands along both coasts and plumes of productive waters extending 500 to 1000 km offshore. Island-inducing upwelling generates highly productive regions around the Galapagos Archipelago (center of left figure).

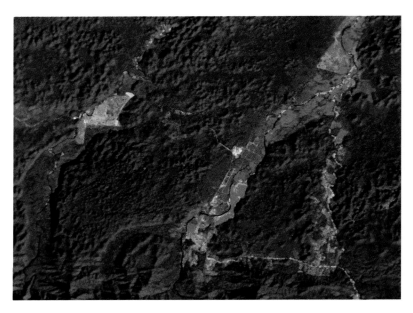

FIGURE 13. SPOT multispectral image of the Hummingbird Highway area in Belize. The highway is depicted by a pale line starting in the upper left corner and terminating in the lower right corner. The highway transects three river systems (depicted by three sinuous vertical lines). Black areas within the two rivers on the left of the image typify rivers with sun-exposed water. (Image provided by Dr. Jack Paris, GeoIPS, California State University, Fresno, CA)

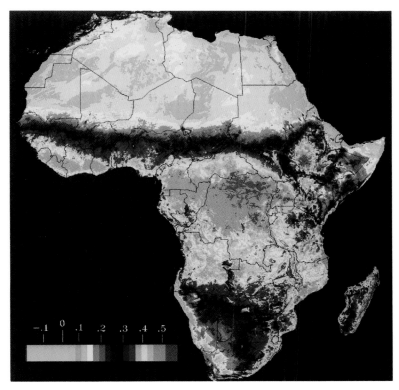

FIGURE 14. This image shows the average Normalized Difference Vegetation Index (NDVI) for Africa for 1987–1989. It is based on data received by instruments on board U.S. National Oceanic and Atmospheric Administration (NOAA) satellites. Colors correlate with photosynthetic activity of plants, rainfall, and the drying power of the atmosphere and integrate several environmental factors that affect disease-transmitting insect vectors. (Reprinted with permission from Dr. D. J. Rogers, Department of Zoology, University of Oxford)

Vector-borne Emerging Pathogens

Introduction

The members of the workshop on vector-borne pathogens sought to identify features peculiar to these organisms that promote their emergence and limit their distribution.

Vector-borne agents of disease tend to be more genetically constant than are those that cycle through only one kind of host because few major variants would thrive in the demanding requirement imposed by an alternating series of dissimilar hosts. A successful variant must be adapted both to an arthropod vector and a vertebrate reservoir host. The workshop participants discussed examples of *de novo* "mutation" of a vector-borne pathogen. Only one apparent case was identified, that of the observed increase in virulence for horses that appeared in the 1993 epizootic of Venezuelan equine encephalitis in Chiapas, Mexico. Although the virus had been enzootic in the region for many years, no mortality in horses had been noted until this outbreak struck. Changes in virulence appear to be more frequent in such directly transmitted agents as the influenza viruses. The 1968 outbreak of Hong Kong influenza, for example, resulted from an apparent viral recombination event leading to enhanced virulence and to pandemic influenza.

Although increased virulence may enhance transmission of a respiratory virus to new hosts, pathogenicity and transmissibility of vector-borne agents generally vary independently. Continuous exposure of Australian rabbits to myxomavirus, for example, selected less pathogenic viruses as well as rabbit populations that became less susceptible to myxoma disease. The agent, however, continued to perpetuate without interruption. This event argues against the recently phrased idea that such pathogens as the malaria parasites evolve toward virulence. The relatively benevolent thrombocytopenia that accompanies infection by the vector-borne viruses, rickettsiae, and protozoa facilitates transmission by helping vector arthropods feed more rapidly. Transmission would be inhibited if infection affected survival.

Pathogens that induce sterilizing immunity tend to be unstable in host populations that are small and isolated. The available supply of potentially susceptible reservoir hosts tends to become exhausted, thereby interrupting transmission and resulting in pathogen reemergence after sufficient susceptible hosts have once again accumulated. Vector-borne infections, because they generally are exceptionally transmissible, would be particularly volatile in such restricted populations. Malaria transmission, in contrast, would be stable in small host populations because infection is chronic.

Enhanced genetic variation in malaria parasites would facilitate emergence of drug resistance. Such a situation may occur along the Thai-Cambodia border where numerous infected gem-miners congregate from diverse malarious sites. Where the force of transmission is great, superinfection would follow. The resulting enhanced diversity would promote reassortment and variation in the parasite population. Selective pressure due to

123

irregular patterns of drug administration would readily select resistant parasites.

Vector and vertebrate reservoir hosts interact dynamically. Each of these sexual populations would vary owing to mutation, recombination and reassortment. Natural or artificial selection would potentiate emergence.

Emergence of a vector-borne infection may follow introduction of exotic organisms from some remote site or invasion of a pathogen from an enzootic cycle. Emergence may also derive from a nonsustainable intervention that causes herd immunity to wane. Travel of people, vectors, and domestic animals may lead to importation of an agent into new sites. If suitable vector and reservoir hosts are present in the new site, the imported infection may perpetuate in the new site and will become "introduced."

Changes in human behavior frequently favor emergence of vector-borne pathogens. Transmission of Oropouche virus, for example, was facilitated by the cacao husks that farmers discarded. These formed ideal breeding sites for the biting midges that transmit this arbovirus. Lyme disease transmission was favored by human behavior that led to increased deer abundance, and the proliferation of deer permitted vector ticks to increase. Dengue fever became more prevalent as urbanization proceeded and local economies advanced. The advent of the automobile thereby rendered used tires ubiquitous; provision of village wells encouraged people to store water in their homes; and the "throw-away" ethic placed vast quantities of discarded food- and beverage-containers around many tropical homes. The resulting accumulation of water-containing artifacts provides an unprecedented mass of breeding sites for the *Aedes aegypti* vector of this virus.

Demographic factors also promote emergence. Urbanization, for example, is associated with outbreaks of dengue. Human settlement of newly deforested areas is associated with emergence of malaria and leishmaniasis.

The genetic background of a host may favor emergence. Small, isolated populations, which have restricted gene pools, may thereby be more prone to debilitating disease than are genetically diverse populations. Island residents also are particularly vulnerable to vector-borne disease owing to the restricted biodiversity that characterizes such geographic sites. Vectors would focus their bites on human or other reservoir populations in the absence of alternative zooprophylactic hosts.

Human immunosuppression may lead to particularly severe pathogenic consequences as in the case of leishmaniasis and Chagas disease but apparently not in the case of malaria. Immunosuppression may be due to coinfection, as in the case of HIV, or to iatrogenic effects, as occurs with chemotherapy.

Apparent but artifactual emergence may follow some technical diagnostic advance or improved monitoring or reporting procedure. The recent widespread replacement of traditional malaria diagnostic microscopy with QBC technology has increased sensitivity and may result in more frequent case-reporting. Reporting artifacts, in turn, may be influenced by physician perceptions. The epidemic curve representing the incidence of Lyme disease in the United States, for example, was deformed in 1989 due to an extraordinary number of reports from one state. This one-time event, which increased national incidence by a tenth, suggested in 1989 that human Lyme disease in the United States was increasing exponentially, and in 1990 that it had plateaued. An objective case-definition is crucial in determining whether an infection is emergent.

The workshop group concluded that vector-borne infections tend to be silent where transmission is stable and long-standing. Emergence tends to follow environmental change that promotes vector abundance or a change in the density or mix of nonhuman vertebrates. Malaria, perversely, might become apparent after herd-immunity is diminished. Because of their extreme communicability, outbreaks of vector-borne infections tend to emerge explosively.

Vector-borne Emergent Disease

THOMAS P. MONATH

ORAVAX, Inc.
230 Albany Street
Cambridge, Massachusetts 02139

In the course of introducing this session on vector-borne emergent diseases, I shall describe the circumstances that surrounded the appearance, in 1951, of a new viral infection on the Macondy Plateau in the East African country that was then known as Tanganyika. A Swahili name, *chikungunya,* meaning "that which bends up" was used to designate the resulting joint and muscle pains associated with that disease, and the virus is now known by that name. Fortunately, a group of particularly effective investigators were then in residence at the East African Virus Research Institute in Entebbe in Uganda, and they investigated this outbreak. They isolated a virus, recognized it as new and began to ask questions about the emergence of the novel epidemic. They learned that the virus probably originated in the surrounding forested region and was only recently introduced onto this treeless plateau. The responsible vectors were *Aedes aegypti* mosquitoes, which develop in the earthen jars in which the local residents store water. The precise causes of this emergence, however, remained elusive.

The recognition of this particular disease episode was facilitated by an existing surveillance mechanism staffed by a group of informed investigators working in well-equipped laboratories. They addressed appropriate questions to this novel situation, and the resulting observations were correctly interpreted. We may not be as prepared today to deal with such an outbreak as we were 40 years ago.

Although vector-borne diseases generally appear with a marked seasonal periodicity, arboviral infections such as St. Louis encephalitis reappear irregularly over many years. Such reemergent or recurrent events require longitudinal programs of research in order to identify the factors responsible for such occurrences.

Numerous examples exist of the transient *de novo* appearance of a truly new arboviral disease. Rocio virus in Brazil, for example, appeared and disappeared and has not been heard of since. The design of a surveillance system suitable for detecting such one-time events requires careful consideration.

Vector-borne infections have been a favorite topic for those interested in emerging diseases because they are so complex. Virus, vector, and one or more kinds of vertebrate host all contribute to the cycle of transmission. Human factors, the landscape, and the climate all play crucial roles in the complex interactions that precipitate such events, and these factors are central to our discussions here today. In an effort to reduce complexity, let us list the issues that generally arise in an analysis of disease emergence and reemergence. 1) The pathogen may have been introduced from afar into an area

126

where transmission may be amplified because appropriate vectors and reservoir hosts are present. 2) Alternatively, the vector may have been transported artificially or by natural means into the area in question. 3) Susceptible hosts may have migrated into the area. During periods of war and turmoil, for example, military populations or refugees have been the victims of enormous outbreaks of sandfly fever and other vector-borne diseases. 4) Most frequently, environmental change in an enzootic site may increase the force of transmission of a pathogen. 5) Finally, the pathogen itself may have evolved.

Because many of the vector-borne viruses are RNA viruses and have segmented genomes, they mutate frequently, and can readily reassort, thereby leading to new variants. Such viral variation is now a subject of intense laboratory study. The relevance of this laboratory work to the situation in nature remains problematic.

In the case of the arboviruses, a genetic change can have a variety of effects. Virulence for human or animal hosts may change and result in an increased ratio of apparent-to-inapparent infection. Antigenic changes may occur permitting the agent to escape the host's immune response. Alternatively, increased virulence of an agent for a silent intermediate vertebrate host might increase the level of viremia and consequently increase infectivity to vectors. Changing virulence can influence infectivity to the vector by some other mechanism. Because these various possibilities are testable, the present challenge is to go from the study of virus variation to an examination of model systems in which each of these elements is addressed. This remains a problem for the future.

A series of outbreaks of St. Louis encephalitis in Memphis, Tennessee in 1975 and 1976 provides an example of this process. Longitudinal studies were set up to identify the factors responsible. Although support for the project ended after a few years, some data were obtained, including estimates of monthly minimum infection rates in the *Culex pipiens* vector for a span of epidemic as well as non-epidemic years. In the non-epidemic years, for example, virus transmission seemed to begin later than in epidemic years and at a lower level. This circumstance may have been a function of vector density or differences in the timing of virus introduction from afar—for example by or from a local reservoir (*e.g.,* overwintering mosquito). Of course, some recurrent change in the virus may have affected the force of its transmission. Our present phase of descriptive epidemiology has impeded many attempts to explain emergent disease events.

Climate may be an important factor in disease emergence. Rainfall, in particular, provides water for aquatic breeding vectors such as mosquitoes. In the case of yellow fever in Africa, epidemics generally occur in the moist savannah zone. Satellite remote sensing indicates that rainfall correlates with a vegetation index (see FIG. 14 in Remote Sensing section), and that the epidemic of 1987 occurred in one year after a sharp change in this index. The challenge is to be alert to such relationships and to recognize patterns. If the pattern were to be recognized over a period of decades, surveillance mechanisms might be put in place that would help explain the anatomy of these epidemic events.

Most important in the multifactorial nature of vector-borne infections are the human factors, particularly human alteration of the environment. One example is the introduction of an exotic vector, *Aedes albopictus*, from Asia into North as well as South America in the mid-1980s. Their larvae entered in artificial containers—used tires that were imported from Asia. This mosquito is capable of transmitting at least 5 different viruses that are endemic to the Americas, including dengue fever and eastern equine encephalitis.

The distribution of *Aedes aegypti* has also changed markedly in recent years. This domesticated mosquito is similarly dependent on human factors for its breeding and distribution. Its reinvasion of Latin America over a short period of time is responsible for the reemergence of dengue and dengue hemorrhagic fever in that part of the world. The causes of this event are complex, including economic changes that promote trash accumulation near people's homes and an increase in the density of the human population.

An underlying theme of this conference revolves around the establishment of systems for detecting and dealing with emerging and reemerging infections. The number of arboviruses isolated by year has steadily increased since the "previrologic" era through the period of "ignorance" during the 1930s and 1940s when nobody was looking, into the period of "exploration" in the 1950s through the early 1970s when the interest in detecting the new arboviruses was intense. This era too has passed. The decline in the number of isolates in recent years is not due to a lack of biodiversity of the arboviruses, but rather to the absence of a surveillance system.

Competing programs have eliminated the resources necessary to permit health policy planners to continue such surveillance efforts. Our situation has deteriorated. I shall conclude by quoting from the introduction to an article published in 1906 describing the yellow fever epidemic in New Orleans during the previous year, the last outbreak of urban yellow fever in the United States. "This large city of 330,000 inhabitants suddenly realizing that it was face to face with a serious outbreak, determined without hesitation and put into force the most recent prophylactic measures to rigidly exclude all the older methods and theories and have proceeded to complete extermination of the vector. In adopting this plan, there was never any hesitation or misgiving. The necessary funds were at once forthcoming and all classes of the community heartily joined the medical authorities in attack." This should stand as a model for the present.

The Emerging Epidemiology of Venezuelan Hemorrhagic Fever and Oropouche Fever in Tropical South America [a]

ROBERT B. TESH

Yale Arbovirus Research Unit
Department of Epidemiology & Public Health
Yale University School of Medicine
P.O.Box 208034
New Haven, Connecticut 06520-8034

The topic for discussion in this section, events leading to the emergence of human pathogens, is an extremely complex subject. First, each human pathogen is distinct with its own unique ecology; the specific factors or events which lead to its first appearance or reappearance are different. Second, the factors responsible for the emergence of a given pathogen may vary from time to time or from place to place. Despite our best intentions and models, it is difficult to predict in advance precisely when or where a particular pathogen will emerge. In the case of yet unknown disease agents, it is impossible.

To begin, let us acknowledge that the emergence of human pathogens is not a new phenomenon; it has been occurring since *Homo sapiens* first appeared on the earth. The medical historian William McNeill has suggested that humans and their disease organisms live in a sort of ecologic equilibrium, and that each time humans have caused disequilibrium in this system, epidemics or emerging diseases have occurred.[1] The devastating epidemics of introduced diseases that occurred in native American populations when the European colonists first arrived in the New World are an example of such a disequilibrium. McNeill further suggests that the only difference between now and 10,000 years ago is that today the human population is much larger and our ability to cause major ecological disturbances is much greater than ever before. In addition, our technical ability to detect new disease agents is now also much better than ever before, so some of the emerging human pathogens probably have been with us for a long time, but were just not recognized before. With this introduction, I would like to describe two emerging viral diseases in tropical South America, which illustrate some of these concepts.

[a] Work reported in this paper was supported by grants AI-10984 and AI-33983 from the National Institutes of Health.

VENEZUELAN HEMORRHAGIC FEVER

In September 1989, an outbreak of a severe hemorrhagic illness, initially thought to be dengue hemorrhagic fever, was first recognized by local physicians in the Municipality of Guanarito, Portuguesa State, Venezuela.[2] The Municipality of Guanarito is located in the central plains (*llanos*) of Venezuela; it occupies about 2,481 km² in total area and makes up most of the southeastern portion of Portuguesa State. The climate is tropical with a mean annual temperature of 28°C and an annual rainfall of 1,300 mm. This region is characterized by marked wet and dry seasons. The present landscape of the region is a patchwork of savannah, gallery forest, and cultivated lands.

Most of the 24,000 human inhabitants of the municipality live in rural areas and are involved in agriculture and cattle raising. The principal crops are corn, sorghum, cotton, sunflowers and melons. Although the town of Guanarito recently celebrated its bicentennial, new agricultural lands are still being developed in the region and the remaining forest is being cut. During the past 10 years, the human population of the municipality has doubled, mainly from migration into the area from other parts of Venezuela and nearby regions of Colombia. In addition to the resident population, a large number of temporary agricultural workers come to the municipality to work during the planting and harvesting seasons.

The etiologic agent of Venezuelan hemorrhagic fever (VHF) is Guanarito virus, a newly recognized member of the Tacaribe complex of the family Arenaviridae.[3] VHF is characterized by the gradual onset of chills, fever, headache, myalgia, sore throat, weakness, anorexia, nausea, and vomiting.[2] Hemorrhagic manifestations, neurologic symptoms, and shock may or may not occur. Typically, these symptoms last about 10 to 14 days and then terminate with complete recovery or death. To date, about 33% of reported cases of VHF have died. Preliminary data suggest that subclinical or asymptomatic infections are not common.

FIGURE 1 shows the monthly number of cases of VHF reported to the Venezuelan Ministry of Health between September 1989 and August 1993.[4] To date, a total of 96 cases have been reported. Most of the cases have occurred in adults, with a male : female ratio of 2 : 1. All cases of the disease have occurred among persons living or working in the Municipality of Guanarito or in adjacent areas of Barinas State. Most of the affected individuals have been agricultural workers; however, much of the rural population living in this area of Venezuela is involved in farming, so occupational exposure is difficult to evaluate.

The temporal pattern of cases suggests that VHF is an endemic disease (FIG. 1). Between September 1989, when the disease was first recognized, until February 1992, an average of 3 cases was reported each month. Although cases have been reported in every month of the year, almost half of them occurred during the dry season in December, January, February and March. Another interesting finding is that the number of reported VHF cases has dropped dramatically since March 1992. The reason for this decrease is unknown.

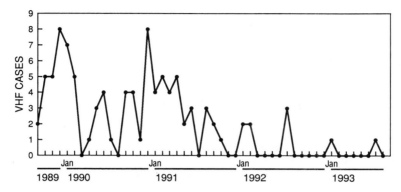

FIGURE 1. Reported cases of Venezuelan hemorrhagic fever, September 1989–August 1993.[4]

The available epidemiologic data suggest that VHF, like the other arenavirus hemorrhagic fevers,[5] is rodent-borne. Humans probably become infected by direct contact with infected rodents or their excreta. In February 1992, we collected wild rodents in several rural communities in the Municipality of Guanarito, where cases of VHF had occurred. These studies implicated the cotton rat, *Sigmodon alstoni*, as the principal reservoir of Guanarito virus.[6] Almost half (48%) of 40 *S. alstoni* that were trapped in the endemic area yielded Guanarito virus. In contrast, only 5% of these rodents had antibodies to the virus. These findings are similar to those reported with other arenaviruses in their natural rodent hosts and suggest that most *S. alstoni* develop a persistent nonimmunizing infection with Guanarito virus.[5] These chronically infected rodents in turn probably serve as the source of infection for humans. Experimental studies are now in progress with cotton rats and Guanarito virus to confirm our field observations.

From this brief review of the epidemiology of VHF, several questions are obvious. First, why was the disease not recognized until 1989? We assume that Guanarito virus has existed in the local rodent population for a long time. There is fossil evidence of *Sigmodon*-like rodents present in the Americas since the late Pliocene epoch.[7] Furthermore, molecular phylogenetic comparison of Guanarito and the 10 other known New World arenaviruses indicates that these agents are genetically very different one from another, suggesting that they probably evolved long ago with their respective natural rodent hosts.[6,8,9] We also know that people have lived in the VHF-endemic area for at least 200 years. Then why weren't cases of the disease recognized earlier?

There are a number of possible explanations: 1) The relatively small human population in the past and the low prevalence of infection allowed sporadic cases to occur before, without their recognition as a distinct entity. Local physicians in Guanare have told us that they recall seeing clinically similar cases before 1989, which were diagnosed as "idiopathic thrombocytopenic purpura." In earlier times, VHF might also have been diagnosed as yellow fever, since the clinical and pathological findings in the two diseases are similar.[9] The natural reluctance of clinicians to suggest a new disease is also illustrated by the fact that the first laboratory confirmed cases of VHF were initially diagnosed as "dengue hemorrhagic fever." 2) Increasing human migration into the endemic region and the development of new agricultural lands may have placed more people in contact with infected rodents. We know that the human population of the region has doubled in the past decade. 3) Recent land-use changes in the region (deforestation and/or large-scale cultivation of corn, sorghum, sunflowers, *etc.*) have provided more favorable habitats and food for a grassland, granivorous species such as *Sigmodon alstoni*, thus allowing populations of these rodents to increase significantly. The latter situation presumably would increase the risk of human contact with infected rodents. It is also possible that Guanarito virus was only recently introduced into the region; however, this seems less likely, given the enzootic nature of the virus maintenance cycle.

Another unanswered question is why the frequency of VHF apparently decreased after February 1992? As far as we can determine, the ecology of the human population did not change during this period and no attempt was made to control wild rodents. Furthermore, serological surveys[6] done on human residents of the region indicate that relatively few people have antibodies to Guanarito virus, thus subclinical infection and herd immunity cannot explain the decrease in VHF cases. The most likely explanations would appear to involve natural changes in the rodent population: either a reduction in the density of *S. alstoni* due to disease or increased predation, or a decrease in the number of virus-infected rodents.

The third question involves the geographic distribution of Guanarito virus and its potential for spread. One of the characteristics of the New World arenaviruses is their focal distribution. To date, 11 different Tacaribe complex arenaviruses have been described from the Americas; each of these agents has a unique and quite limited geographic distribution.[3] In general, these viruses have not been observed to expand their distribution. In the case of Guanarito virus, all isolates until now have come from humans or rodents living within a small area of Venezuela in the southern part of Portuguesa State or in adjacent regions of Barinas State.[2,6] However, no one has yet looked for the virus outside of the known VHF-endemic area. *S. alstoni*, the presumed rodent reservoir, occurs in savannah areas of eastern Colombia, Venezuela, Guyana, Surinam and adjacent territory of northern Brazil.[7] Much of this region of South America is still sparsely populated by humans, so it is conceivable that the virus could be present there and be unrecognized. We are now attempting to define the distribution of Guanarito virus in Venezuela and to determine if other rodent species might be involved in its ecology. Hopefully this information will give some indication of the potential of VHF to appear in other localities.

OROPOUCHE FEVER

A second example of an emerging zoonotic viral disease is Oropouche fever. During the past 30 years, Oropouche fever has emerged as an increasing public health problem in tropical regions of South America. The causative agent, Oropouche (ORO) virus, is a member of the Simbu serogroup of the genus *Bunyavirus*. ORO virus was first isolated from the blood of a febrile forest worker during arbovirus studies in Trinidad in 1955.[10] A few sporadic isolations of the virus were subsequently made in Trinidad and in northern Brazil from sylvan mosquitoes and from a sloth, but it was not until 1961 that the epidemic potential and public health importance of ORO virus were recognized. In that year, the first documented epidemic of ORO fever occurred in Belém, Brazil, a major port city at the mouth of the Amazon River.[10] An estimated 11,000 persons were infected during that outbreak. Since 1961, a total of 26 outbreaks of ORO fever has been reported from the Amazon regions of Brazil and Peru and from the Isthmus of Panama (TABLE 1). The number of persons affected has varied with each outbreak, but the two largest recorded epidemics (Belém and Manaus in 1980–81) involved about 100,000 people each. The most recent reported outbreak occurred in Iquitos, Peru in early 1992; the number of persons infected was not calculated, since the outbreak occurred simultaneously with an epidemic of dengue.

ORO fever in humans is characterized by the abrupt onset of fever, chills, severe headache, generalized myalgia, arthralgia, anorexia, nausea, vomiting, weakness, dizziness, and photophobia.[10] Some ORO fever patients also exhibit meningitic symptoms. The acute clinical illness usually lasts 2 to 5 days, although a period of asthenia and occasionally dizziness may persist for up to a month. No fatalities have been reported with the disease, and life-long immunity follows recovery. However, a significant percentage of patients (as high as 60% in some outbreaks) develop a recurrence of their original symptoms within 2 to 10 days after they become afebrile.

It has been postulated that ORO virus is maintained in two distinct cycles: a) an epidemic urban cycle in which humans are the primary host, and the biting midge *Culicoides paraensis* is the vector; and b) a silent maintenance cycle in which forest animals (probably sloths) are the vertebrate hosts, and a yet unidentified arthropod serves as the vector.[10] It is assumed that humans entering the jungle occasionally become infected with the virus; when they return to their village or town, if conditions are right, temporary urban transmission occurs and an epidemic ensues. This hypothetical model assumes that urban transmission of ORO virus is temporary and sporadic, similar to the epidemiologic model proposed for yellow fever. However, the current working hypothesis to explain the epidemiology of ORO fever may be incomplete. Because of the non-specific nature of this disease, it seems quite possible that the virus could also be maintained for longer periods of time (or even continuously) at a relatively low level of activity in some communities and not be recognized.

TABLE 1. Reported Outbreaks of Oropouche Fever in Tropical America, 1961–1992

Country City/State[a]	Date of Outbreak	Estimated Number of Persons Infected[b]
BRAZIL		
Belém, PA	Feb–May 1961	11,000
Caratateua, PA	Feb–March 1967	400
Braganca, PA	March–July 1967	6,000
Belém, PA	Feb–July 1968	>100
Baiao, PA	June–Sept 1972	≥85
Mojui dos Compos, PA	Dec 1974–April 1975	600
Palhal, PA	Feb–April 1975	420
Santarem, PA	April–July 1975	14,000
Belterra, PA	April–July 1975	1,600
Alter-do-Chao, PA	July–Aug 1975	280
Itupiranga, PA	May–June 1975	420
Varias, PA	June–Oct 1978	2,000
Belém, PA	April–June 1979	16,000
Varias, PA	March–Nov 1979	9,000
Belém, PA	Feb–Oct 1980	102,000
Varias, PA	March–Aug 1980	37,000
Mazagao, AP	1980	?
Manaus, AM	Nov 1980–March 1981	97,000
Barcelos, AM	May–June 1980	171
Porto Franco, MA	Jan–March 1988	>128
Tocantinopolis, TO	Jan–March 1988	?
Ariquemes, RO	Feb–March 1991	58,574
Oro Preto do Oeste, RO	Feb–March 1991	35,413
PANAMA		
Chame/San Miguelito, PN	Sept 1989	?
Chilibre, PN	1990	
PERU		
Iquitos, LO	Jan–April 1992	?

[a] PA = Para, AP = Amapa, AM = Amazonas, MA = Maranhao, TO = Tocantins, RO = Rondonia, PN = Panama, LO = Loreto.

[b] The total number of persons infected in a given epidemic was estimated, based on virus isolations, results of retrospective serologic studies, and the total human population living at the site.

This alternative model is suggested by the circumstances of the two recent outbreaks of ORO fever in Peru and Panama (TABLE 1). The Oro virus isolates in Iquitos were made incidentally from the sera of febrile patients who were bled during an investigation of a dengue epidemic which occurred in that Amazonian port city in early 1992.[11] The ORO virus isolates from the Isthmus of Panama (1989–1990) were made under similar circumstances. In 1985, the mosquito *Aedes aegypti* was reintroduced into Panama; by 1989 it had reached high densities around Panama City. Because of epidemic dengue activity in a number of neighboring countries at that time, the Panamanian Ministry of Health, in collaboration with the Gorgas Memorial Laboratory, began an intensive dengue surveillance program in the greater metropolitan area of Panama City. Residents of the area with febrile illnesses were interviewed and bled. During that one year period (1989), no isolations of dengue virus were made, but 14 ORO virus isolates were obtained from people with suspicious (dengue-like) illnesses.[12] At the time, ORO virus was not known to occur in Panama; however, a retrospective examination of sera that had been collected from residents of one of the affected communities in 1968 and in 1978 indicated that 25% of the samples had preexisting ORO virus antibodies.[12] This serologic evidence confirmed that human infection with the virus had occurred (unrecognized) before.

Because of the non-specific nature of ORO fever and the paucity of diagnostic virus laboratories in the ORO-endemic region, it seems likely that the disease is frequently unrecognized. A review of the localities where ORO outbreaks have been recognized and where the virus has been isolated support this hypothesis. To date, all isolations of ORO virus have come from four arbovirus laboratories in Belém, Lima, Panama City, and Port-of-Spain (FIG. 2).[10–12] These virus isolates were obtained from insects or mammals during arbovirus field studies or from sick people during epidemiologic investigations of outbreaks of febrile illness. Based on these reported isolations, it is apparent that ORO virus has a wide geographic distribution in tropical South America. It also seems likely that human infection and illness due to ORO virus is much more common than is currently reported. Much of the ORO-endemic area is still sparsely populated; but as human settlement and development of the region increase, one would expect epidemics of ORO fever to become more frequent.

Other factors which have probably contributed to the emergence of ORO fever as a human pathogen are deforestation, urbanization and agricultural development. This has to do with the breeding habits of the presumed peridomestic vector, *Culicoides paraensis*. Two of the favorite larval habitats of this biting midge are rotting cacao husks and banana stumps.[10] Such decomposing plant material remains moist even during dry periods and serves as an excellent

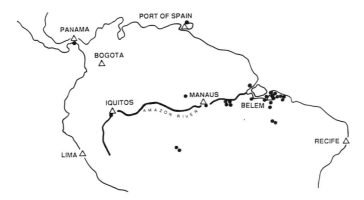

FIGURE 2. Map of northern South America, showing sites (black dots) where Oropouche virus has been isolated.

medium for the microorganisms on which the *Culicoides* larvae feed. As a consequence, very dense populations of *Culicoides paraensis* are often found in rural communities near cacao or banana plantations. Furthermore, since these and other ceratopogonids serve as pollinators of the cacao flowers, farmers often place rotting plant material among the cacao plants to intentionally increase the ceratopogonid population in order to enhance pollination and improve their fruit yield. Even in urban areas of the neotropics, many people have banana trees in their gardens, which can serve as breeding places for the insects.

Thus in the case of ORO fever, as with Venezuelan hemorrhagic fever, we are probably not dealing with a new pathogen; instead an existing virus infection is being recognized more frequently as a result of a growing human population, changing land use patterns, and improved diagnostic facilities. These are just two examples, but it seems inevitable that other zoonotic viruses of this type will continue to emerge as human pathogens, as we upset the ecologic equilibrium. Although we may anticipate such events, it is unlikely that we can predict their occurrence with any certainty. Consequently, the best defense against future pathogens of this type would appear to be 1) an active surveillance network for the early recognition of emerging agents, and 2) trained field teams (a sort of international epidemiologic intelligence service) which could be quickly deployed to define the epidemiology of new disease outbreaks, so that appropriate intervention/control measures can be initiated. Several models for such a surveillance system have been proposed recently.[13,14]

REFERENCES

1. McNeill, W. H. 1993. Patterns of disease emergence in history. *In* Emerging Viruses. S. S. Morse, Ed.: 29–36. New York: Oxford University Press.
2. Salas, R., N. de Manzione, R. B. Tesh, R. Rico-Hesse, R. E. Shope, A. Betancourt, O. Godoy, R. Bruzual, M. E. Pacheco, B. Ramos, M. E. Taibo, J. G. Tamayo, E. Jaimes, C. Vasquez, F. Araoz & J. Querales. 1991. Venezuelan haemorrhagic fever. Lancet **338:** 1033–1036.
3. Tesh, R. B., P. B. Jahrling, R. Salas & R. E. Shope. 1994. Description of Guanarito virus (Arenaviridae: *Arenavirus*), the etiologic agent of Venezuelan hemorrhagic fever. Am. J. Trop. Med. Hyg. **50:** 452–459.
4. Salas, R. 1993. National Institute of Hygiene, Ministry of Health and Social Assistance, Caracas, Venezuela. Personal communication.
5. Childs, J. E. & C. J. Peters. 1993. Ecology and epidemiology of arenaviruses and their hosts. *In* The Arenaviridae. M. S. Salvato, Ed.: 331–384. New York: Plenum Press.
6. Tesh, R. B., M. L. Wilson, R. Salas, N. M. C. de Manzione, D. Tovar, T. G. Ksiazek & C. J. Peters. 1993. Field studies on the epidemiology of Venezuelan hemorrhagic fever: Implication of the cotton rat *Sigmodon alstoni* as the probable rodent reservoir. Am. J. Trop. Med. Hyg. **49:** 227–235.
7. Voss, R. S. 1992. A revision of the South American species of *Sigmodon* (Mammalia: Muridae) with notes on their natural history and biogeography. Am. Mus. Novitates, No. 3050. New York: American Museum of Natural History.
8. Rico-Hesse, R. & J-P. Gonzalez. 1993. Yale University School of Medicine, Department of Epidemiology and Public Health. Personal communication.
9. Coimbra, T. L. M., E. S. Nassar, M. N. Burattini, L. T. M.de Souza, I. B.Ferreira, I. M. Rocco, A. P. A. Travassos da Rosa, P. F. C. Vasconcelos, F. P. Pinheiro,

J. W. LeDuc, R. Rico-Hesse, J-P. Gonzalez, P. B. Jahrling & R. B. Tesh. 1994. A new arenavirus isolated from a fatal case of haemorrhagic fever in Brazil. Lancet. **343:** 391–392.

10. LeDuc, J. W. & F. P. Pinheiro. 1989. Oropouche fever. *In* The Arboviruses: Epidemiology and Ecology. T. P. Monath, Ed. Vol. 4: 1–14. Boca Raton, FL: CRC Press.

11. Wood, O. L. 1992. Naval Medical Research Institute, National Naval Medical Center, Bethesda, MD. Personal communication.

12. Peralta, P. H. & B. E. Dutary. 1990. Gorgas Memorial Laboratory, Panama, Republic of Panama. Personal communication.

13. Lederberg, J., R. E. Shope & S. C. Oaks, Eds. 1992. Emerging Infections: Microbial Threats to Health in the United States. Washington, DC: National Academy Press.

14. Henderson, D. A. 1993. Surveillance systems and intergovernmental cooperation. *In* Emerging Viruses. S. S. Morse, Ed.: 283–289. New York: Oxford University Press.

The Discovery of Arbovirus Diseases [a]

ROBERT E. SHOPE

Yale Arbovirus Research Unit
Department of Epidemiology and Public Health
Yale University School of Medicine
New Haven, Connecticut 06520-8034

In 1930 only three arthropod-borne virus (arbovirus) human diseases were known[1]—yellow fever, dengue fever, and pappataci fever. Today, over a hundred arboviruses cause human disease.[2] How were these viruses and their diseases discovered, and more importantly, how can we improve our chances of finding new emerging arbovirus diseases?

Before these questions are answered, it is helpful to review the ecologic circumstances in which arboviruses replicate and maintain their transmission cycles. With few exceptions, the arboviruses under consideration are zoonotic, that is they are maintained in a cycle of nonhuman vertebrates and arthropods. These arthropods are mosquitoes, phlebotomine sandflies, midges, or ticks. Some arboviruses do not need the vertebrate component and are maintained in the arthropod by passage through the egg—transovarial transmission—and immature stages; the arthropod can transmit these viruses to humans or other vertebrates when it takes its first blood meal. Viremia is transient, lasting only days or rarely weeks. Infection of the arthropod is followed by a period of replication of the virus in the arthropod gut, then the virus passes to the salivary gland. The period from ingestion of the bloodmeal by the arthropod until virus reaches the salivary gland and is excreted in sufficient quantity to be transmitted to the vertebrate host is called the extrinsic incubation period. The extrinsic incubation period may be a few days or two or more weeks. The arthropod, once infected, is infected for life.

People are usually accidental hosts, *i.e.* they are not necessary to maintain the virus in nature. The natural vertebrate host of the arbovirus generally does not become ill, and infections in people are generally inapparent.

Arbovirus disease is seasonal, depending directly or indirectly on the season during which the arthropod takes its blood meals. Many factors influence the prevalence and season of disease, including climate (rainfall, temperature), vector competence, length of extrinsic and intrinsic incubation, density of vectors, transport of virus to distant places, and level of immunity in the vertebrate population.

Techniques to isolate arboviruses have evolved gradually over the years since 1930. Most early attempts were from sick people or animals. Early virologists used a) large domestic animals such as sheep,[3] b) adult mice,[4,5]

---

[a] Studies of Rocio, Cache Valley, Rift Valley fever, and Sindbis viruses reported herein were conducted in part at the Yale Arbovirus Research Unit under support of the World Health Organization, NIH Grant AI 10984, and U.S. Army Grant DAMD 17-90-Z-0020.

138

and later c) embryonated eggs.[6] After the demonstration in 1948 that Coxsackie virus killed baby mice,[7] this method was adopted for arboviruses, and in the early 1950s there was a proliferation of newly recognized arboviruses isolated in baby mice. In the late 1950s vertebrate tissue culture was used extensively in parallel with baby mice, and some investigators employed hamsters. At this time, also, Whitman inoculated mosquitoes by the intrathoracic route as a tool to propagate arboviruses,[8] but this technique did not gain general usage until the early 1970s.[9] At the same time, the use of mosquito cell culture, especially the *Aedes albopictus* line of Singh[10] and the C6/36 clone of Igarashi[11] gained favor; these methods, including baby mice, vertebrate cell culture, mosquitoes, and mosquito cell culture are used today.

Arbovirus disease was also diagnosed serologically. Arboviruses were found to cluster into serogroups (later recognized as belonging mostly to the families Togaviridae, Flaviviridae, Bunyaviridae, Reoviridae, and Rhabdoviridae). It is axiomatic that viruses have relatives. The discovery by Casals that the hemagglutination-inhibition test for Togaviridae and Flaviviridae, and later the complement-fixation test for Bunyaviridae, were relatively broadly cross-reactive, facilitated the detection of antibody to related viruses[12,13] and hence the recognition of the probable identity of agents causing new diseases in the absence of isolation of the causative virus.

The collection, characterization, classification, and diagnosis of arboviruses and their corresponding diseases would not have been possible without a world network of field laboratories and regional reference centers. This network included The Rockefeller Foundation laboratories in India, Nigeria, South Africa, Colombia, Brazil, Trinidad, and California, each collaborating with a local government laboratory and referring field materials to The Rockefeller Foundation Virus Laboratories in New York, later to become the Yale Arbovirus Research Unit.[14] The network also included the Centers for Disease Control (CDC), Cornell University, the University of California at Berkeley, the University of Wisconsin, the system of the Institut Pasteur in New Caledonia, French Guiana, Paris, Senegal, Cote d'Ivoire, Central African Republic, Iran, and Cameroon, the U.S. Navy and Army laboratories, The Ivanovsky Institute of Virology and its network in the USSR, and several other national laboratories in the United Kingdom, Japan, Korea, Taiwan, Brazil, Australia, and other nations. Missing from the network were China and small focal areas either geographically or politically isolated. In its heyday, this network was a formidable system for monitoring arboviruses and for discovering emerging diseases. The World Health Organization has played a coordinating role since 1958 when it instituted the Collaborating Centres for Arbovirus Research and Reference.[15]

Diagnostic reagents are a key factor in identification of viruses and diagnosis of disease. The WHO Centres made reagents available on a reference basis; they also received viruses for identification, and offered training in rapid diagnosis to field scientists. During the 1960s and 1970s the U.S. National Institutes of Health (NIH) maintained a program to produce reference reagents to human disease-causing arboviruses. Especially useful was the provision by the NIH of arbovirus-grouping mouse ascitic fluids so that field laboratories could group new viruses very rapidly using serologic methods.[16]

The decade of the 1930s was characterized as an era in which arboviruses were isolated during epidemics and epizootics directly from blood and/or necropsy materials. These were inoculated into embryonated eggs (Murray Valley encephalitis), sheep (Rift Valley fever), monkeys and mice (St. Louis encephalitis), and adult mice (western encephalitis, eastern encephalitis, Venezuelan encephalitis, Japanese encephalitis, tick-borne encephalitis). During WW II, dengue-1, dengue-2, sandfly fever Naples, and sandfly fever Sicilian viruses were isolated initially in human volunteers; then the viruses were later adapted to adult mice by serial passage.[17]

After the second world war, a new approach was adopted, mainly by the CDC, the U.S. military, and The Rockefeller Foundation laboratories. In addition to looking for disease, scientists of these laboratories searched for viruses in arthropods and wild vertebrate animals by subculturing into baby mice or tissue culture. They also exposed sentinel laboratory animals to biting arthropods in the field, and tested the blood of these animals for viremia. Because arthropods do not become ill when infected, and because many infected vertebrate hosts show no signs of arboviral disease, the approach increased the chances of finding naturally occurring arboviruses. In fact, more than 500 new viruses were found,[18] and their discovery can be credited in large part to this concept. Most of these were orphan viruses—viruses that were not known to cause disease. Now the game became to use these mostly orphan viruses to search for corresponding disease. This game continues today. Of course, not all orphan viruses will match to a disease.

TABLES 1–4 list some epidemic arbovirus diseases that have emerged or reemerged during the past 50 years. How were these viruses and their diseases discovered?

I joined The Rockefeller Foundation arbovirus program in 1958. The director of the New York laboratories, Dr. Max Theiler, handed me a small package of human sera received from Dr. S.G. Anderson of Australia. The sera were from patients of the 1956 Mildura outbreak of epidemic polyarthritis and rash. Hundreds of persons had taken ill while vacationing along the Murray River, and Dr. Anderson had noted that mosquitoes were especially numerous that year. The disease resembled an African malady that had earlier been named chikungunya fever caused by an alphavirus of the same name. What Dr. Theiler did not tell me was that a similar set of acute and convalescent sera had been tested for chikungunya antibody by neutralization test and found negative at The Foundation's laboratory in South Africa.

I tested the sera by hemagglutination-inhibition (HI) with antigens of several alphaviruses; some like chikungunya caused disease, others were orphan viruses. Eight of 12 convalescent sera from the Mildura epidemic reacted with one or more of the alphavirus antigens. Titers were relatively low, and none of the antigens reacted in a diagnostic pattern. We published the results, predicting that the Mildura epidemic was caused by an alphavirus, probably a new virus yet to be discovered.[19] In 1963, seven years after the Mildura outbreak, A. K. O'Gower isolated the causative agent, Ross River virus, from mosquitoes collected at Townsville, Queensland. This was an early suggestion that orphan viruses may cause epidemics, and it was an important demonstration that diagnosticians should use broadly cross-reactive tests such as the HI when searching for the cause of unknown diseases.

Oropouche virus was isolated in 1955 in Trinidad from a febrile forester who also had malaria parasites in his blood.[20] The virus was subsequently recovered from forest mosquitoes in Trinidad, and from mosquitoes and blood of a sloth at a construction site on the Belém-Brasilia Highway, Brazil. The link to human disease was slim, and Oropouche was among the viruses seeking a significant disease. In 1961, an epidemic of Oropouche fever involving over 7,000 cases was detected in Belém, Brazil,[21] and outbreaks in hundreds of thousands of persons subsequently have been found in the Amazon basin. More recently the disease occurred in Panama. A virus was isolated by inoculation of suckling mice from 16 persons in the 1961 Belém epidemic, and the virus was identified using immune sera prepared from the Trinidad human isolate. This is an example of diagnosis of an emerging arboviral disease using reference reagents from an orphan virus (new disease/old virus) (TABLE 1).

A disease variously called Ockelbo disease in Sweden, Pogosta disease in Finland, and Karelian fever in Russia was characterized by fever, rash, and arthritis.[22] There were sporadic cases in the 1960s, but the disease was first noted as widespread epidemics in 1981 and 1982 when it was epidemiologically linked to a greatly increased abundance of mosquitoes (6 to 10 times). A subtype of Sindbis virus was isolated by inoculation of Vero cell culture in Sweden from mosquitoes in 1982, and shown by serology presumptively to be the cause of Ockelbo fever. Although the disease does not differ substantially from that caused by Sindbis virus in Africa, the newly recognized geographic location was noteworthy. This is an example of a known disease and virus emerging in a new location (old disease/old virus/new location) (TABLE 2).

In 1959 a virus was isolated from mosquitoes collected at Akabane in the rural Kanto Plain area of Japan. Akabane virus was brought by Akira Oya to The Rockefeller Foundation Virus Laboratories in New York where it was classified in the Simbu serogroup, but remained as an orphan virus. In the early 1970s epizootics of arthrogryposis and hydranencephaly (AGH), congenital abnormalities in sheep and cattle, were linked by Japanese scientists to infection *in utero* during the early gestation (old virus/new disease).[23] These findings were confirmed by Australian workers, and the disease was reproduced in sheep by inoculation of Akabane virus at the fifth week of gestation.[24]

TABLE 1. Emerging Arbovirus Disease—New Disease/Old Virus

Disease	Virus	Location of Emerging Disease	Year Emerged
Oropouche fever	Oropouche	Brazil	1961

TABLE 2. Reemerging Arbovirus Disease—New Disease/Old Virus

Disease	Virus	Location of Emerging Disease	Year Emerged
Yellow fever	Yellow fever	Kenya	1993
Rift Valley fever	Rift Valley fever	Egypt	1977
Rift Valley fever	Rift Valley fever	Mauritania	1987
Ockelbo disease (Karelian fever) (Pogosta disease)	Sindbis	Sweden	1981–2
Dengue hemorrhagic fever	Dengue	Cuba	1981
Venezuelan encephalitis	Venezuelan encephalitis	Mexico	1993

This was not the end of the story, however. In 1987 the U.S. Department of Agriculture Animal and Plant Health Inspection Service was notified of AGH disease in Nebraska and Texas. They suspected that Akabane virus had been introduced to Texas in an infected ram, then spread to Nebraska. Concerted collaborative efforts at the U.S.D.A. quarantine facility at Plum Island, NY, with scientists at the University of Texas and Yale University established that the disease was caused not by Akabane virus, but rather by Cache Valley virus, an indigenous mosquito-borne virus, widespread in North America (R. Yedloutsnig, personal communication).[25] Cache Valley virus was previously known to cause mild fever in sheep and cattle, but not known to cause AGH. The initial clue to the link of AGH with Cache Valley virus occurred fortuitously when Cache Valley antigen and antibody were included as a control in testing for antibody to the suspected Simbu group viruses. This is an example of old disease/old orphan virus/new location (TABLE 3). This is also a reminder that mother nature does not use a pathogenetic mechanism only once. Let us pause to consider if Cache Valley virus might be linked to abnormalities in other species, including humans.

TABLE 4 lists several examples where new arboviruses were isolated directly in mice or tissue culture from cases of a new disease (new disease/new virus). Kyasanur Forest disease was discovered in Karnataka State, India in 1957 in patients with hemorrhagic fever in an area undergoing deforestation and rapid ecologic change.[26] The group C and Guama viruses were isolated in 1955–56 directly from blood of Brazilian colonists in the Amazon region where the forest was being cut to plant rubber trees.[27] O'nyong-nyong virus was isolated in 1959 from cases of fever, arthralgia, and rash in East Africa during an epidemic involving millions of people.[28] This virus disappeared

TABLE 3. Emerging Arbovirus Disease—New Disease/Old Virus

Disease	Virus	Location of Emerging Disease	Year Emerged
Arthrogryposis & hydranencephaly	Cache Valley	USA	1989

TABLE 4. Emerging Arbovirus Disease—New Disease/Old Virus

Disease	Virus	Location of Emerging Disease	Year Emerged
Kysanur Forest disease	Kysanur Forest disease	India	1957
Rocio encephalitis	Rocio	Brazil	1975–6
O'nyong-nyong	O'nyong-nyong	East Africa	1959
Epidemic polyarthritis & rash	Ross River	Australia	1956
Groups C & Guama fever	Group C & Guama	Brazil	1954
LaCrosse encephalitis	LaCrosse	Wisconsin	1960

and cases have not been seen since. Rocio virus was isolated in 1975 from brain of a fatal case of encephalitis in the Ribeira Valley of coastal São Paulo State, Brazil.[29] This disease affected about a thousand patients with a 10% case fatality rate. It persisted through 1976, then disappeared and has not been seen since.

TABLE 2 lists diseases remerging in new places (old virus/old disease/new location). Dengue hemorrhagic fever appeared in Cuba for the first time in epidemic form in the New World in 1981,[30] Venezuelan equine encephalitis in horses in Mexico in 1993 after an absence of 20 years, yellow fever in Kenya in humans in 1993 for the first time there in epidemic form,[31] and Rift Valley fever in Egypt in 1977[32] and in Mauritania in 1987[33] outside of its usually recognized range. In each epidemic the virus was isolated in cell culture or mice directly from cases.

How can we improve our chances of finding new arbovirus diseases? The historical record tells us that new arbovirus diseases consistently appear, that old diseases appear in new places, and that if we look, we find diseases to match orphan viruses. One of the first priorities should be to search in those areas of the world neglected in the past. China, especially western China for instance, has a wide variety of ecosystems, some completely unexplored.

A 1992 report of the Institute of Medicine on "Emerging Infections" recommended worldwide monitoring for diseases, especially acute respiratory, encephalitis and aseptic meningitis, hemorrhagic fever, acute diarrhea, and febrile exanthema.[34] WHO, CDC, and the Association of American Scientists have independently endorsed and initiated plans to establish (or reestablish) world surveillance for infectious diseases.

The emphasis of current proposals is on case-finding. In our enthusiasm to establish monitoring, we should not forget the historical record which tells us that orphan viruses are also an important component for identifying the cause of diseases. Unfortunately, grant support for case-finding is much more likely to materialize than for collecting orphan viruses. Virus collection has virtually ceased. We need to find a politically acceptable way to return to the collecting business, perhaps in the name of basic science or preservation of biological diversity.

Molecular technology also works against collecting. Some laboratories involved in arbovirus surveillance in arthropods and wild animals are switching to immunological and molecular probes to replace virus isolation. A probe will only find the virus one is looking for. It will never find an entirely new virus. Are we thus doomed in the future to finding only the causes of the old diseases/old viruses, and new diseases/old viruses?

REFERENCES

1. ANONYMOUS. 1930. A System of Bacteriology in Relation to Medicine, Vol. VII. His Majesty's Stationery Office, London.
2. BENENSON, A., Ed. 1990. Control of Communicable Diseases in Man, 15th edition. Washington, DC: APHA.
3. DAUBNEY, R., J. R. HUDSON & P. C. GARNHAM. 1931. Enzootic hepatitis or Rift Valley fever. An undescribed virus disease of sheep, cattle and man from East Africa. J. Pathol. & Bacteriol. **34:** 545–579.
4. THEILER, M. 1930. Studies on the action of yellow fever virus in mice. Ann. Trop. Med. Parasitol. **24:** 249–272.
5. WEBSTER, L. T. & G. L. FITE. 1933. A virus encountered in the study of material from cases of encephalitis in the St. Louis and Kansas City epidemic of 1933. Science **78:** 463–465.
6. FRENCH, E. L. 1952. Murray Valley encephalitis: Isolation and characterization of the etiological agent. Med. J. Aust. **39:** 100–103.
7. DALLDORF, G. & G. M. SICKLES. 1948. An unidentified, filterable agent isolated from the feces of children with paralysis. Science **108:** 61–62.
8. WHITMAN, L., data cited in M. Theiler & W. G. Downs, Eds. 1973. Arthropod-borne Viruses of Vertebrates: 103. New Haven, CT: Yale University Press.
9. ROSEN, L. & D. GUBLER. 1974. The use of mosquitoes to detect and propagate dengue viruses. Am. J. Trop. Med. Hyg. **23:** 1153–1160.
10. SINGH, K. R. P. 1967. Cell cultures derived from larvae of *Aedes albopictus* (Skuse) and *Aedes aegypti* (L.) Curr. Sci. **36:** 506–508.
11. IGARASHI, A. 1978. Isolation of a Singh's *Aedes albopictus* cell clone sensitive to dengue and chikungunya virus. J. Gen. Virol. **40:** 531–544.
12. CASALS, J. & L. V. BROWN. 1954. Hemagglutination with arthropod-borne viruses. J. Exp. Med. **99:** 429–449.
13. CASALS, J. & L. WHITMAN. 1960. A new antigenic group of arthropod-borne viruses. The Bunyamwera group. Am. J. Trop. Med. Hyg. **9:** 73–77.
14. DOWNS, W. G. 1982. The Rockefeller Foundation Virus Program 1951-1971 with update to 1981. Ann. Rev. Med **33:** 1–29.
15. COCKBURN, W. C. 1973. The programme of the World Health Organization in medical virology. Progr. Med. Virol. **15:** 159–204. Basel: Karger.
16. CUNNINGHAM, S., Ed. 1978. NIAID Catalog of Research Reagents 1978-1980. DHEW Publ. No. (NIH) 78-899. Washington, DC: US DHEW.
17. SABIN, A. B. 1951. Experimental studies on phlebotomus (pappataci, sandfly) fever during World War II. Arch. Gesamte Virusforsch. **4:** 367–410.
18. KARABATSOS, N., Ed. 1985. Catalogue of Arthropod-Borne Viruses of the World. San Antonio, TX: Am. Soc. Trop. Med. Hyg.
19. SHOPE, R. E. & S. G. ANDERSON. 1960. The virus etiology of epidemic exanthem and polyarthritis. Med. J. Aust. **47:** 156–158.
20. ANDERSON, C. R., L. P. SPENCE, W. G. DOWNS, & T. H. G. AITKEN. 1961. Oropouche virus: A new human disease agent from Trinidad, W.I. Am. J. Trop. Med. Hyg. **10:** 574–578.
21. PINHEIRO, F. E., M. PINHEIRO, G. BENSABATH, O. R. CAUSEY & R. E. SHOPE. 1962. Epidemia de virus Oropouche. Rev. Serv. Espec. Saude Publica **12:** 15–23.
22. ESPMARK, A. & B. NIKLASSON. 1984. Ockelbo disease in Sweden: Epidemiological, clinical, and virological data from the 1982 outbreak. Am. J. Trop. Med. Hyg. **33:** 1203–1211.
23. KUROGI, H., Y. INABA, E. TAKAHASHI, K. SATO, T. OMORI, Y. MIURA, Y. GOTO,

Y. FUJIWARA, Y. HATANO, *et al.* 1976. Epizootic congenital arthrogryposis-hydranencephaly syndrome in cattle: Isolation of Akabane virus from affected fetuses. Arch. Virol. **51:** 67–74.

24. PARSONSON, I. M., A. J. DELLA-PORTA & W. A. SNOWDEN. 1975. Congential abnormalities in foetal lambs after inoculation of pregnant ewes with Akabane virus. Aust. Vet. J. **51:** 585–586.

25. CHUNG, S. I., C. W. LIVINGSTON, JR., J. F. EDWARDS, R. W. CRANDELL, R. E. SHOPE, S. A. SHELTON & E. W. COLLISSON. 1990. Evidence that Cache Valley virus induces congenital malformations in sheep. Vet. Microbiol. **21:** 297–307.

26. WORK, T. H. & H. TRAPIDO. 1957. Summary of preliminary report of investigations of the Virus Research Centre on an epidemic disease affecting forest villagers and wild monkeys of Shimoga District, Mysore. Ind. J. Med. Sci. **11:** 340–341.

27. CAUSEY, O. R., C. E. CAUSEY, O. M. MAROJA & D. G. MACEDO. 1961. The isolation of arthropod-borne viruses including members of two hitherto undescribed serological groups, in the Amazon region of Brazil. Am. J. Trop. Med. Hyg. **10:** 227–249.

28. HADDOW, A. J., C. W. DAVIES & A. J. WALKER. 1960. O'nyong-nyong fever: An epidemic virus disease in East Africa. I. Introduction. Trans. Roy. Soc. Trop. Med. Hyg. **54:** 517–522.

29. LOPES, O., T. L. M. COIMBRA, L. SACCHETTA DE A., *et al.* 1978. Emergence of a new arbovirus disease in Brazil. I. Isolation and characterization of the etiologic agent, Rocio virus. Am. J. Epidemiol. **107:** 444–449.

30. KOURI, G., M. G. GUZMAN & J. BRAVO. 1986. Hemorrhagic dengue in Cuba: History of an epidemic. Bull. Pan. Am. Health. Org. **20:** 24–30.

31. WORLD HEALTH ORGANIZATION. 1993. Yellow fever, Kenya. Weekly Epidem. Record. **68:** 159–160.

32. MEEGAN, J. M. & R. E. SHOPE. 1981. Emerging concepts on Rift Valley fever. *In* Perspectives in Virology XI, edited by M. Pollard, pp. 267–287. New York: Alan R. Liss.

33. DIGOUTTE, J. P. & C. J. PETERS. 1989. General aspects of the 1987 Rift Valley fever epidemic in Mauritania. Res. Virol. **140:** 27–30.

34. LEDERBERG, J., R. E. SHOPE & S. C. OAKS, JR., Eds. 1992. Emerging Infections: Microbial Threats to Health in the United States. Washington, DC: National Academy Press.

The Emergence of Lyme Disease and Human Babesiosis in a Changing Environment[a]

ANDREW SPIELMAN

Department of Tropical Public Health
Harvard School of Public Health
665 Huntington Avenue
Boston, Massachusetts 02115

Two zoonoses that emerged in North America and Europe during the 1970s have continued to assume increasing importance in human health. *Ixodes* ticks transmit both infections. Lyme disease, a spirochetosis due to *Borrelia burgdorferi*, may produce a debilitating chronic illness affecting diverse organsystems. Human babesiosis, an occasionally fatal malaria-like infection due to *Babesia microti*, may occur alone or as a companion to Lyme disease. An arboviral infection, tick-borne encephalitis, can be cotransmitted with the Lyme disease spirochete in Eurasia. Interpretation of clinical findings can be difficult because an individual *Ixodes* tick can transmit each pathogen alone or in combination with other pathogens, resulting in human disease that varies in incubation period and in clinical signs and symptoms. The objective of the following discussion is to examine the evidence indicating that the borrelial and babesial zoonoses are "new" and to review the factors that may affect risk of human infection.

EARLY SPORADIC INFECTIONS

Lyme disease, then known as erythema migrans (EM), was originally thought to be a rare condition that mainly affected Europeans who had been exposed to ticks.[1] In North America, the first recognized case of Lyme disease involved a Wisconsin resident, who became ill in 1969.[2] The earliest known American infection was recognized retrospectively in a resident of Cape Cod, Massachusetts, who appeared to have been infected there in 1962.[3] Human infection is frequent across much of the northern portion of the Eurasian land-mass.

The history of human babesiosis parallels that of Lyme disease. The condition was first diagnosed in a resident of Yugoslavia in 1957 (probably due to infection by the bovine parasite, *Ba. divergens*) and in several other residents of Europe and North America during the following decade.[4] *Ba. microti* was first recognized as zoonotic in North America in 1969,[5] coincident

[a] Supported in part by Grant AI19693 from the National Institutes of Health.

with the first report of American Lyme disease. This malaria-like infection was acquired on Nantucket Island, in Massachusetts, only about 20 km from the site on Cape Cod in which the earliest case of human Lyme disease was recorded. Before 1973, babesiosis and erythema migrans (= Lyme disease) appeared only rarely to affect human health.

FIRST OUTBREAKS

The appearance, in 1973, of a second case of babesiosis on Nantucket Island in a neighbor of the first patient indicated that residents of that site may be subject to some measurable risk of infection.[6] A comprehensive epizootiological-epidemiological study on Nantucket was, therefore, begun. *Ba. microti* infection was soon discovered in numerous Nantucket *Peromyscus leucopus* mice,[7] and a newly described tick (designated as *Ixodes dammini*)[8] was implicated as the vector.[9] Although the tick had been abundant in the 1920s on the Elizabeth Islands, a virtually uninhabited group of islands some 20 km to the west of Nantucket, it had not been reported elsewhere until 1961.[10] During the mid-1930s, *I. muris*, but not *I. dammini*, was abundant on Nantucket Island as well as on Martha's Vineyard, an island located between Nantucket and the Elizabeth Islands.[11] The environmental conditions for the spread of this zoonosis apparently had emerged during the years immediately following World War II. Both infections may have existed there in an enzootic rather than a zoonotic cycle.

Human babesiosis attracted extraordinary attention on Nantucket Island during the summer of 1975, 2 years after the second Nantucket case was recognized.[6] Some 7 cases were diagnosed, all but one affecting summer residents of this vacation resort. Public notices were posted in prominent places to advise visitors of this emerging hazard to their health. Thereafter, a gradually increasing trend in incidence of "Nantucket fever" became evident, reaching a total of 17 cases in 1991. About twice that number of human infections has been diagnosed each year at the eastern end of Long Island in New York.

The first recognized outbreak of Lyme disease occurred in coastal Connecticut in 1975, nearly coincident with the first recognized cluster of Nantucket babesial infections.[12] Since 1972, 51 residents of several affluent suburban communities were recognized as suffering from an atypical oligoarthritis that first was tentatively diagnosed as juvenile rheumatoid arthritis. The term, "Lyme arthritis," was coined in recognition of one of the main affected sites, the town of Old Lyme, Connecticut. An association with erythema migrans was established in 1976. In accordance with the enlarged spectrum of pathogenesis of this disease, the term "Lyme disease" soon replaced "Lyme arthritis."

EVOLVING DISTRIBUTION OF DISEASE

The place-focused nature of their vernacular names may initially have prompted health authorities to include a relevant travel history in the differential diagnoses both for Nantucket fever and Lyme disease, a requirement that continued until the early 1980s. For this reason, Lyme disease was not diagnosed in residents of Massachusetts until 1982, and the erythema migrans-like rashes that commonly were seen on residents of Martha's Vineyard, Massachusetts, were attributed to spider-bite. The EM-like rashes that were evident on various of the Nantucket patients were ascribed to babesiosis rather than Lyme disease. In retrospect, it seems evident that Lyme disease had been zoonotic in certain sites during the 1970s along with babesiosis.

Once established in a community, risk of human infection by the agent of Lyme disease increases rapidly. The various vacation communities located on Fire Island, in New York, were massively affected during the late 1970s,[13] as was Great Island on Cape Cod, in Massachusetts.[3] Within a few years after the first cases were noted, annual incidence exceeded 5%. The well-documented Ipswich epidemic, in northeastern Massachusetts, developed similarly.[14] The first human cases occurred in 1980, one year after the vector *Ixodes* ticks first were discovered on the carcasses of deer. Incidence exceeded 10% by 1986, particularly affecting people who lived where deer were most abundant. A similar pattern of explosive epidemiological growth was noted in communities in Westchester County, New York, and in various sites in New Jersey, Pennsylvania and in Wisconsin and Minnesota.

The pattern of increase of Lyme disease in the United States is suggested by the trend in cases officially reported to the CDC. The curve sweeps upward from a few cases in 1980 to some 10,000 in 1992.[15] A leveling trend is suggested by the data for the 1990s, perhaps due to reporting artifacts. Experience in Massachusetts suggests that primary care physicians under-report Lyme disease (personal observation). Although reporting is mandatory, fewer than 100 cases are listed for the State each year. On Nantucket Island alone, however, at least 76 cases were diagnosed in 1990 and 126 in 1991 (S.R. Telford, III, personal communication). We find that many physicians who frequently see cases of Lyme disease seem to regard such diagnoses as routine. Indeed, reporting efficiency seems to decline with time. Certain of these infections may be over-diagnosed, however, as in the case of patients who were referred to a specialty clinic because of presumed Lyme disease; only 43% were confirmed.[16] Because more cases would be under-reported at the primary care level than are over-referred to specialty clinics, the shape of the official epidemic curve should be viewed as a conservative reflection of the actual societal disease burden.

Incidence of clinical human babesiosis on Nantucket Island appeared to increase from nil in the 1960s, to some 5 per year in the 1970s, to 10 in the 1980s and 15 in the 1990s (personal observation). The rates on Shelter Island appeared to run a parallel course at about twice the magnitude of those on Nantucket. The distribution of human *Ba. microti* infection, however, appears to have increased more slowly than did that of the agent of Lyme disease. No babesial infection was found in mice during the 1970s,[17] and no human cases were diagnosed in residents of Connecticut until 1990. Human infections began to appear in mainland situations in Massachusetts and Connecticut during the late 1980s.[18] Although no formal temporal trend could be documented for Connecticut, no evidence of infection, either in mice or people, could be detected some dozen years earlier.[19] Interestingly, 2 cases of human babesiosis were demonstrated in 1985 in the part of Wisconsin in which Lyme disease first appeared.[20] We find that *I. dammini* ticks acquire borrelial infection more readily than babesial infection, and that about as many vector ticks are naturally carriers of babesial as borrelial infection. This difference in competence may explain why one of these infections is spreading more rapidly than the other.

DEVELOPMENT OF THE ZOONOSES IN THE OLD WORLD

Lyme disease began to be diagnosed in numerous Europeans during the mid-1980s, a few years after the epidemic was recognized in the United States.[21] The European epidemic curve, subsequently, seems to have risen more steeply than that of North America, rising to about twice the American level. At least 1,000 new human cases occur annually in Sweden.[22] Similar estimates have been cited for such countries as Switzerland and Austria. The comparable estimate for Germany, however, is 30,000 to 60,000 cases.[21] Indeed, *Borrelia*-specific antibody is said to be detectable in some 7% of German residents. The epidemic of Lyme disease in Europe appears to be increasing.

Elsewhere, human Lyme disease infections have been reported from northeastern China, Japan, South Africa, and Australia.[22] Although no tropical or South American cases of Lyme disease or human babesiosis have been confirmed, clinical diagnoses are said to be made in certain locations. Their validity remains to be determined.

DIRECT EVIDENCE OF ANTIQUITY

Direct evidence of the presence of the agent of Lyme disease in North America extends back only to the 1950s. Spirochete-specific DNA sequences were recognized in *Ixodes dammini* ticks that were collected on Long Island at that time and preserved in museum collections.[23] Evidence of *Ba. microti* infection had been recorded somewhat earlier, in the 1930s, in the blood of a rodent captured on Martha's Vineyard.[24]

EPIZOOTIOLOGY

The agents of Lyme disease and of human babesiosis are transmitted by a variety of *Ixodes* ticks, but mainly those in the *I. ricinus* complex of species. In addition, certain rabbit-feeding *I. dentatus* may maintain enzootic transmission. Of these, the northern deer tick (*I. dammini*) of the northeastern US, the wood tick of Europe (*I. ricinus*) and the Taiga tick of Eurasia (*I. persulcatus*) are responsible for most of the known episodes of transmission. Similar ticks

(*I. pacificus*) serve as vectors in the western United States.[25] Only sporadic cases seem to be transmitted by black-legged ticks (*I. scapularis*) of the southeastern U.S.

Deer are the main definitive hosts for the various members of the *I. ricinus* complex of ticks.[26] Although diverse host-related names, such as "sheep tick" and "bear tick," have locally been applied to them, such designations tend to be misleading. The adult stage of these ticks is most abundant on deer, and these animals are the most abundant large animals in infested sites. This deer-tick relationship has been studied most extensively in Massachusetts. To test the hypothesis that deer are essential to a dense infestation of these ticks, deer were virtually eliminated from a 300 ha peninsula in Massachusetts.[27] These ticks thereafter became scarce, while increasing in comparison sites on Nantucket Island. Ecological observations are consistent with this conclusion. Indeed, self-perpetuating *I. dammini* infestations occur solely where deer are abundant, and the abundance of these vector ticks appears to be determined by the abundance of deer.

Various mice (particularly *Peromyscus leucopus* in eastern North America) are the reservoir hosts both for the agent of babesiosis and of Lyme disease.[28] Ecologically analogous European mice (*Apodemus agrarius*) are important reservoirs of infection in peridomestic sites in which they are abundant.[29] These rodents are competent hosts, abundant in nature, abundantly parasitized by the vector tick and abundant wherever deer are abundant. They never serve as host for adult *I. ricinus*-like ticks.

Birds transport the agent of Lyme disease and of human babesiosis into remote sites. Although certain birds may be competent as hosts for the spirochete, others also support infection. In any event, the abundance of birds does not approach that of mice, and their vagility would serve to dilute a focal infestation. Birds never serve as host for adult *I. ricinus*-like ticks.

ENVIRONMENTAL CHANGE IN EASTERN UNITED STATES

The landscape of the eastern portion of the United States has changed radically since the arrival of European immigrants.[30] In 1602, for example, Brevet described an uninhabited island near Cape Cod in Massachusetts as "The chiefest trees of this Island, are Beeches and Cedars; the outward parts all overgrown with lowe bushie trees, three or foure feet in height, . . . an incredible store of Vines, as well in the woodie part of the island; where they run upon every tree, as on the outward parts, that we could not goe for treading upon them; . . . Here also in this island, great store of Deere, which we saw, and other beasts as appeared by their tracks . . . also, great store of Pease, which grow in certeine plots all the Island over."[31] In contrast to this pristine site, Brevet described nearby inhabited regions in these terms: "we stood a while like men ravished by the beautie and delicacie of this sweet soile; for besides divers cleare Lakes of fresh water (whereof we saw no end) Meadowes very large and full of greene grasse; even the most woody places . . . doe grow so distinct and apart, one tree from another, upon grassie ground." In mainland sites, Morton in 1632 stated that "the Salvages are accostomed to set fire of the country in all places where they come; and burn it, twize a yeare, vixe, at the Spring, and at the fall of the leafe. The reason that moves them to do so, is because it would be otherwise so overgrown with underweedes that it would be all copice wood, and the people could not be able in any wise to passe through the country out of a beaten path . . . And this custome of firing the country is the means to make it passable, and by that meanes the trees growe here and there as in our parks; and that makes the country very beautiful, and commodius."[32] The first European settlers described the inhabited environment as park-like, comprised of open meadows interspersed with groves of stately trees, an environment that was shaped by fire and the human hand.

During the following 200 years, the eastern segment of the United States was rendered virtually treeless.[33] Prodigious quantities of wood were used as domestic fuel, as much as 20 cords per year for a house heated by open fireplaces. Other wood was converted into charcoal for smelting iron ore dredged from bogs and for manufacturing glass. Extensive wheat farming kept much of the region free of trees. The "woods" in which Thoreau[34] lived in 1845 were then a last remnant left by the new railroad's requirement for fuel. His famous protests were most directly stimulated by the steam engine.

The extent of woodland in 1860 was less than 20% of that present in 1992[35] when "about three-quarters of New England is covered with woodland or forest, and the remaining quarter includes all the cities and their surrounding suburbs."[36] The transfer of agriculture from the eastern seaboard to the Great Plains resulted in the reforestation of vast regions of eastern North America. This new brush-choked woodland resembles that which covered the uninhabited, deer-infested, island first visited by Brereton in 1604.

Europe too, recently became reforested, but over a much shorter span of time than in North America. European forests were exploited as fuel during the 1940s, and few trees remained when the economy began to rebound during the 1950s. Impenetrable stands of deer-infested new growth now lie interspersed with houses in much of Central Europe.

ABUNDANCE OF DEER

The white-tailed deer of eastern North America (*Odocoileus virginianus*), originally, was scarce in the more northern states because large predators too easily destroyed them where snow accumulated and became crusted.[37] The southern New England coast and islands, therefore, provided favorable habitat due to the warming influence of the Gulf stream. These animals inhabit the forest's edge and are most abundant near meadows that are about 1 or 2 ha in extent. They browse (on brush) rather than graze (on grass). Although deer will feed on grass, they prefer to feed on the leaves and buds of woody plants. Poison ivy is frequently eaten.

Deer abundance, in the eastern United States, has changed in parallel with that of the woodland. These large animals became virtually extinct during the 1600s and remained vanishingly scarce until the early 1900s. Thoreau[34] never saw a deer on the Massachusetts mainland and described them in terms of a local tradition dating back to the mid-1700s. Indeed, any sighting of a deer in the northeastern United States was regarded as a "headline event" at the turn of the present century.

European deer were virtually exterminated during the 1940s along with large tracts of forest.[29] These animals provided a much needed source of animal protein during this period of economic stress, and the trees provided fuel. European deer became as scarce in 1950 as those in eastern North America were a half century earlier. The European deer management system, that had evolved over the centuries did not reestablish itself in time to prevent the resulting explosive overgrowth of deer; in Central Europe, at least, few people could own hunting weapons. In addition, the housing pattern became increasingly dispersed, encroaching on long-standing deer habitat.

The deer herd of the eastern United States began to rebound during the early 1900s, and since 1960 has expanded explosively (FIG. 1). These records of hunter-killed deer suggest a gradual phase of increase in density during 1900–1955 followed by a more rapid phase after 1970. Differing deer management practices prevent any direct comparison of these phases. Collisions with automobiles, as in Europe, have become commonplace. Like deer, people favor a meadow environment, such that close proximity is a daily event. The European deer herd also began to increase explosively during the 1960s. A brush-choked forest had rapidly developed and deer multiplied unchecked.

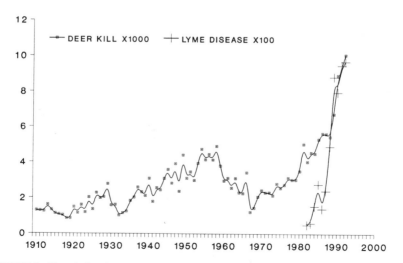

FIGURE 1. Correlation between deer density during the 20th century and the incidence of human Lyme disease. The pattern of increasing density of deer in the northeastern United States is indicated by the total number of these animals killed by hunters in Massachusetts, and the incidence of Lyme disease by the number of cases reported to the CDC.

The process of reforestation simultaneously created a new environment both in North America and Europe in which deer now thrive.

ABUNDANCE OF THE VECTOR TICK

Northern *I. dammini* were recognized as morphologically distinct and geographically isolated from their southern *I. scapularis* siblings in 1979.[8] Laboratory cultures of these ticks isolated from Georgia and from Massachusetts at that time could not be hybridized.[38] The ranges of these ticks have subsequently merged, and similar laboratory cultures of such ticks recently proved to be fully interfertile and "morphometrically" similar.[39] Although these cultures may have been contaminated, this evidence was taken as evidence that the populations in nature are fully interfertile. Additional evidence of conspecificity was interpreted from a nondifferentiated nuclear rDNA sequence.[40] *I. dammini* should continue to be considered as distinct from *I. scapularis*, however, because neither of these recent studies accounted for the morphological divergence of these ticks and their original geographical isolation.

The oldest known collections of *I. dammini* date back to the early 1920s. Preserved specimens of *I. "scapularis,"* collected at that time, correspond to *I. dammini* specimens collected in 1944 and in 1979. Self-perpetuating infestations by these ticks were discovered in Rhode Island in the early 1960s and on Long Island a few years later. A peninsula (Long Point) projecting from the Canadian shore of Lake Ontario was the site of the first reported intense infestation of this tick in an inland location. This infestation dated from about the mid-1960s. Soon thereafter, an intense infestation was recognized in northwestern Wisconsin, centering around the town of Spooner. Beginning in the early 1970s, *I. dammini* infestations came to span much of the northeastern quadrant of the United States.[28] During the 1980s, intense foci developed in many locations, apparently spreading southward from the original foci in Spooner, Long Point, and the Elizabeth Islands. By the 1990s, the range of the northern array of tick populations had extended toward the South.

In the western United States, another tick, *I. pacificus*, was recognized as the cause of numerous clusters of Lyme disease.[41] This tick, too, depends on deer as its definitive host. But, deer density in northern California and Oregon, where these foci became apparent, seems to have been more stable than in the eastern United States and in Europe. It may be that the emergence of Lyme disease in western North America is an artifact due to publicity rather than changes in the force of transmission of the pathogen.

European *I. ricinus* have long been known as parasites of sheep and cattle.[29] They have been implicated as the vectors of such viral infections as tick-borne encephalitis (TBE), and protozoal infections as *B. divergens*. Until recently, however, their presence correlated strongly with the presence of domestic ungulates. As a result, people who were exposed to the bites of wood ticks, and were thereby at risk of acquiring TBE or babesiosis, mainly were limited to members of certain occupational groups such as farmers and soldiers. The population at risk changed during the 1980s. Wood ticks now attack people in London in Richmond Park, near Paris at Versailles, and in Berlin around the Wannsee. As in *I. dammini*-infested sites in the United States, long-term residents of these and other European sites regard the presence of these ticks with alarm and consider them to be something new.

SUMMARY

This pattern of spread of Lyme disease and its vectors in the northeastern United States and Europe derives from the recent proliferation of deer, and the abundance of deer derives from the process of reforestation now taking place throughout the North Temperate Zone of the world. Residential development seems to favor small tree-enclosed meadows interspersed with strips of woodland, a "patchiness" much prized by deer, mice, and humans. As a result, increasingly large numbers of people live where risk of Lyme disease and babesiosis is intense. The agents of these infections, that once were transmitted enzootically by an exclusively rodent-feeding vector, have become zoonotic.

REFERENCES

1. AFZELIUS, A. 1921. Erythema chronicum migrans. Acta Derm. Venereol. **2:** 120–125.
2. SCRIMENTI, R. J. 1970. Erythema chronicum migrans. Arch. Dermatol. **102:** 104–105.
3. STEERE, A. C., E. TAYLOR, M. L. WILSON, J. F. LEVINE & A. SPIELMAN. 1986. Longitudinal assessment of the clinical and epidemiological features of Lyme disease in a defined population. J. Infect. Dis. **154:** 295–300.
4. TELFORD, S. R. III, A. GORENFLOT, P. BRASSEUR & A. SPIELMAN. 1993. Babesial infestations in man and wildlife. *In* Parasitic Protozoa, Vol. 2: 1–47. J. P. Krier, Ed. New York: Academic Press.
5. WESTERN, K. A., G. D. BENSON, G. R. HEALY & M. G. SCHULZE. 1969. Babesiosis in a Massachusetts resident. N. Engl. J. Med. **283:** 854–856.
6. DAMMIN, G. J., A. SPIELMAN, J. L. BENACH & J. PIESMAN. 1981. The rising incidence of clinical *Babesia microti* infection. Hum. Pathol. **12:** 398–400.
7. HEALY, G. R., A. SPIELMAN & N. GLEASON. 1976. Human babesiosis: Reservoir of infection on Nantucket Island. Science **192:** 479–480.
8. SPIELMAN, A., C. M. CLIFFORD, J. PIESMAN & M. D. CORWIN. 1979. Human babesiosis on Nantucket Island, USA: Description of vector, Ixodes (Ixodes) *dammini*, n. sp. (Acarina: Ixodidae). J. Med. Entomol. **15:** 218–234.
9. SPIELMAN, A. 1976. Human babesiosis on Nantucket Island: Transmission by nymphal *Ixodes* ticks. Am. J. Trop. Med. Hyg. **25:** 784–787.
10. HYLAND, K. E. & J. A. MATHEWSON. 1961. The exoparasites of Rhode Island mammals. I. The tick fauna. Wildl. Dis. **11:** 1–14.
11. SMITH, C. N. 1944. Biology of *Ixodes muris*. Ann. Entomol. Soc. Am. **37:** 221–34.
12. STEERE, A. C., S. E. MALAWISTA, D. E. SNYDMAN, R. L. SHOPE, W. A. ANDIMAN, M. R. ROSS & F. M. STEELE. 1977. Lyme arthritis: An epidemic of oligoarticular arthritis in children and adults in three Connecticut communities. Arth. Rheum. **20:** 7–17.
13. HANRAHAN, J. P., J. L. BENACH, J. L. COLEMAN, E. M. BOSLER, D. L. MORSE, D. J. CAMERON, R. EDELMAN & R. KASLOW. 1984. Incidence and cumulative frequency of endemic Lyme disease in a community. J. Infect. Dis. **150:** 489–496.

14. LASTAVICA, C. C., M. L. WILSON, V. P. BARARDI, A. SPIELMAN & R. D. DEBLINGER. 1989. Rapid emergence of a focal epidemic of Lyme disease in coastal Massachusetts. New England J. Med. **320:** 133–137.
15. CENTER FOR DISEASE CONTROL. 1993. Lyme disease surveillance—United States, 1991–1992. Lyme Dis. Surveillance Summary **4:** 1–4.
16. STEERE, A. C., E. TAYLOR, G. L. MCHUGH & E. L. LOGIGIAN. 1993. The overdiagnosis of Lyme disease. JAMA **269:** 1812–1816.
17. ANDERSON, J. F., R. C. JOHNSON, L. A. MAGNARELLI, F. W. HYDE & J. E. MYERS. 1987. Prevalence of *Borrelia burgdorferi* and *Babesia microti* in mice on islands inhabited by white-tailed deer. App. Environ. Microbiol. **53:** 892–894.
18. KRAUSE, P. J., S. R. TELFORD II, R. RYAN, A. B. HURTA, I. KWASNIK, S. LUGER, J. NIEDERMAN, M. GERBER & A. SPIELMAN. 1991. Geographical and temporal distribution of babesial infection in Connecticut. J. Clin. Microbiol. **29:** 1–4.
19. ANDERSON, J. F., L. A. MAGNARELLI & J. KURZ. 1979. Intraerythorocytic parasites in rodent populations of Connecticut: *Babesia* and *Grahamella* species. J. Parasitol. **65:** 599–604.
20. STEKETEE, R. W., M. R. ECKMAN, E. C. BURGESS, J. N. KURITSKY, J. DICKERSON, W. L. SCHELL, M. S. GODSEY, JR. & J. P. DAVIS. 1985. Babesiosis in Wisconsin: A new focus of disease transmission. JAMA **253:** 2675–2678.
21. MATUSCHKA, F. R. & A. SPIELMAN. 1986. The emergence of Lyme disease in a changing environment in North America and Central Europe. Exp. Appl. Acar. **2:** 337–353.
22. JAENSON, T. G. T. 1991. The epidemiology of Lyme borreliosis. Parasitol. Today **7:** 39–45.
23. PERSING, D. H., S. R. TELFORD III, P. N. RYS, D. E. DODGE, T. J. WHITE, S. E. MALAWISTA & A. SPIELMAN. 1990. Detection of *Borrelia burgdorferi* DNA in museum specimens of *Ixodes dammini* ticks. Science **249:** 1420–1423.
24. TYZZER, E. E. 1938. *Cytoecetes microti* n. g. n. sp.; a parasite developing in granulocytes and infective for small rodents. Parasitology **30:** 247–257.
25. LANE, R. S. & J. E. LOYE. 1991. Lyme disease in California: Interrelationship of Ixodid ticks (Acari), rodents, and *Borrelia burgdorferi*. J. Med. Entomol. **28:** 719–725.
26. WILSON, M. L., T. S. LITWIN, T. A. GAVIN, M. C. CAPKANIS, D. C. MACLEAN & A. SPIELMAN. 1990. Host-dependent differences in feeding and reproduction of *Ixodes dammini* (Acari: Ixodidae). J. Med. Entomol. **27:** 945–954.
27. WILSON, M. L., S. R. TELFORD III, J. PIESMAN & A. SPIELMAN. 1988. Reduced abundance of immature *Ixodes dammini* (Acari: Ixodidae) following elimination of deer. J. Med. Ent. **25:** 224–228.
28. SPIELMAN, A., M. L. WILSON, J. F. LEVINE & J. PIESMAN. 1985. Ecology of *Ixodes dammini*-borne human babesiosis and Lyme disease. Ann. Rev. Entomol. **30:** 439–460.
29. MATUSCHKA, F. R. & A. SPIELMAN. 1989. Lyme Krankheit durch Zecken: Der verhaengnisvolle Biss. Bild der Wissenschaft. **8:** 54–64.
30. CRONON, W. 1983. Changes in the Land: Indians, Colonists, and the Ecology of New England. New York: Hill and Wang.
31. BORLAND, H. 1965. Our Natural World. Garden City, NY: Doubleday.
32. BROMLEY, S. J. 1935. The original forest types of New England. Ecol. Monog. **5:** 61–89.
33. JORGENSEN, N. 1971. A Guide to New England's Landscape. Barre Publication. Barre, MA.
34. THOREAU, H. D. 1854. Walden; or, Life in the Woods. Boston, MA: Ticknor and Fields.
35. FOSTER, D. R. 1992. Land-use history (1730–1990) and vegetation dynamics in central New England. J. Ecol. **80:** 753–771.
36. THOMSON, B. F. 1977. The Changing Face of New England. Boston, MA: Houghton Mifflin.
37. ALLEN, G. 1929. History of the Virginia deer in New England. Proc. New Engl. Game Conf. **1:** 19–38.
38. GOWAN, T. D. 1978. Some aspects of the reproductive biology of the black-legged tick, *Ixodes scapularis* (Acari:Ixodidae). Thesis, Master of Science, Georgia Southern College, Statesboro, GA.
39. OLIVER, J. H. JR., M. R. OWSLEY, H. J. HUTCHESON, A. M. JAMES, C-S. CHEN, W.

S. IRBY, E. M. DOTSON & D. K. MCLAIN. 1993. Conspecificity of the ticks *Ixodes scapularis* and *I. dammini* (Acari: Ixodidae). J. Med. Entomol. **30:** 54–63.

40.   WESSON, D. M., D. K. MCLAIN, J. H. OLIVER, J. OIESMAN & F. H. COLLINS. 1993. Investigation of the validity of species status of *Ixodes dammini* (Acari: Ixodidae) using rDNA. Proc. Natl. Acad. USA **90:** 10221–10225.

41.   BURGDORFER, W., R. S. LANE, A. G. BARBOUR, R. A. GRESBRINK & J. R. ANDERSON. 1985. The western black-legged tick, *Ixodes pacificus*: A vector of *Borrelia burgdorferi*. Am. J. Trop. Med. Hyg. **34:** 925–930.

Emergence of Eastern Encephalitis in Massachusetts [a]

NICHOLAS KOMAR AND ANDREW SPIELMAN

Department of Tropical Public Health
Harvard School of Public Health
665 Huntington Avenue
Boston, Massachusetts 02115

INTRODUCTION

The recent history of eastern encephalitis (EE) dates back 60 years. The agent of this mosquito-borne ornithosis was described in the early 1930s[1] and soon became the first arbovirus to be implicated in the etiology of human encephalitis.[2] In September of 1938, a searing outbreak struck Massachusetts, hospitalizing at least 34 people, almost all of whom died.[3,4] A similar epidemic struck New Jersey in 1959, resulting in 32 recorded human cases, of which 22 were fatal.[5] More limited outbreaks occurred in Massachusetts in 1955 and 1956,[2] and massive aerial applications of insecticide appear to have prevented anticipated outbreaks in 1973[6] and 1990. Some 72 human cases have been recorded in Massachusetts since 1938[7], and 190 are known from the eastern United States since 1955.[8] The alarming case fatality rate of this disease and the tragic neurological sequelae that frequently cripple its survivors stimulate more alarm among the residents of Massachusetts than its actual risk might warrant. Even the threat of an outbreak disrupts society.

Although equine disease consistent with EE was described as early as 1831,[9] the nature of these early outbreaks remains speculative. Equine EE disease was first demonstrated in 1933, in the mid-Atlantic states.[10] Hundreds of EE-infected horses died in each of the major outbreaks.[4,5,8] These events suggest a transmission hiatus followed by a recent re-emergence of EE virus infection.

Environmental change in the eastern United States may have created conditions that caused EE to wane and later reemerge as a prominent zoonosis. To explore this hypothesis, we analyzed the natural history of the various vector and reservoir hosts of EE virus and rationalized this information in terms of landscape changes and the known distribution of EE infection in Massachusetts.

[a] Supported in part by a grant (AI 19693) from the National Institute of Allergy and Infectious Disease.

VECTORS

The mosquito vector that perpetuates EE virus (FIG. 1), *Culiseta melanura*, feeds on birds almost exclusively. Its larvae breed in the enclosed pockets of water that form beneath buttressed swamp trees or under those that have partially been wind-thrown such that water puddles deep beneath their roots.[11] Its extreme host-specificity[12] provides this mosquito with extraordinary capacity as a vector. At least a tenth of these mosquitoes live long enough to become infectious.[13]

In Massachusetts, underground bodies of water suitable for larval *Cs. melanura* occur mainly in mature Atlantic white cedar (*Chamaecyparis thyoides*) and red maple (*Acer rubrum*) swamps. This swamp habitat (forested wetland) constitutes the venue for enzootic transmission of EE virus.[14] *Cs. melanura* mosquitoes can be exceedingly abundant there. Adults of this species predominate in the collections taken in light traps set near swamps. Their density is more a function of the level of accumulated ground-water than of recent rainfall.

The abundance of *Cs. melanura* during the transmission season is largely determined by precipitation patterns during the previous fall.[15] These mosquitoes overwinter as nearly mature larvae diapausing in their underground breeding sites, provided that ground-water is sufficient; they resume develop-

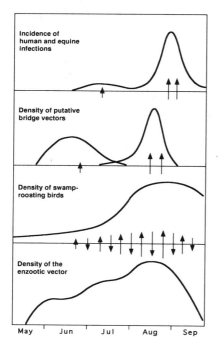

FIGURE 1. The natural cycle of EE virus between birds and bird-feeding *Culiseta melanura* mosquitoes. Occasional equine or human infections follow midsummer contact between infected birds and certain *Aedes* or *Coquillettidia* mosquitoes that feed indiscriminately. Outbreaks of EE in mammals result from such late summer contact with *Aedes vexans* mosquitoes. (Arrows indicate virus transmission.)

ment with the onset of warm weather in May.[11] These mosquitoes continue to proliferate until a period of drought or cold weather intervenes. Although EE virus amplifies solely where mature swamp trees are abundant, epidemics occur solely when precipitation has followed a certain long-term pattern.

Mosquitoes that feed readily both on birds and mammals are directly responsible for human or equine EE virus infection. *Aedes vexans*, for example, breeds during warm weather in open meadows that are flooded by heavy rains and oviposits where puddled water recedes. Because their eggs accumulate on the ground, larval density would be greatest following a period of heavy August or September rainfall that follows some weeks without rain. These mosquitoes appear to provide the main epidemic bridge in Massachusetts.[16] Drought that is intense enough to deplete ground-water, however, would abort any zoonotic outbreak by interrupting the development of *Cs. melanura*.

Another mosquito, *Ae. sollicitans*, appears to serve this bridge function in the vicinity of tidal marshes.[17] The ubiquitous system of ditches that presently disfigures such sites were installed during the early 1900s to relieve the annoyance caused by these mosquitoes[18]. These ditches may have been effective. If so, these vector-competent mosquitoes would have been abundant in the region when *Cs. melanura* appears to have been scarce. The absence of EE-suggestive outbreaks prior to the 1930s, therefore, supports the idea that little virus was then circulating.

RESERVOIRS

EE virus appears to perpetuate solely in birds;[19] mammalian hosts fail to develop a viremia that is sufficiently intense to infect vector mosquitoes.[20] An effective reservoir host for EE virus in Massachusetts would be a bird that is abundant at night during mid- and late summer in or near *Cs. melanura*-infested swamps. Various kinds of birds nest sparsely in swamps, but only a few roost there massively. American robins (*Turdus migratorius*) are the most prominent tree-roosting birds in such sites, and they roost colonially in the summer after nesting ceases.[21] Common grackles (*Quiscalus quiscula*), European starlings (*Sturnus vulgaris*), and red-winged blackbirds (*Agelaius phoeniceus*) form large roosts in the reeds that grow nearby, but not in trees. Thousands of such birds may return on subsequent August or September nights to the same cluster of trees or reeds. Such birds leave their roosting sites during the daytime to search for food, frequently on lawns where *Ae. vexans* may be questing for hosts. We have identified 11 robin and 6 mixed blackbird roosts in southeastern Massachusetts and believe that few have been overlooked.

Many diverse wild birds become exposed to EE virus,[22] and some may transport the virus between enzootic sites. Such wading birds as snowy egrets (*Egretta thula*) or glossy ibis (*Plegadis falcinellus*) are frequently infected and may serve this transport function (W. Crans, personal communication). Although these birds migrate along much of the Atlantic Coast of the Americas, South American isolates seem genetically distinct from those taken in the North.[23] The early-summer wanderings of egrets, however, may serve annually to reintroduce the virus into Massachusetts from more southerly sites. Although the discovery of a virus-infected pool of larval and another of male *Cs. melanura* suggest inherited transmission, no vehicle for local hibernal survival of EE virus in Massachusetts has yet been identified.

THE VIRUS

EE virus is most intensely transmitted in Massachusetts during mid- or late summer. Infected mosquitoes generally become evident in August, with occasional isolates as early as June. Birds, too, most frequently become viremic during August and September.[22] Occasional equine or human infections have occurred as early as July; but clusters of cases associated in place and time occur solely in August or September. Outbreaks of EE occur just before the onset of cold weather.

Although forested wetlands occur throughout New England, a particularly large swamp complex is situated in Plymouth and Bristol Counties in southeastern Massachusetts. The largest of these swamps, the Hockomock, appears to be a perennial focus of transmission in the region; virus is present there every summer.

A "companion agent," Highlands J virus, which produces an apparently benign infection in people and horses, appears to infect the same vector and reservoir hosts as EE virus, but tends to be more abundant. The presence of this additional virus suggests that a cluster of arboviral pathogens may simultaneously emerge in the same environment.

GENERAL LANDSCAPE CHANGES

The European settlers who first colonized Massachusetts found an idyllic landscape.[24] Isolated groves of large trees were interspersed with grassy meadows. Brushy vegetation was scarce due to the fires that the aboriginal people regularly set whenever the undergrowth became sufficiently flammable.[25] Corn was grown in numerous large fields. Mature trees were then abundant.

The colonists depended on the forests for essential resources.[26] The mother country having largely been denuded, forest products found an immediate market, particularly the giant white pines (*Pinus strobus*) that were harvested as masts for the British navy. Exploitation of forests for lumber, firewood, charcoal and for cropland and pasture resources stripped virtually the entire Massachusetts countryside of its forest cover by the mid-1800s. The resulting treeless landscape that Thoreau witnessed in the 1840s represented the maximum of deforestation in eastern Massachusetts.

The original cedar swamps of the region largely were destroyed. Their wood was in great demand for shingles, posts, poles and barrels.[27] The traditional New England house was shingled as well as roofed in cedar. Before the 1880s, many of the cedar swamps that remained in southeastern Massachusetts (especially Cape Cod) were converted into open cranberry bogs, a novel agricultural industry that remains prominent in the region.[28] Howe and Allen,[29] in describing the distribution of the rare pileated woodpecker in Massachusetts, noted that "in Plymouth County, fresh peck-holes were seen in a heavy cedar swamp in 1896." This spectacular bird depends upon mature trees. A 1918 forest survey in Plymouth County notes that "quite a little of this species [cedar] is found in isolated sections of the county, and generally in swamps,"[27] and mentions that "several swamps of large area also occur, the Great Cedar Swamps of Bridgewater and Middleborough being the most important." Cedar forest, however, was not included in the six categories of forest surveyed: white pine, pine and oak, pine and maple, oak, pitch pine, and red maple. Although cedar swamps were severely reduced by the turn of the century, they never completely disappeared.

Mature red maple also provides underground pools suitable for mosquito breeding. The 1918 survey found that nearly pure stands of red maple covered more than 10% of Plymouth County, or 19,021 ha.[27] Between the mid-1800s when deforestation was at its height and 1918, much Massachusetts land had reverted to forest. In 1918, forest covered about 70% of the county. Only 16% of the red maple forest, however, included mature trees, whose trunk diameter at breast height averaged 20 cm or greater and were 15 to 24 m tall.

Because eastern North America was largely deforested by the mid-1800s, few trees were mature enough to become buttressed or wind-thrown until the mid-1900s. Such trees now cover much of the region for the first time in a century, and their present density is unprecedented.[30] The relatively recent discovery of *Cs. melanura*,[31] supported by comments in the early entomological literature,[32] suggests that suitable breeding sites were scarce during the 19th century. In New Jersey in 1902, these mosquitoes were considered as scarce and local.[18] The present EE surveillance program operated by the Massachusetts Department of Public Health indicates that *Cs. melanura* is now the most abundant mosquito collected in southeastern Massachusetts.[33] Both the precolonial and modern landscapes of southeastern Massachusetts appear to have been permissive for these insects.

WETLAND CHANGES

Until recently, wetlands were viewed as undesirable, and their removal was regarded as a sign of progress during the 1920s and 1930s (C. L. Best, personal communication). As early as 1918, legislation was passed in Massachusetts designed to "promote the improvement of lowlands."[34] A State Drainage Board was created, becoming the State Reclamation Board in 1932. Its objective was to "reclaim" wetlands for cultivation. Federal and state drainage operations focused almost exclusively, however, on coastal salt marshes due to lobbying by the Anti-Mosquito Association of Massachu-

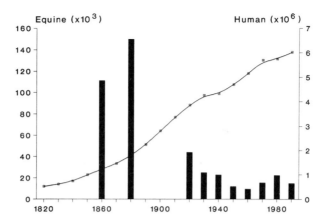

FIGURE 2. Changes in the availability of mammals as hosts for EE virus in Massachusetts. (Abundance of horses and mules[49-54] is indicated by bars and that of people[55,56] by a curve.)

setts.[35] Federal agencies such as the Works Progress Administration under President Franklin Delano Roosevelt drained vast salt marshes in order to reduce annoyance due to brackish-water breeding *Ae. sollicitans* mosquitoes. The Great Depression primed these projects with available labor, and drainage work extended inland as well. Mosquito abatement, after the 1930s, no longer was used to justify removal of wetlands, although the newly organized county mosquito control projects continued to maintain ditches previously created by farmers and the W.P.A. (D. Henley and A. de Castro, personal communication).

New drainage and filling projects, however, were undertaken in inland regions for the purpose of reclaiming land for a variety of purposes including agriculture, commercial development, recreation, housing, and roadbuilding.[36] In southeastern Massachusetts, where wetlands still comprise one-fifth of the land surface, the rate of loss of palustrine wetland (including forested wetland) is about 60 ha per year. The overall extent of wetland in Massachusetts decreased by almost 30% during the last 200 years.[37]

Urban and suburban development continuously reduced the area of Massachusetts covered by forested wetland. Such development is closely associated with dense human populations (FIG. 2). Residential patterns in southeastern Massachusetts, however, increasingly expose numerous people to the threat of EE infection. Housing developments now interdigitate with wetlands, such that linear exurban communities extend along the narrow ridges that penetrate wetlands. New England land considered to be developed nearly tripled from 0.65 million ha in 1945[38] to 1.62 million ha in 1980.[39] Residential and commercial developers, who sought to "reclaim" wetlands, generally were able to acquire these sites at low cost. Wetland development ended in the 1960s when the conservation movement gained state, and later federal, support for protecting these sites.

CONSERVATION TRENDS

The modern conservation movement in Massachusetts began early in the 20th century with official recognition that natural resources are essential and should be protected and managed for the economic welfare of the State. Thus, the Department of Conservation was created in 1918 to protect forest resources, fish and game, and domestic animals.[40] The rapid disappearance of quality timber resources in the early 1900s, and the increasing dependance on imported wood products, demonstrated the need for reforestation and a managed approach to forestry. Beginning in the 1920s, the forestry industry refrained from clear-cutting large tracts of land, owing to the perceived need to preserve the forests as a sustainable resource. The impact of conservationist thinking is reflected by reduced lumber production in the early part of this century (FIG. 3).

The strength of the growing conservation ethic was demonstrated by the creation of the Civilian Conservation Corps that employed millions of people between 1933 and 1942 for forest management and dam building. The conservation movement ignored wetlands, however, until 1963, when the Jones Act was passed in Massachusetts to protect coastal wetlands. Inland wetlands acquired protection in 1965 with the Hatch Act. Such legislation was combined and expanded with the Wetlands Protection Act of 1974.[41] The unique and fragile ecology of wetlands, and their importance to a healthy water supply and flood protection was then recognized. Wetland reclamation has become severely restricted in Massachusetts, and violations are penalized by heavy fines.

Wetlands conservation almost inevitably promotes mosquito abundance, particularly that of *Cs. melanura*, and provides refuge for diverse wildlife that includes reservoir hosts for EE virus.

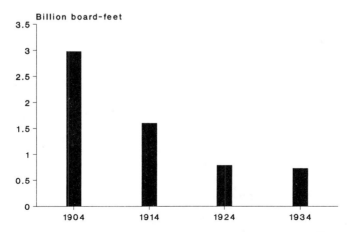

FIGURE 3. Trends in lumber production in Massachusetts.[38]

CHANGES IN BIRD POPULATIONS

Today's Massachusetts avifauna differs markedly from that of colonial times. Transient masses of passenger pigeons (*Ectopistes migratorius*), for example, were then prominent. Wherever their massive flocks appeared during the early years of the Republic, entire towns would turn out to hunt them. An industry developed that was based on the flesh, feathers, and oil derived from these birds. The last of the pigeon marketing companies, the pigeon traders and the pigeon trappers and hunters, known as "pigeoners," died out with these wild doves in the earliest years of the 20th century. The last great flocks of New England disappeared in the late 1870s,[42] well after the eastern forest reached its nadir. Because of their vagility, passenger pigeons would have diluted the force of transmission of EE virus. The virus acquired during one night's residence in a swamp might produce a viremia during another night's residence in an upland location where *Cs. melanura* are scarce.

The snowy egret, as well, became virtually extinct at about the time that passenger pigeons disappeared. Although once abundant (at least in the Southeast), these wetland residents were destroyed because of the Victorian millinery trade, which generated a lucrative market for their plumes. They "bred in millions in southern swamps" during colonial times,[43] and were "an accidental visitor in Massachusetts" in the 19th century. Only three specimens were recorded between 1917 and 1925. They became evident once again in the mid-1900s, coincident with the recognition of zoonotic EE.[44] Snowy egrets are now an abundant feature of the coastal New England landscape, and these wide-ranging birds may reintroduce EE virus annually. Glossy ibis, which are now common in similar wetland habitats, were once "one of the rarest of occasional southern visitors" to New Jersey[44] and a "mere straggler here from the tropics" in Massachusetts.[43] These, as well as other now-thriving avian populations may increasingly contribute as transport hosts for EE virus.

Robins also thrived, increasingly exploiting the changing landscape of eastern North America. Writing in 1937, Stone[44] observed that "Originally there were probably few if any summer Robins [in southern New Jersey]..., but the wonderful development of shade trees...and the steady increase in dwellings with gardens and shrubbery and well-kept lawns have caused a corresponding increase in Robins." In 1905, it was regarded as "the most generally common bird in Massachusetts...Its custom of seeking the vicinity of human dwellings, lawns, gardens, and cultivated fields, all have resulted in its increasing in numbers. As the forests were cleared, the planting of fruit trees furnished it food and nesting places; and so the Robin became part and parcel of our rural civilization."[45] The extraordinary 19th century robin roosts that included tens of thousands of birds[21] probably derived from the restricted nature of the forest rather than a superabundance of these birds. This continuing proliferation of wetland-roosting birds and their close day-time association with human habitations provides an ideal present potential for the development of outbreaks of equine and human EE.

Although commercial hunting eliminated certain native birds, the needs of recreational hunters increased the abundance of other non-native species.

The Ring-necked pheasant (*Phasianus colchicus*), in particular, was introduced into the eastern United States in 1887[42] and became established there as an abundant game bird in fields and marshes. EE virus activity has often been noted in farm-reared flocks of these birds.[46] Although this virus generally produces a silent infection in native birds, it tends to be so pathogenic in pheasants that they die before many mosquitoes can imbibe virus from them.

EE virus is similarly lethal in other introduced birds, including domestic pigeons (*Columba livia*) and house sparrows (*Passer domesticus*).[47,48] Both birds are abundant around human habitations, but do not normally frequent swamps. Their deaths accompany increased levels of enzootic transmission. House sparrows first became established in Boston in 1869,[45] and rapidly overwhelmed the native avifauna but subsequently diminished in density when horses were replaced by motor vehicles. Undigested seeds in horse feces were an important food source for these birds. The European starling was successfully introduced into New York City's Central Park in 1890.[42] They were evident in Massachusetts by 1916, and in the 1920s, massive flocks of starlings commonly roosted at night in open wetlands. Roosting starlings, however, are less exposed to the bites of *Cs. melanura* mosquitoes than are robins. A bird that dies of EE before it can infect mosquitoes would be as zooprophylactic as passenger pigeons that would carry the virus to a remote location.

The force of transmission of EE virus depends on the density of virus-susceptible reservoir birds. Immune robins, for example, would be particularly zooprophylactic because they are so frequently bitten by *Cs. melanura*. Indeed, antivirus antibody has been detected during 1959-1970 in southeastern Massachusetts in 25% of resident robins.[22] If EE virus has emerged recently, the severity of the notorious EE outbreak of 1938 may have been due in part to the consequent scarcity of immune reservoir birds.

The native birds of the eastern United States are better adapted to this virus than are the more recently imported animals, and this argues for the antiquity of EE virus in Massachusetts. *Cs. melanura* mosquitoes would have transmitted the virus there among a previously rich avifauna before the ancestral forests were destroyed.

CHANGES IN MAMMAL POPULATIONS

Although the presence of mammals appears not to affect the force of transmission of EE virus, the resulting disease in people and horses signals an outbreak. The presence of numerous nonvaccinated horses serves a particularly sensitive sentinel function because mosquitoes so frequently feed on these animals and the disease is so spectacular and the findings pathognomonic. It seems meaningful, therefore, that no equine outbreaks such as those noted in 1831 were recorded for the next 100 years even though horses were vastly more abundant than at present (FIG. 2). We take this to mean that little or no virus was then being transmitted in Massachusetts. The veterinary vaccine became available in 1974. The increasing density of people in southeastern

Massachusetts progressively increases the likelihood of human disease while the absolute number of equine infections is diminishing.

SUMMARY

The 20th century emergence in Massachusetts of zoonotic eastern encephalitis was interpreted in terms of recorded environmental change. The main mosquito vector of the infection, *Cs. melanura*, appears to have been scarce in eastern North America before the 1930s. Its relative scarcity resulted from destruction of the swamps that had been lumbered or drained for farming in the 18th and 19th centuries. When swamps matured once again early in the 1900s, the formation of subsurface pools of water beneath mature trees would have increased the availability of breeding sites for this mosquito. Transmission would have further been enhanced by the simultaneous proliferation of wetland-roosting robins and the extinction of such vagile birds as the passenger pigeon. Although numerous horses were maintained in Massachusetts at the time, no outbreaks of "equine sleeping sickness" came to public notice between the 1830s and the 1930s, when mature trees were scarce and the fauna was most disturbed. The severity of the first major outbreak in 1938 may have been potentiated by the absence of herd-immunity in a rapidly proliferating population of reservoir birds. These considerations suggest that recent landscape and faunal changes caused zoonotic EE to emerge in Massachusetts after waning for a century.

ACKNOWLEDGEMENTS

We thank Gary Gonyea of the Massachusetts Department of Environmental Protection for supplying useful research materials and Mary Wilson of Mt. Auburn Hospital, Cambridge and Kathleen S. Anderson for helpful comments.

REFERENCES

1. TEN BROECK, C. & M. H. MERRILL. 1933. A serological difference between eastern and western encephalomyelitis virus. Proc. Soc. Exp. Biol. Med. **31**: 217–220.
2. FEEMSTER, R. F. 1957. Equine encephalitis in New England. N. Engl. J. Med. **257**: 701–704.
3. FEEMSTER, R. F. 1938. Outbreak of encephalitis in man due to the eastern virus of equine encephalomyelitis. Am. J. Pub. Health **28**: 1403–1410.
4. AYRES, J. C. & R. F. FEEMSTER. 1949. The sequelae of eastern equine encephalomyelitis. N. Engl. J. Med. **240**: 960–962.
5. GOLDFIELD, M. & O. SUSSMAN. 1966. The 1959 outbreak of eastern encephalitis in New Jersey. 1. Introduction and desciption of outbreak. Am. J. Epidemiol. **87**: 1–57.
6. GRADY, G. F., H. K. MAXFIELD, S. W. HILDRETH, R. J. TIMPERI, JR., R. F. GILFILLAN, B. J. ROSENAU, D. B. FRANCY, C. H. CALISHER, L. C. MARCUS & M. A. MADOFF. 1978. Eastern equine encephalitis in Massachusetts, 1957–1976: A prospective study centered upon analyses of mosquitoes. Am. J. Epidemiol **107**: 170–178.

7. EDMAN, J. D., R. TIMPERI & B. WERNER. 1994. Epidemiology of eastern equine encephalitis in Massachusetts. Proc. Fla. Mosq. Control Assoc. **64:** 84–96.

8. LETSON, G. W., R. E. BAILEY, J. PEARSON & T. F. TSAI. 1993. Eastern equine encephalitis (EEE): A description of the 1989 outbreak, recent epidemiological trends, and the association of rainfall with EEE occurrence. Am. J. Trop. Med. Hyg. **49:** 677–685.

9. HANSON, R. P. 1957. An epizootic of equine encephalomyelitis that occurred in Massachusetts in 1831. Am. J. Trop. Med. Hyg. **6:** 858–862.

10. TEN BROECK, C., E. W. HURST & E. TRAUB. 1935. Epidemiology of equine encephalomyelitis in the eastern U.S. J. Exp. Med. **62:** 677–685.

11. HAYES, R. O. & H. K. MAXFIELD. 1967. Interruption of diapause and rearing larvae of *Culiseta melanura* (Coq.). Mosq. News **27:** 458–461.

12. NASCI, R. S. & J. D. EDMAN. 1981. Blood feeding patterns of *Culiseta melanura* (Diptera: Culicidae) and associated sylvan mosquitoes in southeastern Massachusetts eastern equine encephalitis enzootic foci. J. Med. Entomol. **18:** 493–500.

13. MORRIS, C. D. 1989. Phenology of trophic and gonobiologic states in *Culiseta morsitans* and *Culiseta melanura* (Diptera: Culicidae). J. Med. Entomol. **21:** 38–51.

14. HAYES, R. O., L. C. LaMOTTE & A. D. HESS. 1960. Enzootic eastern encephalitis activity in Massachusetts. Mosq. News. **20:** 85–87.

15. HAYES, R. O. & A. D. HESS. 1964. Climatological conditions associated with outbreaks of eastern encephalitis. Am. J. Trop. Med. Hyg. **13:** 851–858.

16. FEEMSTER, R. F. & G. A. GETTING. 1941. Distribution of the vectors of equine encephalomyelitis in Massachusetts. Am. J. Pub. Health **31:** 791–802.

17. CRANS, W. J., J. McNELLY, T. L. SCHULZE & A. MAIN. 1986. Isolation of eastern equine encephalitis virus from *Aedes sollicitans* during an epizootic in southern New Jersey. J. Am. Mosq. Cont. Assoc. **2:** 68–72.

18. SMITH, J. B. 1904. Report of the New Jersey State Agricultural Experiment Station upon the Mosquitoes Ocurring within the State, their Habits, Life History, etc. Trenton, NJ: MacCrellish & Quigley, Trenton.

19. DAVIS, W. A. 1940. A study of birds and mosquitoes as hosts for the virus of eastern equine encephalitis. Am. J. Hyg. **32:** 45–59.

20. CHAMBERLAIN, R. W., R. K. SIKES, D. B. NELSON & W. D. SUDIA. 1954. Studies on the North American arthropod-borne encephalitides. VI. Quantitative determination of virus-vector relationships. Am. J. Hyg. **60:** 278–285.

21. BREWSTER, W. 1890. Summer robin roosts. Auk **7:** 360–373.

22. MAIN, A. J., K. S. ANDERSON, H. K. MAXFIELD, B. ROSENAU & C. OLIVER. 1988. Duration of alphavirus neutralizing antibody in naturally infected birds. Am. J. Trop. Med. Hyg. **38:** 208–217.

23. CALISHER, C. H., K. S. C. MANESS, R. D. LORD & P. H. COLEMAN. 1971. Identification of two South American strains of eastern equine encephalomyelitis virus from migrant birds captured on the Mississippi Delta. Am. J. Epidemiol. **94:** 172–178.

24. BROMLEY, S. W. 1935. The original forest types of southern New England. Ecological Monographs **5:** 61–89.

25. DAY, G. M. 1953. The Indian as an ecological factor in the Northeastern forest. Ecology **34:** 329–343.

26. CARROLL, C. F. 1973. The Timber Economy of Puritan New England. Providence, RI: Brown University Press.

27. MORRIS, J. J. 1919. The Forests of Plymouth County. Boston: Massachusetts State Forester. Published by subscription.

28. THOMAS, J. D. 1990. Cranberry Harvest: A History of Cranberry Growing in Massachusetts. New Bedford, MA: Spinner Publications, Inc.

29. HOWE, R. H. & G. M. ALLEN. 1901. The Birds of Massachusetts. Cambridge, MA.

30. FOSTER, D. R. 1992. Land-use history (1730–1990) and vegetation dynamics in central New England. J. Ecol. **80:** 753–771.

31. COQUILLETT, D. W. 1902. New forms of Culicidae from North America. J. N. Y. Ent. Soc. **10:** 191–194.

32. MATHESON, R. 1929. A Handbook of the Mosquitoes of North America. London: Bailliere, Tindall & Cook.
33. ANONYMOUS. 1993. Summary of EE surveillance program. Massachusetts Department of Public Health, 10/1/93.
34. ANONYMOUS. 1922. Draining of Bay State swamps is hailed as great public benefit. Sunday Herald, Boston, February 13, 1922.
35. WHIPPLE, G. C. 1922. Mosquito control in Massachusetts. Boston Society of Civil Engineers, Papers and Discussions 9: 249–268.
36. TINER, R. W. JR. & W. ZINNI. 1988. Recent Wetland Trends in Southeastern Massachusetts. Newton Corner, MA: U.S. Fish and Wildlife Service, National Wetlands Inventory Project.
37. DAHL, T. E. 1990. Wetlands losses in the United States 1780's to 1980's. Washington, DC: U.S. Department of the Interior, Fish and Wildlife Service.
38. BALDWIN, H. I. 1949. Wooden Dollars. Boston, MA: Federal Reserve Bank of Boston.
39. IRLAND, L. C. 1982. Woodlands and Woodlots, the Story of New England's Forests. Hanover, NH: University of New England Press.
40. BAZELEY, W. A. L. 1920. Annual Report of the Commissioner of Conservation and State Forester for the Year Ending November 30, 1920. Commonwealth of Massachusetts Public Document No. 73. Boston: Wright & Potter Printing Co.
41. ANONYMOUS. 1991. Wetlands White Paper: A report on the protection of wetlands in Massachusetts. Massachusetts Department of Environmental Protection, February 1991.
42. FORBUSH, E. H. 1927. Birds of Massachusetts and Other New England States Part II. Land Birds from Bob-whites to Grackles. Massachusetts Department of Agriculture, Boston.
43. FORBUSH, E. H. 1925. Birds of Massachusetts and other New England States Part I. Water birds, marsh birds and shore birds. Massachusetts Department of Agriculture, Boston.
44. STONE, W. 1937. Bird Studies at Old Cape May. Vol. I. New York: Dover Publications, Inc.
45. FORBUSH, E. H. 1929. Birds of Massachusetts and other New England States Part III. Land birds from sparrows to thrushes. Massachusetts Department of Agriculture, Boston.
46. BEADLE, L. D. 1952. Eastern equine encephalitis in the United States. Mosq. News 12: 102–107.
47. FOTHERGILL, L. D. & J. H. DINGLE. 1938. A fatal disease of pigeons caused by the virus of the eastern variety of equine encephalomyelitis. N. Engl. J. Med. 219: 411.
48. LOCKE, L. N., J. E. SCANLON, R. J. BYRNE & J. O. KNISLEY, JR. 1962. Occurrence of eastern encephalitis virus in house sparrows. Wilson Bull. 74: 263–266.
49. UNITED STATES DEPARTMENT OF AGRICULTURE. 1863. Annual Report of the Commissioner of Agriculture for the Year 1862. Government Printing Office, Washington, DC.
50. UNITED STATES DEPARTMENT OF AGRICULTURE. 1881. Annual Report of the Commissioner of Agriculture for the Year 1880. Government Printing Office, Washington, DC.
51. UNITED STATES DEPARTMENT OF COMMERCE BUREAU OF THE CENSUS. 1927. United States Census of Agriculture: 1925 Part I. The Northern States. Government Printing Office. Washington, DC.
52. UNITED STATES DEPARTMENT OF COMMERCE BUREAU OF THE CENSUS. 1937. United States Census of Agriculture: 1935 Vol. I. Statistics by Counties with State and U.S. Summaries Part I. The Northern States. Government Printing Office, Washington, DC.
53. UNITED STATES DEPARTMENT OF AGRICULTURE. 1940. Agricultural Statistics 1940. Government Printing Office, Washington, DC.
54. UNITED STATES DEPARTMENT OF COMMERCE BUREAU OF THE CENSUS. 1982. 1982 Census of Agriculture Vol. 1 Part 21. Massachusetts State and County Data. Government Printing Office. Washington, DC.
55. WILKIE, R. W. & J. TAGER, Eds. 1991. Historical Atlas of Massachusetts. Amherst, MA: University of Massachusetts Press.
56. UNITED STATES DEPARTMENT OF COMMERCE BUREAU OF THE CENSUS. 1991. 1990 Census of Population and Housing—Massachusetts. Government Printing Office, Washington, DC.

Rift Valley Fever Virus Ecology and the Epidemiology of Disease Emergence[a]

MARK L. WILSON[b]

Yale Arbovirus Research Unit
Department of Epidemiology and Public Health
Yale University School of Medicine
60 College Street
New Haven, Connecticut 06520-8034

Since 1930 when it was first described during an epizootic among domestic ungulates in Kenya,[1] Rift Valley fever (RVF) has appeared in dozens of temporally and spatially punctuated animal and human outbreaks that even today defy prediction. Sudden and severe epizootics, sometimes accompanied by epidemic human disease, have occurred throughout sub-Saharan Africa.[2] An acute viral infection producing inapparent or mild disease in adult sheep and cattle, RVF provokes abortion among pregnant ungulates and often is fatal to young animals.[3,4] Human disease is characterized initially by abrupt onset of high fever, severe headache, myalgia, conjunctival injection and incapacitating prostration of several days duration.[5] Some patients develop fatal hemorrhagic fever or encephalitis, and those who survive may experience ocular disease (primarily retinal vasculitis). Serological evidence suggests that low-level endemic transmission occurs regularly throughout much of the African continent, but most of this remains unrecognized due to inadequate surveillance and health care facilities.[2]

Transmission of RVF virus (a phlebovirus of the family *Bunyaviridae*) is principally mosquito-borne to both animals and people.[6–8] Potential mosquito vectors include more than 30 species from which RVF virus has been isolated.[2] Experimental and field studies suggest that certain floodwater *Aedes* spp. which emerge from temporary ground pools following seasonal rains are important enzootic vectors.[9–12] Epizootic transmission correlates temporally with periods of heavy rainfall in East Africa,[13] when particular *Culex* species become infected.[6,8] Then, and perhaps also during enzootic transmission, human infections may result from exposure to infected animal tissues.[14–16] The risk factors associated with human exposure have not yet been completely defined.[17]

Some of the main interactions of RVF virus cycles are represented schematically in FIGURE 1.

[a] Supported by a grant from the MacArthur Foundation (9008073 Health).
[b] Tel: 203-785-2904; Fax: 203-785-4782.

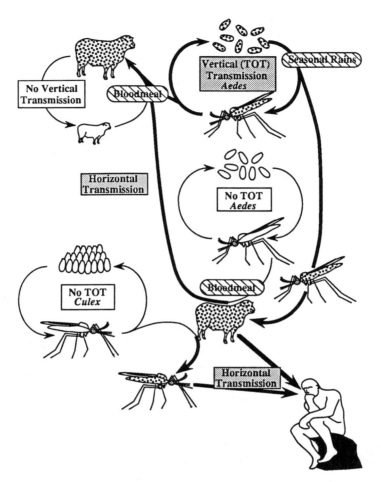

FIGURE 1. Schematic diagram of the principal routes of transmission of Rift Valley fever (RVF) virus. Heavy lines indicate virus transfer while light lines represent the continuation of cycles that do not involve RVF virus. Interactions producing horizontal transmission, vertical transmission (transovarial transmission, TOT) or no transmission are indicated.

RVF occurs sporadically in time and space throughout sub-Saharan Africa, with documented disease or evidence of RVF virus coming from at least 24 countries.[2] In addition to the outbreaks that have been recognized in eastern Africa since the 1930s[18] and in southern parts of the continent since the 1950s,[3,4] the first documented West African epizootic/epidemic to be reported occurred during 1987 along the Senegal-Mauritania border.[19–21] An earlier epidemic that surfaced north of the Sahara in the Egyptian Nile delta during 1977–78[22] seemed peculiar as the virus was previously unknown there and subsequent transmission ceased. It now appears that introduction of RVF virus into sites not exhibiting sustained transmission may occur more often than once believed, as another Egyptian outbreak began in July 1993.[23]

What characteristics of this mosquito-borne, viral, zoonotic disease predispose it to intense anthroponotic/epizootic activity, seeming disappearance, then sudden, unpredicted reactivation? How might an analysis of this agent's transmission dynamics, and of the ecology and epidemiology of associated human disease, help us to predict the appearance of other agents and diseases with similar characteristics? The following discussion addresses various aspects of the natural transmission cycle of RVF virus, as well as the manner in which human activity and ecological events may influence the likelihood of RVF emergence. First, the characteristics of the RVF virus transmission cycle that potentiate outbreaks will be outlined. Second, the ecological changes that initiate transmission will be identified. Finally, the likelihood of future outbreaks will be addressed in terms of recent experience.

ECOLOGY OF RVF VIRUS TRANSMISSION

The force of transmission of RVF virus depends on complex interactions among mosquito vectors, non-human vertebrates, and human hosts (TABLE 1).

Mosquitoes perpetuate transmission either by a) vertical or transovarial transmission directly to the next mosquito generation, or b) horizontal transmission to vertebrates which then infect other blood-feeding mosquitoes (FIG. 1). The relative importance of vertical versus horizontal transmission either in maintaining virus transmission or in RVF outbreaks remains speculative. Various animals produce viremias sufficient to infect engorging mosquitoes, suggesting that horizontal amplification supplements the vertical mode; vertical transmission under some ecological conditions is not adequate to maintain viral foci. The densities of certain vertebrates, particularly domestic ungulates, therefore appear crucial in potentiating zoonotic outbreaks. Such animals may be abundant locally, are bitten frequently by various presumed vector species, and develop high viremias prior to producing antibody.

The development of neutralizing antibody following infection introduces another factor that contributes to the spatial and temporal instability of RVF. Subsequent to epizootic transmission, herd immunity in domestic ungulates will be elevated, perhaps reaching a prevalence of more than two-thirds (personal observation). Antibody appears to be life-long with passive transfer via milk from mothers to their offspring protecting these young animals for months. Thus, risk of local epizootic transmission is decreased following intense transmission as the pool of susceptible animals becomes reduced. Horizontal transmission, therefore, would not perpetuate the virus. The complex relationship among various RVF virus-competent mosquito species, their biting habits, the availability of different vertebrate hosts, and the immune status of such populations provokes instability (TABLE 1).

TABLE 1. Principal Characteristics of Rift Valley Fever Virus Transmission and Infection That May Lead to Spatio-Temporal Instability, Resurgence or New Emergence of Disease

Characteristic	Ecological or Epidemiological Event	Effect on Virus Transmission or Disease Appearance
Transmission by vector		
Transovarial	*Aedes* emergence following seasonal rains	Maintenance and over-wintering
Enzootic	*Aedes* (?*Culex*) feeding on susceptible animals	Amplification; increased local prevalence
Epizootic	Flooding and extreme *Culex* abundance; widespread feeding	Amplification; spillover to humans; expansion
Infected domestic ungulates		
Distribution	Migration or export	Expansion of range
Susceptibility	Viral or animal population genetic change	Increased transmission or disease
Concentration	Improved pasturage or sale	Greater transmission
Human disease		
Endemic	Association with domestic animals	Resurgence during transmission periods
Epidemic	Settlements or work near dams and irrigation	New foci of intense transmission
	Urbanization and crowding	Introduction/expansion

Human infection, nevertheless, contributes little to the maintenance of RVF virus transmission. *Aedes* mosquitoes of the *Aedimorphus* and *Neomelaniconion* subgenera are competent vectors, but they rarely bite humans.[9,12] In particular, *Aedes* (*Neomelaniconion*) *mcintoshi* (= *Ae. lineatopennis*) appears to efficiently transmit RVF virus transovarially, thereby maintaining enzootic transmission when infected adults emerge from temporary ground pools that form after periods of heavy rainfall. Anthroponotic transmission would not be directly affected unless other "bridge" vector mosquitoes that bite both domestic animals and humans were present. Certain *Culex* species, particularly *Cx. pipiens* may serve this role, because they are RVF virus-competent and often abundant when and where RVF virus is circulating.[2] The absence of observations prior to and during outbreaks severely limits our ability to interpret relevant ecological conditions.

ENVIRONMENTAL CHANGE AND RVF EMERGENCE

Whether as "natural" events, or those that constitute or result from human activity, ecological and environmental factors may affect the RVF virus transmission cycle. These events, as classified by Lederburg *et al.*,[24] include a)

economic development and changing land use (*e.g.*, dams and irrigation, better health care and surveillance, improvement of pasturage); b) **human demography and behavior** (*e.g.*, increased urbanization and crowding, living with and slaughtering domestic ungulates); c) **international travel and commerce** (*e.g.*, exportation of domestic ungulates, human travel, nomadism and migration); and d) **biological adaptation and change** (*e.g.*, increased virus infectivity, vectorial capacity or animal susceptibility). In addition, e) **climatic events** such as periods of unusual rainfall are considered (TABLE 2).

Four categories of change that indicate emergence of human RVF are those producing a) increased endemic disease, b) more frequent periods of elevated transmission, c) greater severity or intensity of epidemics and d) expansion of RVF endemic areas or invasion into unaffected regions (TABLE 2). Accordingly, RVF is considered to be emerging where **endemic prevalence** increases, *i.e.* where the percentage of persons within an endemic area exhibiting anti-RVF virus antibody grows. Secondly, greater **epidemic frequency** constitutes emerging RVF when periods of excessive incident cases occur more commonly. Thirdly, RVF emerges when **epidemic intensity** is heightened, *i.e.* when the proportion of a population or size of an area experiencing epidemic disease becomes greater. Finally, the **expansion or**

TABLE 2. Comparison of the Relative Contribution of Various Factors to the Potential for Emergence of Human Rift Valley Fever[a]

Factors in Emergence	Relative Increase in Type[b] of Emergence			
	Endemic Prevalence	Epidemic Frequency	Epidemic Intensity	Expansion/invasion
Economic Development/Land Use				
Dams and irrigation	+	0	+	+
Surveillance/health care	0	+	+	+
Improvement of pasturage	+	−	+	−
Human Demography and Behavior				
Urbanization and crowding	−	+	+	0
Living with domestic ungulates	+	+	+	0
Slaughter of sick animals	0	+	0	0
Vaccination of healthy animals	−	−	−	−
International Travel/Commerce				
Domestic ungulate export	−	+	0	+
Human travel/migration	0	0	0	+
Biological Adaptation and Change				
Increased viral virulence	+	0	+	0
Improved vector competence	+	+	+	0
Greater animal susceptibility	+	0	+	+
Climatic Events				
Excessive rainfall	0	+	0	+

[a] The factors in emergence are categorized by the scheme of Lederberg *et al.*, 1992.

[b] **Endemic prevalence** is the proportion of persons within an endemic area exhibiting antibody against RVF virus; **Epidemic frequency** is the frequency of occurrence of periods of elevated incidence; **Epidemic intensity** is the proportion of population or size of area experiencing infection during an epidemic; **Expansion/invasion** is the appearance of incident cases in an area where none had occurred previously.

invasion of RVF virus represents disease emergence when incident cases appear in an area where none had occurred previously. The contributions of various factors to each type of RVF emergence are outlined below.

Economic Development and Changing Land Use

The importance of mosquitoes as vectors and reservoirs of RVF virus is central to the influence of environment on emergence of this disease. Changing patterns of water storage and use that alter the breeding and larval development of vector species affect intensity of transmission. Particular patterns of standing water following damming of rivers and irrigation of surrounding land may encourage reproduction of certain *Culex* mosquitoes; impact on floodwater *Aedes*, however, seems less likely. Thus, increased populations of *Culex* species that enhance transmission among animals and to humans would increase local endemic prevalence without impacting on the frequency of such epidemics. The intensity of epidemics, however, may be expanded as in the Mauritanian outbreak. Finally, damming and irrigation alone should not cause the distribution of RVF virus to change, although habitats could be created that support eventual virus introductions (TABLE 2).

Improved access to health care facilities and/or increased surveillance may uncover new cases of RVF, effecting emergence through increased awareness. Although prevalence of infection should not become greater, the recognition of epidemic disease, including diagnosis of mild cases, would increase with improved surveillance and access to care. Furthermore, increased availability of clinics would enhance recognition of expansion into areas where RVF had not been found previously.

Economic development in Africa taking the form of improved pasturage often leads to greater concentrations of ungulates and decreased nomadic grazing, thereby increasing the risk of enzootic and epizootic RVF. Accordingly, prevalence of human RVF would rise, as might the intensity of human epidemics. The frequency of recurring epidemics, but not of epizootics, however, might actually decline if human antibody prevalence were to increase to high levels. In addition, more sedentary sheep and cattle rearing could reduce the chances that long-distance grazing would introduce RVF virus into new areas, unless this new system of animal production led to increased export (see below).

Human Demography and Behavior

A second group of factors influencing emergence of RVF involves socio-cultural patterns of habitation and of interaction with domestic animals (TABLE 2). As human populations grow and economic incentives attract increasingly more people into larger villages and cities, most vector-borne disease transmission mounts. Increased abundance and density of humans, combined with decreased average age of the population, initially would reduce antibody prevalence in humans, a measure of previous RVF exposure. Conversely, the frequency and intensity of epidemic RVF would increase owing to the greater proportion of people lacking protective antibodies. While little impact of urbanization on expansion or invasion by this virus would be anticipated, humans migrating with their animals into communities where RVF virus is not known could introduce the agent into such sites.

During migration into towns or cities, people typically transport both domestic animals and traditional husbandry and butchering techniques. The practice of living near their animals, sometimes sleeping a short distance away, often continues under these new, more crowded conditions. Such close proximity permits multiple bloodmeals by mosquitoes that may mechanically transfer RVF virus from viremic sheep or goats to nearby humans. This may encourage the emergence of RVF if there is increased endemic prevalence and possibly epidemic frequency in regions where transmission already occurs. The intensity of epidemics will be enhanced as neighbors become infected. Such proximity to animals should not play a role, however, in the expansion of RVF.

Muslim practice prohibits the consumption of meat from animals that have died before they could be slaughtered. Impoverished Africans face the loss of one of their most valuable resources when a sheep, goat or cow becomes moribund. These animals are likely to be slaughtered immediately in order to be consumed correctly. If they are ill from RVF virus infection, humans may be exposed to aerosol contamination during slaughter or to infection by contact during butchering or meat preparation. Such practices could increase human disease during epizootic/epidemic activity, but probably have little or no impact on endemic prevalence, epidemic intensity, or expansion.

Vaccination of domestic ungulates against RVF virus has been practiced in various settings and represents a potentially important impact on transmission. Evaluation of the effects is complicated by coverage, because the number and proportion of animals that are effectively protected varies among different RVF vaccination campaigns. In general, protection of vertebrates infecting vectors that also feed on people should reduce all categories of RVF emergence. This assumes that a live-attenuated vaccine does not revert to virulence and provoke disease, and that the reuse of needles while vaccinating animals during an epizootic does not increase transmission. Once undertaken, however, vaccination in a highly enzootic region eventually may increase epidemic intensity if not practiced yearly on all newborns; decreased transmission leaves a large cohort of unvaccinated animals unprotected.

International Travel and Commerce

Long-distance movement of humans and transport of animals creates opportunities for the introduction of infectious agents into regions where they were not present previously (TABLE 2). Export of domestic ungulates may permit RVF virus to expand in distribution, emerging where numerous susceptible hosts reside. This appears to have occurred on at least two occasions in the Nile delta.[22,23] In addition to encouraging invasion into new areas, such commerce also may increase the frequency of epidemic RVF if viremic animals are introduced into herds with a low prevalence of immunity. The intensity of epidemics, however, should not be influenced by long-distance transport of this sort. Interestingly, the proportion of antibody-positive animals that remains after export may decline as younger animals typically constitute the majority of those that are exported; endemic prevalence would appear to decline accordingly.

Human travel, nomadism and migration probably have little effect on the emergence of this zoonosis. Even when viremic humans visit non-endemic sites, the probability seems remote that a mosquito will become infected, then later will feed on a susceptible animal, and that animal will infect other vectors, and finally establish a local transmission cycle. However, humans that become viremic after flying to uninfected countries where animal quarantine nevertheless is strict may represent the rare but important means of long-distance introduction of RVF to other continents. Regardless, neither the local prevalence of RVF nor the frequency or severity of epidemics should be influenced by such human travel.

Biological Adaptation and Change

Genotypic change that alters any aspect of the virus-vector-host interface may lead to enhanced transmission efficiency and emergence of RVF. Although this represents an accepted mechanism for other arboviruses, emergence of RVF through such genetic change remains speculative. The most likely scenario would involve the coevolution of RVF virus infectivity, vertebrate susceptibility, and vector competence. Increased infectivity, pathogenicity, or virulence of the virus should enhance endemic prevalence (more successful human infections) and epidemic intensity (increased infection and more severe disease). However, little direct impact on the frequency of infection or expansion of range would be envisioned (TABLE 2).

Evolutionary change that improves mosquito vector competence in transmitting RVF virus should increase the prevalence of human infection, the frequency of epidemics, and epidemic intensity. The magnitude of such change, however, would depend on the biting tendencies of the mosquitoes, and on their capacity for transovarial transmission. Little influence on RVF emergence through expansion or invasion is likely from this type of genetic change.

Selection that increases sheep or cattle susceptibility to RVF virus could increase viremia or decrease the minimum infective dose for these animals, thus elevating the risk of certain kinds of human exposure. Increased animal susceptibility might affect prevalence of human RVF by permitting greater infection of mosquitoes that could later transmit to people. The frequency of epidemics should not, however, be increased. The number of people affected during an outbreak and the likelihood that transmission might extend to other regions also would mount if domestic animal susceptibility increased.

Climatic Events

Climatic fluctuations (including precipitation, temperature and humidity), as distinct from the hypothetical "global warming" changes, are likely to affect the emergence of RVF (TABLE 2). For example, periods of extreme rainfall directly increase egg hatching and larval survival of *Aedes* floodwater species. Enhanced seasonal rainfall fills depressions, stimulating egg hatching and larval development. If already infected by vertical transmission, these mosquitoes can induce or enhance horizontal transmission, producing more frequent epidemics, and possibly importation into new regions. Little or no increase in the intensity of epidemics or in the prevalence of antibody in humans should be observed where these periods of excessive seasonal rainfall occur regularly. Extended periods of excessive rains could, however, allow intense buildup of *Culex* populations that might potentiate the emergence of human RVF. *Culex* species are believed to be important horizontal transmission vectors as at least six common species are competent, and various members of this genus often are abundant during epidemics.[2]

EMERGENCE AND FUTURE REEMERGENCE

How might emerging RVF today influence the process of continued emergence or resurgence tomorrow? Can analyses of transmission dynamics that consider conditions underlying the appearance of RVF be used to predict changes likely to take place in the future? Although the complexity, uncertainty, and spatio-temporal nonlinearity of RVF virus transmission would seem to make it nearly intractable, some generalities are proposed that should help guide such analysis. These predictions are offered to stimulate thinking about the relevant ecological and epidemiological processes that affect RVF emergence.

The four classes of change that indicate emerging RVF have been evaluated for their future impact on the above-mentioned measures (TABLE 3). Increasing **endemic prevalence** of human RVF is not likely to augment either future endemic prevalence or expansion/invasion. As with most zoonoses, the rate of incident human infection is largely independent of past human

TABLE 3. The Influence of Various Categories of Emergence of Human Rift Valley Fever on Future Reemergence

Past or Present Increase In	Effect on Future Increase in			
	Endemic Prevalence	Epidemic Frequency	Epidemic Intensity	Expansion Invasion
Endemic prevalence	0	−	−	0
Epidemic frequency	+	−	0	0
Epidemic intensity	+	−	−	+
Expansion invasion	−	+	+	+

infections. Thus, human antibody prevalence will vary with changes in RVF virus-infected vertebrate or vector populations, and human birth/death rates. Similarly, the ability of RVF virus to expand or invade new areas should not be enhanced by human disease. Indeed, increased endemic prevalence could lower the frequency and intensity of future epidemics if susceptibility declined as herd immunity increased.

Previously elevated **epidemic frequency** will increase future RVF emergence that is measured by endemic prevalence since antibody prevalence which remains evident for many years will have increased. For this same reason, however, the future frequency of epidemics may actually decline. No impact on subsequent intensity of epidemics nor on the range of RVF should result (TABLE 3).

Past increases in **epidemic intensity** also should affect future endemicity because more people from a larger area would be immune to RVF viral infection. For these same reasons, successive epidemics should be both less frequent and less intense.

Finally, the **expansion or invasion** of RVF into new sites may result in progressive invasion of contiguous sites and subsequent further expansion. The range of the virus is likely to increase unevenly, with some regions experiencing undetectable epizootic activity.

HYPOTHESIS TESTING AND FURTHER STUDY

What can these theoretical relationships and hypothetical interactions inform us about the risk of RVF emergence and resurgence? Can this information be used to predict future events accurately, or is it solely useful in developing *post hoc* explanations? The hypothetical effects proposed here cannot be confirmed experimentally. An alternative, that of retrospective epidemiological analysis, has been undertaken following a few RVF epizootics/epidemics, but analysis is limited by sparse comparative data. These studies indicate that RVF emerges rapidly and without discernible warning.

Using basic epidemiological and ecological information, the RVF epidemic along the Senegal River following the closing of the Dialmo dam was predicted more than a decade in advance of its occurrence.[19,25] Likewise, using information from the earlier Egyptian outbreak, simple deduction led to the prediction that RVF would eventually resurge there (Dr. Robert E. Shope, personal communication). While the precise times and places that RVF will emerge cannot be defined, enough information concerning the conditions that favor such change is now available to allow for general predictions that should increase awareness and responsiveness.

Prospective studies of emerging RVF will require surveillance and readiness coordinated among numerous sites. This discussion may help guide surveillance efforts designed to monitor the future emergence of RVF. Teams of entomologists, virologists, and epidemiologists should be capable of responding quickly to outbreaks that occur. Government advisors should have the understanding or advice necessary to make rapid and informed decisions on intervention at sites where RVF emerges. Similar approaches might help predict outbreaks of other arboviral agents.

REFERENCES

1. DAUBNEY, R., J. R. HUDSON & P. C. GARNHAM. 1931. Enzootic hepatitis or Rift Valley fever: An undescribed disease of sheep, cattle and man from East Africa. J. Pathol. Bacteriol. **89**: 545-579

2. MEEGAN, J. M. & C. L. BAILEY. 1988. Rift Valley fever. In Arboviruses Epidemiology and Ecology, T. P. Monath, Ed. Vol. IV: 51–76. Boca Raton, FL: C.R.C. Press.

3. EASTERDAY, B. C. 1965. Rift Valley fever. Adv. Vet. Sci. **10**: 65–127.

4. SHIMSHONY, A. & R. BARZILAI. 1983. Rift Valley fever. Adv. Vet. Sci. Comp. Med. **27**: 347–425.

5. PETERS, C. J. & J. M. MEEGAN. 1981. Rift Valley fever. In CRC Handbook Series in Zoonoses. J. H. Steele, Ed.:403-420. Boca Raton, FL: C.R.C. Press.

6. MEEGAN, J. M., G. M. KHALIL, H. HOOGSTRAAL & F. K. ADHAM. 1980. Experimental transmission and field isolation studies implicating Culex pipiens as a vector of Rift Valley fever in Egypt. Am. J. Trop. Med. Hyg. **29**: 1405–1410.

7. McINTOSH, B. M. & P. G. JUPP. 1981. Epidemiological aspects of Rift Valley fever in South Africa with references to vectors. Contrib. Epidemiol. Biostat. **3**: 92–99.

8. McINTOSH, B. M., P. G. JUPP, I. DOS SANTOS & A. C. ROWE. 1983. Field and laboratory evidence implicating Culex zombaensis and Aedes circumluteolus as vectors of Rift Valley fever virus in coastal South Africa. S. Afr. J. Sci. **79**: 61–64.

9. LINTHICUM, K. J., F. G. DAVIES, C. L. BAILEY & A. KAIRO. 1983. Mosquito species succession in a dambo in an East African forest. Mosq. News **43**: 464–470.

10. LINTHICUM, K. J., F. G. DAVIES, C. L. BAILEY & A. KAIRO. 1984. Mosquito species encountered in a flooded grassland dambo in Kenya. Mosq. News **44**: 228–232.

11. LINTHICUM, K. J., F. G. DAVIES & A. KAIRO. 1984. Observations of the biting activity of mosquitoes at a flooded dambo in Kenya. Mosq. News **44**: 595–598.

12. LINTHICUM, K. J., F. G. DAVIES, A. KAIRO & C. L. BAILEY. 1985. Rift Valley fever virus (family Bunyaviridae, genus Phlebovirus). Isolations from Diptera collected during an inter-epizootic period in Kenya. J. Hyg. Camb. **95**: 197–209.

13. DAVIES, F. G, K. J. LINTHICUM & A. D. JAMES. 1985. Rainfall and epizootic Rift Valley fever. Bull. W.H.O. **63**: 941–963.

14. SMITHBURN, K. C., A. F. MAHAFFY, A. J. HADDOW, S. F. KITCHEN & J. F. SMITH. 1949. Rift Valley fever: Accidental infections among laboratory workers. J. Immunol. **62**: 213–227.

15. CHAMBERS, P. G. & R. SWANEPOEL. 1980. Rift Valley fever in abattoir workers. Cent. Afr. J. Med. **26**: 122–126.

16. VAN VELDEN, D. J. J., J. D. MEYER, J. OLIVER, J. H. S. GEAR & B. McINTOSH. 1977. Rift Valley fever affecting humans in South Africa: A clinicopathological study. S. Afr. Med. J. **51**: 867–871.

17. WILSON, M. L., L. E. CHAPMAN, D. B. HALL, E. A. DYKSTRA, K. BA, H. G. ZELLER, M. TRAORE-LAMIZANA, J. P. HERVY, K. J. LINTHICUM & C. J. PETERS. Rift Valley fever in rural northern Senegal: Human risk factors and potential vectors. Am. J. Trop. Med. Hyg. **50**: 663–675.

18. DAVIES, F. G. 1975. Observations on the epidemiology of Rift Valley fever in Kenya. J. Hyg. Camb. **75**: 219–230.

19. DIGOUTTE, J. P. & C. J. PETERS. 1989. General aspects of the 1987 Rift Valley fever epidemic in Mauritania. Res. Virol. **140**: 27–30.

20. JOUAN, A., I. COULIBALY, F. ADAM, B. PHILIPPE, O. RIOU, B. LEGUENNO, R. CHRISTIE, N. O. MERZOUG, T. KSIAZEK & J. P. DIGOUTTE. 1989. Analytical study of a Rift Valley fever epidemic. Res. Virol. **140**: 175–186.

21. KSIAZEK, T. G., A. JOUAN, J. M. MEEGAN, B. LeGUENNO, M. L. WILSON, C. J. PETERS, J. P. DIGOUTTE, M. GUILLAUD, N. O. MERZOUG & O. I. TOURAY. 1989.

Rift Valley fever among domestic animals in the recent West African outbreak. Res. Virol. **140:** 67–77.

22. MEEGAN, J. M. 1979. Rift Valley fever in Egypt. An overview of the epizootic in 1977 and 1978. Contrib. Epidemiol. Biostat. **3:** 100–113.

23. ARTHUR, R. R., M. S. EL-SHARKAWY, S. E. COPE, B. A. BOTROS, S. OUN, J. C. MORRILL, R. E. SHOPE, R. G. HIBBS, M. A. DARWISH & I. Z. E. IMAM. 1993. Recurrence of Rift Valley fever in Egypt. Lancet **342:** 1149–1150.

24. LEDERBERG, J., R. E. SHOPE & S. C. OAKS, Eds. 1992. Emerging Infections, Microbial Threats to Health in the United States. Washington, DC: National Academy Press.

25. TIRRELL, S., R. E. SHOPE, J. M. MEEGAN & C. J. PETERS. 1985. Rift Valley fever diagnosis, surveillance, and control. Fourth International Conference on the Impact of Viral Diseases on the Development of African and the Middle East Countries. Rabat, Morocco, April 14-19.

The Emergence of New Plant Diseases

The Case of Insect-transmitted Plant Viruses

P. K. ANDERSON

Agricultural Institute of Canada (AIC)
Field Project on Insect-Transmitted Plant Pathogens
Universidad Nacional Agraria Apartado OR-8
Managua, Nicaragua

F. J. MORALES

Virology Research Unit
Centro Internacional de Agricultura Tropical (CIAT)
Apartado 6713
Cali, Colombia

INTRODUCTION

Diseases caused by plant pathogens are a principal constraint to agricultural production. The etiological agents causing plant disease include fungi, bacteria, mycoplasmas, spiroplasmas, viruses and viroids. Although accurate global figures for crop loss assessment are not available, it is generally accepted that, of the various plant pathogens, viruses rank second only to fungi with respect to the yield losses they cause [1].

The viruses are currently classified into 35 groups or families [2] (FIG. 1). The majority (25) of the classified virus taxa are transmitted by invertebrate vectors, primarily insects (TABLE 1). Harris [3] reviewed the arthropod and nematode species confirmed as competent vectors (TABLE 2). However, these numbers, accepted as given, can be somewhat misleading. For example, in the case of the whiteflies (Aleyrodidae), of the 1156 identified whitefly species, only three species have been confirmed as competent vectors of plant viruses. Yet, the sweet potato whitefly, *Bemisia tabaci* (Gennadius) is known to transmit at least 9 distinct geminiviruses in crops in the Americas, [4] and the damage caused by these viruses each year often reaches millions of dollars. The six insect families considered to be most important as insect vectors of plant viruses are the Aphididae (aphids), Cicadellidae (leafhoppers), Delphacidae (planthoppers), Aleyrodidae (whiteflies), Chrysomelidae (leaf beetles) and Thripidae (thrips).

The best available source for crop loss estimates is Cramer [5] who compiled crop loss estimates from available sources to cover world crops. Even with the limited knowledge that existed in virology thirty years ago, a significant proportion of crop loss could be attributed to insect-transmitted viruses (TABLE 3). And, numerous epidemics caused by insect-transmitted viruses during the first three-quarters of this century are well documented. Planthopper-transmitted Fiji reovirus threatened the sugar industry in the early 1900s and caused epidemics in Fiji and Australia in the 1950s, 1960s and 1970s. [6]

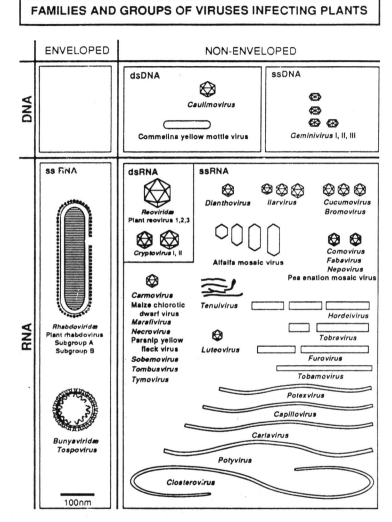

FIGURE 1. The families and groups of plant viruses (from Francki *et al.* 1991[2], used with permission from Springer-Verlag).

Likewise, the sugarbeet industry in the western United States was almost destroyed by the leafhopper-transmitted beet curly top geminivirus in the 1920s. The planthopper-transmitted rice hoja blanca tenuivirus caused a 25% and 50% loss of the total rice crop in Cuba and Venezuela in 1956[7] and complete loss of many rice fields in Colombia in 1958.[8] After two separate epidemics in the 1950s and 1960s the disease virtually disappeared from the

TABLE 1. Principal Modes of Transmission for the Virus Families and Groups

Virus Family or Group	Principal Mode of Transmission
Alfalfa mosaic virus	aphids; seed
Badnavirus	mealybugs; leafhoppers; seed; pollen
Bromovirus	beetles; seed
Bunyaviridae (Tospovirus)	thrips; seed
Capillovirus	contamination[a]
Carlavirus	aphids; whiteflies
Carmovirus	contamination; beetles
Caulimovirus	aphids
Closterovirus	aphids; seed
Comovirus	beetles; seed
Cryptovirus	seed; pollen
Cucumovirus	aphids; seed
Dianthovirus	soil-borne
Fabavirus	aphids
Furovirus	fungi
Geminivirus	whiteflies; leafhoppers
Hordeivirus	contamination; seed
Ilarvirus	seed; pollen
Luteovirus	aphids
Maize chlorotic dwarf virus	leafhoppers
Marafivirus	leafhoppers
Necrovirus	fungus; seed
Nepovirus	nematodes; seed
Parsnip yellow fleckvirus	aphid
Pea enation mosaic virus	aphids; seed
Potexvirus	contamination
Potyvirus	aphids; mites; whiteflies; fungi; seed
Reoviridae	leafhoppers; planthoppers
Rhabdoviridae	aphids; leafhoppers
Sobemovirus	beetles; seed
Tenuivirus	planthoppers
Tobamovirus	contamination
Tobravirus	nematodes; seed
Tombusvirus	contamination; seed
Tymovirus	beetles; seed

[a] Contamination refers to viruses readily transmitted following passive inoculation of suscepti-ble hosts (*e.g.*, natural contact with infected plants in the field; people, animals or tools brushing against infected and healthy plants).

region for almost 15 years. In 1981, serious, widespread outbreaks recurred in Colombia, Ecuador, and Venezuela causing losses of up to 100%.[9] By 1977, 162 million cacao trees had been lost in Ghana owing to the mealybug-transmitted cacao swollen shoot badnavirus, and tree eradication continued at a rate of 15 million trees per year.[10]

CONDITIONS GIVING RISE TO DISEASE

Levins *et al.*[11] have identified numerous conditions which they believe may give rise to diseases of humans. The same conditions may be considered to explain the emergence of insect-transmitted plant viruses.

TABLE 2. Systematic Classification of Nematode and Arthropod Species Known to be Vectors of Plant Pathogens[a]

Class	Order	Family Name	Common Name	Number of Species
Nematodea	Dorylaimida	Trichodorida	nematodes	13
		Longidoridae	nematodes	15
Aracnida	Acarina	Eriophyidae	mites	2
Insecta	Homoptera	Aphididae	aphids	193
		Cicadellidae	leafhoppers	36
		Delphacidae	planthoppers	22
		Pseudococcidae	mealybugs	18
		Aleyrodidae	whiteflies	3
		Membraciadae	membracids	1
	Hemiptera	Lygaeidae	lygaeids	2
		Piesmidae	lacebugs	1
		Miridae	mirids	1
	Thysanoptera	Thripidae	thrips	4
	Coleoptera	Curculionidae	weevils	11
		Chrysomelidae	leafbeetles, flea beetles	6
		Coccinellidae	coccinelids	2
		Meloidae	blister beetles	1
	Diptera	Agromyzidae	leafminers	2

[a] After Harris, 1981.[3]

Ecological or Social Change Brings Host (Plant Species) into Contact with Unknown Vector or Pathogen

Cacao is native to South America. It was introduced into West Africa where most of the cacao is currently produced. The first introductions of cacao into West Africa occurred in the latter part of the 19th century. In Ghana, for instance, cacao production increased from 0.3 tons of cacao beans

TABLE 3. Estimated Damage Attributable to Insect-transmitted Plant Pathogens (ITPPs) in the United States[a]

Crop	% Damage Attributable to All Pests[b]	% Damage Attributable to ITPPs
Wheat	25.4%	0.8%
Oats	30.6%	2.7%
Barley	25.4%	3.9%
Potato	28.8%	4.4%
Sugarbeet	30.2%	5.2%
Sugarcane	33.7%	9.7%
Pear	19.5%	10.3%
Cherries	23.9%	9.6%
Strawberries	46.6%	3.0%
Orange	21.2%	5.0%
Grapes	35.5%	10.8%

[a] Based on data from Cramer.[5]
[b] Insects, weeds, fungi, bacteria, viruses, *etc.*

in 1891, to over 40,000 tons in 1911. The swollen shoot disease was first noticed in 1936[12] after the virus had been introduced into cacao plantations by mealybugs from indigenous trees.[13] Since that year, over 160 million trees, affected by cacao swollen shoot virus, have died or have been eradicated in West Africa.[14]

New Habitats Are Created Which Permit a Rare or Remote Microorganism (Virus) to Become Abundant and in Contact with Plants

Rice yellow mottle sobemovirus was originally restricted to the Kisumu district of Kenya.[15] Following large irrigation projects in East Africa, rice and other grasses became extensively cultivated or disseminated, respectively, in the region, persisting through dry seasons. These intensive rice cultivation practices and an abundance of diverse grass species led to a build up of the virus and its beetle vectors in the irrigated areas, resulting in the dissemination of the virus throughout West Africa.[16]

The Pathogen Is Introduced into Previously Unexposed Populations

Citrus tristeza closterovirus (CTV) was probably introduced into South America (via Argentina) from Africa, between 1927 and 1930.[17] The presence of an efficient aphid vector, *Toxoptera citricidus* (Kirkaldy), also introduced from Asia into South America, accelerated the dissemination of CTV in this continent. The vectors occurring in the United States, *Aphis gossypii* Glover and *A. spiraecola* Patch, are inefficient by comparison. By 1950, over 6 million citrus trees had been destroyed in a single state of Brazil (São Paulo), and several million more citrus trees have died or declined in South America and the United States (California, Florida) since 1930.[18]

Population Movements Bring Non-resistant (Plant) Populations into Contact with Populations That Harbor Pathogens without Severe Morbidity

Potato Y potyvirus (PVY) is common in commercial potato-growing areas, where this virus is found with the absence of noticeable symptoms. These PVY strains are readily transmitted by aphids from potatoes to several non-cultivated hosts. The wild PVY sources are responsible for the severe epidemics that have occurred in commercial plantings of tobacco, tomato, and pepper in areas with a history of potato production.[19]

(Plant) Populations Become More Vulnerable to Disease through Drugs, Malnutrition, or Environmental Stresses

Bean common mosaic is the most widely distributed disease of the common bean *Phaseolus vulgaris*. Pathogenic variability is represented by at least

10 well-characterized bean common mosaic potyvirus (BCMV) strains, which interact with specific recessive genes present in some bean genotypes in a gene-for-gene fashion. Disease (common mosaic) occurs when the virus strain possesses matching pathogenicity genes or when bean genotypes do not possess genes for resistance to the virus. However, incorporation of a single non-specific dominant gene effectively prevents the chronic systemic infection of all bean genotypes by any of the known strains of the virus. Furthermore, the virus cannot become seed-borne in bean genotypes possessing the dominant gene. Because BCMV has a restricted host range outside *Phaseolus vulgaris*, the monoculture of bean cultivars possessing monogenic dominant resistance should result in the eradication of the disease. However, this type of resistance can "break down" when common mosaic-resistant cultivars are grown under high temperature conditions, characteristic of tropical summertime seasons as well as some marginal areas where beans have been displaced by more profitable cash crops. When challenged by certain BCMV strains, the bean common mosaic-resistant plants grown under high-temperature stress develop systemic necrosis (hypersensitivity) that results in total yield loss (plant death).[20]

Pathogens Spill Over from Other Species

Cucumoviruses are multi-component isometric plant viruses that contain genomic, subgenomic, and sometimes other RNA species known as satellite RNAs, which may significantly modify pathogenicity. Cucumoviruses have a broad pathogenicity spectrum, infecting no less than 775 species in different plant families, particularly species of the Cucurbitaceae.[21] Since the 1970s, several cucumoviruses have been isolated from severely affected species of the Fabaceae. The pathogenic specialization of cucumoviruses to legumes is now a well-documented phenomenon, which continues to grow in complexity due to the seed-transmission of cucumoviruses and continuous attack of cultivated legumes by cucumoviruses transmitted by aphids from other crops, mainly cucurbits.

Pathogens Evolve towards Greater Virulence

Plant pathogens in general have demonstrated their ability to overcome vertical resistance conditioned by single resistance genes in plants. A gene-for-gene relationship has been demonstrated for bean common mosaic virus (BCMV) and its host *Phaseolus vulgaris*, the common bean. Briefly, pathogenic variants of BCMV have been arising as a result of the cultivation of bean genotypes possessing strain-specific recessive genes for BCMV resistance. The most recently characterized strains of BCMV have the ability to attack most recessive resistance genes present in bean cultivars. Additionally, necrosis-inducing BCMV strains capable of challenging non-specific dominant resistance are now predominant in certain bean-growing regions, particularly in East Africa.

Mixed Pathogen Communities Allow for Hybridization or Recombination Creating New Pathogenic Types

The possibility of creating infectious pseudo-recombinants between the DNA A and B components of the bean golden mosaic, African cassava mosaic and tomato golden mosaic geminiviruses has already been demonstrated.[22-24]

Bioengineered Organisms Escape or Are Released into the Environment and Evolve

The introduction of an avirulent mutant (strain 1) of tomato mosaic tobamovirus in northern England, during 1972-1974, in order to protect tomato seedlings from more virulent strains (cross-protection phenomenon), resulted in the appearance of virulent forms of strain 1 in all commercial plantings where the mutant had been released.[25,26]

EPIDEMIOLOGICAL POTENTIAL FOR NEW PLANT DISEASE

It is clear, that under appropriate conditions, new diseases have emerged and will continue to emerge. The critical issue is not the emergence of new diseases, but rather the rate of emergence of new diseases. Over the last two decades, epidemics caused by insect-transmitted plant viruses, in crops of economic and nutritional importance, have increased in frequency and severity.

In the case of Nicaragua, for example, during a survey conducted in the mid-1950s in 21 localities, Litzenberger and Stevenson[27] observed virus infection in 19 crop plants, but no plant virus epidemics were reported in the country prior to 1980. Since 1980, four separate virus epidemics have affected cropping systems in Nicaragua. In the 1984–85 production cycle, the Nicaraguan tobacco company, TANIC, reported yield losses ranging from 17–64% in their production fields due to the necrotic strain of potato Y potyvirus, transmitted by aphids. A complex of plant pathogens (corn stunt spiroplasma, maize bushy stunt mycoplasma, maize rayado fino virus), all transmitted by the leafhopper *Dalbulus maidis* (DeLong and Wolcott), caused disease in maize plantings which attained epidemic levels in Nicaragua by the mid-1980s with damage fluctuating between 60–100%, where damage is defined as reduction in crop yield. In 1986, yield losses due to these pathogens totaled 29,445 T, representing an economic loss of US $5,005,700.[28] And, in 1987, the maize pathogens were responsible for damage of up to 60% over a 12,000 ha area in Nicaragua.[29] In the 1990 production cycle, an unidentified whitefly-transmitted geminivirus reduced average tomato yields by 25% in the principal tomato-producing zone of Nicaragua.[30] By the following production cycle, 1991, the virus epidemic had become so severe that many tomato fields were 100% infected and producers were abandoning their fields.[31] And, since 1990, one of the principal bean-producing zones reports that bean yields have dropped 82%, from 508 kg/ha to 91 kg/ha, owing to infection by a whitefly-transmitted geminivirus.[32]

Traditionally, Latin America has produced its own staple crops (maize, beans, rice, cassava, potatoes) and a limited number of export crops—cotton and the so-called dessert crops (coffee, tea, chocolate, bananas, sugar cane)—to generate foreign exchange. Export crops were cultivated in fairly well-defined areas and cropping cycles, under rain-fed conditions. The pressure to increase production, in order to generate the foreign exchange for ever-increasing foreign debts in the face of falling world market prices for traditional export crops, has led to dramatic changes in agricultural production in Latin America. Cultivation of traditional exports has expanded in space (increased acreage) and time (irrigated year-round cultivation). And, export crops have become more diverse, giving rise to the current tendency to cultivate non-traditional exports (*e.g.,* melons, mangos, papaya, passion-fruit, Tahiti lime, vegetables) for North American and European off-season markets. The demands of the economic world order are changing the face of agriculture in Latin America, and concurrently creating the conditions which are leading to an ever-increasing rate of emergence of new plant diseases.

CONFRONTING UNCERTAINTY: THE CASE OF BEAN GOLDEN MOSAIC VIRUS IN LATIN AMERICA

Perhaps the single most illustrative example of changing agricultural environments and their effect on the incidence of viral diseases is that of a whitefly-transmitted geminivirus in the lowlands of Latin America. This is the bean golden mosaic virus (BGMV) transmitted by the sweet potato whitefly, *Bemisia tabaci* (Gennadius). The common bean (*Phaseolus vulgaris* L.) is one of the main staple foods in Latin America, particularly among the rural and urban poor. Brazil alone grows over five million hectares of dry beans, which contribute 6.7% and 16.0% of the calories and proteins, respectively, consumed by the urban poor. In Central America, beans are equally important in the diet of all people in the region often being consumed three times a day. Despite its small area (489,368 km^2) Central America devotes twice as much of its geographical area to the cultivation of beans (735,000 ha) as does Brazil. Beans are also produced in some Caribbean islands, such as Cuba (26,000 metric tons [MT]), the Dominican Republic (55,000 MT) and Haiti (56,000 MT), where they also play an important nutritional role in the diet of the lower socio-economic classes.

Despite the large area planted with beans in Central America, productivity is low (495 kg/ha) compared to the average expected yield (over 1,500 kg/ha) in most bean-producing regions of the United States and other temperate countries in the world. Biotic constraints, particularly diseases, are the main factors responsible for the low productivity of the common bean in Latin America. While the number of fungal and bacterial pathogens of beans has remained relatively stable in the past decades, the number of viruses affecting beans has been steadily increasing, owing to the introduction of new germplasm and, more importantly, to the commercial expansion of export commodities, causing changes in the population dynamics of insect vectors and the number of plant viruses recorded.

BGMV is the most devastating viral pathogen of beans in tropical Latin America. It is estimated that over 2,500,000 ha of beans are currently under attack by BGMV, and that at least an additional one million hectares cannot be planted every year due to the possibility of total yield losses, mainly during the dry seasons of the year, when whitefly populations peak. BGMV has become a widespread problem and is now known to cause epidemics in at least 13 Latin American countries; it is considered to be the limiting biotic factor to bean production in Latin America.[33]

As a general rule, crop plants must be protected from viral infection during the first, vegetative stages of plant development. The earlier the infection the greater the resulting damage. Early infection of BGMV in susceptible red bean varieties results in 100% yield reduction due to high incidence of flower abortion and pod deformation.[34] By the time that virus symptoms manifest in the plant, the infection has become systemic and actions taken by the producers have little impact.

The occurrence of BGMV epidemics is unpredictable as a result of the close association that exists between climatic conditions, the population dynamics of the insect vector, and the survival of virus reservoirs in nature. The two tactics most frequently implemented by producers to protect their crops from the uncertainty of BGMV infection are the use of BGMV-tolerant[a] bean varieties and insecticides to reduce populations of vectors. The use of insecticides for managing vector populations is problematic. Populations of *B. tabaci* have become so resistant that most insecticides are no longer effective. This ineffectiveness is resulting in a series of expensive and damaging practices to the producers and the environment: increased number of insecticide applications, use of more costly and more toxic systemic insecticides, the use of insecticides not registered for crop production, and the use of untested alternative pesticides.

Despite the continual screening of bean germplasm since 1972, not a single BGMV-immune bean genotype has been found to date. Nonetheless, some black-seed genotypes have been intensively used as sources of tolerance. And, over the last two decades, CIAT has liberated more than 20 bean varieties demonstrating increasingly greater resistance to BGMV. However, the level of tolerance achieved does not prevent the occurrence of significant yield losses in situations of high disease pressure. Additional mechanisms of resistance have been recently identified in different bean genotypes, and their recombination has yielded promising results. It is apparent that none of the new BGMV-tolerant genotypes developed can be deployed in regions where they may be exposed to high virus/vector pressure without additional protective measures.

---

[a] Tolerance in plant pathology is defined as the ability to endure disease without serious injury or crop loss.

Plant disease forecasting, based on the use of mathematical modeling, represents a strategy to confront uncertainty of plant disease infection, and has been shown to be successful for numerous pathosystems[b] in Europe, North America and Australia.[35] A successful forecasting system is characterized by importance, usefulness, cost effectiveness, multi-purpose applicability, reliability, simplicity and availability.[36] The BGMV pathosystem possesses basic attributes that suggest it is a good candidate for the development of a successful forecasting system. Bean golden mosaic is a significant constraint to crop protection when it appears, but it is not continually present; it is important but sporadic in time and space. Detection technology and effective crop management methods for BGMV are available; thus, a forecast would be useful. Given that BGMV infection often results in total crop loss, investing in a forecasting system would be cost effective for most producers. And, a forecasting system for the whitefly-transmitted BGMV would serve the development of forecasting efforts for the other whitefly-transmitted viruses which are affecting tomatoes, melons, cotton and tobacco in Latin America. The challenge, then is to assure that the forecasting system which is developed is based on sound biological and environmental data (reliable), easily implemented by growers and technicians (simple) and uses data collection and communication technology which are appropriate and accessible to the growers and technicians (available).

For the BGMV system, the most important epidemiological characteristic is the number of vectors immigrating into the bean fields. An analytical system model exists which can predict crop damage caused by BGMV when whitefly immigration into bean fields is measured (Levins and Anderson, unpublished manuscript, 1991).[37] One of the advantages of a systems model is that it can be readily adapted from one location or environment to another. This is an important feature for a pathosystem, such as BGMV, which is distributed over a broad geographical/ecological range, or for a local disease which has the epidemiological potential to become widespread.

However, by the time that levels of immigrating whiteflies are actually measured, the infections have occurred and it is too late for the producer to plan or take action. The forecasters of greatest value are positive pre-planting forecasters,[35] *i.e.*, a model that predicts, before planting takes place, that an outbreak is likely to occur. Depending on the forecast, producers can then select from a menu of options. For example, if predicted damage is too high, growers may choose to plant an alternative crop. With an intermediate level damage, use of available BGMV-tolerant bean varieties would provide adequate crop protection. When little damage is forecast, producers may choose to increase acreage and use a less tolerant, more preferred bean variety.

For that reason, the existing analytical system model must be linked to a simple empirical model which will predict the number of whiteflies coming

---

[b] Pathosystem is defined here as a pathogen and the biological organisms (*e.g.*, pathogen hosts, pathogen reservoirs, vector, reproductive hosts of vectors) involved in the reproduction, transmission and survival of the pathogen.

into the field sufficiently ahead of the planting to allow producers to make their choices. Empirical data exist that suggest that whitefly abundance is correlated with the extensive cultivation of reproductive hosts of *Bemisia tabaci* and rainfall. A collaborative research effort (Morales and Anderson, unpublished) is being set up to conduct and coordinate research and data collection which is expected to lead to an empirical-systems model to predict BGMV epidemics and form the basis for a BGMV warning system.

CONCLUSIONS

The study of plant virus epidemics, including the monitoring, modeling and prediction of epidemics of recognized plant viruses as well as new plant viruses, has been a totally neglected science in Latin America and is only an emerging area of pursuit in the developed-economy countries. One of the current challenges of virology is to move forward not only in molecular virology but also in virus epidemiology. Continued advances in molecular techniques will result in the generation of data that will answer academic questions regarding virus systematics as well as provide tools that will allow for easier detection and diagnosis of new diseases. However, advances in the area of botanical (virus) epidemiology are as important as the continued development of molecular virology. While it is not possible to study diseases before they appear, it is possible to develop general frameworks, analytical tools and a menu of strategies to deal with diseases once they have appeared. The case study of bean golden mosaic virus illustrates a disease which took almost two decades to emerge but for which tools still do not exist to adequately confront the problem.

Levins *et al.*[11] consider that once a disease appears and is recognized, the existing array of molecular, immunological, physiological and epidemiological tools can be mobilized to confront it. This may be true in the context of developed-economy contexts, or even internationally supported health programs in the developing-economy countries. However, as new plant virus problems come to the attention of producers and scientists in Latin American agricultural research institutions, it is evident that the capacity to identify, characterize and manage plant viruses in this part of the world, has actually diminished in relation to previous decades, owing to the deteriorated economic situation of most Latin American nations. Thus, Latin America is currently struggling with complex virus problems caused by the changing agricultural environments, which affect both export and staple commodities but unfortunately lacks sufficient human and financial resources to confront these problems.[38]

Quarantine programs which may prevent, or slow down, the introduction of new plant pathogens are not in place in most Latin American countries because of lack of trained personnel and finances to maintain the programs. Laboratory facilities to diagnose viruses once new viral diseases are observed are limited to the International Agricultural Centers or the wealthier universities in the region who can afford to purchase, service and maintain expensive equipment and pay salaries that will retain trained scientists and technicians. Few scientists are trained to study plant virus epidemiology and implement virus management strategies from a conceptual framework of virus epidemiology.

The economics which drive environmental/agricultural changes and lead to new virus epidemics are intimately linked to the emergence of new human epidemics as well. The displacement of traditional food staples by the expansion of traditional exports and the introduction of non-traditional exports have exposed the staple crops to new stresses commonly found in areas marginal for agricultural production. The virus epidemics affecting people's staple foods create conditions for malnutrition which then become part of the environment and pre-condition for the emergence of new human disease and human epidemics.

The science of epidemiology has, to-date, developed within the fields of human, veterinary and botanical epidemiology in an independent and compartmentalized fashion. The study of epidemiology across fields has the potential to inform and enrich studies in each field. Recent theoretical work on plant virus epidemiology[39] has borrowed heavily from concepts developed in human epidemiology (*e.g.*, MacDonald's conceptual framework, vectorial capacity, reservoir potential). Study across the fields of epidemiology has enriched the development and application of virus epidemiology. Conversely, scientists working in human epidemiology may find that research with plant pathosystems, where experiments are easier to establish and hosts may be manipulated without ethical considerations, may allow for the development and testing of concepts which would be difficult to test in human pathosystems. A more integrated approach to the epidemiology of infectious disease would expedite the development of botanical epidemiology and link it more intimately to human epidemiology.

In the face of the alarming rate with which new diseases are emerging both in plant and human communities, there is an urgent need to develop and promote teaching and research programs in integrated disease epidemiology in order to develop appropriate frameworks, tools, and protection strategies as well as to train scientists and field workers who will be called on to further the understanding of and protect human, animal and plant populations from the new diseases that continue to emerge. For the developing-economy countries, it is imperative that the international donor community begin to establish projects and fund work in integrated epidemiology, including botanical/virus epidemiology as readily as they fund and set up projects in molecular biology and biotechnology.

REFERENCES

1. MATTHEWS, R. E. F. 1992. The Fundamentals of Plant Virology. San Diego, CA: Academic Press.
2. FRANCKI, R. I. B., C. FAUQUET, K. L. KNUDSON & L. BROWN. 1991. Classification and Nomenclature of Viruses: Fifth Report of the International Committee for Taxonomy of Viruses (Arch. Virol. Supplementum 2). Vienna: Springer-Verlag.

3. HARRIS, K. F. 1981. Arthropod and nematode vectors of plant viruses. Ann. Rev. Phytopathol. **19**: 391–426.
4. ANDERSON, P. K. 1993. La naturaleza compleja de la problematica de mosca blanca y el reto para la sanidad vegetal. *In* Memoria de Taller Nacional de Mosca Blanca, Managua, Nicaragua, 16 y 17 Julio, 1992. P. K. Anderson, A. Chavarria & F. Guharay, Eds. Managua, Nicaragua: CATIE/MAG-MIP.
5. CRAMER, H. H. 1967. Plant Protection and World Crop Production. Leverkusen, Germany: Bayer (Pflanzenschutz-Nachrichten).
6. RYAN, C. C. 1988. Epidemiology and control of Fiji Disease virus of sugarcane. Adv. Dis. Vector Res. **5**: 163–176.
7. UNITED STATES DEPARTMENT OF AGRICULTURE. 1960. Hoja blanca: Serious threat to rice crops. USDA/Agric. Res. Serv. Bull.
8. GARCES-OREJUELA, C., P. R. JENNINGS & R. L. SKILES. 1958. Hoja blanca of rice and the history of the disease in Colombia. Plant Dis. Rep. **45**: 949–953.
9. ZEIGLER, R. S. & F. J. MORALES. 1990. Genetic determination of replication of rice hoja blanca virus within its planthopper vector, *Sogatodes oryzicola.* Phytopathology **80**: 559–566.
10. BOS, L. 1982. Crop losses caused by viruses. Crop Prot. **1**: 263–282.
11. LEVINS, R., C. ALBUQUERQUE DE POSSAS, T. AWERBUCH, U. BRINKMANN, I. ECKARDT, P. EPSTEIN, N. MAKHOUL, C. PUCCIA, A. SPIELMAN & M. E. WILSON. 1993. Preparing for new infectious diseases. Harvard School of Public Health. Boston, MA (Working Paper No. 8).
12. STEPHEN, W. F. 1937. A new disease of cacao in the Gold Coast. Trop. Agric. (Trinidad) **14**: 84.
13. POSNETTE, A. F. 1947. Virus diseases of cacao in West Africa. I. Cacao viruses IA-1D. Ann. Appl. Biol. **34**: 388–402.
14. LEGG, J. T. 1979. The campaign to control the spread of cacao swollen shoot in Ghana. *In* Plant Health: The Scientific Basis for Administrative Control of Plant Parasites. D. L. Ebbels & J. E. King, Eds. Blackwell Scientific Publications. Oxford, UK.
15. BAKKER, W. 1970. Rice yellow mottle, a mechanically transmissible virus disease of rice in Kenya. Neth. J. Plant Pathol. **76**: 53–63.
16. BAKKER, W. 1974. Characterization and ecological aspects of rice yellow mottle virus in Kenya. Agric. Res. Reports 829, 152 pp.
17. MENEGHINI, M. 1946. Sobre a natureza e transmisibilidade da doen a 'Tristeza' dos citrus. O Biologico **12**: 285–287.
18. BAR-JOSEPH, M., S. M. GARNSEY & D. GONSALVES. 1979. The closteroviruses: A distinct group of elongated plant viruses. Adv. Virus Res. **25**: 93–168.
19. SIMONS, J. N., R. A. CONOVER & J. M. WALTER. 1956. Correlation of occurrence of potato virus Y with areas of potato production in Florida. Plant Dis. Rep. **40**: 531–533.
20. DRIJFHOUT, E. 1978. Genetic Interaction between Phaseolus vulgaris and Bean Common Mosaic Virus with Implications for Strain Identification and Breeding for Resistance. Doctoral Thesis. Wageningen Agricultural University, Wageningen, the Netherlands.
21. PALUKAITIS, P., M. J. ROSSINCK, R. G. DIETZGEN & R. I. B. FRANCKI. 1992. Cucumber mosaic virus. Adv. Virus Res. **41**: 281–348.
22. GILBERTSON, R. L., S. H. HIDAYAT, J. P. EPAMINODAS, M. R. ROJAS, Y. M. HOU & D. P. MAXWELL. 1993. Pseudorecombination between infectious cloned DNA components of tomato mottle and bean dwarf mosaic geminiviruses. J. Gen. Virol. **74**: 23–31.
23. STANLEY, J., R. TOWNSEND & S. J. CURSON. 1985. Pseudorecombinants between cloned DNAs of two isolates of cassava latent virus. J. Gen. Virol. **66**: 1055–1061.
24. VON ARNIM, A. & J. STANLEY. 1992. Determinants of tomato golden mosaic virus symptom development located on DNA-B. Virology **186**: 286–293.
25. FLETCHER, J. T. & J. M. ROME. 1975. Observations and experiments on the use of an avirulent mutent strain of tobacco mosaic as a means of controlling tomato mosaic. Ann. App. Biol. **81**: 171–179.
26. FLETCHER, J. T. & D. BUTTLET. 1975. Strain changes in populations of tobacco mosaic virus from tomato crops. Ann. Appl. Biol. **81**: 409–412.

27. LITZENBERGER, S. C. & J. A. STEVENSON. 1957. A preliminary list of Nicaraguan plant diseases. Plant Dis. Rep. (Suppl.) **243:** 1–19.
28. URBINA, R. 1986. Incidencia del achaparramiento en el cultivo de maiz y su impacto en el pais. Ministerio de Agricultura y Reforma Agraria (MIDINRA). Managua, Nicaragua.
29. CIMMYT. 1990. CIMMYT 1989 Annual Report (International Maize and Wheat Improvement Center). Beyond Subsistence: New Options for Asian Farmers. Mexico, DF: CIMMYT.
30. SIMAN, J., D. GOMEZ, P. ROSSET, I. RIVAS, B. GUERRERO & R. DAVILA. 1992. Diagnostico de los factores que incidieron en el rendimiento y en la rentabilidad de tomate en la sexta region. *In* Avances Tecnicas: Abril 1990–Marzo 1992. Managua, Nicaragua: CATIE/MAG-MIP.
31. GOMEZ, D. & J. SIMAN. 1992. Diagnostico fitosanitario de invierno sobre tomate en la sexta Region, Matagalpa, Nicaragua, 1991. *In* Avances Tecnicas: Abril 1990-Marzo 1992. Managua, Nicaragua: CATIE/MAG-MIP.
32. ANDERSON, P. K., A. CHAVARRIA & F. GUHARAY, Eds. 1993. Memoria de Taller Nacional de Mosca Blanca, Managua, Nicaragua, 16 y 17 Julio 1992. Managua, Nicaragua: CATIE/MAG-MIP.
33. GALVEZ, G. & F. J. MORALES. 1989. Whitefly-transmitted viruses. *In* Bean Production Problems in the Tropics. H. F. Schwartz & M. A. Pastor-Corrales, Eds. Cali, Colombia: CIAT.
34. MORALES, F. J. & A. I. NIESSEN. 1988. Comparative response of selected *Phaseolus vulgaris* germ plasm inoculated artificially and naturally with bean golden mosaic virus. Plant Dis. **72:** 1020–1023.
35. THRESH, J. M. 1986. Plant virus disease forecasting. *In* Plant Virus Epidemics: Monitoring, Modelling and Predicting Outbreaks. G. D. McLean, R. G. Garrett & W. F. Ruesink, Eds. Sydney, Australia: Academic Press.
36. CAMPBELL, C. L. & L. V. MADDEN. 1990. Plant Disease Epidemiology. New York: John Wiley & Sons.
37. ANDERSON, P. K. 1994. El insecto vector: *Bemisia* sp. *In* Bean Golden Mosaic Research Advances. F. J. Morales, Ed.: 125–143. Cali, Colombia: CIAT.
38. MORALES, F. J. 1992. Viruses and the changing agricultural environment in the lowlands of Latin America. *In* Fifth International Plant Virus Epidemiology Symposium on Viruses, Vectors and the Environment, Bari, Italy, 27–31 July 1992, pp. 67–68.
39. ANDERSON, P. K. 1991. Epidemiology of Insect-transmitted Plant Pathogens. Doctoral Thesis. Harvard School of Public Health, Boston, MA.

Vector-borne Emerging Pathogens

General Discussion

THOMAS MONATH: I shall take the chairman's prerogative and pose the first question to Dr. Anderson. Host abundance may determine vector density, and this is fundamental to the dynamics of transmission. This interaction is complex if such hosts are incompetent as reservoirs of the pathogen in question. The hosts that permit the vector to flourish may, therefore, actually diminish the force of its transmission. The case of St. Louis and western equine encephalitis transmitted by *Culex tarsalis* in the western United States is instructive. During the summer the vector shifts from feeding on birds to large mammals and is diverted from the main reservoir in the transmission cycle. This suggests a dynamic interplay involving different hosts as sources of blood and of virus.

Because plants provide food for vectors, particular agricultural practices might influence transmission of vector-borne infection. This year, for example, rodent-borne hantavirus infection gained prominence because of an outbreak in the western United States, and the availability of piñon nuts as food for the rodent reservoir seems to have played a role in this outbreak. Plants similarly provide nutrients for mosquitoes and other vectors. Would you comment on the role of agriculture in these trophic resources.

PAMELA K. ANDERSON: Similar events characterize the relationships between plants, their pathogens, and vectors. When certain non-cultivated host plants invade a field and come to predominate, those vector insects that preferentially feed on them tend to concentrate in their vicinity. Such plants can actually be manipulated as refugia that divert pests from the crop-system. This provides a kind of trap-crop strategy for protecting economically valuable crops. Indeed, host-pathogen-vector relationships are complex.

Your comment on rodent density and plant availability is similarly intriguing. Changes in agricultural practice frequently permit rodents to proliferate, and they, in turn, may serve as reservoirs for human pathogens.

STEPHEN MORSE: This raises the interesting possibility that large nonhuman mammals near an endemic focus may serve a zooprophylactic role. Are there examples in which removal of a particular host precipitates an outbreak of human disease?

RICHARD LEVINS: Uwe Brinkmann spoke of such a situation that affected a community in Africa. The residents originally raised pigs; but when they converted to Islam, these animals were destroyed. The mosquitoes then turned their attention to people. These are complex situations in which common sense may not apply because reservoir density may increase as well as decrease the problem. If a smaller proportion of a larger population bites people, the resulting epidemic is difficult to predict.

RICHARD CASH: Another example of zooprophylaxis occurred in Pakistan, where David Nalen showed that a coating of mud diverted anopheline mosquitoes from feeding on water buffalo. When the mud was washed off by rain, the malaria vectors would feed on these preferred hosts instead of entering houses where they bite people and transmit malaria. A buffalo washing system might be used to reduce risk of malaria. Lyme disease presents an interesting system in which any number of interventions against the transmission of the agent of Lyme disease seem possible. These might include changing ecology, eliminating voles, mice, or deer, ensuring that people wear proper clothing and examine themselves for ticks and so on. How does one decide on an appropriate intervention where there are so many different possibilities?

ANDREW SPIELMAN: Although various kinds of interventions are available for use against Lyme disease, each generally requires the active participation of local property owners. An almost universal failure of the general population to understand risk, however, constitutes a major obstacle to effective implementation of interventions. Even the well-educated residents of the enzootic sites near the site of this conference seem unsatisfied with any environmental action that offers less than a promise of complete protection. People often refuse to invest in tick-suppression efforts on their own properties, for example, because their neighbors may fail to act similarly. They frequently express the fear that they may acquire infection on their neighbor's neglected property in spite of their own efforts. Few people seem to conceive of community level of risk. A partially effective vaccine, paradoxically, would readily be accepted.

Deer elimination effectively reduces risk of Lyme disease by reducing the abundance of vector ticks. Mouse reduction may also limit risk. There is a short-term danger to public health in these activities, however, because vector ticks may concentrate their feeding on people if they fail to be swept up by wild animals. Brush removal, especially by fire, seems useful. Insecticidal applications also are useful, either when applied in impregnated surrogate nesting material or by direct application. Communities debate the use of these measures with vehemence, but as yet, with little direction.

LEONARDO MATA: Although, for many years, Costa Rica appeared to be free of *Aedes aegypti*, I suspect that remote foci continued to be present there. In any event, this vector of dengue virus has now become abundant enough to be the cause of a catastrophic epidemic that began on October 7, 1993. More then 4,000 cases have been recognized so far, and the epidemic continues. The resulting level of criticism of the government has been so intense that the next presidential elections may be affected.

This experience leads me to identify a series of research objectives that are particularly relevant to this emergent disease. We should ask: How rapidly can these vector mosquitoes proliferate in a tropical environment? How rapidly can an apparently dengue-free region become vulnerable to outbreaks of this disease? What interventions can be used to reduce such an ongoing outbreak? Can the density of these mosquitoes be reduced to a level at which risk is slight? It is interesting that in Latin America, only Argentina and Panama presently appear to be risk-free, although the vector is present in Panama.

MONATH: I agree that these are the crucial research questions that should be applied to such a situation. We could spend the entire symposium discussing the series of questions that you've raised.

TAMARA AWERBUCH: Many of these vector-borne infections emerge and reemerge owing to diverse factors. Changes in the land produce new water sources and landscapes that permit reservoir hosts to proliferate. Each may contribute to the emergence of disease. An understanding of these processes requires a system that combines these many components into a synthetic structure that lends itself to qualitative and quantitative analysis. These many components should be studied not in isolation but together as an integrated system. The use of mathematical modeling would facilitate resolution of such complex interactions.

MONATH: This issue of complexity bears on the choice of surveillance methods for emergent infections and intervention strategies. Landscape changes may produce a profound effect on human health, as in the case of Lyme disease and Oropouche and Guanarito virus. Such changes have long intrigued health scientists. Landscapes have been transformed by economic development projects, as by the construction of the Volta Dam, the opening of the transAmazon highway and the creation of the vast Sudanese and Sri Lankan irrigation schemes, and numerous integrated programs of study have been set up to evaluate their impact on human health. Although certain development projects caused no obvious health problems, others were the source of major epidemics. Certain projects exacerbated malaria, others caused schistosomiasis, *etc.* In many instances the studies were interesting, viruses and other agents were isolated, and much was learned. But because such studies generally lacked a mechanism for linkage to relevant interventions, this approach has tended to become senescent.

A section of the United States Public Health Service once dealt with water management and its impact on human disease. Although this Centers for Disease Control unit was entirely devoted to the study of the health impact of environmental change, that infrastructure no longer exists. In the event that such long-term environmental changes should occur, no governmental structure exists for dealing with the problem. How will health policy planners identify appropriate and cost-effective interventions against future threats of vector-borne disease or other disease outbreaks?

RITA COLWELL: In the case of cholera, for example, policy planners should receive the following information. Exposed people can benefit from a personal protection measure that is used to curb river blindness (onchocerciasis). Drinking water should be filtered through swatches of cloth during appropriate times of year in order to reduce the number of copepods that are ingested. These minute arthropods carry numerous vibrios. If the massive ingestion of these pathogens were reduced, epidemics would be averted, although the pathogen would not be eliminated.

There is a hubris in the statement that smallpox is eradicated because it carries the assumption that the virus will never reappear. Perhaps many members of this group are not fully convinced that smallpox is permanently eradicated. In spite of this doubt, other eradication-directed decisions are being made that create the potential for long-term damage to the public health.

GARY SMITH: I agree that we should not be thinking about eradication of infection nearly as much as reduction of ill-health. Our goal should be to ameliorate disease, and this can be greatly facilitated using modeling. Modeling can help in advising policy planners because it reduces confusing detail. The first comments should be simple, and complexity added as necessary. The patterns that occur in nature generally can, thereby, be reproduced quickly because only a few significant factors generally influence the system. Once that degree of understanding is attained, the advice should be couched as follows, "We think this group of things, this very small group of things, should probably be attacked first because in our opinion it's what accounts for most of what one sees. I'm not trying to describe all the little ups and downs that there are, but the main thrust of it."

ANDERSON: A mathematical model that has been developed to analyze insect-transmitted plant pathogens in Nicaragua includes 13 kinds of intervention strategies. Thereby, we identified certain essential features of a major epidemic in corn that occurred in the mid-1980s as well as others that require further explanation. This model helps provide a rational basis for research. It is particularly useful in fund-raising efforts because the logic of our program can readily be demonstrated. It has profoundly influenced the planning of our field work.

CHARLES PUCCIA: Can we anticipate that new diseases may emerge more rapidly in certain kinds of environments than in others? Changes in tropical habitats, for example, may be more persistent than changes of similar magnitude in temperate environments and this may promote disease outbreaks.

SPIELMAN: Indeed tropical environments tend to be vulnerable to vector-borne disease because they are so seasonally constant. The seasonal changes that occur in temperate regions limits the duration of any infestation of vector arthropods. These inherently changeable environments enjoy a certain resilience when they are subject to artificial change. Vector arthropods generally flourish where the environment is unstable. Therefore when an appropriate disturbance occurs in a tropical environment, it tends to cascade over many years. Any change is magnified more in a tropical environment than in a temperate environment simply because of the absence of seasons.

PUCCIA: Although seasonal changes in the tropics are less marked than in temperate regions, seasonality generally is pronounced. Even a marine environment fluctuates with season.

SPIELMAN: Outbreaks of Rift Valley fever virus in Egypt appear to be anthroponotic, and this provides an interesting example of changing land-use practices and the emergence of disease. Houses in the Nile Valley have been built increasingly close to the water table following construction of the Aswan Dam, and this has resulted in the proliferation of *Culex pipiens* mosquitoes. This has permitted a marked increase in the prevalence of human lymphatic filariasis. The resulting microfilaremias increase the competence of these mosquitoes for many viruses, including Rift Valley fever virus. This complex chain of causation seems to have led to the emergence of anthroponotic Rift Valley fever, now in its second invasion of Egypt.

Hantaviruses and the Hantavirus Outbreak in the United States

A Case Study in Disease Emergence[a]

STEPHEN S. MORSE[b]

The Rockefeller University
1230 York Avenue, Box 120
New York, New York 10021

In the summer of 1993, patients, mostly young and previously healthy adults, were admitted to hospitals in New Mexico, Arizona, and Colorado with fever and acute respiratory distress syndrome (ARDS); a number subsequently died from pulmonary edema and respiratory failure. Serology and detection of genetic sequences by polymerase chain reaction (PCR) provided evidence that a previously unrecognized hantavirus was the cause of the outbreak (the condition is now called Hantavirus Pulmonary Syndrome).[1] By PCR, the same sequences were identified in tissues taken at autopsy from several of the patients and in tissue samples from local rodents. The major reservoir was *Peromyscus maniculatus*, the deer mouse, which was also the rodent most commonly trapped near houses in the area. A high proportion (20–30%) of captured *Peromyscus maniculatus* proved positive by serology or PCR.

Hantaviruses are naturally occurring viruses of rodents.[2–5] Human disease is zoonotic, as a result of contact with infected rodents or their secretions. (Human infection probably occurs most commonly through inhaling virus shed by the infected mouse in its urine; for those with possible exposure to rodents in the field, the CDC has recently issued recommendations for protective measures.[6]) Anecdotal reports from the Four Corners area suggested that the winter had been unusually wet, resulting in a large crop of nuts and other rodent food, and, in turn, an exceptionally large rodent population, and thereby offering more opportunities for people to come in contact with infected rodents (and, hence, the virus). This has apparently been confirmed by the ecological research station at Sevilleta, New Mexico, which documented a tenfold increase in area rodent populations between May 1992 and May 1993. The abnormally high precipitation has been attributed to climatic events caused by the western Pacific phenomenon known as El Niño.

Since the start of the current outbreak in the Southwest this year (and including a few cases occurring before the outbreak and confirmed retrospectively), the federal Centers for Disease Control and Prevention (CDC) tabulated 45 confirmed cases in 12 states (as of November 16, 1993), with 27

[a] Supported by grant R01 RR03121 and, in part, by grant RR01180, from the National Institutes of Health, US DHHS.
[b] Tel.: (212) 327-7722; FAX: (212) 327-7974 or 327-7172.

199

deaths (60% mortality) (figures are from ref. 1, with update by personal communication). Of the 45 cases confirmed by November 1993, 32 were in New Mexico, Arizona, and Colorado, in the Four Corners area. The current outbreak began in late 1992, with cases peaking in May through July 1993. After peaking in the summer, cases appear to have dropped off sharply since August. Earlier cases so far confirmed (retrospectively) include a case from July 1991; one person in Oregon (outside the Four Corners area) was identified as having been infected in July 1992. In June 1993, a man in Louisiana died of a similar acute respiratory distress syndrome. Preliminary results on the hantaviral sequences detected in lung tissue from this patient indicates another hantavirus, apparently quite distinct from the "Four Corners" virus but in the same evolutionary lineage. The rodent reservoir in this case is unknown but may be *Peromyscus gossypinus*, the cotton mouse.

It is very likely that re-examination of earlier cases of respiratory distress will identify sporadic occurrences of hantaviral infection, and that this and other hantaviruses will be found when stored tissue samples from rodents are tested. Indeed, although cases of disease were not identified in California until this year, PCR examination of tissues from deer mice collected in August 1983 in Sweetwater Canyon, Mono County, California yielded viral genetic sequences that appear closely related to the Four Corners virus.[7] In another study, published in 1985, hantavirus-seropositive *Peromyscus* were also identified in California, New Mexico, and Colorado in 1983;[8] the virus thus identified was probably Four Corners, although more specific characterization was not possible with the tests then available. These results suggest that the viruses that cause hantavirus pulmonary syndrome have been present in rodent hosts for some time (and might even be as ancient as the host species itself), but are newly recognized as a cause of human disease.

Several references give sequence data and some construct phylogenies (refs. 9–14, and abstract by Schmaljohn *et al.*, American Society for Virology annual meeting 1993). As a very rough generalization, the viruses tend to group by species of reservoir (rodent) host (viruses from the same or closely related hosts tend to be more closely related, suggesting possible coevolution), and secondarily by geography. The considerable diversity of the hantaviruses, and the apparent number of geographic variants, could be the result of high evolutionary rates or of long evolutionary history; it is most likely the result of both. The number of different rodent species that harbor hantaviruses and the wide distribution of these viruses suggest a long history. The range of North American hantaviruses is presently unknown, but, on the basis of present evidence, they appear to be numerous and widely distributed.[8] The host *Peromyscus spp.* are ubiquitous in North America, the range of *P. maniculatus* covering virtually all of the United States (and much of North America, even extending into parts of Mexico) except for portions of the southeast and south central United States (in some parts of which *P. gossypinus* is found). The only North American hantavirus known previously, Prospect Hill, was first identified in meadow voles (*Microtus pennsylvanicus*), originally in Maryland and later also in the Midwest, but has not been associated with human disease. *Microtus pennsylvanicus*, the reservoir host for Prospect Hill, is found across North America (except for extreme northern portions) approximately to the latitude of northern Georgia. Detection of Prospect Hill virus in voles from both the East and the Midwest suggests that the virus is likely to be widespread in populations of that rodent. As additional sequences from the North American viruses become available,[14] there will be important refinements in the phylogenetic analysis. From presently available data, both of the newly recognized peromyscine hantaviruses (Four Corners and the Louisiana virus) are distinct from hantaviruses previously identified, but appear to group with Prospect Hill.[7,14] There would appear to be about 30% divergence between Prospect Hill and Four Corners at both the nucleotide and amino acid levels.[7,14] Molecular comparisons of Prospect Hill, which appears to have low virulence for humans, with the highly virulent hantaviruses causing the pulmonary syndrome will be of interest, for the insights such comparisons may give into understanding the genetic basis for the virulence, host range, and tissue tropism of these newly recognized viruses (that is, why these viruses are so virulent in humans and why they cause clinical manifestations different from other hantaviruses). Molecular comparisons ("molecular epidemiology", as Myers termed it[15,16]) have already been useful for identifying source and geographic locale of infection.[14]

The pulmonary syndrome seen in North America is a non-classical manifestation of hantavirus infection, which classically involves a hemorrhagic fever with renal syndrome. Hantaviruses constitute a genus in the family Bunyaviridae; other members include Hantaan (the cause of Korean hemorrhagic fever), and Puumala and others in Europe, all of which classically cause hemorrhagic fevers with renal syndrome (fever, bleeding, kidney damage, and shock) (TABLE 1). Numerous hantaviruses are found worldwide in various rodent species (TABLE 1), and a given hantavirus is often closely associated with a particular rodent host. The type member of the genus is Hantaan,[17] whose major natural host in Asia is the striped field mouse, *Apodemus agrarius* (an alternative host, found in the Balkans, is *Apodemus flavicollis*). At present, some 100,000–150,000 cases of Korean hemorrhagic fever (Hantaan infection) are diagnosed annually in China alone;[3,4] numbers have increased over the years as rice planting (a good environment for *Apodemus agrarius*) has become more extensive,[5] leading to both more mice and greater opportunities for human contact. A related virus, Seoul, was originally described in rats in Korea; viruses closely related to Seoul have since been identified in urban rats living in American cities[3,4,18] and elsewhere.[19] It has been suggested that rats carried on ships from Asia may have introduced Seoul virus into the United States. In Korea, Seoul virus has caused hemorrhagic fever with renal syndrome similar to Hantaan virus, but usually considerably milder. In the United States, seropositive individuals have been found in some inner city areas, and there is some evidence for a possible association with chronic renal disease, including renal hypertension[4,18] Since hantaviruses follow the distribution of their reservoir hosts, it is likely that the rat-borne hantaviruses

TABLE 1. Some Hantaviruses and Their Rodent Reservoirs[a]

Virus[b]	Primary Host	Distribution	Disease
Hantaan	*Apodemus agrarius*	Asia (China, Korea, E. Russia)	Epidemic hemorrhagic fever; Korean hemorrhagic fever; classic HFRS[c]
	Apodemus flavicollis	S. Europe	Severe HFRS[c]
Rat-borne (Seoul, etc.)	*Rattus*	Worldwide	Acute epidemic hemorrhagic fever (Asia); ?chronic renal disease
Puumala	*Clethrionomys glareolus*	N. and E. Europe	Nephropathia epidemica
Prospect Hill	*Microtus pennsylvanicus*	USA	None known
Leakey[d]	*Mus musculus*	USA (Texas)	None known
"Four Corners"[e]	*Peromyscus spp.*	USA (west, south)	Hantavirus Pulmonary Syndrome (fever with acute respiratory distress)

[a] From LeDuc *et al.* (ref. 3), modified.
[b] Each named virus is likely to represent a group containing geographic and other variants; a number of specific names have been proposed for some of the individual isolates.
[c] Hemorrhagic fever with renal syndrome.
[d] Status uncertain.
[e] Informal name. The North American hantaviruses found in *Peromyscus spp.* have not yet received names; the number of related viruses and their distribution are unknown. "Four Corners" virus was originally identified in *Peromyscus maniculatus* in the southwestern United States, and the same or closely related viruses have been identified in *Peromyscus maniculatus* in other parts of the United States. A distinct virus has been identified in Louisiana; the rodent host is unknown. Another hantavirus has been reported in *Sigmodon hispidus* (Cotton rat, in Florida).

(Seoul virus and its close relatives) are as universal and cosmopolitan as domestic rats themselves.

In Europe, in addition to classic Hantaan in *Apodemus* species in eastern Europe, there is also the less severe nephropathia epidemica, associated with Puumala virus; the vole *Clethrionomys glareolus*, widespread in Europe, is the usual reservoir host.[2] Periodic reports from Europe of new isolates,[13,20,21] and of cases from new areas[22–24] suggest that there are undoubtedly other hantaviruses in geographically isolated populations of rodents, and in other rodent species. As suggested by the recent identification of the "Four Corners" and related U.S. hantaviruses, and by the earlier serosurveys of rodents in the United States,[8] this will be equally true here (and probably worldwide).[19] The identification of Puumala virus (normally found in voles) in wild *Mus musculus* (house mouse) in Yugoslavia[21] suggests that, under suitable conditions, interspecies transfer of hantaviruses among different rodent species can occur, and has probably occurred in the past.

What are the lessons for students of emerging diseases? First of all, as with other emerging viruses, this virus is not new. Periodic discoveries of "new" zoonoses (*e.g.*, Guanarito, the cause of Venezuelan hemorrhagic fever,[25] a newly recognized rodent-borne virus related to other arenaviruses such as Junin) also suggest that the known viruses are only a fraction of the total number that exist in nature.

Emerging infections can be defined as infections that either are newly appeared in the population, or are rapidly increasing their incidence or expanding their geographic range.[26–28] Re-emerging diseases are those that were previously decreasing but are now rapidly increasing again. Many examples of disease emergence involve the introduction of a virus into a human population, typically from a zoonotic (animal) reservoir, followed by dissemination. "Viral traffic" (or more generally, "microbial traffic"), the mechanisms that allow or facilitate the introduction of existing viruses into new settings, such as new host species or new host populations, seems to underlie most instances of disease emergence: with rare exceptions, most outbreaks of "new" viruses, and many other emerging infections, appear to be caused by microbial traffic. Viral (or microbial) traffic can serve to introduce viruses into a human population from a zoonotic source or to spread a previously isolated virus to new hosts.[26–28]

Changing environmental conditions are often responsible for viral traffic. Because people are major agents of ecological change, often these changes are brought about by human activities. As one example involving another species, bovine spongiform encephalopathy (BSE) appeared in Britain within the last few years as a probable interspecies transfer of scrapie from sheep to cattle.[29] Changes in rendering processes, allowing incomplete inactivation of scrapie agent, were probably responsible.[30]

Introduction of viruses into the human population is often the result of human activities, such as agriculture, that cause changes in natural environments. Often, these changes place humans in contact with previously inaccessible viruses. Some of the activities that can precipitate emergence include specific types of agricultural practices, or changes in agricultural practices. The example given earlier with Hantaan, in which rice planting increases zoonotic transmission both by causing increases in the population of the virus' natural host, *Apodemus agrarius*, and also by providing a setting for contact between zoonotic host and people, is not an isolated instance. Junin virus, the cause of Argentine hemorrhagic fever, is an Arenavirus normally maintained in the rodent *Calomys musculinus*. Conversion of grassland to maize cultivation favored a rodent that was the natural host for this virus, and human cases increased in proportion with expansion of maize agriculture[5,31] Other viruses with similar life histories are known, *e.g.* the other arenaviruses and hantaviruses, and more are likely to appear as new areas are placed under cultivation.

I have previously suggested[27,28] that disease emergence could be viewed as a two-step process, first introduction and then dissemination, and that emphasis should therefore be placed on understanding the conditions that affect each of these steps. One might speculate that evolution may be especially important in the transition from step 1 to step 2, where adaptedness to the new host may be critical to the eventual success of a newly introduced virus.[27,28] The success of a new virus depends on its ability to spread within the human population after introduction.[26–28,32–34] Here, too, human intervention is providing increasing opportunities for dissemination of previously localized viruses. As with HIV, human activities can be especially important in disseminating newly introduced viruses that may not yet be well adapted to the human host and may not be efficiently transmitted from person to person. A similar situation would apply to viruses already present for some time in a limited or isolated human population. Human population movements, upheavals caused by migration or war, can greatly affect this process. Human migration to cities can introduce remote viruses to a larger population. Migrations from rural areas to cities continue unabated. The United Nations has estimated that by the year 2025, 65% of the world's population (including 61% of the population in less-developed regions) will live in cities.[35] Similar opportunities are offered on a global scale by rapid air travel, as suggested by studies modeling the spread of influenza epidemics[36] and of HIV.[37,38] Thus, in many of its aspects, the problems of understanding the appearance and control of emerging diseases are often as much social as scientific, and the social sciences must be included in approaches to emerging diseases.

The hantavirus outbreak in the United States was identified because an alert clinician noticed something unusual. The CDC, thus alerted, carried out field investigations in cooperation with the states, and instituted appropriate responses. Once the cause was identified, such relatively simple measures as rodent control could greatly reduce risk. But all of this depended on the initial recognition of an unusual event and on having some system to respond appropriately. Thus, effective disease surveillance, to provide early warning of emerging infections, is the essential first step,[26,39,40] and must be backed by a commitment to an appropriate rapid response. It is widely agreed that world surveillance capabilities are critically in need of improvement.[39,40] As a result of financial constraints and diminished interest, surveillance capabilities are weaker today than they were in 1968, when the World Health Assembly held preliminary discussions on global surveillance.

To summarize, the emergence of the hantaviruses illustrates a number of key points about emerging infections.[27,28] Most have probably existed for many years, and perhaps caused occasional cases of disease but (as in the Four Corners) were unrecognized until environmental conditions precipitated an outbreak large enough to be noticed. To judge from their numbers and distribution (both geographically and in numbers of rodent species involved), hantaviruses probably diversified many years ago, and periodic human outbreaks are now due to human exposure to mostly previously evolved viruses carried in natural hosts. Human activities can precipitate the emergence of a "new" disease by causing environmental disruption or other conditions that favor a natural host (*e.g.,* rice planting causes increased local populations of *Apodemus agrarius*). Human activities, such as environmental disruption, agriculture, population migration and rural urbanization, now offer greater opportunities for dissemination of infectious agents and natural hosts or vectors that have hitherto been geographically isolated, thus increasing opportunities for new infections.[27,28] Finally, as probably happened with the rat-borne hantaviruses, some may be disseminated by human activities and may establish themselves in new settings far from home. These patterns of course are not unique to the hantaviruses. Other rodent-borne pathogens, such as the Arenaviruses, have quite similar ecology, and even the primate retroviruses show some parallels,[15,41] suggesting these mechanisms as quite general causes of emerging diseases.[27,28] Early warning systems (refs. 26–28, 39, and Bryan *et al.*, pages 346–361 in this volume), based on networks for surveillance of "new" infections, are an essential and greatly needed defense against emerging infections.

ACKNOWLEDGMENTS

I thank Drs. Gerald Myers, Ho Wang Lee, Stuart Nichol, C. J. Peters, James Le Duc, Pierre Rollin, and James Childs for discussions and for sharing unpublished data on hantaviruses.

REFERENCES

1. CDC. 1993. Update: Hantavirus pulmonary syndrome—United States, 1993. MMWR [Morbidity and Mortality Weekly Reports] **42**: 816–820, October 29, 1993.
2. LeDuc, J. W. 1987. Epidemiology of Hantaan and related viruses. Lab. Anim. Sci. **37**: 413–418.
3. LeDuc, J. W., J. E. Childs & G. E. Glass. 1992. The Hantaviruses, etiologic agents of hemorrhagic fever with renal syndrome: a possible cause of hypertension and chronic renal disease in the United States. Annu. Rev. Public Health **13**: 79–98.
4. LeDuc, J. W., J. E. Childs, G. E. Glass & A. J. Watson. 1993. Hantaan (Korean hemorrhagic fever) and related rodent zoonoses. *In* Emerging Viruses. S. S. Morse, Ed.: 149–158. New York: Oxford University Press.
5. Johnson, K. M. 1993. Emerging viruses in context: An overview of viral hemorrhagic fevers. *In* Emerging Viruses. S. S. Morse, Ed.: 46–57. New York: Oxford University Press.
6. CDC. 1993. Hantavirus infection—Southwestern United States: Interim recommendations for risk reduction. MMWR **42** (No. RR-11): 1–13.
7. Nerurkar, V. R., K.-J. Soong, D. C. Gajdusek & R. Yanagihara. 1993. Genetically distinct hantavirus in deer mice. Lancet **342**: 1058–1059.
8. Tsai, T. F., S. P. Bauer, D. R. Sasso, S. G. Whitfield, J. B. McCormick, T. C. Caraway, L. McFarland, H. Bradford & T. Kurata. 1985. Serological and virological evidence of a Hantaan virus-related enzootic in the United States. J. Infect. Dis. **152**: 126–136.
9. Xiao, S.-Y., R. Yanagihara, M. S. Godec, Z. A. Eldadah, B. K. Johnson, D. C. Gajdusek & D. M. Asher. 1991. Detection of hantavirus RNA in tissues of experimentally infected mice using reverse transcriptase-directed polymerase chain reaction. J. Med. Virol. **33**: 277–282.
10. Arthur, R. R., R. S. Lofts, J. Gomez, G. E. Glass, J. W. LeDuc & J. E. Childs. 1992. Grouping of hantaviruses by small (S) genome segment polymerase chain reaction and amplification of viral RNA from wild-caught rats. Am. J. Trop. Med. Hyg. **47**: 210–224.
11. Grankvist, O., P. Juto, B. Settergren, C. Ahlm, L. Bjermer, M. Linderholm, A. Tärnvik & G. Wadell. 1992. Detection of nephropathia epidemica virus RNA in patient samples using a nested primer-based polymerase chain reaction. J. Infect. Dis. **165**: 934–937.
12. Antic, D., C. Y. Kang, K. Spik, C. Schmaljohn, O. Vapalahti & A. Vaheri. 1992. Comparison of the deduced gene products of the L, M and S genome segments of hantaviruses. Virus Res. **24**: 35–46.

13. XIAO, S.-Y., G. DIGLISIC, T. AVSIC-ZUPANC & J. W. LEDUC. 1993. Dobrava virus as a new hantavirus: Evidenced by comparative sequence analysis. J. Med. Virol. **39:** 152–155.
14. NICHOL, S. T., C. F. SPIROPOULOU, S. MORZUNOV, P. E. ROLLIN, T. G. KSIAZEK, H. FELDMANN, A. SANCHEZ, J. CHILDS, S. ZAKI & C. J. PETERS. 1993. Genetic identification of a hantavirus associated with an outbreak of acute respiratory illness. Science **262:**914–917.
15. MYERS, G., K. MACINNES & B. KORBER. 1992. The emergence of simian/human immunodeficiency viruses. AIDS Res. Hum. Retroviruses **8:** 373–386.
16. OU, C.-Y., C. A. CIESIELSKI, G. MYERS, et al. 1992. Molecular epidemiology of HIV transmission in a dental practice. Science **256:** 1165–1171.
17. LEE, H. W. 1982. Korean hemorrhagic fever. Progr. Med. Virol. **28:** 96–113.
18. GLASS, G. E., A. J. WATSON, J. W. LEDUC, G. D. KELEN, T. C. QUINN & J. E. CHILDS. 1993. Infection with a ratborne hantavirus in US residents is consistently associated with hypertensive renal disease. J. Infect. Dis. **167:** 614–620.
19. LEDUC, J. W., G. A. SMITH, J. E. CHILDS, F. P. PINHEIRO, J. I. MAIZTEGUI, B. NIKLASSON, A. ANTONIADIS, D. M. ROBINSON, M. KHIN, K. F. SHORTRIDGE, M. T. WOOSTER, M. R. ELWELL, P. L. T. ILBERY, D. KOECH, E. ROSA, T. SALBE & L. ROSEN. 1986. Global survey of antibody to Hantaan related viruses among peridomestic rodents. Bull. WHO **64:** 139–144.
20. GLGIC, A., N. DIMKOVIC, S.-Y. XIAO, G. J. BUCKLE, D. JOVANOVIC, D. VELIMIROVIC, R. STOJANOVIC, M. OBRADOVIC, G. DIGLISIC, J. MICIC, D. M. ASHER, J. W. LEDUC, R. YANAGIHARA & D. C. GAJDUSEK. 1992. Belgrade virus: A new hantavirus causing severe hemorrhagic fever with renal syndrome in Yugoslavia. J. Infect. Dis. **166:** 113–120.
21. DIGLISIC, G., S.-Y. XIAO, A. GLIGIC, M. OBRADOVIC, R. STOJANOVIC, D. VELIMIROVIC, V. LUKAC, C. A. ROSSI & J. W. LEDUC. 1994. Isolation of a Puumala-like virus from *Mus musculus* captured in Yugoslavia and its association with severe hemorrhagic fever with renal syndrome. J. Infect. Dis. **169:** 204–207.
22. PETHER, J. V. S., N. JONES & G. LLOYD. 1991. Acute hantavirus infection. Lancet **338:** 1025.
23. PHILLIPS, M. J., S. A. N. JOHNSON, R. K. THOMSON & J. V. S. PETHER. 1991. Further UK case of acute hantavirus infection. Lancet **338:** 1530–1531.
24. KULZER, P., R. M. SCHAEFER, E. HEIDBREDER & A. HEIDLAND. 1992. Retrospective diagnosis of small epidemic of haemorrhagic fever with renal syndrome. Lancet **339:** 940–941.
25. SALAS, R., N. DE MANZIONE, R. B. TESH, R. RICO-HESSE, R. E. SHOPE, A. BETANCOURT, O. GODOY, R. BRUZUAL, M. E. PACHECO, B. RAMOS, M. E. TAIBO, J. G. TAMAYO, E. JAIMES, C. VASQUEZ, F. ARAOZ & J. QUERALES. 1991. Venezuelan haemorrhagic fever. Lancet **338:** 1033–1036.
26. MORSE, S. S. 1990. Regulating viral traffic. Issues Sci. Technol. [Natl. Acad. Sci.] 7: 81–84.
27. MORSE, S. S. 1991. Emerging viruses: Defining the rules for viral traffic. Perspect. Biol. Med. **34:** 387–409.
28. MORSE, S. S. 1993. Examining the origins of emerging viruses. *In* Emerging Viruses. S. S. Morse, Ed.: 10–28. New York: Oxford University Press.
29. MORSE, S. S. 1990. Looking for a link. Nature **344:** 297.
30. WILESMITH, J. W., J. B. M. RYAN & M. J. ATKINSON. 1991. Bovine spongiform encephalopathy: Epidemiological studies on the origin. Vet. Rec. **128:** 199–203.
31. DE VILLAFAÑE, G., F. O. KRAVETZ, O. DONADIO, R. PERCICH, L. KNECHER, M. P. TORRES & N. FERNANDEZ. 1977. Dinámica de las comunidades de roedores en agro-ecosistemas pampásicos. Medicina (B. Aires) **37** (Suppl. 3): 128–140.
32. SHOPE, R. E. & A. L. EVANS. 1993. Assessing geographic and transport factors, and recognition of new viruses. *In* Emerging Viruses. S. S. Morse, Ed.: 109–119. New York: Oxford University Press.
33. ANDERSON, R. M. & R. M. MAY. 1979. Population biology of infectious diseases. Nature **280:** 361–367 & 455–461.
34. ANDERSON, R. M. & R. M. MAY. 1991. Infectious Diseases of Humans: Transmission and Control. Oxford, UK: Oxford University Press.

35. UNITED NATIONS. 1991. World Urbanization Prospects, 1990. New York: United Nations.
36. LONGINI, I. M. JR., P. E. M. FINE & S. B. THACKER. 1986. Predicting the global spread of new infectious agents. Am. J. Epidemiol. 123: 383–391.
37. FLAHAULT, A. & A.-J. VALLERON. 1990. HIV and travel, no rationale for restrictions. Lancet 336: 1197–1198.
38. FLAHAULT, A. & A.-J. VALLERON. 1992. A method for assessing the global spread of HIV-1 infection based on air travel. Mathemat. Pop. Stud. 3: 161–171.
39. HENDERSON, D. A. 1993. Surveillance systems and intergovernmental cooperation. In Emerging Viruses. S. S. Morse, Ed.: 283–289. New York: Oxford University Press.
40. MORSE, S. S. 1992. Global microbial traffic and the interchange of disease. Am. J. Publ. Health 82: 1326–1327.
41. GAO, F., L. YUE, A. T. WHITE, et al. 1992. Human infection by genetically diverse SIV$_{SM}$-related HIV-2 in West Africa. Nature 358: 495–499.

Disease in Evolution: Hantavirus[a]

General Discussion

Moderator and editor, James LeDuc; Main Speakers, James LeDuc,
Ruth Berkelman and Stephen S. Morse

JAMES LeDuc: I would first like to thank Mary for inviting me to participate in this symposium. The topic is timely. I am always anxious to have an
opportunity to talk about my favorite group of viruses, the hantaviruses. I
want to discuss seven items: recognition, virus characteristics, the disease
itself, the hosts, time, chronic disease, and what I have called "more to come."

Recognition

Hantaan virus, when grown in VERO E-6 cells, shows characteristic
cytoplasmic fluorescence that is typical of that seen with all members of this
group of viruses. The isolation of Hantaan virus, and its adaptation to growth
in cell culture, is the key advance that allowed this entire cascade of recognition
of the hantaviruses to start. The disease itself, Korean hemorrhagic fever or
hemorrhagic fever with renal syndrome, had been known in medical communities for many years, at least since the Korean War for western clinicians and
probably for centuries for Asian investigators. But there was never a tool to
provide a specific diagnosis. With the isolation of prototype Hantaan virus
in 1976 by Ho Wang Lee, a tool became available to establish an etiologic
diagnosis. In many ways we were fortunate that the test which was first used
was not very specific, but was quite sensitive. Consequently we were able to
recognize a number of related viruses through serological cross reactions.

Virus Characteristics

Given the isolation of prototype Hantaan virus, we were quickly able to
recognize many other related viruses, including Seoul virus, maintained by
Rattus norvegicus, Puumala virus, the cause of nephropathia epidemica in
Scandinavia and western Europe, Prospect Hill virus, which has been in the
news recently as the most closely related virus to the new "Four Corners"
virus, a virus from Thailand, which we isolated several years ago, and Thottopa-
layam, a virus that had been isolated in the 1960s in India and was never
really classified. In addition to these viruses, there is the Four Corners virus,
and also another virus called Dobrava or Belgrade.

Once we had the original Hantaan virus isolate, we could look at it

---

[a] This version also edited by M. Wilson 3/94.

virologically. It quickly became apparent that this was a bunyavirus (Family Bunyaviridae). Knowing that these were bunyaviruses told us a lot about what we should expect from this group. The bunyaviruses are characterized by a number of genetically and antigenically closely related viruses, but each of these viruses occupies a distinct ecological niche. Some examples are California encephalitis group viruses, comprising a dozen or so different viruses, each maintained by a specific mosquito vector and each occupying a distinct niche. Another group is the phleboviruses with 30 or 40 distinct strains, all antigenically and genetically similar, but ecologically, each fills a distinct niche.

The Disease

In moderate and severe disease, there are five distinct phases; a febrile phase, a hypotensive phase, an oliguric phase, a diuretic phase, and a prolonged convalescence. Some of the clinical presentations are fever, shock, renal impairment, hemorrhages, relative hypervolemia and fluid and electrolyte imbalances. These classic five stages are more or less present in many hantavirus diseases. If we look at the Four Corners virus infections, we see that the pulmonary problems are really part of the classic hypotensive phase. After a febrile onset, patients quickly go into the hypotensive phase. Instead of bleeding into the gut, which is typical of some hantavirus infections, they have vascular leakage into the lungs. Many hantavirus infections can skip some phases, but generally these five phases are characteristic of this group of viruses.

The Hosts

A critical point that is key to understanding the epidemiology of the entire group involves the rodent hosts. Several years ago Ho Wang Lee found that virus or antigen was present in blood, lungs, parotid glands, kidney, saliva, feces, and urine following experimental infection of susceptible rodents, and that neutralizing and immunofluorescent antibodies (IFA) were produced following infection. After animals were infected, they had a short viremia, but then virus was recoverable from their tissues, probably for life. The virus was shed in saliva, feces and especially urine, probably also for the duration of life. Virus persists in the presence of both IFA and neutralizing antibody. As far as we know, there is no clinical disease in rodents following infection. It appears that they reproduce the same as uninfected rodents, they live the same length of time, and they appear to have no adverse effects from infection.

Time

Cases of Korean hemorrhagic fever seen in Korea cluster dramatically in late fall and early winter. By the second week in January, cases almost disappear, although scattered cases may occur throughout the year. This is in part because of the behavior of the people at risk, and in part due to the basic biology of the rodent host. During harvest season, people may go out and live in the fields, where there is ample opportunity for exposure to rodents. Alternatively, the rodents come to humans, as seen during rodent population explosions, or in inner cities.

If we consider rodent hosts and time, a good example is the population density of *Clethrionomys glareolus* in northern Sweden, which is cyclical. There are not only seasonal changes, but also dramatic population fluctuations annually. There can be as much as 1,000 fold difference in population abundance between peak years and immediately following crashes. As might be expected, there is a strong correlation between the incidence of human disease and changes in rodent population densities.

Chronic Disease

We did a lot of work in Baltimore over the past several years looking at an association between past exposure to hantaviruses and subsequent development of chronic renal disease, specifically hypertensive renal disease. A clear, significant association was found between past hantaviral infection, based on the presence of specific antibody to a local strain of hantavirus, and a specific chronic renal disease. Two different populations were examined and compared to the general population of Baltimore, a proteinuria group, where an odds ratio of 11.14 (for hypertensive renal disease) was found, and a dialysis group, where a highly significant p value was seen. These associations were specific for hypertensive renal disease, and unrelated to other causes of chronic renal disease. These observations challenge some of the dogma about infectious diseases and their association with long-term chronic diseases. This is an area that clearly deserves additional attention.

More to Come

There is evidence that acute hemorrhagic fever with renal syndrome exists in parts of the world that are not now considered to be endemic for this disease. For example, among humans in Argentina, where we did some work a couple of years ago in association with a vaccine efficacy trial for Argentine hemorrhagic fever (AHF), we found patients with a clinical diagnosis of mild Argentine hemorrhagic fever, but who were serologically negative for AHF. These patients did, however, possess specific antibodies to hantaviruses. For example, one patient admitted to the hospital with a diagnosis of mild AHF had elevated titers by enzyme immunoassay for IgM and IgG for Hantaan and Puumala viruses, with the IgM titer dropping over time, but the IgG titers persisting. We confirmed these results by both IFA, and more importantly by plaque neutralization tests. It is clear that there are more hantaviruses waiting to be discovered.

. . .

RUTH BERKELMAN: I will describe what happened earlier this year in the

Four Corners area. In early May, a physician took care of a young man who collapsed on the way to the funeral of his girlfriend, who had become sick about five days previously. The physician became curious about what was going on, made phone calls, and came up with five similar cases that had occurred recently, each one seeing a different physician. He notified public health officials, including epidemiologists with the Indian Health Service, the New Mexico Department of Health, and the Office of Medical Investigation in New Mexico. They responded promptly. They originally thought the disease was plague, as plague exists in the area, but the New Mexico State Laboratory did not identify plague as the cause. They also looked for flu and sent specimens to the influenza laboratories at CDC.

About two weeks into the outbreak, the Thursday before Memorial Day, the regional director of the Indian Health Service called CDC and requested assistance. The Department of Health also requested CDC's assistance. We immediately met with our senior virologists and bacteriologists, as well as toxicologists, and developed a lengthy list of possible causes. The disease affected predominantly young adults, who had flu-like symptoms, with fever accompanied by muscle aches; within hours, several of them developed rapid respiratory distress and many died. We also had a girl who collapsed on the dance floor, with no prior symptoms. Questions arose, such as whether all of the cases were related. What would be called a case?

On the Saturday of Memorial Day weekend, we [CDC] sent people to join a New Mexico Department of Health and Indian Health Service Team. Soon there were four state health departments working along with the Indian Health Service, the Navajo Nation Division of Health, the University of New Mexico and CDC. We screened for a broad array of agents, including toxins. We talked about what could it be, but the syndrome did not really match any of the agents well. Most scientists said, for each of many organisms, "It could be, but I don't think so." The high rodent population was discussed along with many other things. About 15 classes of pathogens were being looked at. The serology first signaled that the cause might be a hantavirus.

We had reagents [to look for hantaviruses] because of the earlier work that had been done by the Army on hantaviruses. Without those, it would have taken CDC longer to identify a hantavirus as the etiology. Paired sera from people that had survived showed a rise in antibody to hantavirus. Scientists at CDC immediately did PCR and sequencing. Because sequencing had been done by the Army, we were able to establish that this was a hantavirus. Immunohistochemistry pulled it together, providing evidence that antigen was present in the lung tissues. The [hantavirus] antigen could be seen in the lining of the vessels, which matched the clinical finding of non-cardiogenic pulmonary edema. The capillaries in the lung were leaking.

A phylogenetic tree showed that this hantavirus was not one of the known hantaviruses. It was closest to the Prospect Hill virus, but it was distinct. We knew it was a new virus at that point. Because we knew hantaviruses were associated with rodents, we immediately sent a field team out to trap rodents. Jamie Childs and others trapped rodents around the case homes and found over 60% of their rodent captures were the deer mouse, *Peromyscus maniculatus*. Everywhere they put a trap, they found rodents. Of the *Peromyscus maniculatus* 33% were positive for hantavirus, and by nucleotide sequencing, the virus in the rodents matched the virus found in humans. Over 80% of the rodents captured in the homes were *Peromyscus maniculatus*. We caught more rodents around the case homes than the control homes.

The distribution of the deer mouse extends well into North America. We have no deer mice in the Southeast, but the rest of the United States does. We have found human cases of hantavirus in twelve states to date. We have also found cases outside the range of *Peromyscus maniculatus*, so we believe that there may be different reservoir hosts for the virus. The clinical syndrome in these cases was the same as those in the Southwest. Forty-two cases, with 26 deaths have now been confirmed. Cases tapered off in late summer, but we are concerned that cold weather will bring rodents back into the homes. We have put out a call to physicians to notify public health officials in their states if they have cases of unexplained acute respiratory distress. We are now beginning to figure out the geographic distribution, the magnitude, and the spectrum of this disease. There are still a lot of unanswered questions at this point.

· · ·

STEPHEN MORSE: The range of *Peromyscus maniculatus* and closely related *Peromyscus* species is over much of the United States and covers other portions of North America and Central America. This is the potential distribution of cases of the hantavirus pulmonary syndrome. Most, but not all, cases to date coincide with the distribution of *Peromyscus maniculatus* and are caused by what has unofficially been called Four Corners virus.

BERKELMAN: We are calling the disease hantavirus pulmonary syndrome (HPS). The name of the virus is still being discussed.

MORSE: For now, I'll call it colloquially "Four Corners virus." Hantaviruses represent a virus group found in a number of different rodents. The distribution of a hantavirus will generally follow that of its reservoir rodent host or hosts. Seoul virus, for example, which is rat-borne, has a cosmopolitan worldwide distribution following that of its rat host. Rat-borne hantavirus is in Brazil (South America) and probably every place else with rats.

In the United States there have been cases of HPS outside the range of *Peromyscus maniculatus*. It is not known at this point what the natural host is for these other viruses, for example in cases in Louisiana. It could possibly be another *Peromyscus*. *Peromyscus gossypinus*, for example, is found in a number of places in the Southeast, where *Peromyscus maniculatus* is not found. Or it could be some other rodent. Genetic sequence work done by Stuart Nichol and colleagues at CDC suggests that the virus in the Southeast is likely to be another virus distinct from the Four Corners (hantavirus pulmonary syndrome) virus.

Before the events of 1994, we knew of one naturally occurring, widespread hantavirus in the United States and North America, the Prospect Hill virus, which is not known to cause human disease. It is carried by *Microtus pennsylvanicus*, the meadow vole, a rodent found in the northern portion of North

America. I suspect that the virus can probably be found throughout much of the range of *Microtus*, although we do not really know. There have been identifications of this virus in places as far apart as the Great Lakes area and Maryland's "Prospect Hill," the farm belonging to Carleton Gajdusek of NIH, where the virus was first identified.

Tools are now available to do phylogenetic analysis. One can line up sequences, as Stuart Nichol and his colleagues have done, and look at the evolutionary, if you will, the phylogenetic relationships of these viruses. The hantaviruses are presently split essentially into two major branches, one consisting of Hantaan and Seoul (which you could call the Old World hantaviruses), and another major branch with the European viruses such as Puumala. Grouped with these but branching off separately at different times are the North American viruses, such as Prospect Hill, Four Corners, and others.

Another virus that fits on this phylogenetic tree probably in about the same place as the Four Corners virus is called Sweetwater Canyon. It was identified recently by Rick Yanagihara and colleagues in Gajdusek's laboratory, again by PCR. It probably groups with the Four Corners virus, although, to the best of my knowledge, it has not yet been formally compared to the Four Corners virus. But, on the phylogenetic tree, it seems to be about as far from Prospect Hill as Four Corners is. Interestingly, this virus was identified from a sample taken from *Peromyscus* in California in 1983. That is of significance because there was a case of fatal hantavirus pulmonary syndrome recently in a graduate student at Mammoth Lakes, California. Although sequences are not yet, to the best of my knowledge, fully available from that isolate for comparison with the Sweetwater Canyon virus, it seems very similar. This is suggestive evidence that these viruses have probably been here for a long time in these natural rodent host populations.

Another piece of evidence supporting the relative antiquity of these viruses comes from serosurveys. Work by both Jim LeDuc and by Ted Tsai showed hantavirus reactivity in *Peromyscus* populations from North America using Hantaan as an antigen. Thus, we have seen a tremendous diversification of hantaviruses all over the world, with no evidence at this point of an evolutionary change in virulence.

Molecular epidemiology has been valuable in analyzing this outbreak. Segments of the viruses from a number of the patients from the Four Corners area have been sequenced by PCR. It turns out those sequences, in those segments at least, are essentially identical to corresponding segments in the virus carried by the mice in the same area. The few exceptions are instructive. For example, one person who fell sick in Arizona turned out to have a strain with sequences that grouped exactly with Colorado strains, specifically sequences from Grand Junction. In fact, the patient had been in Colorado. These results indicated that he became infected in Colorado, but did not become sick until he returned to Arizona. Without the benefit of molecular epidemiology his infection probably would have been misclassified. Molecular epidemiology is also useful for being able to tell if a viral strain is a new virus, or has been here for some time. For example, the apparently identical nature of the viral sequences from both—human cases and local mice (including samples at least 10 years old)—all suggest that we are not seeing anything new.

So why now? The short answer, which may or may not be right, is that this was a very good year for the rodent. Cases may have existed sporadically in the past; these may be identified retrospectively with evaluation of stored sera from individuals who have had acute respiratory distress syndrome of unknown etiology.

There have been some claims that this was a result of El Niño, which led to increased rainfall, and more piñon nuts for the rodents to eat. There was indeed a population increase both in *Peromyscus* and in the wood rats in that area. The short explanation is simply a change in the ecology, more rodents, and more opportunity for people to get infected. Why hasn't this been seen in the past? I think one reason is just perhaps the cases were too scattered, too sporadic, and there wasn't a sufficiently high index of suspicion. Ten years ago it might have been possible to identify this virus, but twenty years ago it would not have been possible, simply because the antigens, and other tools, were not available.

What does this portend for the future? There is a very wide distribution of *Peromyscus maniculatus* in North America. It is likely that a number of populations of *Peromyscus* in different parts of the country do indeed have this virus. I think an important question is to know what other populations of *Peromyscus* in what other areas might also harbor the same or a similar virus. The closest relative of this virus is Prospect Hill virus, which is, as far as anyone knows, nonpathogenic for humans. (That is to say, no human disease has been identified.) Although they are fairly close relatives, there is considerable sequence divergence between Prospect Hill and the viruses causing hantavirus pulmonary syndrome. Even in a comparatively well-conserved region, there is still about 35–40% sequence difference. I think it will be instructive to compare, in terms of looking at pathogenesis, the differences in sequences between this virus and its other close relatives. This may help to answer the question about this non-classic presentation of a hantavirus infection. Hantaviruses classically cause hemorrhagic fevers with renal syndrome. With hantavirus pulmonary syndrome, there are limited hemorrhagic manifestations. We are still far from understanding the genetics of virulence in these viruses, and what is responsible for these different expressions of virulence. In some ways, hantaviruses are good examples of emerging viruses because they are diversified, they're worldwide, and in many cases they represent the situation frequently seen with emerging viruses, an ecological change that allows a virus already existing to be introduced into the human population. In some cases, their reservoir hosts are well distributed, but many emerging viruses have also been spread through human activities, as in the case of the rat-borne hantaviruses.

There are many questions about rodent population dynamics that are still unanswered. Data about the transmission of the virus within *Peromyscus* from individual to individual, and the population dynamics of the rodent might allow us to model and better predict the appearance of these diseases.

General Discussion

LeDuc: Are there any questions for any of our presenters?

QUESTION: How is the reservoir maintained in nature and is there any transplacental transmission in the mice population?

LeDuc: We've looked fairly carefully for vertical transmission from infected rodent mother to offspring. That does not appear to happen, at least prior to birth. We have also looked at wounding in free ranging rats in Baltimore, and there seems to be a very nice correlation between antibody prevalence and increased frequency of wounding and also increased mass, indicating older ages. So there's clearly transmission between rats, at least in the inner city. We could make an argument that part of the transmission is saliva based. That is not to exclude aerosol transmission. Certainly humans get infected most often by the aerosol route. There are very good incidental observations, for example, of people walking into contaminated rodent colonies, spending a very short time there, not touching anything, just breathing the air, and subsequently becoming infected.

LAURIE GARRETT: It seems like just about every place where anybody's made a concerted effort to look for it in the rodent population, some kind of hantavirus has been found all over the world. This interesting pattern of evolving a chronic disease cycle in human beings may somehow be a wise evolutionary direction, if you will, for a viral population, instead of causing an acute disease, acute viremia, and possibly die-off of the host. To cause a long chronic disease state would seem to make sense. Do you have any speculations, Jim, on what this means as evolution, when you look at the whole hantavirus family.

LeDuc: In human disease, I do not think that there is a chronic shedding of virus, or that humans in anyway assist in the maintenance of the virus. I think humans are by and large a dead-end host as far as maintenance of the virus is concerned. I think the chronic disease that we are seeing is probably the result of the initial insult of the infection, and that predisposes people to subsequent development of these chronic conditions. And again, that's all speculation. We do not have any real data on that, apart from the associations I mentioned. However, the fact that rodents become infected and apparently live a perfectly healthy normal life, including reproduction, while harboring this virus, indicates a very well-established parasite-host relationship, which would indicate a very longstanding condition.

BERKELMAN: With the hantavirus pulmonary syndrome, those who recover (and about $1/3$ do) have no evidence of long-term effects.

MORSE: There is no denying that hantaviruses are a very successful group of viruses that have probably been evolving for a very long time, given their worldwide distribution and diversity. They would seem to have been diversifying and coevolving with their rodent hosts, possibly over eons.

RICHARD CASH: If I'm not mistaken, most of the cases at the beginning were young men. What is your explanation for that? What is your explanation for the fact that most of these cases are in the Native American population in the Four Corner area, given the distribution of the virus and the distribution of the rodent. Maybe you might speculate on both of those.

BERKELMAN: Usually, if one looks at cases in China and other geographic areas, the distribution is predominantly young male. Actually, in this outbreak it is about even among women and men.

CASH: But they are still of the same age group. It is not children, it is not the elderly. Why is that?

BERKELMAN: Among cases identified to date, the age range is about 11 to 65 years with no one younger, and that's been typical of other hantaviruses as well. I don't have the explanation for that. It may well be that your healthier host can set up an intensive immune reaction, and it may be that this is causing some of the capillary leakiness, but this is only speculation. We checked blood samples of family members of patients; none showed evidence of infection. Are they not around the rodents as much?

CASH: I would think in fact they would be around the rodents more, out there playing in the fields. And why in this particular area? I mean there are lots of communities in the United States that are in close proximity to these rodents. Why in this particular area, in this particular Native American population, which I believe was all Navajo, if I'm not mistaken.

BERKELMAN: It was mainly Navajo, but also Hopi.

CASH: Well they are right in the middle of the Navajo reserves.

BERKELMAN: Yes, and again if you look at the confirmed cases right now, a little under half of the cases are Native American. If you think about the hogans and where people live, that may be part of the explanation; certainly rodents are in places where many of the cases have been living.

CASH: Are there any co-factors? Is there any genetic co-factor in this population? Are there other co-factors, maybe something in the other practices that they carry out, that may relate to their susceptibility?

BERKELMAN: Well, we've looked at a number of things, for example different activities, and have not found much in that arena. Mainly what is being trapped in the home and around the home differentiates risk.

MORSE: Is altitude a factor at all?

BERKELMAN: The issue of altitude has been raised, but I do not think it has been resolved.

QUESTION: Would you like to speculate on whether you believe this could have been predicted? Put it more generally, is there a system of analysis or understanding that you believe could now be put into place that would enable closer prediction about the likelihood of new outbreaks with hantavirus?

MORSE: I see these as two different questions. In answer to the first question, others may feel differently, but I would say "no." When we were on the Institute of Medicine (IOM) committee, thinking up various hypothetical scenarios for diseases threatening the United States, we would have thought it too far fetched to suggest that a relatively ecologically stable area like the Four Corners region would have an outbreak of a new disease, with a totally different pathogenesis from the classic forms of disease caused by that group of viruses, happening in the United States, with high mortality: it would have seemed too much like fiction. So I don't think the events could have been anticipated *a priori*. I think we now have information that allows us to anticipate better. Secondly, I would say that this argues for the value of surveillance. Chance does favor the prepared mind, and if you can't anticipate every possible disease emergence, the least you can do is try to identify it as soon as possible, and act appropriately, as was done here. I can't think of any theoretical basis though, in answer to your question, on which this could have been predicted, specifically. It would have seemed too unlikely, which is what makes it interesting.

BERKELMAN: I also think that an important point here is that this easily could have been missed.

ROBERT E. SHOPE: I cannot claim a special reason for it, but the table in the IOM report which lists the conditions in which the committee thought surveillance should be maintained, number one on the list is acute respiratory disease. So in that sense, perhaps we've predicted it, but I don't think we really did.

MORSE: I suppose I've been as guilty as everyone else in speculating that, had we had adequate surveillance in place, we might have caught HIV sooner. But, in reality, you have to temper that with the thought that HIV, if it had been identified 25 years ago, would have seemed like the least likely pathogen to succeed. It wasn't until we saw its unfortunate success at our great expense that we became aware that you didn't necessarily have to have all the best qualities of a pathogen, high transmissibility for example, to be able to be a successful pathogen and spread through the human population causing serious disease. Political will and social factors are often as important as recognition in controlling disease. This is a lesson we have to remember.

BERKELMAN: Something to note also might be that there may have been epidemics of this in the past. In the southwestern United States in 1918 and 1933, they actually describe something very similar to this. Since 1918 was also the year of the influenza pandemic, it could have just been flu; we don't know. But 1933 has no other explanation. Both were also years of the piñon nut.

NICHOLAS KOMAR: Have any attempts been made to locate cases in Mexico? What types of intervention strategies are possible to prevent this type of outbreak, or to stem the outbreak?

BERKELMAN: Both Canadian and Mexican health authorities were notified. To date we have heard nothing from those areas, but they are on the lookout for it, and have notified their staffs. In terms of what was done to control the outbreak, CDC brought in a number of experts on a couple of different occasions. One group was primarily mammalogists who looked at what control strategies could be used. The first strategy, to get rid of the reservoir host, was discarded because this deer mouse is one of the most common small mammals in North America. The best control strategy is to try to decrease exposure of the human to rodents. To do that, we have worked with the state health departments, the Navajo Nation, and others, and have published guidelines on how to deal with rodents in different settings, how to disinfect, how to clean up. There are programs going on to try to plug up holes in houses. There are educational campaigns for physicians in the area and some nationwide. Both physician/health-care provider education and public education are needed.

When you have an outbreak like this, there is a lot of hysteria, a lot of panic. We had 20 people taking phone calls from the public and physicians for a couple of months. It finally died down, but we had questions like "could my patients possibly have this?" "What do I do?" People wanting to know if they could go camping in the area. Plus, we had questions from all the people in the laboratory and from field workers. It was a fairly substantial undertaking, to say the least.

LeDuc: Ruth, didn't you have a case from Argentina, at least a suspect case?

Berkelman: Yes, C. J. Peters is heading this investigation. C. J. Peters is Chief of our Special Pathogens Branch, and he sent a copy of the MMWR to someone he knows in Argentina, who replied and sent an abstract that said that they had some evidence of pulmonary problems in several of their patients. We still do not know whether this is a hantavirus that's similar to that in the United States. It was just a couple of patients.

Richard Levins: I'm not sure exactly how this might apply to this particular case, but recognizing that rodents are a major reservoir for human viruses, and that the ectoparasites of rodents and the feces are important elements, I would start out by looking at the ecology of rodent feces. Now the exposure to anything carried by the feces depends not only on the production of the feces, but also its survival. There are a number of groups of insects, including the scarab beetles, which are dung beetles, that collect the feces. There are also some ants that do that. So, one possibility is that the production of feces may have increased with the rodent population increase. Another possibility is a decline in the collecting. For instance, the rodents may have increased too rapidly for the ants and the scarab beetles to respond, and therefore the residence time on the ground and exposure would be greater. I am not guaranteeing this because I don't know the scarabs of the Southwest, but I think that instead of focusing on the disease as the object of study, which the CDC has to do, at academic institutions the approach would be to look at the ecology of the rodents in relation to their pathogens and their byproducts, as they cycle through the ecosystem.

LeDuc: The question was raised earlier—could this have been predicted? I think with perfect hindsight that there are indicators here that at least would have given us clues. The known association of both hantaviruses and arenaviruses with rodent populations would lead one to be suspicious whenever there is an increase in a population of rodents. I think that monitoring rodent populations, perhaps could have given us an indication of potential problems. I showed the data from Scandinavia with this cyclic pattern of *Clethrionomys glareolus*, the host of Puumala virus, which is a good example of how it is possible to systematically monitor and predict rodent population fluctuation. So I think, given a very bright group of ecologists that set their minds to this, perhaps it could have been predicted.

SHOPE: Jim, I think what could have been predicted was that there was infection in the rodents. I don't think that any of us would have set up a monitoring program for acute respiratory disease and used hantaan antigens.

LEDUC: Yes, I agree. If one had looked, one would have found virus in the rodents, but one wouldn't have known that it was connected to any disease.

BERKELMAN: Jim, in fact, was a skeptic at first when we came up with the serology. He knew the pulmonary syndrome didn't fit with hanta-viruses.

MORSE: It's a non-classic presentation. But I think the point is well taken. If there's an ecological change that results in an increase in species that are natural hosts for zoonotic infections, even if there isn't a known infection, it's worth keeping an eye on that.

GARRETT: I think the CDC people are being a little modest here. The fact of the matter is, your colleagues in Fort Collins had tipped people off that the ecological conditions looked ripe for an increase in the rodent population, and put out alerts for a watch on plague. So somebody did have their eyes open, and that's probably part of the reason everybody was so well prepared this time.

BERKELMAN: We were all prepared for plague when this first happened. But I will also make a case that if you get into cost effectiveness, your surveillance in response to this kind of situation is going to be far more cost effective than trying to anticipate this kind of event. Keeping track of our rodent populations and hantaviruses in those populations is going to be important at this point, but I think it's almost a black hole to think you're going to anticipate this type of thing.

QUESTION: As a chronic disease epidemiologist, I was actually much more amazed by your chronic renal disease data, which showed a lot more deaths. Did you calculate the population attributable for action? Are you basically telling us all the renal disease in inner city Baltimore is due to hantavirus infections?

LEDUC: No, only a very small part of the renal disease might be associated with past hantaviral infection. The study involved looking at a "normal" population to get a background antibody prevalence rate, which we then age stratified. That sample was drawn primarily from the emergency room at Hopkins Medical Center. Overall antibody prevalence was 0.25% in the "normal" population, as compared to 2.76% among dialysis patients with end-stage renal disease. (ref: Glass, G. E. et al. 1993. Infection with a ratborne hantavirus in US residents is consistently associated with hypertensive renal disease. J. Infect. Dis. 167: 614–620.)

QUESTION: So you don't think it's a good case-control study.

LEDUC: Well, it is a difficult population to work with, but the bottom line is that around 3% of the people that were into end-stage renal disease had antibody to a hantavirus, versus well less then 1% in the normal population.

BERKELMAN: We think it is worth some study.

LEDUC: From a cost-benefit analysis, as a nation we spend a tremendous amount of money on maintenance of end-stage renal disease patients. Three percent of a billion dollars is a lot of money.

PAUL EPSTEIN: I'd like to come back to the question of surveillance for a moment, and whether you think that monitoring vulnerable populations and regions, critical regions, is justified. I know Steve, in the *New York Times* article back in July, talked about ecological conditions, and the six years of drought and one year of rain. There was also a Chief from the Navajo Nation quoted as saying that we've lost our balance with nature. I think it's telling in terms of what that region is. It has been identified as critical by some people who are trying to look at critical regions where diseases may emerge.

MORSE: What criteria? It would be helpful if we set up criteria for identifying critical regions. One obvious one is areas of high biodiversity that are also undergoing ecological change. What other criteria could we establish that would enable us to target the right areas?

EPSTEIN: There is a book that's in manuscript coming out of Clark University looking at nine critical regions, looking at basic life support systems such as water, soil fertility, forest cover.

DONALD ROBERTS: With Lyme disease, we seem to be concerned mostly with *Peromyscus leucopus,* and now with these viruses we're concerned with *Peromyscus maniculatus.* As I recall, these two species are morphologically very similar, and they occur in the same locations in many parts of the United States. Was *Peromyscus* found in the Maryland area?

LEDUC: Prospect Hill virus was originally found in *Microtus.* We did find some antibody-positive *Peromyscus* in Baltimore in park settings. I don't know the species either, but the rates were quite low. I think that's in George Korch's paper (1989. Am. J. Trop. Med. Hyg. **41:** 230–240).

BERKELMAN: We have found hantavirus in other rodents, though the *Peromyscus maniculatus* is the one that has the highest seropositivity rate; quantitatively, it probably has a higher amount of virus than positive rodents from other species.

ROBERTS: The point of my curiosity is has anyone looked at *Peromyscus leucopus* specifically?

LEDUC: Not that I'm aware of.

QUESTIONS: Do any of these homes have cats? Are cats affected by this virus? Bob, you were once giving us a nice example of when the cats were killed and the rats then moved from the forest into the city. So are cats involved? Could cats be used as a way of keeping mice at least away from the houses?

BERKELMAN: I think there was a study in Asia on this, and cat ownership doubled the risk of getting Hantaan virus. But whether it was the cats bringing the mice to the owner, or what the mechanism was is speculation. In a study in Great Britain, stray cats were much more likely to have antibody to hantavirus than pet cats, and sick cats were more likely to have antibody than healthy cats. So they certainly can become infected, but whether they're excreting the virus, we don't know. In a case-control study in the Four Corners area, there was no association with cat ownership. I do know that there was the case in Nevada where the surviving woman told the story of having thrown out the mouse that the cat had brought to her. I'm still not sure that cat ownership may not play a role, but currently there's no association statistically.

MORSE: Have there been any serosurveys of cats in the Four Corners area?

BERKELMAN: Not that I'm aware of.

LEDUC: I think that the Chinese isolated a hantavirus from cats.

QUESTION: I'm wondering whether the excess deaths in the routine mortality surveillance would have shown up, given the number of deaths in the age and sex profile. In other words, if it hadn't been for the sentinel sensitivity of the physicians, would this have shown up in the normal mortality statistical collections in the Southwest or the states?

BERKELMAN: We have not looked at it. I think that one of the issues is that this would not have been found unless you were looking for it, and the vital statistics records are often pretty delayed. Unless you start to look at it, and stratify by age, you may not find it using vital statistics. But it is an interesting question. You can go back and find evidence of HIV before we found it, because you find it in pneumonia mortality in certain cities.

QUESTION: This is going to lead to the second part of my question, which is, how many other diseases are out there emerging, particularly in the high risk groups which are vulnerable, for example the aged? It's very difficult to pick up the emerging viruses. Really what we're looking at, is the mortality pattern, which would be a summation of these individual episodes. What we're seeing is really the sensitivity of detection system in this case.

GARRETT: Along that line, I know C. J. Peters was saying that as soon as he got a chance to catch his breath, he was going to go through archive tissue on the rodents from the area that had been collected annually for the plague surveys. Do you know yet whether this was like an epidemic in the rodent population this year or whether this was just the endemic level with a surge in rodents?

BERKELMAN: I don't know.

GARRETT: Has anybody had a chance to look at archive ARDS tissue from human patients?

BERKELMAN: Well, only back to 1991.

GARRETT: And there were no hantavirus positives before?

BERKELMAN: We do not have specimens before 1991. We haven't looked at any before 1991 that I'm aware of. Of the first 50 cases that came in with a diagnosis of unexplained acute pulmonary syndrome from all over the United States, outside the Four Corners area, three were positive for hantavirus.

GARRETT: I know also that C. J. Peters was saying he expected that there was a high probability of *Peromyscus* in the Northeast being found infected. He thought that if there was someplace else he was going to find another hantavirus, it would be in the Lyme zone, as he put it.

BERKELMAN: I think he's found evidence of hantavirus in *Peromyscus* in Virginia.

ANDREW SPIELMAN: The question was asked whether other agents of this kind are around. We're living in an ocean of microbial agents; there is

Jamestown Canyon virus, which is a virus of deer. It is a mosquito-transmitted virus that infects about half of the deer population in the Northeast. There's Hart Park virus, another mosquito-borne agent of rabbits, with a significant amount of seropositivity in this region. LaCrosse virus is right across the line in New York in the Albany area. There's Powassan virus around us, there's hemobartonella in mice and ticks, and there's ehrlichia in this area. There's also rickettsiae of various other kinds, such as *Rickettsia montana*. An enormous pool of agents are in our environment, sitting and waiting for a person to initiate a disease process in.

KOMAR: Is there evidence of either natural or laboratory infection of arthropods with hantavirus? If urine-transmitted infections or aerosol-transmitted infections could be controlled, is this the type of agent that we should be on the look out for potential vector-borne transmission.

LEDUC: I think the consensus opinion is that if vector-borne transmission exists, it's not critical for the long-term maintenance of the virus or for infection in humans. This is a unique characteristic of the hantaviruses among the family Bunyaviridae, in that most viruses of this family are transmitted by a vector. It was somewhat of a surprise when we finally classified Hantaan virus and found it to be in the family Bunyaviridae. Nonetheless, I think there have been ample studies now to clearly show that vector transmission is probably not significant in the transmission of these viruses to humans.

SHOPE: This is a continuation of the answer to Lincoln Chen's question. Andy has given us a litany of agents which we know are out there. The other side of the coin is that, in some of the best series, only about 50% of encephalitis cases are diagnosed. We should be asking the question, what's causing the other 50%? The same thing is true in dengue epidemics. If you get 40% of the people in a dengue epidemic seroconverting, that's normal. What are the other 60%? I think in almost any epidemic we have, there are excess cases that we can't explain, and those must be caused by something.

QUESTION: Bob, would you answer a question about the IOM recommending that respiratory disease is the disease that is the best sentinel signal for epidemic disease. What is the basis of that?

SHOPE: I don't remember. Maybe somebody else does. Andy, do you remember why respiratory disease was first on our list?

SPIELMAN: I'll venture a guess. It was probably because of the high transmissibility and difficulty of intervention with most respiratory and respiratorily transmitted infections. It would raise a warning signal, like the 1918–1919 [influenza] pandemic which spread so rapidly. What interventions do you have to keep ahead of it unless you're well prepared? I don't recall if that was exactly our reason.

MARY WILSON: What do we know about duration of persistence of the virus in the environment?

BERKELMAN: Sunlight kills it.

LEDUC: It is a Bunyavirus, and by and large these viruses are not especially stable in the environment, so I think it must be protected in a microenvironment.

MORSE: I could share a comment that came up at an earlier meeting, which was the question about the shedding of virus in urine. What is the pH of rodent urine? I think, Bob, you had an answer that this has actually been studied, and that it varies seasonally depending on diet. That could very well influence the survivability and transmissibility of the virus, or the ability of the virus to be shed in the urine. I don't know in *Peromyscus* if that's a factor with this virus. That is one of the things that has not really been studied.

SPIELMAN: Is there much inapparent infection in humans?

BERKELMAN: When Jay and others were out in the Four Corners area, they wanted to know if there was subclinical infection. One of the ways they looked was to take blood samples from about 500 people who came in with fever and flu-like symptoms. There was no evidence of infection in these patients. Now, if you look at background studies, just seroprevalence studies, you find about a 1% background rate. But we really think that what we're seeing is the whole iceberg, not just the tip.

LEDUC: We have some data that was never published, but an outbreak of Korean hemorrhagic fever occurred in marines that deployed as a group to Korea from Okinawa. Some of their members became sick in Korea. When they then returned in a group, several more became ill. I don't remember exactly how many were sick, but the total population was about 2,000 individuals. We bled each and every one of those people. It turned out that the only people infected were those that had been clinically ill; there were no asymptomatic infections. That may be a unique group, but it certainly indicates that with classic prototype Hantaan virus, the majority of infections lead to overt disease.

ROBERTS: I'd like to follow up on what Andy was saying, and give not a litany so much of agents, but a comment on the vertebrate animals that are found in our suburban/urban areas. I have really been amazed at the density of a variety of vertebrates in the suburban areas of Washington DC. I teach a course in medical acarology, and to obtain specimens of *Peromyscus* for my class, I trap them in my backyard. If I want to see raccoons and possums and rabbits and squirrels, I look in my backyard. I think we probably have a problem within our urban areas that is largely being ignored, probably because there's nothing we can do about it. It would not surprise me, as a matter of fact, to find that the density of many of these vertebrates is higher on an area basis in our urban areas, than in the rural areas.

GARRETT: Now that you have said that, I have to point out that the federal commitment to rat control in urban areas of the United States has declined radically in the last 10 years to the degree that there is now no federal funding whatsoever for rat control in New York City. All rat control that does go on in New York City is done under city and state funds, which have greatly diminished. Personnel is down by 60% as compared to a decade ago. Is the rat population bigger? All we know is that most urban centers in the United States have also had a decline in the amount of garbage collection. Instead of collecting 3 days a week, it's down to 2 or 1 day a week. More garbage sits on sidewalks in American cities now than a decade ago, because of the recession and federal cutbacks and so on. So given the combined effect of a decrease in rat control plus accumulating garbage, one could assume that there is an increase in the population. But, rat control efforts are so down that nobody is counting anymore, so we don't know what is really happening.

BERKELMAN: That's right. As an addendum to what you're saying, when we figured out this was a hantavirus, and we needed to trap rodents in different states, we found many of the rodent control programs had been dismantled by the states in the early 1980s. A number of these states have no programs at all at this point. People just didn't think about rodent control in the 1980s.

Models for New and Resurgent Diseases

CHARLES J. PUCCIA, TAMARA AWERBUCH, AND
RICHARD LEVINS

Department of Population and International Health
Harvard School of Public Health
665 Huntington Avenue
Boston, Massachusetts 02115

MODELING STRATEGY FOR NEW AND RESURGENT DISEASES

As disciplines emerge, coalesce and diverge, particular methodologies gain favor. The emerging study of new and resurgent disease requires the examination of systems of increasing complexity. That is, we have to consider many variables at the same time and these may themselves be very different kinds and even belong to different biological and social disciplines. Models are constructs which we make to study directly instead of the objects of real interest. Making a model requires making theoretical and practical choices in which tradeoffs are necessary among goals such as achieving generality, realism, precision, manageability, cost, and intelligibility.

Models can be divided into two categories: tactical models and strategic models. In well-established disciplines tactical models (*sensu* May, 1983. *Stability and Complexity of Model Ecosystems,* Princeton University Press) are widespread. These rely on specific information, detailed knowledge, accurate measurements and aim to give precise results. For example, a tactical model of striped bass population size would give a lot of detail to the precise growth and reproductive parameters of striped bass in order to help the fisheries managers determine the level of fishing activity consistent with avoiding overfishing.

New disciplines can benefit by employing strategic models, even though they are also associated with established disciplines that have accumulated knowledge over long periods. Strategic models are characterized by their wide applicability, describe qualitative behaviors, and yield broad generalizations; they depend less on precise assumptions and data. They are often of a qualitative nature and reach qualitative conclusions. For example, even the simple verbal model that proposes that the prevalence of a disease is the result of the opposing processes of contagion and recovery or death suggests that it is not necessary to reduce transmission to zero to eliminate an infection, but only to bring it below some threshold. The strategic models apply in cases where the questions of interest arise from general characteristics, such as whether nutrient loading determines the stability of the system, or if pesticide use to control malaria will cause greater fluctuations in the occurrence of the disease.

225

Modeling approaches that gain favor sometimes ignore the state of knowledge of a discipline, and reflect the urgency of real problems. The greater the sense of urgency, the greater is the appeal to pragmatism that insists on using tactical, precise models. This notion misunderstands the requirements of modeling. Strategic, general models provide practical insight when a) the current state of disciplinary knowledge is insufficient for precise parameter measurements, or b) the kinds of questions being asked are global or general or cross disciplinary boundaries.

The study of new and resurgent infectious disease (hereafter, New Disease) is an emergent discipline. We can build on an already rich tradition of epidemiological modeling (see Tamara Awerbuch's review in this volume). The demands for a coherent theoretical framework for true interdisciplinary investigation suggest these needs among others:

   i. Identify the close link between ecological change and disease;
  ii. Investigate the evolutionary response of hosts and parasites to changes in the environment;
 iii. Recognize the need to understand variability and uncertainty, both in nature, in data, and in response of organisms;
 iv. Consider the relationships between multiple infections and alternative responses of the host and agent;
  v. Develop an understanding of physiological and behavioral responses by humans to disease and the influences this has to the outcome. For example, the knowledge about AIDS within a community could reduce the transmission rate.

The present workshop develops along the lines of tuning the questions without promise of immediate answers. Strategic models provide answers to simple questions based on sketchy knowledge. The simplicity of questions belies the complexity of the problem. Answers from strategic models provide insight, give direction to future investigation, and lend structure to knowledge. Strategic models deal with complexity in ways that would be intractable for tactical models because of their requirement for precise numbers and detailed interactions. Incorporating aspects of complexity into models can lead to unexpected outcomes.

Tactical models enable action: intervention, management, surveillance, or sponsorship. The place for these models in the New Disease discipline depends on the specific domain and disease. Modification or incorporation of models from a specific specialty can be appropriate. Destruction of forests leading to new sites for breeding mosquitoes and the resurgence of malaria might be addressed by examination of existing malaria models and identification of parameters affected by deforestation. The study of legionellosis and the probability of occurrence depends on the human actions that change the environment in ways that alter virulence, frequency, modes of transmission and the ecological habitat of the *Legionellae* bacteria. In this case the use of classical respiratory models modified to include parameters specific to the bacteria and human host contact might be sufficient. Specific prescriptions for the best use of tactical or strategic models very much depend on the questions at hand. A viable approach would combine strategic and tactical modeling.

This section proposes initial questions for the study of New Disease and the relevant models and modeling approaches. Among these are the following:

1. Ecological Change, Complexity, Models, and Disease

   Deforestation, irrigation, agricultural expansion, urbanization, migration, nutrient enrichment of marine ecosystems and temperature changes all act to change the abundance of vectors and reservoirs or their contact with people. But these changes take place in the context of communities of species, not as the direct effect of environmental change on the physiology of single species. Temperature, for example, may act directly on the rate of reproduction of mosquitoes, but the effect of temperature change percolates through the network along pathways that amplify or buffer the impact.

   Models depict organismic interactions through parametric relationships. Climatic change, human transformation of the environment, and geomorphological change alter the parametric relationships and may eliminate or create new relations among the organisms and between the organisms and the physical environment. These changes percolate through a network of interactions, being amplified along some pathways and damped out along others. The number of potential pairwise and higher-order interactions increases more rapidly than the number of variables, even though not all possible interactions occur. The network reveals a complexity that makes a single, seemingly simple event, like deforestation, have multiple consequences: new breeding grounds for mosquitoes, habitation of lands previously void of human settlement, and shifts in rainfall pattern or water-soil relationships.

   We are concerned with the sensitivity of the species' abundances and disease prevalence to changes in external conditions. Sometimes small external changes may have large effects; impacts may be several steps removed from the direct point of entry into the systems; big changes in the environment may be passed along to "sink" variables, leaving the directly affected species unchanged.

2. The Coexistence of Disease

   People typically carry more than one infection at a time. These pathogens interact at the level of the individual host—competing for nutrients, stimulating or suppressing the immune system, altering their shared environment. One may increase transmission of another (*e.g.*, by causing sneezing) or reduce transmission by immobilization. At the population level, one disease may mask or draw attention to another, and therapy aimed at one disease may facilitate or reduce the spread of another. As a result, some genotypes of pathogens may be mutually exclusive. For example, classical and El Tor cholera usually replace each other rather than coexist, while AIDS facilitates the reproduction of many pathogens, and other STDs facilitate the spread of AIDS. The pathogens may exchange genes and affect natural selection. Areas in the southeastern United States that are infested with mosquitoes that can transmit dengue remain free of dengue. Models aid in explaining general conditions as well as specific cases for the establishment of multiple stable states, like the occurrence or non-occurrence of disease.

3. Evolutionary Responses

    Pathogens respond to changing environments that place different demands on their fitness and give rise to opportunities for exchanges of genes. This may result in microevolutionary changes in virulence, symptoms, or mode of transmission. Evolving organisms interact with existing organisms and environments, changing the relationship among them and altering the local environment. Coevolution among organisms and selective pressures on the pathogens depend on the human host and frequently on an outside environment for those pathogens that have a cycle outside the human host; this can lead to the adaptation of pathogens to new hosts and the adoption of the parasitic way of life by free-living microorganisms.

4. Behavioral and Physiological Responses

    Hosts can have behavioral and physiological responses to pathogens. This includes the role of knowledge as an epidemiological factor and of the behavior of the public health sector as part of the dynamics. The differential vulnerability of hosts in different social settings has to be taken into account.

5. Uncertainty and Variability

    All models should include or account for the uncertainty and variability that arises in biological systems.

6. Spatial and Temporal Conditions

    Diseases must be studied and modeled in space as well as time. The conditions which favor the increasing prevalence of an infection in a given locality are not identical with those that favor its geographic spread.

Ecological change appears in the model as changes in parameters. A study of understanding environmental changes or behavioral changes on various parameters requires knowing which parameters influence the infectious diseases. This includes the characteristics of the various organisms involved in the processes of transmission, infection of the host and maintenance in reservoir agents. There are consequences for every change. Small changes may produce small outcomes; small changes may lead to a threshold effect; small changes may shift a pattern from periodicity to chaos.

RATIONALITY OF MODELING PLANT, ANIMAL, AND HUMAN DISEASES

Disease is a general biological phenomenon, and most of the issues referred to above are relevant to plants and domestic and wild animals as well as to people.

A unified theory of parasitism should include all these hosts. The differences among them sometimes require different models but also can be used to advantage. Plant pathologists work with hundreds of cultivated plants, so that changes in parasite ranges, symptoms, and hosts are common occurrences. The immobility of plants makes some spatial processes more apparent. Plant and animal breeding makes it relatively easy to examine genetic aspects of resistance. On the other hand, people can talk about how they feel so that morbidity can be described more completely than in other species. And medicine has provided more complete physiological knowledge of humans than of any other animals.

Taxonomic differences obscure the fact that plants and animals have similarities in an ecological context. Disease patterns show similarities among plants, animals and humans that models may be able to identify as part of the structural similarity of living organisms.

However, differences in biology, either across ecological trophic levels or by social interactions, will produce differences in disease patterns. Models of the way social consciousness influences disease recognition, for example, may show that certain patterns of disease spread seen in humans cannot be viewed in plants.

Natural selection patterns will also vary among plants and animal hosts and their parasites. Evolutionary changes include changes in the pathogen and changes in the vector. Different time-scales of evolutionary change will reveal different consequences. Elucidating various host or parasite defenses against either natural or manufactured chemicals can be sharpened by models for animals, plants, and humans. The feedback from host to parasite becomes an important area of research and study, and each taxonomic group reveals aspects of this mechanism. Models provide a means to explore and understand feedback mechanisms.

MODELS: THE GOAL TO UNDERSTAND AND PROTECT AGAINST NEW AND RESURGENT DISEASES

Whatever else may be said about the program of new and resurgent disease, certainly there is the feeling of being overwhelmed—overwhelmed by the number of measurements, the number of decisions, the number of possible outcomes, and the number of variables and parameters. Models provide a means to reduce the numbers, yet not to reduce the problem by becoming simplistic. Models can remain holistic by using techniques of lumping or redefining variables, combining parameters and defining boundaries. At later stages, the parameters can be recombined, boundaries redefined, and variables re-organized.

Models enable the identification of components that are most sensitive to alterations. For humans, the behavioral response to disease is an important component. For humans, individual behavior and intervention policies affect the disease dynamics and pathogen evolution. Crop diseases also evolve in response to agricultural technology and social relations. The species cohabiting an area alter the presence of vectors, reservoirs and natural enemies of both. Certain parameters may be revealed for some diseases as crucial to control, as in the contact rate. We should understand the difference between sensitivity as related to the infection rate in a population versus the sensitivity that influences health care.

Models used to identify early indicators of new and resurgent diseases are powerful tools for disease prevention. Knowing the consequence of rainfall on malaria, or the size of nutrient runoff during the spring from rivers into the marine environment for the outbreak of cholera would be a great advance.

Models may prove useful to show how delays in intervention affect the ability to control disease or demonstrate the effectiveness of alternative intervention modes. Models aid policy, but also policies may become part of the models, as variables. They are necessary because in the complex systems we are using common sense is an inadequate guide.

Common mathematical tools are one link among plant, animal and human epidemiologists. These include the following, roughly descending from tactical modeling strategies to strategic strategies:

1. Simultaneous differential and difference equations (with or without delays) for the prevalence of infections and the abundances of vectors and reservoirs. When solved for their equilibrium values we can determine conditions for permanent endemism, episodic outbreaks or exclusion. Some of these models are aimed at specific infections in particular places, *e.g.*, Lyme Disease in New England, and include great detail. They usually cannot be solved analytically; numerical methods, like computer simulation, can give expected trajectories that depend on the accuracy of the data and the realism of the assumptions. These are the most common models used in epidemiology and are often what is meant by modeling.

2. Statistical models correlate observations of interest to factors that may be important by means of regression, analysis of variance and covariance, contingency tables and other familiar techniques. These methods minimize the epidemiological and clinical assumptions about a disease and simply describe quantitative relations among variables. They are useful for short-term projection and also to identify possible influences but do not provide understanding of the dynamics or anticipate what would happen in altered circumstances.

3. Sensitivity analysis is both a tool for validation of results and an exploration of how outcomes would be different if parameters such as contagion rates or duration of immunity change. It indicates when crude estimates are adequate for our purposes or when more precise data are required. Sensitivity is defined as the derivative of some outcome with respect to a given parameter. Sometimes it is useful also to examine the sensitivity of the sensitivity, that is, in what circumstances are the outcomes more or less sensitive to small changes. An extreme type of sensitivity arises in chaotic equations where even arbitrarily close estimates of a variable can lead to quite divergent outcomes.

4. Qualitative analysis using methods such as signed digraphs and time averaging explore the directions of changing outcomes in response to changing conditions. They examine the "what if" questions about the roles of particular factors, anticipate the changes caused by interventions, develop

indicators of types of dynamics and pose problems that can then be studied by other means.

5. Spatial models such as cellular automata are at present studied mostly by computer simulation, in which grids in the computer represent a geographic pattern formed by local dynamics and "migration."

Mathematical modeling of disease problems should be integrated into a coherent research program during preliminary definition of a problem, as part of experimental design and in the interpretation of results. It should also inform all proposals for intervention. In order to do this, a mutual education process is needed in which biologists and public health scientists learn enough about models to be able to know what they can do, how they are developed, and how to evaluate them. Modelers need to work closely enough with the other researchers to be able to propose relevant modeling approaches and also to develop new modeling tools appropriate to the complex, dynamical and diverse problems of new diseases.

Evolution of Mathematical Models of Epidemics

TAMARA AWERBUCH

Department of Population and International Health
Harvard School of Public Health
665 Huntington Avenue
Boston, Massachusetts 02115
and
Dana-Farber Cancer Institute
44 Binney Street
Boston, Massachusetts 02115

BEGINNINGS

It was not until the end of the last century, with the publication of Ross's work on malaria, that the realization that epidemics emerge and persist due to the interaction of many ecological factors gave birth to the field of Mathematical Epidemiology. But already in the 17th century there was considerable interest in patterns of the spread of epidemics. The increasing mobility of the upper and mercantile classes motivated the development of an alarm system that would alert them with some precision when to move away from epicenters of emerging infectious diseases. For this purpose the Bills of Mortality was published in London as early as the 1600s (FIG. 1). In this document, mortality due to a variety of causes was systematically recorded, informing the people of the city of the patterns in the rise and fall of particular epidemics.

In 1665, the year of the great plague, people (mostly from the nobility and mercantile class) left the city when the numbers of deaths due to this illness increased. As the number of deaths sharply declined, suggesting that the epidemic was over, they returned with the expectation that the danger was over as well. But it was soon discovered that mortality increased again, and that the new victims were chiefly among the very people that had left and returned.[1,2] The lesson was that the inspection of numbers and the analysis of statistical data were not enough to predict the future course of an epidemic. It became obvious that the dynamics of the socio-economic characteristics of the London population in those times played an important role in determining the patterns of spread.

The regular patterns in which epidemics rose and declined were the focus of Farr's work on smallpox in 1840 and Brownlee's studies on outbreaks of plague in 1906.[3,4] They modeled the data for particular epidemics in terms of mathematical curves that were compatible with the observations. It turned out that when the equations describing the curves were used to make predictions, there was little overlap between the predictions and the actual data, indicating that other strategies were needed for understanding and predicting the course of epidemics.

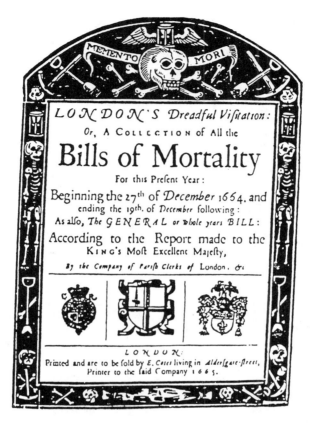

FIGURE 1. Title page of the London Bills of Mortality for 1665, the year of the great plague. (From H. W. Haggard[1])

ROSS'S MODELS

In the course of his research in India, while trying to understand the role of mosquitoes in the transmission of malaria, Ross constructed the first deterministic models for describing epidemics. These models were based on the underlying mechanisms governing epidemics, and described in mathematical notation the processes involved in their emergence, maintenance, and spread.[5,6] Ross's models kept evolving as he acquired more mathematical sophistication and knowledge of the biology involved in the transmission process.

The first models were simple: he laid out in a linear fashion the biological steps involved in transmission.[7] Thus, the number of new malaria infections per month in an endemic area were described as:

$$\text{Number of New Infections} = P \times M \times I \times A \times B \times S \times F$$

where: P = size of population in a particular location
        M = proportion of infected people
        I = proportion of infected people that are infectious
        A = average number of mosquitoes per person per month
        B = proportion of uninfected mosquitoes feeding on people
        S = proportion of mosquitoes surviving the extrinsic incubation period
        F = proportion of infected mosquitoes feeding on people

The number of recoveries per months were formulated as:

$$\text{Number of Recoveries} = R \times M \times P$$

where: R = recovery rate

For the purpose of analyzing an endemic situation Ross made the logical assumption that the recovery rate equals the rate at which new infections are introduced:

$$R \times M \times P = P \times M \times I \times A \times B \times S \times F$$

Assuming that the human-biting habits of infectious and non-infectious mosquitoes are the same (B = F), it can be readily seen from this equation that:

$$A = R/(B^2 \times I \times S)$$

where A would be interpreted as the critical mosquito density below which malaria cannot be maintained. Using parameter values based on intuition and experience, Ross estimated A to be approximately 40.[7]

Ross expanded his models and introduced the use of difference equations to represent changes in the prevalence of infection per unit time:

$$X_{(t+1)} = X_{(t)} + h \times X_{(t)} \times (1 - X)_{(t)} - r \times X_{(t)}$$

where: $X_{(t+1)}$ = prevalence of infection at time (t + 1).
        $X_{(t)}$ = prevalence of infection at time t.
        $(1 - X)_{(t)}$ = proportion of uninfected people at time t.
        h = transmission rate which is a function of parameters describing interactions between mosquitoes and humans.
        r = recovery rate which is a function of interactions between the parasite and the immune system.

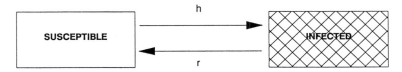

FIGURE 2. Schematic representation of compartmental model for the Theory of Happenings (Ross, 1916[6]).

The infection prevalence at a particular time $(t + 1)$ is a sum of three terms; the middle term, representing the prevalence rate of new infections is proportional to the prevalence rates of existing susceptibles and infectives.

This idea was later translated in terms of a differential equation and expanded into the Theory of Happenings:[6]

$$dX/dt = h \times (1 - X) - r \times X$$

where in the general case of infectious diseases:

X = prevalence of infection at time t.
dX/dt = the change in prevalence per unit time.

The process is represented schematically in FIGURE 2:

The equation is integrated analytically, yielding a functional relationship between the prevalence rate and time, as illustrated in FIGURE 3. This is basically an age-prevalence curve for a population living under defined endemic conditions: $h = 0.005$ and $r = 0.005$ with the initial condition that $X_0 = 0$ at $t = 0$. Under this scenario children in the endemic area become infected at a rate h as soon as they are born, recovering at a rate r, and reaching a maximum prevalence defined by $h/(h + r)$.

CLASSICAL MODELS

Ross's models served as an inspiration to persons developing many subsequent epidemic models of infectious diseases.

In all classical models the central assumption is that epidemics are spread by transmission of the parasite from infected to susceptible individuals in the population; assuming that humans are the reservoir, the population is divided into distinct classes according to the infection status of its members. In their early classical work on the theory of epidemics Kermack and McKendrick (1927) subdivided the total population (N) into Susceptibles (S), Infective (I) and Removed (R), as presented schematically in FIGURE 4a.[8] Susceptible individuals in the first compartment (S) can move to the second one (I) once they become infected; those who recover with immunity, or are removed from exposure or die, move from the second compartment to the third one (R). This system can be represented by a set of three differential equations

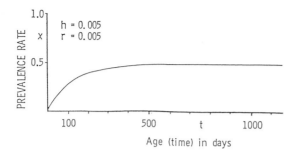

FIGURE 3. Malaria prevalence (Pr) as a function of age. $Pr = \{h/(h + r)\}\{1 - e^{-(h+r)t}\}$.

representing the transitions among the various compartments. Although the equations are non-linear, it was possible to solve them analytically once mathematical approximations had been made. When plotted with the right parameter values, there was a good fit between the model and data for death by plague in Bombay during an epidemic in 1906. In FIGURE 4b an additional term was included to account for loss of immunity, allowing for recovered individuals to reenter the compartment of susceptibles. Since natural births and deaths in a population can have a considerable effect on the spread of an epidemic, vital dynamics was later added (FIG. 4c), further increasing the level of complexity.

Compartmental models with various degrees of complexity have been used to describe and analyze the course of specific epidemics such as AIDS, measles, malaria, and leishmaniasis. An AIDS model representing the transition of the population from susceptibles to infectious and from infectious to symptomatic, and fitted to the number of cases among homosexuals in Boston revealed a pattern of progression presented in FIGURE 5.[9] Here the model parameters were assumed to be constant. A more realistic model for a particular population would take into account behavioral and social changes that would make the contagion parameter a function of these changes. As a result we expect to introduce oscillations in the pattern of spread.

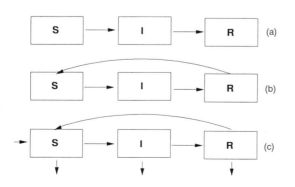

FIGURE 4. Schematic representation of SIR (Susceptible, Infectious, Removed) models with increasing complexity.

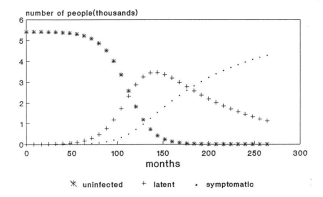

FIGURE 5. Simulated progression of the AIDS epidemic among homosexuals in Massachusetts. (From Sandberg *et al.*[9])

STEADY STATES

Methods for exploring steady states were instrumental in providing information on the circumstances under which an epidemic can grow, decline, or become established. Thus, it was possible to discover the threshold effect and define the Basic Reproductive Number (R_0), the number of secondary infections produced by introducing an infectious individual into a population of susceptibles, in terms of the model parameters.[10] In the case of the model represented in FIGURE 4b, it has two theoretical steady states, one when the whole population is in the compartment of susceptibles and the disease is eradicated, and the other determined by the model parameters resulting in:

$$R_0 = (S + I + R) \times h/r$$

The approach to this steady state can be oscillatory.[11] The equilibrium association between the infectious agent and its host fluctuates at times, leading to periodic oscillations. Some conditions such as high transmission efficiency and a short-lived infection will favor oscillations. Seasonal variations in transmission rates induced by biological and social factors will produce also oscillations in the incidence of infection.

As models increase in complexity, their equations become harder or impossible to solve analytically. In this case one can resort to high power computing for numerical solution; most of the studies in mathematical epidemiology today use this approach since adequate computer programs are available for this purpose. For many examples, see the 1991 book of Anderson and May.[12] Stability of steady states of complex systems can be analyzed using Routh-Hurwitz criteria;[2] however, this approach becomes cumbersome for very large systems. The problem can then be treated productively with qualitative methods that require almost no computation.[13] For an example, see the chapter by Richard Levins in this volume (pp. 260–270).

STOCHASTICITY IN EPIDEMIC MODELS

Most of the existing models of infectious diseases are primarily deterministic with some of the parameters, such as the contagion and the recovery rates, having probabilistic meanings. In such a context for example we talk about the average probability of becoming infected; however there are many factors determining infectivity which are different from individual to individual and the probabilities will have distributions. In order to simulate this variability it is possible to introduce stochastic components into the models. They may play an important role in determining whether an epidemic will take off when the size of the community is small.[12,14] Stochastic effects may lead to the disappearance of an infection in the initial phase of an epidemic when the parasite tries to become established, thus preventing it from progressing to an endemic state.

Reed and Frost introduced one of the first stochastic models of epidemics as part of a course they taught in John Hopkins University in 1928.[15] In this model a closed population of susceptibles was exposed to one or two infectious individuals; each person had a random probability of contacting every other person, and the new infected individuals appearing at each time interval were counted. By running the simulation many times a distribution of epidemic sizes was obtained and analyzed with the appropriate statistics, thus enabling us to follow a simulated emerging infectious disease. This simple model was extended by Elveback and Fox to study competition between viral agents in a community of families.[16,17] With stochastic models it was also possible to show a positive relationship between the size of the initial number of infectives in a population and the size of outbreak of one of two competing infections.[18] The effect of distance between infectives and susceptibles can be also explored with spatial stochastic simulations using cellular automata (see chapter by Kiszewski and Spielman in this volume, pp. 249–259).

If one wants to study the effect of many factors on the progression of an epidemic (for example by introducing high levels of demographic and geographic detail), stochastic models are impractical and have no advantage over deterministic models that deal with large populations; deterministic models can include many parameters, making them valuable for identifying the components that are most vulnerable to control.

MALARIA MODELS AFTER ROSS

Ross's models were simple and described the main characteristics of the epidemic. Later they were expanded by other researchers to capture the further features involved in the process of malaria transmission. These models grew along with the further understanding of the biological mechanisms of vector-host-parasite interactions and were tailored to describe epidemics in different parts of the world. For example, superinfection, acquisition of immunity, and seasonal variation in mosquito populations were all introduced in later malaria models.[19–21] The best known is the one developed with WHO support as part of the Garki project between the years 1969 and 1976 in the savanna of West Africa.[21] This model was tested in the field and was used to explore the expected effects of possible interventions. It consisted of a set of seven difference equations, each describing the change in the proportion of people in each compartment of the model. This level of complexity required computer support that was already available at the time the study was carried out. The solution of difference and differential equations no longer depended on analytical methods, and the equations were solved numerically with the aid of the computer.

As the world experiences environmental change, the many factors contributing to the spread of malaria will change as well; malaria models will hence have to have a corresponding flexibility that incorporates these changes. For example, a problem particular to the Brazilian Amazon is the migration of non-immune persons to this area and the destruction of the rain forest, which create new ecological conditions favoring the spread of malaria in the region. Human factors, such as the response to epidemics at the individual and the community level, will have to be taken into account as an integral part of the models. A problem particular to Thailand at the Cambodian border is the migration of opportunistic gem miners to the area and the development of malaria strains resistant to therapies owing to wide use of anti-malaria drugs. Although the Thai and Brazilian sites may share some common features, such as the basic vector-host-parasite interactions, they will differ, for example, in migration patterns and in the process leading to the development of resistant strains. The similarities and differences will have to be captured by the structure of the models.

The analysis of the models will depend on the questions that we ask. In general we will want to run computer simulations of differential equations to explore the change in the variables as a function of time. We will want to use signed digraphs (see Levins chapter in this volume) to find the sensitivity of the average equilibrium levels to parameter change and to identify factors affecting the stability, resilience and resistance of the equilibrium, and the sources of endogenous oscillations.

MODELS WHEN HUMANS ARE NOT THE RESERVOIR

Most of the existing mathematical models represent epidemics where humans are the reservoir. However, there are epidemics caused by transmission of the parasite from animal reservoirs to humans. For example, the virus of eastern encephalitis resides mostly in birds and is transmitted to humans by a bite of a mosquito (see chapter by Komar and Spielman, pp. 157–168); in another example the agent of Lyme disease is a spirochete that cycles in nature in small rodents and is transmitted to humans by a bite of the deer tick taking a blood meal in the process of going through its life cycle. Models for these diseases will be more complex and will have to combine various mathematical methodologies.

In the case of Lyme disease the seasonality of the life cycle of the tick is crucial to transmission; thus a multiple matrix model was constructed to represent this cycle and to explore the role of host abundance in the propagation of the tick.[22,23] The Lyme disease modeling will progress in modular fashion and in parallel to research that is being conducted in the field. In the next step, transmission of infection will be incorporated, and as a further step this ecological model will be combined with a probabilistic one that describes transmission to humans. Modeling will also make use of new computer methodologies, such as cellular automata, making it possible to explore new features of epidemics (see chapter by Kiszewski and Spielman).

REFERENCES

1. HAGGARD, H. W. 1957. Devils, Drugs and Doctors. New York: Harper & Row.
2. EDELSTEIN-KESHET, L. 1988. Mathematical Models in Biology. New York: Random House.
3. FARR, W. 1840. Progress of Epidemics. Second Report of the Registrar General of England and Wales.
4. BROWNLEE, J. 1906. Statistical studies in immunity: The theory of an epidemic. Proc. R. Soc. of Edinburgh 26: 484–521.
5. ROSS, R. 1911. The Prevention of Malaria, 2nd edition. London: John Murray.
6. ROSS, R. 1916. An application of the theory of probabilities to the study of *a priori* pathometry, Part I. Proc. R. Soc., Ser. A 92: 204–230.
7. FINE, P. E. M. 1975. Ross's *a priori* Pathometry—a Perspective. Proc. R. Soc. Med. 68: 547–551.
8. KERMACK, W. O. & A. G. MCKENDRICK. 1927. Contributions to the Mathematical Theory of Epidemics. R. Statistical Soc. J. 115: 700–721.
9. SANDBERG, S., T. AWERBUCH & R. GONIN. Simplicity vs. complexity in deterministic models: An application to AIDS data. Submitted for publication, 1994.
10. MAY, R. M. 1983. Parasitic infections as regulators of animal populations. Am. Sci. 71: 36–45.
11. HETHCOTE, H. W. 1976. Qualitative analyses of communicative disease models. Math. Biosci. 28: 335–356.
12. ANDERSON, R. M. & R. M. MAY. 1991. Infectious Diseases of Humans: Dynamics and Control. Oxford: Oxford University Press.
13. PUCCIA, C. & R. LEVINS. 1986. Qualitative Modeling of Complex Systems: An Introduction to Loop Analysis and Time Averaging. Cambridge, MA: Harvard University Press.
14. BARTLETT, M. S. 1957. Measles periodicity and community size. J. R. Statistical Soc. A 120: 48–70.
15. ABBEY, H. 1952. An examination of the Reed-Frost theory of epidemics. Hum. Biol. 24: 201–233.
16. ELVEBACK, L., J. P. FOX & A. VARMA. 1964. An extension of the Reed-Frost epidemic model for the study of competition between viral agents in the presence of interference. Am. J. Hyg. 80: 356–364.
17. ELVEBACK, L., E. ACKERMAN, G. YOUNG & J. P. FOX. 1971. Stochastic two agent epidemic simulation models for a community of families. Am. J. Epidemiol 87: 373–384.
18. KENDALL, W. S. & I. W. SAUNDERS. 1983. Epidemics in competition, II: The general epidemic. J. R. Statistical Soc. B 45: 238–244.
19. MACDONALD, A. 1957. The Epidemiology and Control of Malaria. London: Oxford University Press.
20. STRUCHINER, C. J., M. E. HALLORAN & A. SPIELMAN. 1989. Modeling malaria vaccines, I: New uses for old ideas. Math. Biosci. 94: 87–113.

21. DIETZ, K., L. MOLINEAUX & A. THOMAS. 1974. A malaria model tested in African savannah. Bull. WHO **50:** 347–357.
22. SANDBERG, S., T. E. AWERBUCH & A. SPIELMAN. 1992. A comprehensive multiple matrix model representing the life cycle of the tick that transmits the agent of Lyme disease. J. Theor. Biol. **157:** 203–220.
23. AWERBUCH, T. E. & A. SPIELMAN. 1992. Host abundance and tick dynamics: the case of Lyme Disease. *In* Proceedings of the Workshop on Modelling of Vector-Borne and Other Parasitic Diseases, Nairobi.

Characteristics of Host-Parasite Interactions That Promote Parasite Persistence

GARY SMITH

University of Pennsylvania
School of Veterinary Medicine
New Bolton Center
382 W. Street Road
Kennett Square, Pennsylvania 19348

INTRODUCTION

Mathematical models of infectious diseases have helped us understand how the disease-causing organism persists and spreads in host populations. Many of these insights have come from generic models that apply equally well to infectious diseases in animals or humans. Nevertheless, we have often been able to collect data for animal diseases that it would be impossible or unethical to collect for human diseases, and several of the important insights have arisen specifically as a result of modeling infections in animals. Anderson and May's analysis of viral and bacterial infections in mice is a classic example.[1,2]

This paper concentrates on what properties of the infection ensure that the newly introduced pathogen manages to persist in the host population, and what properties of the infection enhance or impede the spread of a pathogen within and between host populations. Finally, the future development of mathematical models of emerging diseases is discussed.

The paper begins by describing the properties of a parameter called the basic reproduction ratio (formerly called the basic reproductive rate or the contact number[3,4]). This parameter will be used to compare the effect of different evolutionary strategies on an infection's ability to persist.

THE BASIC REPRODUCTION RATIO (R_0)

The properties of the basic reproductive rate will be illustrated by reference to an elementary model of an endemic infection involving viruses or bacteria.[4] The main assumptions of the model are as follows: the host population density (N) is constant, that is births equal deaths (μ) (this assumption does not apply to wildlife populations but is a good approximation for many domestic species and for human populations in industrialized, developed countries), susceptible hosts (X) move into the infected/infectious class (Y) at a per capita rate, βY (where βY is the incidence of disease or the "force of infection"[3,5] and infected hosts move into the recovered/immune class

242

(Z) at a per capita rate δ (where $1/\delta$ is the mean expected time spent in the infected class). These assumptions lead to

$$\frac{dX}{dt} = \mu N - \mu X - \beta XY \tag{1}$$

$$\frac{dY}{dt} = \beta XY - \mu Y - \delta Y \tag{2}$$

$$\frac{dZ}{dt} = \delta Y - \mu Z \tag{3}$$

A local stability analysis of this model indicates that a newly introduced infection will persist provided:

$$\frac{\beta N}{(\mu + \delta)} \geq 1 \tag{4}$$

The ratio on the left hand side of inequality (4) is called the basic reproduction ratio (R_0). It can be rearranged to demonstrate that there is a critical minimum threshold initial density of hosts required for disease persistence, *i.e.*

$$N > \frac{(\mu + \delta)}{\beta} \tag{5}$$

The basic reproduction ratio of microparasitic infections is defined as "average number of secondary infections produced when one infected individual is introduced into a host population where every host is susceptible."[3] The power of R_0 is that it is an index of the degree of difficulty we may have in implementing effective disease control measures at any given population density. Any evolutionary strategy that increases the value of R_0 makes the disease more difficult to eradicate (or, conversely, increases the infection's ability to persist in small, patchy populations of host). Examples include any infection-induced changes in host behavior that increase β, the likelihood of transmission (furious rabies comes to mind; see also Dobson[6]).

I shall now elaborate Eqs. (1)–(3) in incremental steps to illustrate how vertical transmission, asymptomatic carrier states, recrudescent infections, long-lived free-living stages, sexual transmission and intermediate host phases (for macroparasites) affect R_0. The general methodology follows that of Anderson and Trewhella[7] and Smith and Grenfell.[8] There are some caveats to the generalizations listed below and the interested reader is referred to Anderson.[2]

Vertical Transmission

There are two types of vertical transmission: in one, offspring are infected before birth. Examples include bovine viral diarrhea (BVD), venereal spirochetosis in rabbits, African swine fever virus in soft ticks, La Crosse virus in mosquitoes and *Toxocara canis* in dogs.[9-11] In the other (pseudovertical transmission), offspring are infected almost immediately after birth. Examples include tuberculosis in possums and lungworms (*Filaroides*) in dogs.[11,12] We can represent both types by modifying Eqs. (1) and (2) as follows:

$$\frac{dX}{dt} = \mu(X + (1 - p)Y + Z) - \beta XY - \mu X$$

$$\frac{dY}{dt} = \mu pY + \beta XY - (\mu + \delta)Y$$

(6)

where p is the proportion of all births to infected mothers that involve vertical transmission. If we let the basic reproduction ratio for Eqs (1)–(3) be R, the basic reproduction ratio of the new model is given by

$$R_0 = R + \frac{\mu p}{(\mu + \delta)}$$

(7)

It will be typical of the examples that follow that the original value for the basic reproduction ratio (R) will be increased by some factor.

Asymptomatic Carriers

We modify the basic Eqs. (1) and (2) to incorporate a new infectious group (Y_2) that become asymptomatic carriers for their entire lifetime. Examples of this kind of asymptomatic carrier state include BVD and *Trypanosoma equiperdum* in equines.[9] The proportion of all infections that enter this state is given by the parameter $(1 - f)$.

$$\frac{dX}{dt} = \mu N - \beta Y_1 X - \beta Y_2 X - \mu X$$

$$\frac{dY_1}{dt} = f(\beta Y_1 X + \beta Y_2 X) - (\mu + \delta)Y_1$$

(8)

$$\frac{dY_2}{dt} = (1 - f)(\beta Y_1 X + \beta Y_2 X) - \mu Y_2$$

The increase in the basic reproduction ratio is directly proportional to $(1 - f)$, *i.e.*

$$R_0 = R \left(\frac{\mu + \delta(1 - f)}{\mu} \right)$$

(9)

Recrudescent Infections and Long-lived, Free-living Infective Stages

In this model we imagine a disease like infectious laryngotracheitis (ILT) in broiler chickens, which is maintained in intensive rearing conditions.[13]

Recovered animals contain inactive infections that recrudesce at a per capita rate, γ. Susceptible animals can also become infected when they come into contact with an environmental source of virus (E). The virus has a mean life span in the environment of $1/\tau$ days.

$$\frac{dX}{dt} = \mu N - \beta XY - \beta_2 XE - \mu X$$

$$\frac{dY}{dt} = \beta XY + \beta_2 XE - (\mu + \delta)Y + \gamma Z$$

$$\frac{dZ}{dt} = \delta Y\gamma Z - \mu Z \tag{10}$$

$$\frac{dE}{dt} = \alpha Y - \tau E$$

The basic reproduction ratio is[8]

$$R_0 = \frac{N(\gamma + \mu)\left(\beta + \beta_2 \dfrac{\alpha}{\tau}\right)}{\mu(\mu + \delta + \gamma)} \tag{11}$$

If there is no environmental contamination ($\alpha = 0$) the increase in the basic reproduction ratio is due entirely to recrudescent infections:

$$R_0 = R\frac{(\mu + \delta)(\gamma + \mu)}{\mu(\mu + \delta + \gamma)} \tag{12}$$

If there is no recrudescent infection ($\gamma = 0$) the increase in the basic reproduction ratio is due entirely to environmental contamination.

$$R_0 = R\left(1 + \beta_2\frac{\alpha}{\tau}\right) \tag{13}$$

Other Mechanisms for Persistent Infections

So far the models have dealt with infections in which the basic reproduction ratio is critically dependent upon the host population density. There remains that class of microparasitic infections that are sexually transmitted. In this case, R_0 depends not on host population density but rather on the mean number of sexual partners per host and its associated variance. It is characteristic of sexually transmitted infections that they are maintained by a core of highly active individuals. This high variance associated with the mean number of sexual partners keeps R_0 at high levels and allows sexually transmitted diseases to be maintained in very low density populations (see Anderson and May[3] and Smith and Dobson[9], for further discussion).

Macroparasitic infections of animals share many of the strategies set out above in the context of viral and bacterial disease. In addition, many of them require one or more intermediate hosts in their life cycle. This has been shown to have a buffering effect. The basic reproduction ratio depends in part upon the product of the respective host densities, thus an intermediate host which exists at high densities will permit the persistence of the infection of a definitive host which normally occurs in low density patches.[14]

A PERSISTENT MISCONCEPTION

One often hears that a newly introduced pathogen, though it may be highly pathogenic to begin with, will evolve to a state of lower pathogenicity and so, by preserving its host population, also ensure its own persistence. It is necessary to point out that this is only one of several evolutionary pathways that a pathogen may follow. For example, if there is an association between virulence and transmission, as there seems to be in the case of myxoma virus infections in rabbits, then the predominant viral strains tend towards an intermediate degree of pathogenicity.[1,15] Ewald[16] provides a more detailed discussion of the evolution of virulence.

MODEL DYNAMICS

So far I have concentrated on the static aspects of animal models. However, the evolutionary strategies listed above also have a profound effect on the dynamics of infectious disease (the patterns we see in the field). I note in passing, for example, that carriers and recrudescent infections may severely damp the oscillatory behavior that is so typical of many microparasitic infections.[7,17]

THE SPREAD OF INFECTIONS

The spatial spread of infections is receiving increasing attention, particularly as interest grows in the population dynamics of AIDS. The spread of animal infections has also been examined (see Murray[18] for a review). I shall simply allude to a study by Dobson and May[19] who used a model by Kallen et al.[20] to examine the spread of rinderpest in ungulates in Africa. The velocity of spread (c) was found to depend upon the mortality caused by the pathogen (μ), the basic reproduction ratio (R_0) and a diffusion coefficient (D, an estimate of the area covered by a wandering animal in a given time interval).

$$c = 2[\mu D(R_0 - 1)]^{1/2} \tag{14}$$

The interesting feature of Eq. (14) is that it illustrates once more the importance of estimating the basic reproduction ratio.

THE USE OF MODELS IN THE STUDY OF EMERGING DISEASES

It may appear from the preceding sections that I am suggesting that we attempt to measure the basic reproduction ratio for emerging diseases and use it as some kind of predictor as to whether the infection is likely to persist and how difficult it might be to eliminate. Unfortunately, measuring the basic reproduction ratio of even established endemic infections is a process fraught with difficulty and these problems will probably multiply prohibitively in the case of an emerging disease. In fact it may not be possible to use models to predict very much at all about emerging diseases because, by definition, our experience, and therefore our knowledge, of the infection is too limited. Nevertheless, previous models of established infections in humans and domestic animals *can guide our thinking* about what is likely to happen, and models of emerging diseases can be used to explore the potentials and pitfalls of proposed control strategies. The formal representation of the formula for the basic reproduction ratio serves to focus our attention on what is important, and the analysis of the behavior of even incomplete models gives pause for thought. Two models serve as examples. Poco's model[21] of Lyme borreliosis indicated that moderate reductions in the density of white-tailed deer could decrease or increase the proportion of infected ticks depending on the prevailing circumstances. This ambiguous result is important because it reveals the power of models to highlight the counterintuitive point that planned reductions in deer density may have exactly the opposite effect to the one desired. The second example concerns Aujezsky's disease in pigs. Early vaccines against Aujezsky's disease protected against clinical signs but not infection. Thus vaccinated animals that later became infected still shed virus, and vaccination was not recommended as a virus-elimination strategy. Nevertheless, vaccinates were harder to infect and, once infected, shed virus for a shorter time than non-vaccinates. A mathematical model of this system was able to show that vaccination was sufficient to eliminate the virus from an infected herd provided certain conditions pertained and, indeed, field trials seem to suggest the same thing.[8] This somewhat arcane example may have more central relevance in the case of putative vaccines against AIDS.

There is much we do not know about the important emerging diseases. But, while it is not necessary to know all there is to know about a system in order to answer useful questions, it is necessary to have a rational framework for making the best use of the information to hand. This is the principal value of models.

Finally, it is worth reflecting on the future of models in the context of new and reemerging diseases. Most new or reemerging diseases of importance tend to be microparasitic infections (principally viruses) and in consequence, the models elaborated here have followed the usual format for microparasitic infections in which hosts are distinguished according to whether or not they are infected. In concentrating on infection rather than disease the models narrow our focus and limit the control options we can examine within these very powerful frameworks. Perhaps it is time microparasitic models were elaborated to further distinguish hosts with repect to whether or not infection leads to disease (like some models of macroparasitic infections[22]). Disease is multicausal and infection is a neccessary but not necessarily sufficient cause of morbidity or death. By writing models which encompass the other component causes of disease we may enhance our ability to devise control strategies for dealing with new and reemerging infections.

REFERENCES

1. ANDERSON, R. M. & R. M. MAY. 1979. Population biology of infectious diseases: Part I. Nature **280**: 361–367.
2. ANDERSON, R. M. 1979. The persistence of direct life cycle infectious diseases with populations of hosts. Lect. Math. Life Sci. **12**: 1–67.
3. ANDERSON, R. M. & R. M. MAY. 1991. Infectious Diseases of Humans: Dynamics and control. Oxford: Oxford University Press.
4. HETHCOTE, H. W. 1989. Three basic epidemiological models, *In* Applied Mathematical Ecology, Biomathematics. S. A. Levin, T. G. Hallam & J. L. Gross, Eds. Vol. **18.** 119–144. Berlin: Springer-Verlag.
5. ROTHMAN, K. J. 1986. Modern Epidemiology. Boston: Little, Brown and Company.
6. DOBSON, A. P. 1988. The population biology of parasite induced changes in host behaviour. Quart. Rev. Biol. **63**: 140–164.
7. ANDERSON, R. M. & W. TREWHELLA. 1985. Population dynamics of the badger (*Meles meles*) and the epidemiology of bovine tuberculosis (*Myobacterium bovis*). Phil. Trans. R. Soc., London, B **310**: 327–381.
8. SMITH, G. & B. T. GRENFELL. 1990. Population biology of pseudorabies in swine. Am. J. Vet. Res. **51**: 148–155.
9. SMITH, G. & A. P. DOBSON. 1992. Sexually transmitted diseases in animals. Parasitol. Today **8**: 159–166.
10. BOLIN, S. R. 1990. The current understanding about the pathogenesis and clinical forms of BVD. Vet. Med., October 1990: 1124–1131.
11. NOBLE, E. R., G. A. NOBLE, G. A. SCHAD & A. J. MacINNES. 1989. Parasitology, then biology of animal parasites. Philadelphia: Lea and Febiger.
12. ROBERTS, M. G. 1990. The dynamics and control of bovine tuberculosis in possums. IMA Journal of Mathematics Applied in Medicine and Biology **9**: 19–28.
13. DAVISON, S., G. SMITH & R. J. ECKROADE. 1989. Laryngotracheitis in chickens: The length of the preinfectious and infectious periods. Avian Dis. **33**: 18–23.
14. KEYMER, A. E. 1982. Tapeworm infections. *In* Population Dynamics of Infectious Disease: Theory and Applications. R. M. Anderson, Ed.: 109–138. London: Chapman and Hall.
15. MAY, R. M. & R. M. ANDERSON. 1983. Epidemiology and genetics in the coevolution of parasites and hosts. Proc. R. Soc., London, B **219**: 281–313.
16. EWALD, P. W. 1993. The evolution of virulence. Sci. Am. **268** (April): 86–93.
17. COYNE, M. J., G. SMITH & F. E. MacALLISTER. 1989. Mathematical model for the population biology of rabies in raccoons in the mid-Atlantic states. Am. J. Vet. Res. **50**: 2148–2154.
18. MURRAY, J. D. 1989. Geographical spread of epidemics. *In* Mathematical Biology, Biomathematics, Vol. **19.** 651–696. Berlin: Springer-Verlag.
19. DOBSON, A. P. & R. M. MAY. 1986. Disease and conservation. *In* Conservation Biology: The Science of Scarcity and Diversity. M. E. Soule, Ed.: 345–365. Sinauer Associates Inc.
20. KALLEN, A., P. ARCURI & J. D. MURRAY. 1985. A simple model for the spatial spread and control of rabies. J. Theor. Biol. **116**: 377–393.
21. PORCO, T. C. 1991. A model of the enzootiology of Lyme disease in the Atlantic North East of the United States. Nat. Resources Model **5**: 469–505.
22. MEDLEY, G. F., H. L. GUATT & D. A. P. BUNDY. 1993. A quantitative framework for evaluation of the effect of community treatment on the morbidity due to ascariasis. Parasitology **106**: 211–221.

Virulence of Vector-borne Pathogens

A Stochastic Automata Model of Perpetuation[a]

ANTHONY E. KISZEWSKI AND ANDREW SPIELMAN

Department of Tropical Public Health
Harvard School of Public Health
665 Huntington Avenue
Boston, Massachusetts 02115

INTRODUCTION

Some authors suggest that the virulence of a pathogen is related to its mode of transmission.[1] If the host is rapidly killed or incapacitated, the pathogen would fail to perpetuate if transmissibility required host motility. Perpetuation of such virulent pathogens, therefore, would be facilitated if some vector carried them "with direction" beyond the immediate contacts of the original host. Indeed, many of the more apocalyptic "plagues" seem to be vector- or water-borne.

Pathogens that perpetuate vertically, passing solely from one host generation to the next, represent the extreme of proximate-passage. The inherited nematode (*Parasitodiplogaster* spp.), parasites of fig wasps (*Pegoscapus* and *Tetrapus* spp.), for example, are less pathogenic than are those that pass horizontally.[2] Indeed, phage-virulence of vertically infected *Escherichia coli* increases more rapidly than in bacteria subjected to horizontal transmission.[3] Thus, morbidity and mortality may vary with the spatial distance over which transmission occurs.

Because fitness of a pathogen is most labile in the case of a new disease, we explored the evolution of virulence in a model that relates transmission-distance to pathogenicity. In particular, we sought to determine whether vector-borne pathogens may tend to become more virulent than pathogens transmitted by direct host-to-host contact.

EXISTING MODELS OF THE EVOLUTION OF VIRULENCE

Mathematical models of the coevolution of hosts and parasites generally are based on the original epidemic equations of Kermack and McKendrick[4] or a later derivative.[5] Assumptions of asexuality permit a simplified set of assumptions. One such model[6] simulated a host population infected with two strains of a pathogen, one more virulent than the other. Although these pathogens were similarly transmitted, the more virulent strain could "steal"

[a] Supported in part by a training grant from the National Institutes of Health (AI 07350-05) and by research grants (AI 19693 and 29724).

249

hosts infected with the less virulent strain. Ultimately, both strains were lethal, with no chance of recovery or host resistance. When a large increase in transmissibility was coupled with a small increase in mortality, the more lethal pathogen predominated. Intermediate values of transmissibility and lethality permitted coexistence. While the results of this model may be directly applicable to some natural systems, the assumptions of total lethality, no immunity and complete replacement of one strain by another are excessively restrictive.

A related model,[7] providing for recovery of infected hosts, found that the most fit parasite is one that is poorly transmissible, nonpathogenic and that permits recovery of the host. Both host and parasite benefit from the light health burden imposed in this model, producing an "evolutionary stable strategy" (designated as ESS). This strategy, however, assumes no linkage between transmissibility and disease burden. The strength of that linkage crucially determines the evolution of virulence.[8]

A STOCHASTIC MODEL OF PATHOGEN COMPETITION

We constructed a stochastic model to determine how a link between virulence and transmissibility may affect the selective fitness of competing pathogens. One pathogen was given a fixed advantage in transmissibility over the other, but was burdened with varying mortality costs. A spatial orientation was used to determine whether transmission distance affects pathogenicity. This stochastic cellular automaton represents an interpretation of the standard SIR epidemic model.[9]

Cellular automata are dynamic systems of matrices consisting of discrete numbers whose values from one time step to the next and are a function of the values of a set of surrounding sites or "neighbors" on the matrix. With stochastic automata,[9] neighborhood values are used to derive a transition probability rather than a specific, deterministic state change. Biological applications of cellular automata have been reviewed by Ermentrout and Edelstein-Keshet.[10] In ecology, they have been used mainly to study the spatial dynamics of competitive interactions between organisms[11-14] or the spatial aspects of genetic exchange in populations.[15-16] Cellular automata have been proposed as an alternative to the use of differential equations in modeling natural phenomena.[17] Their greatest utility lies in their ability to reveal the spatial characteristics of a system. Many spatially oriented questions that would be difficult to model with differential equations can readily be analyzed by means of cellular automata. The spatial dynamics of an oscillating epidemic, including the morphology of epidemic wavefronts, can be examined graphically as demonstrated (FIG. 1).

MODEL ASSUMPTIONS

1. Virulence is defined as the increase in probability of death induced by a pathogen in its host. Transmissibility is represented as the probability

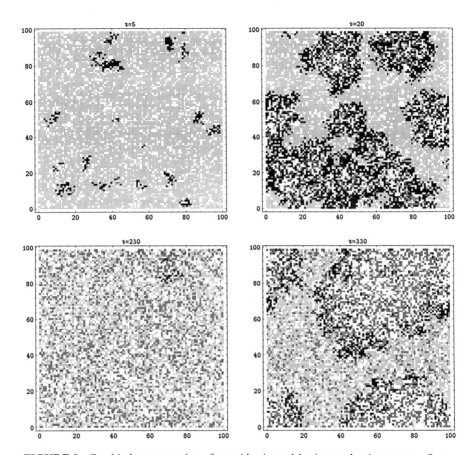

FIGURE 1. Graphical representation of an epidemic model using stochastic automata. Snapshots from the first 2 peaks of an oscillating epidemic are shown (peak one at 5 weeks and 20 weeks, peak 2 at 230 weeks and 330 weeks). Black squares represent infected hosts. Light gray squares represent susceptible hosts. Dark gray squares represent immune hosts. White squares represent unoccupied space.

that an infected host will transmit a pathogen to an uninfected host in its neighborhood.

2. The environment is represented by a matrix of 100 by 100 cells, representing a closed system with each edge contiguous with its opposite edge. The population is represented in the matrix by cells bearing non-zero states. Each cell represents one location which is either empty or occupied by a single individual. The individual is in one of 3 states with respect to each of the 2 pathogens: susceptible, infected or immune. Thus, there are 8 possible states for each cell. The population is dynamic and evolves as a function of a set of transition probabilities among these 8 states.

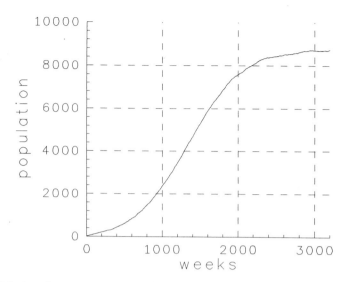

FIGURE 2. Population growth curve for hosts in the absence of epidemic pathogens in a matrix of 10,000 cells.

3. A probabilistic algorithm is used to simulate births. Successful births are conditional on both the outcomes of random draws at each site as well as whether the sites are occupied. The probability of a successful draw at each site is weighted linearly by the global population size. The probability of births is thus density-dependent and is positively regulated by the size of the host population and negatively regulated by the amount of unoccupied space present in the matrix. The growth curve of a population free of epidemic pathogens is represented (FIG. 2).

4. The probability of natural mortality, that which is not attributed to the epidemic pathogens, is fixed at 0.04 percent of all individuals per week. In the absence of epidemic pathogens, this gives a mean host lifespan of 48.08 years. The survival curve from a cohort of 100 hosts is represented (FIG. 3).

5. The 2 pathogen strains are assumed to be asexual and microparasitic. They are identical to each other in all respects except for virulence and transmissibility. Hosts can be dually infected with both strains without either gaining dominance over the other. Hosts are uniformly susceptible to both pathogens and are their sole reservoir. For the less virulent pathogen, the average period an infected host is capable of infecting another host, or the mean infective time, is about 4.9 weeks. The mean infective time of the virulent pathogen is a function of its virulence.

6. Immunity occurs at a rate of 20% of infected individuals per week and may occur as early as one week after a host acquires an infection. Immunity is lost at a rate of 2% of immune individuals per week.

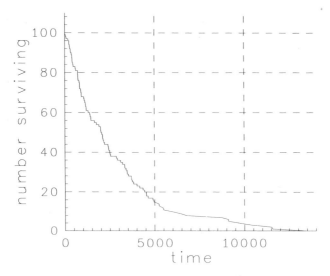

FIGURE 3. Survivorship curve for a cohort of 100 hosts in the absence of epidemic pathogens.

7. Transmission probabilities from an infective source to susceptible individuals are greatest with those adjacent to the source of infection and decrease geometrically with distance. For the greater distance transmission scenario, non-zero infection probabilities extend out into the matrix up to 4 layers in each direction (including diagonals) from the infective source. The probability that a susceptible cell will acquire an infection in a given week depends on the number of infective sources in its neighborhood as well as their distances. For the long-range transmission model, this probability is calculated with:

$$p_{inf} = t_c \left(1 - (1 - w_a)^a (1 - w_b)^b (1 - w_c)^c (1 - w_d)^d\right)$$

Here, t_c is a transmission coefficient representing the number of new infections expected to originate per unit time from a single infected source to its surrounding 9 cell by 9 cell neighborhood. Variables a–d are the numbers of infected individuals present within each of 4 radii surrounding the susceptible cell. The effects of increasing distance on decreasing probability of transmission are simulated through the choice of w_{a-d}, which are weighting factors used to simulate an exponential decrease in infective force with distance. The weighting factors were chosen such that with each step out from a point source of infection on the grid, the probability of an infection for each cell decreased by one half. These weights were normalized such that the maximum infective probability of a neighborhood equals one when t_c equals one ($w_a = 0.038461538$, $w_b = 0.019230769$, $w_c = 0.0096153846$, $w_d = 0.0048076923$). Thus, in non-overlapping infective neighborhoods, the transmission coefficient (t_c) represents the expected number of new infections arising per week per neighborhood.

8. The corresponding equation for short distance transmission is:

$$p_{inf} = t_c \, (1 - (1 - w_a)^a (1 - w_b)^b)$$

In this case, $w_a = 0.0625$ and $w_b = 0.03125$. With this arrangement of weights, any 2 infective sources selected at random from either scenario share an equal probability of producing infections in their neighborhoods each week despite the disparity in neighborhood size.

9. Mixed infections do not permit interactions between pathogens. It is assumed that one always dominates over the other in a mixed infection, and that neither has an advantage over the other. The mean impact of multiply infected hosts over the population is, thus, the average of the 2 mortality rates.

INITIAL CONDITIONS

1. The host population is increasing in size but is at about 95% of the carrying capacity (about 8,000 individuals), which is determined by the density-dependent birth algorithm.

2. All hosts are susceptible and naive except for 20 individuals, 10 infected with pathogen A, and 10 infected with pathogen B. These are dispersed randomly throughout the susceptible population.

3. Hosts infected with the less virulent pathogen (A) have an additional 0.4 percent probability of death over the background mortality rate. This value is held constant over all simulations. The more virulent pathogen (B) has a probability of transmission 50% greater than that of pathogen A. Although this advantage in transmissibility is also held constant over all simulations, the probability of death due to pathogen B is varied over a set of 20 simulations for each scenario (TABLE 1).

SCENARIOS

To examine the effect of a direct linkage between virulence and transmissibility, in all cases, an increase in mortality caused by one pathogen is assumed to be associated with an increase in its probability of transmission. This is modeled over a range of possible costs in greater mortality to the host from no increase in mortality to a level of mortality resulting in the extinction of that pathogen. The hypothesis that mobile virulent pathogens can better persist in a host population than those dependent on host-host transmission will be tested with the following scenarios:

1. Long-range transmission (vector- or water-borne). Non-zero transmission probabilities extend out to 4 cells in each direction (a 9 by 9 cell transmission area). Each infective individual has the potential to directly infect up to 80 other individuals.

TABLE 1. Relationship between Mortality Rate and Mean Infective Time for the More Virulent Pathogen B and Differences in Mean Infective Time from the Less Virulent Pathogen A[a]

Percent Mortality Due to Infection with More Virulent Pathogen B (per week)	Mean Infective Time of Infections with More Virulent Pathogen B (weeks)	Difference in Mean Infective Time Relative to Pathogen A ($mit_b - mit_a$, weeks)
0	4.990	+0.098
0.02	4.985	+0.093
0.05	4.978	+0.085
0.1	4.965	+0.073
0.2	4.941	+0.048
0.4	4.892	0
0.6	4.845	−0.047
0.8	4.799	−0.094
1.0	4.755	−0.137
2.0	4.537	−0.355
3.0	4.340	−0.552
4.0	4.160	−0.733
5.0	3.994	−0.899
7.0	3.698	−1.194
9.0	3.444	−1.449
11.0	3.222	−1.671
13.0	3.027	−1.866
15.0	2.854	−2.038
20.0	2.498	−2.395
40.0	1.666	−3.227

[a] Mortality parameters for pathogen B are listed for each of the 20 simulations conducted for both scenarios. Mortality due to pathogen A was held constant throughout all simulations.

2. Short-range transmission (host-host). Non-zero transmission probabilities extend out to 2 cells in each direction (5 by 5 transmission area). Each infective source can infect up to 24 individuals.

Each simulation was followed to a condition of near equilibrium (500 weeks) and fitness was assessed as the average prevalence of infection of each pathogen strain in the host population.

RESULTS

The outcomes of the remote and proximate scenarios respectively representing the difference in mean infective time for the virulent pathogen (B) ranged from a decrease of 3.5 weeks to an increase of 0.5 weeks (mean infective time was negatively correlated with probability of host mortality) (FIGS. 3 and 4). The pathogen that predominated in the population at 500 weeks depended on this difference in mean duration of infectivity. The virulent pathogen (B) competitively excluded the less virulent (A) solely when its decrease in mean infective time remained below a specific threshold. In all other cases, the less virulent pathogen predominated at the end of the simulation, with the more virulent pathogen usually driven to extinction.

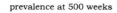

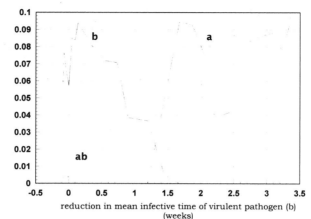

FIGURE 4. Long-distance transmission scenario—prevalence of both pathogens in the host population at 500 weeks is plotted for 20 different levels of impact of the more virulent pathogen (B), expressed as a reduction in mean infective time relative to that of the less virulent pathogen (A). In all cases, pathogen B has a 50% advantage in probability of transmission over pathogen A.

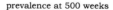

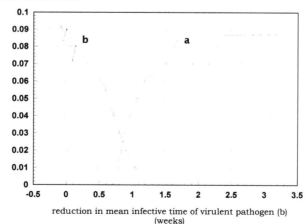

FIGURE 5. Short-distance transmission scenario—prevalence of both pathogens in the host population at 500 weeks is plotted for 20 different levels of impact of the more virulent pathogen (B), expressed as a reduction in mean infective time relative to that of the less virulent pathogen (A). In all cases, pathogen B has a 50% advantage in probability of transmission over pathogen A.

Remote transmission permitted the virulent pathogen to persist in the population with lower mean infective times than in the proximate scenario. Transmission over a great distance also increased the likelihood of the occurrence of mixed infections at equilibrium. Mixed infections never occurred at the end of any of the proximate simulations because one pathogen generally greatly predominated over the other, even when both ultimately were present. In the case of remote transmission, mixed infections were rare except when differences in mean infective time were small. Thus, under certain conditions, mobility enhanced the likelihood that the virulent pathogen would coexist with the less virulent strain in the host population.

The models were relatively insensitive to initial conditions, with small changes in parameters causing little alteration in equilibrium conditions after 500 time steps. All simulations shared an early epidemic peak and a crash of the pathogen population, followed by a rapid damping of oscillations to equilibrium. In two dimensions, this corresponded to a transition from a relatively homogeneous population of naive members to a heterogeneous terrain dotted with islands of susceptibility, which served as predictors of future outbreaks (FIG. 1). Certain pathogens persisted as wandering foci, which moved across the grid through patches dense with susceptibles. The structure of the matrix at equilibrium is coarser in systems with a narrow area of transmission than for those with a wider area of transmission, which tend to become much more mixed and less patchy. This patchiness could be demonstrated quantitatively by comparing coefficients of spatial autocorrelation. These results are analogous to the differences in spatial heterogeneity that result from different neighborhood sizes as reported in isolation-by-distance models of gene flow in populations.[15] Such differences in spatial heterogeneity have directly been observed in the distribution of melanic phenotypes of English moths that have different propensities for long-range flight.[18] Thus, patchiness is often the result of poor mixing caused by limited mobility.

DISCUSSION

Even when a linkage between virulence and transmissibility is assumed, our model demonstrates a limited competitive advantage of increased virulence. A wide parameter-space exists over which a nonvirulent pathogen may outcompete a highly virulent pathogen and even drive it to extinction. In both scenarios, the more virulent and more transmissible pathogen became more prevalent at equilibrium when its negative impact on hosts was low relative to the less virulent strain. This competitive advantage completely disappeared when increasing rates of host mortality caused the mean duration of infectivity to fall below a certain critical value. This threshold may represent the point at which the basic reproduction number of the more virulent pathogen falls below that of the less virulent one.

This model supports the hypothesis that mobile pathogens can withstand a greater level of mortality in their hosts than do less mobile pathogens. The range over which a more virulent pathogen is able to persist without extinction in a competitive situation with a less virulent pathogen was somewhat wider when transmission occurred over longer distances.

The greater persistence of the virulent pathogens in systems where they are transmitted over greater distances may be a function of their ability to disperse more readily to areas where susceptible hosts are more prevalent. In terms of this model, mobile pathogens are able to exploit susceptibility on the fringes of their transmissible range and thus increase the probability of reaching patches in the matrix capable of sustaining replication. This mobility affords greater opportunity for perpetuation over longer periods. Greater mobility may also explain the increased prevalence of mixed infections in the remote transmission scenario by increasing the probability that a singly infected host might be exposed to hosts carrying the other strain.

We conclude that newly emergent vector-borne pathogens may remain highly virulent longer than do those that are directly transmitted. Ultimately, however, both categories of pathogens would evolve toward a less virulent state. Enhanced virulence would be adaptive solely over a narrow range of conditions. When duration of infectivity exceeds duration of host survival, relatively nonvirulent pathogens would ultimately tend to drive other pathogens into extinction.

SUMMARY

To determine how virulence may be perpetuated in populations of vector-borne pathogens, we simulated their fitness in a stochastic simulation based on cellular automata. Thereby, directly transmissible pathogens that differed in virulence were permitted to compete for hosts with similarly virulent pathogens that could infect hosts remotely because they were vector-borne. Fitness was defined as the proportion of the host population infected with each pathogen at equilibrium. Virulent, directly transmitted pathogens prevailed solely when their infectivity was transient. When duration of infectivity exceeded that of host survival, the less virulent pathogen invariably prevailed. Although remotely transmitted virulent pathogens persisted somewhat longer than did virulent pathogens that were transmitted directly, they never perpetuated themselves. We conclude that populations of vector-borne pathogens may retain pathogenicity somewhat longer than do those that are directly transmitted, but that both kinds of pathogens tend to become nonvirulent.

ACKNOWLEDGMENTS

We are greatly indebted to Drs. Tamara Awerbuch and Martin Eichner for their invaluable advice and encouragement. This work was conceived as a project for the course Mathematical Models in Biology taught by Dr. T. Awerbuch.

REFERENCES

1. EWALD, P. W. 1987. Transmission modes and evolution of the parasitism-mutualism continuum. Ann. N.Y. Acad. Sci. **503:** 295–306.
2. HERRE, E. A. 1993. Population structure and evolution of virulence in nematode parasites of fig wasps. Science **259:** 1442–1445.
3. BULL, J. J. & I. J. MOLINEUX. 1992. Molecular genetics of adaptation in an experimental model of cooperation. Evolution **46:** 882–896.
4. KERMACK, W. O. & A. G. McKENDRICK. 1927. A contribution to the mathematical theory of epidemics. Proc. R. Soc. A **115:** 700–721.
5. ANDERSON, R. M. & R. M. MAY. 1979. Population biology of infectious diseases: Part I. Nature **280:** 361–367.
6. LEVIN, S. A. & D. PIMENTEL. 1981. Selection of intermediate rates of increase in parasite-host systems. Am. Nat. **117:** 308–315.
7. BREMERMANN, H. J. 1980. Sex and polymorphism as strategies in host-pathogen interactions. J. Theor. Biol. **87:** 671–702.
8. ANDERSON, R. M. & R. M. MAY. 1982. Coevolution of hosts and parasites. Parasitology. **85:** 411–426.
9. DOBERKAT, E. 1981. Stochastic automata: Stability, nondeterminism, and prediction. Lecture Notes in Computer Science. Berlin, Heidelberg, New York: Springer-Verlag.
10. ERMENTROUT, G. B. & L. EDELSTEIN-KESHET. 1993. Cellular automata approaches to biological modeling. J. Theor. Biol. **160:** 97–133.
11. CRAWLEY, M. J. & R. M. MAY. 1987. Population dynamics and plant community structure: Competition between annuals and perennials. J. Theor. Biol. **125:** 475–489.
12. HASSELL, M. P., H. N. COMINS & R. M. MAY. 1991. Spatial structure and chaos in insect population dynamics. Nature **353:** 255–258.
13. SILVERTOWN, J., S. HOLTIER, J. JOHNSON & P. DALE. 1992. Cellular automaton models of interspecific competition for space—the effect of pattern on process. J. Ecol. **80:** 527–534.
14. COLASANTI, R. L. & J. P. GRIME. 1993. Resource dynamics and vegetation processes: Deterministic model using 2-dimensional cellular automata. Func. Ecol. **7:** 169–176.
15. ROHLF, F. J. & G. D. SCHNELL. 1971. An investigation of the isolation-by-distance model. Am. Nat. **105:** 295–313.
16. DYTHAM, C. & B. SHORROCKS. 1992. Selection, patches and genetic variation: A cellular automaton modeling *Drosophila* populations. Evolut. Ecol. **6:** 342–351.
17. TOFFOLI, T. 1984. Cellular automata as an alternative to (rather than an approximation of) differential equations in modeling physics. Physica **10D:** 117–127.
18. BISHOP, J. A. & L. M. COOK. 1975. Moths, melanism and clean air. Sci. Am. **232:** 90–99.

Natural Selection in Pathogens

RICHARD LEVINS

Department of Population and International Health
Harvard School of Public Health
665 Huntington Avenue
Boston, Massachusetts 02115

Evolution in microbial pathogens depends on the same principles of variation and selection as in higher plants and animals. The dynamics of these processes have been explored in great detail for almost a century and need not be recapitulated here. But there are also some special features, either unique to bacteria and viruses or at least of special importance in these groups.

First, viruses and bacteria are haploids. Therefore questions of the phenotypes of heterozygotes, which have occupied the attention of population geneticists, do not arise. In fungi, heterocaryosis may play a role similar to heterozygosity. Here, direct gene-to-gene interactions among alleles within the cell nucleus do not occur, but their products may interact in the shared cytoplasm.

Second, there are special sources of variation in addition to ordinary random mutation and sexual recombination. Plasmids and phage particles and simple transformation (non-sexual exchange of DNA) allow for new genetic material from other species that are taxonomically remote, either directly or through bridge species. Thus the whole shared habitat may function as a single gene pool under conditions of extremely intense selection. For viruses, a shared habitat means infecting the same cell, but for bacteria it can refer to the domain of a whole flora such as the mouth, gut, female reproductive tract, or blood. Multiple infections from different sources (different species or populations of the same species) create the conditions for recombination and production of new strains of pathogens.

Third, mutation may not be random in the sense that neither the frequency nor the direction of mutation is necessarily independent of the conditions of selection.[1]

But the availablity of genetic variation is not simply a matter of mutation rates. A new variant must be able to increase fitness if it is to be selected. The effect on fitness of a random mutation will depend on the ecological location of the species. If it is already in a highly stressed, low resource environment, there will be few degrees of freedom available for improving fitness. Newly introduced genes in these populations may provide resistance to antibiotics or other stressors in very specific ways that require energy expenditure and therefore detract from the ability to face other challenges. But other kinds of mutations of a less specific sort may increase access to energy or other resources, providing the means to resist the immediate stressor and other threats as well. A species that has a generally low reproductive rate but broad tolerance of environmental variation may be kept in check by competitors and antagonists, but as conditions become more extreme the other species may drop out and it can not only survive but also adapt. Much recent research is focused on the evolutionary potential of species in different ecological niches and habitats (see for example the *American Naturalist* 1993 symposium supplement[2]).

The ecologically determined fraction of new genes that are beneficial in either way, multiplied by the rate of genetic variation, can provide a rough measure of the capacity of species to evolve. We then have to relate this evolution to virulence, contagion, time course within a host or the dynamics of epidemics. If energy is abundant then variants which detoxify an antibiotic may still have the reserves available for reproduction and meeting other challenges.

Fourth, the absence of the relatively sharp separation between the germ cells and somatic cells that we usually assume in multicellular organisms allows for cross-generational transmission (cell size, nutrient and enzyme concentrations), which is neither "genetic" in the usual sense nor "environmental" and therefore erased at reproduction. These transmissions are responsive to the environment. But since the host environment is influenced by the infection, the phenotype will change in regular ways in the course of an infection. Thus the pathogen can alter its own physiology by way of the host, in a sense using the host as an epigenetic factor. The antigenic or morphological characteristics may go through a regular sequence of changes, with the clone as a whole behaving to some extent like an individual organism. The host's response may even be a necessary part of the development of the pathogen, eventually giving rise to the form that can be transmitted. This gives the time course of an infection some of the qualities of "development" as well as of microbial population growth and evolution. Whereas population growth depends on reproduction, the production of like by like but with quantitative increase, and evolution is the irreversible production of unlikes, development is the production of unlikes in a regular sequence of stages eventually giving rise to the type of the original stage.

Fifth, bacteria are very small; their enormous surface-to-volume ratio results in a greater intensity of metabolic interchange among cells than takes place among metazoans. At the same time, the small size allows room only for some 100,000 macromolecules in a bacterium. It is not possible to contain all the enzymes that might be useful or store all the necessary nutrients. Thus different macromolecules, which by themselves may contribute to fitness, are also to some extent competing for space within the microbial cell, creating negative interactions among fitness components.

Despite the relatively easy genetic exchanges among microbes they do not all become one single optimal genotype. Rather their survival depends on the composition of their community of microorganisms, both homo- and heterospecific. Nutrients leak from cells that synthesize them to feed at least a minority of cells that do not. Detoxification of their shared environment is important to their joint survival. When cells die their components become available to their neighbors. This means that density- and frequency-dependent selection are likely to be the norm among bacteria, whereas they have been treated as interesting anomalies (most likely unjustly) in plant and animal population genetics.

Sixth, if an infection of a host results in a serious disease, it means that the host has been changed. The immune system, nutritional state, temperature, and other characteristics of the environment of the pathogen (and therefore the condition of the host) are a product of its own activity. The pathogen may also affect its own environment by way of the behavior of the host and medical intervention. For instance, a variant of an infection which produces a rash earlier than another may provoke earlier diagnosis and treatment. Since different genetic variants affect the host differently, our models must allow that the conditions of natural selection (the host environment, as expressed in selection coefficients) are themselves the outcome of selection.

Seventh, infection implies that the pathogen population is exposed both to the environment of the host and to the environment of transmission from host to host. This environment of transmission may be a vector, some other species, or the air, water or soil. Survival in that habitat may involve passive persistence as a spore or resting stage, but might also require active metabolism and reproduction in both situations. Selection in the host and selection in the environment between hosts may be quite different. Then the evolution of the pathogen will be the result of selection in possibly opposing directions and the outcome can depend on the duration of the two or more phases.

Eighth, people respond to epidemics. As the prevalence or incidence increase, we may see behavioral changes or public health interventions which change contagion, accelerate diagnosis and treatment, affect the vector or reservoir populations or survival habitats. People may panic during the upsurge of a life-threatening disease and take measures which protect or even harm them. When a disease passes its peak, or if it lasts long enough to become just another background hazard, the behavior may revert if protective measures are costly or uncomfortable. The duration of social "memory" and the capacity to take action for future expected outcomes is very sensitive to the social experience and resources of different parts of a population, the experiences that either teach or discourage the belief that people can understand their world and affect what happens to them and that current behavior influences what happens months or years from now. These aspects of social life are co-parameters along with the reproductive rates of pathogens or biting rates of mosquitoes or duration of immunity. This makes issues of equity and empowerment epidemiological issues as well as issues of justice.

It is also possible that the health care system acquires skill and resources during an outbreak, or conversely that it becomes saturated and treatment becomes less available or effective or that contagion increases. All of this dynamic affects the conditions of natural selection, the relative fitnesses of different genotypes, and hence changes in gene frequency. Thus public health policy becomes an evolutionary force.

In modeling these processes it would be ideal to treat in the same model the origins of variation, the identification of the selective values relating pathogen fitness to virulence and symptoms, the dynamics of the selection process itself, and the consequences of selection in the pathogen for the individual host and for the host population. The structure of this framework is shown in FIGURE 1. In most cases we are not ready to carry out the complete analysis, but we can examine parts of the causal network, focusing on those situations where our casual common sense reasoning may be misleading.

Our research program is considering three contexts of natural selection in pathogenic microorganisms and their vectors, operating on different time scales and with different assumptions as to what remains constant: microevolution within an individual host, intermediate level (mesoevolution) change during a period of endemism or recurrent outbreaks, and macroevolutionary and biogeographic changes in hosts and vectors above the species level.

Microevolution within an Infected Host in the Course of an Infection

The responses of the host to the infection (with or without medical intervention) change the environment of the pathogen, so that the infecting population of microbes may change during the course of the infection. Of special interest are the changes of serotype which help the pathogen evade the immune system. These may be induced by the host immune system itself and therefore are not simple "random mutations". Microbial changes can have other consequences besides avoiding the body's defenses. The surface antigens help a pathogen attach to its preferred tissue sites but also make the microbial invader detectable by the antibodies generated by the host. Therefore in the early stages of an infection the more "visible" and aggressive genotypes may have an advantage that is lost as the immune system responds. The altered serotypes may also attach to other host tissues, changing symptoms. Finally, these other sites, such as the central nervous system, may not afford exits to the outside as readily but represent evolutionary dead ends.

Such processes may be important for the clinical picture of an infection.

Evolution during an Outbreak

If a pathogen normally infects another species but may spill over to humans and be transmitted for several cycles among people before dying out, the environment of the human host is unfamiliar to the pathogen at the start

FIGURE 1. Structure of framework for modeling dynamics of the selection process.

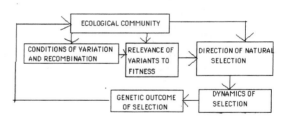

of an outbreak. The pathogens may evolve rapidly in response to these new host conditions so that the first cases will be regularly different from later ones. The sequence may be toward diminishing severity as in Lassa fever or toward increased severity.

New therapeutic practices or patterns of patient behavior can also be the new selective forces acting on familiar pathogens. Ewald[3] has considered some of these situations.

The alternation of conditions between the environment within the host and that outside the host means alternating selection pressures. When infection begins, the invading pathogen population has the makeup that has been selected for the outside environment. It is then selected for reproductive rate in the host. Suppose that an initial inoculum X is multiplied by R within a host. It then faces conditions in the external environment where only a fraction of the pathogens survives each day. Let that fraction be S. Then by the time it infects a new host, the numbers are reduced to RS^t for time t between hosts. One genotype with fitnesses R_1, S_1 will replace another with fitnesses R_2, S_2 if $R_1S_1^t > R_2S_2^t$, or $R_1 > R_2(S_1/S_2)t$.

If $R_1 > R_2$ and $S_1 > S_2$ then genotype 1 will be favored by selection. But there may be a negative relation between reproductive success in the host and survival outside the host. Suppose that $R_1 > R_2$ but $S_1 < S_2$. Then the outcome can depend on t. During the height of an epidemic t may be short and selection favors the rapid reproducer. When the interval t is longer for reasons of changes in the environment or because there are fewer susceptible people, the inequality may be reversed to favor the durable survivors in nature. An alternative genotype with a very high R may still be favored by selection, whereas an only moderately higher rate of reproduction in the host would be selected against. Suppose the genotype in question confers antibiotic resistance at the expense of survival between hosts. It will spread in a population if the prevalence is high enough to reduce the waiting time between hosts below some threshold. Also, different genotypes that confer moderate resistance may be selected against, but a recombinant that combines them may pass the threshold and be favored.

Selection may favor different genotypes in the course of an outbreak or in places with different endemic prevalences. But we still do not know how this affects the symptoms or virulence of a disease. It is often assumed, plausibly but not rigorously, that increased reproduction in the host implies greater virulence. But this is not always the case. In the tristeza disease of citrus, the concentration of strains of benign virus in an infected host tree is not less than that of the more virulent strain. The difference in virulence seems to be related to differential attachment to xylem cells and the consequent blocking of water transport.

The outcome of selection is not necessarily the replacement of one genotype by another or an equilibrium gene frequency. We[4] studied the dynamics of frequency dependent selection that may apply to this situation.

Suppose that there are two serotypes which infect a host, with frequencies x and $1 - x$ and exponential rates of increase r and s, respectively. Assume that each serotype evokes a highly specific antibody which reduces its rate of increase. Let the fitnesses r and s decrease with their abundance because of the antibodies they evoke:

$$r = r_0 - r_1 x$$

$$s = s_0 - s_1(1 - x).$$

Finally, let $\beta = r_0 - s_0 + s_1$ and $a = (r_1 + s_1)/r_0 - s_0 + s_1)$.
Then the new frequency after a cycle of selection will be

$$x_{n+1} = x_n \exp[\beta(1 - ax_n)/\{1 - x_n + x_n \exp[\beta(1 - ax_n)]\}$$

Here β represents the intensity of selection and a is a measure of the asymmetry of selection. If $r_0 = s_0$ and $r_1 = s_1$ then $a = 2$ and the equilibrium gene frequency $1/a$ would be $1/2$. In that case, if $\beta \leq 4$ the equilibrium is stable and will be reached as long as there is some heterogeneity to begin with. If $\beta \geq 4$ the equilibrium is unstable and we would observe sustained oscillations with gene frequency alternating above and below $1/2$. If selection is asymmetric or the production of antibody is slower so that fitness depends on gene frequencies going further back than one cycle, more complicated behaviors are possible. A combination of strong selection and marked asymmetry can result in chaotic trajectories. The serotypes would fluctuate in frequency without obvious pattern.

This is one example of a difference equation. Difference equations arise in a number of situations in epidemiology. In what follows, the behavior of the public health sector is an essential part of the dynamics. Suppose that there is a population of mosquitoes that grows logistically during the rainy season so that at the end of the season an initial abundance in year n, x_n, has become $x_n e^{rt}/(1 - x_n + x_n e^{rt})$. Here t is the fraction of the year suitable for mosquito reproduction.

Now the Health Department or Ministry enters with a mosquito control program so that during the rest of the year, over a period $1 - t$, there is an imposed mosquito mortality rate that depends on the effectiveness of the technology and on the budget. Let the budget be an increasing function of the level of concern, and therefore of the abundance of mosquitoes. Therefore mortality per unit time is some increasing function of x_n, say mx_n, and survival a decreasing function of mortality, $\exp\{-mx_n\}$. At the start of the next rainy season the mosquito population has become

$$x_{n+1} = x_n \exp\{rt - mx_n(1 - t)\}/[1 - x_n + x_n \exp\{rt\}].$$

The outcome depends on the parameters r and m and the duration of the rainy season, t. Roughly, if the mosquito population expands greatly during the rainy season and contracts sharply during the dry due to the intervention, then populations may show erratic fluctuations. Climate change can alter t, the relative duration of the rainy season. Pesticide resistance would reduce m. Therefore both could affect the time course of the populations. Modifications of the assumptions to allow dormant eggs from previous years to hatch give delay equations that we are now studying.

The choice of the functional form for mortality was to some extent arbitrary. The specific model was intended to reveal qualitative relations rather than provide numerical results. Therefore it is necessary to examine the curve $x_{n+1} = g(x_n)$ more generally to determine how different specific situations will depart from the behavior of the initial model. This is done in APPENDIX 1, where we present a new method for interpreting difference equations in a simple intuitive way.

Biogeographic Change

A major current concern is, how might expected climate changes affect the distribution of disease? This requires the linking in a causal network of the following processes:

1) Identify the climatic changes that are relevant to the organism in question, remembering that organisms select, transform and define their environments.[5] Global warming may be relevant as average temperature, as degree days, as daily maximum, as number of hours of daylight below some threshold, as uncertainty of food supply, as gas or salt concentrations in water, *etc.*

2) Determine their physiological effects. For instance, temperature change can be a stressor but also may accelerate development, reduce size of invertebrates and change the developmental synchrony of insect parasites and their hosts.

3) Trace the initial physiological impact through the network of species interactions of an ecological community. The mathematical method as developed in Puccia and Levins[6] is shown in APPENDIX 2. Some qualitative results are that a strong physiological impact does not necessarily imply a large population impact; the effect of a climatic change may be greatest through indirect pathways; the outcome may even be the reverse of what the physiological impact would lead us to expect, depending on the rest of the ecosystem; and all impacts are reduced in communities with strong over-all negative feedback.

4) Consider the direction of natural selection on these parameters and the context of variability and selection that determines evolutionary adjustment. Any evolutionary change will also percolate through the whole network as described in 3) and affect all species in the community.

Conclusions

The evolution of pathosystems involves the multiple interactions among variables in the contexts of variation, selection and the impact of selection in communities of species and with the interventions of the health system.

In this unfamiliar terrain plausible common sense verbal arguments may turn out to be quite misleading. Mosquito populations reduced by larvicides may have more robust individuals and therefore may show increased vectorial capacity. Insecticides may increase the abundance of insect vectors. Antibiotics may lead to increased infection, immunization may increase the severity of disease, health centers may be the foci of infection and diagnosis may lead to victimization. There is no alternative to the broad-based, multilevel and transdisciplinary analysis of epidemiological complexity.

REFERENCES

1. FOSTER, P. L. & J. CAIRNS. 1992. Mechanisms of directed mutation. Genetics **13**(4): 783–789.
2. PARSONS, P. A. (Symposium Organizer). 1993. Evolutionary responses to environmental stress. Am. Nat. **142**: Supplement.
3. EWALD, P. 1987. Transmission modes and the evolution of the parasite mutalism continuum. Ann. N.Y. Acad. Sci. **503**: 295–305.
4. GROVE, E. A., V. L. KOCIC, G. LADAS & R. LEVINS. 1993. Periodicity in a simple genotype selection model. Diff. Equations and Dynam. Sys. **i**(1): 35–50.
5. LEVINS, R. & R. C. LEWONTIN. 1986. The Dialectical Biologist. Cambridge, MA: Harvard University Press.
6. PUCCIA, C. & R. LEVINS. 1986. Qualitative Modeling of Complex Systems: An Introduction to Loop Analysis and Time Averaging. Cambridge, MA: Harvard University Press.

APPENDIX 1: UNDERSTANDING DIFFERENCE EQUATIONS

Suppose that the curve in FIGURE 2 gives the relationship between the prevalence of a disease at two consecutive times:

$$p_{n+1} = g(p_n).$$

Draw the 45° diagonal from the origin. It intersects the curve at the equilibrium value of p, where $p_{n+1} = p_n$. If the slope of $g(p_n)$ is greater than -1 at equilibrium, the equilibrium is locally stable. If it is greater than -1 for all points after the peak, then this equilibrium is globally stable and there are no periodic orbits. The trajectory can be found from any starting point p_n by going vertically to the curve and then horizontally to the diagonal, and repeating the process.

Now identify the landmarks in the graph. First find the largest value of the curve below equilibrium, peak A. Draw a horizontal line to the diagonal. The abscissa of this point is M, the maximum value in the permanent region. Next find the minimum height of the curve above equilibrium but below M. The horizontal line to the diagonal locates m. The variable will eventually remain in the region of permanence [m, M]. From the equilibrium point draw a horizontal line to the curve $g(p)$. This identifies y_{-1}, the "pre-image" of the equilibrium. If $y_{-1} < m$ and the equilibrium is unstable, then p_n will be alternately above and below equilibrium. Now draw a horizontal line from y_{-1} to lower values of the curve. This locates y_{-2}, the pre-image of y_{-1}. If $y_{-2} < m$, the dynamics is chaotic. That is, there are periodic orbits of all periods and also non-periodic trajectories, and initial conditions that are arbitrarily close to each other can give rise to divergent outcomes.

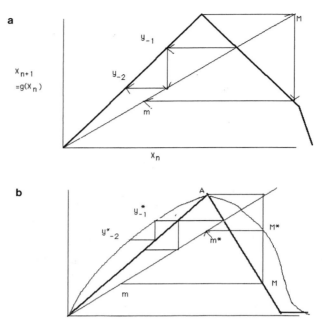

FIGURE 2. Graphical interpretation of a difference equation. **a.** A polygon graph showing how to find the landmark points. **b.** Bulging the graph to the left of the peak shifts y_{-1} and y_{-2} to the left so that they may fall below m. Bulging above the peak shifts m to the right.

The procedure outlined above can be used with or without an equation. It can also tell how the outcome changes with changed assumptions. Suppose that the disease is more contagious when prevalence is low. Then the curve would bulge to the left. The pre-images y_{-1} and y_{-2} will shift to the left while m has not been affected at all. Therefore oscillation and chaos are made more likely. Or suppose that intervention is increased when the incidence is greatest, thus lowering the peak. This reduces M and increases m. Now m can be greater than y_{-1} and y_{-2}, removing chaotic or long oscillations. Or suppose that at high prevalence it is no longer possible to isolate patients so that the right-hand leg of the curve increases. This will not affect the pre-image points but will increase m, reducing the possibility of chaos. Note that the same intervention, increased treatment and lowering $g(p_n)$, will have different effects on the dynamics depending on which prevalences are most affected. Finally, since contagion and recovery both depend on the parameters of the pathogen, even small genetic changes can alter the dynamics. A genotype which is more contagious to some subset of the population will bulge the curve below the peak to the left and may stabilize a chaotic process.

APPENDIX 2: SIGNED DIGRAPHS AND THE SENSITIVITY OF VARIABLES TO PARAMETER CHANGE

The vertices of a graph are the variables of interest. They may be species in a community or the familiar Susceptibles, Exposeds, Infecteds, and Resistants of a standard SEIR epidemiological model with or without variables added for the behavior of the Ministry of Health.

The links between variables show their interactions. A sharp arrowhead indicates a positive effect $\longrightarrow$ and a round arrowhead a negative effect, $\longrightarrow\!\!\circ$. (These are the signs of the first partial derivatives, $\partial(dx_i/dt)/\partial x_j$, the a_{ij} of the Jacobean matrix). A path $P_{ij}^{\,k}$ is a simple path from x_j to x_i passing through k vertices without entering any vertex more than once. The complement of the path is the network of all variables not on the path. The feedback or "gain" of a network is $(-1)^{k+1}$ times the determinant of that matrix of k interacting variables. It can also be expressed in terms of the sums of products $\Sigma(-1)^{m+1}L(m, k)$, where $L(m, j)$ is the product of m disjunct loops with a total of k vertices.

The basic result is

$$\partial x_i/\partial C = \Sigma \partial(dx_j/dt)/\partial x_j \; P_{ij}^{\,k} \; F\{comp(P_{ij}^{\,k})\}/F_n.$$

Summation is over all impacts and paths.

That is, the effect of a parameter change on the equilibrium level of any variable is equal to the sensitivity of the variable receiving the impact times the path from that variable to the target variable times the feedback of the complement divided by the feedback of the whole system. A strongly negative F_n makes all variables less sensitive to environmental or to genetic changes. The complement of a variable may be positive. Then the impact is the reverse of what is expected from the direct impact and the path. A zero complement would result in no change. The magnitude of the change is not necessarily greatest at the point of direct impact.

Signed Digraphs of Model Ecopathosystems

In FIGURE 3, a–d represent a sample of alternative models of the insertion of *Vibrio cholerae* into marine ecosystems. In (a), the relation between the vibrio and algae is mutualistic. Vibrio is self-damped by competition for space on the algal surface. In (a), the vibrios are consumed along with the algae by crustaceans (C) that are consumed by fish predators, which in turn have their own predators. In (b) the top predators have been removed either by over-fishing or pollution. In (c) the vibrio is commensal with the algae and also competes with it for nutrients. The crustacean has only one trophic level above it. In (d) the vibrio is a parasite of the crustacean. In the tables next to each graph the rows represent the direction of change of equilibrium population levels in response to changes entering the system by way of the specified variable. Each column shows the response of a given variable to all the sources of change. Looking down a pair of columns we can see what

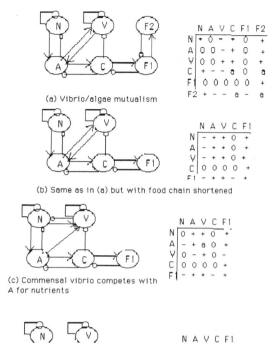

(a) Vibrio/algae mutualism

	N	A	V	C	F1	F2
N	+	0	-	+	0	+
A	0	0	-	+	0	+
V	0	0	+	+	0	+
C	+	-	-	a	0	a
F1	0	0	0	0	0	+
F2	+	-	-	a	-	a

(b) Same as in (a) but with food chain shortened

	N	A	V	C	F1
N	-	+	+	0	+
A	-	+	+	0	+
V	-	+	+	0	+
C	0	0	0	0	+
F1	-	+	+	-	+

FIGURE 3. Models of marine ecosystems with *Vibrio cholerae*.

(c) Commensal vibrio competes with A for nutrients

	N	A	V	C	F1
N	0	+	+	0	+
A	-	+	a	0	+
V	0	-	+	0	-
C	0	0	0	0	+
F1	-	+	+	-	+

(d) Vibrio parasitizes crustaceans

	N	A	V	C	F1
N	0	+	0	0	+
A	-	+	0	0	+
V	0	0	+	0	-
C	0	0	0	0	+
F1	-	+	-	-	+

correlation patterns to expect between any two variables in response to changes entering by way of any variable. The tables are all different, and therefore appropriate observations could differentiate among models. The removal of the top predator from (a) to (b) changes almost all relations. In (a), despite the mutualism between the vibrio and algae, they will be uncorrelated in response to nutrient changes. In (b) they show a strong positive correlation, but both will be negatively correlated with nutrients, although positively correlated with nutrient input. The anomalous response of nutrient level to nutrient input is a consequence of the positive (mutualist) feedback between A and V that appears in the complement of N. An increased input of nutrient results in an amplified increase in the algae/vibrio mutualist subsystem that then consumes more nutrient to below its original level. This positive feedback makes the whole system more labile, and along with the negative three-variable loop A, C, V can cause oscillations.

Mathematical Modeling

Concept Paper

INTRODUCTION

The study of the emergence of new diseases is a complex area requiring an interdisciplinary approach. Mathematical models allow the integration of the multiple factors involved in the appearance and spread of new infectious diseases. This methodology can incorporate biological, social, behavioral, economic, and political factors into structures that lend themselves to quantitative and qualitative analyses.

USES OF MATHEMATICAL MODELS

1. Understanding conditions under which infectious diseases emerge and spread. This includes the identification of epidemiological characteristics, such as the basic reproductive rate and vectorial capacity, which become objects of study in their own right, and the impacts of phenomena such as asymptomatic carriers, long latency, transovarial transmission in vectors and the dynamic consequences of the heterogeneity of populations. It also includes the modeling of the vulnerability of populations, which requires the integration of social variables into previously narrowly defined biological models.

2. The development of diagnostic indicators based on the dynamics of outbreaks. Such characteristics as the rates of increase and decrease of prevalence, the shape of the spatial spread, the constancy or variability of times between outbreaks and their magnitudes will eventually become as familiar as the fevers, rashes and hematological indicators in puzzling out anomalous health problems.

3. Prediction of possible outbreaks of known infections. We understand prediction not as the definitive specification of time and place for an epidemic, but as a reduction of uncertainty about future events through the identification of processes and signs of increasing risk.

4. Prediction of most likely geographic sites and types of new infections combining models of the community ecology of microorganisms, the dynamics of natural selection, and the patterns of host susceptibility.

5. Evaluating potential intervention strategies by taking into account the behavior of the intervenor as co-variable with that of the vectors, hosts and parasites.

6. Development of research strategies by identifying what we need to know and creating new objects of research.

EXAMPLES[a]

Examples of mathematical models that have had an important influence on disease control policies include the Ross malaria model,[1,2] the MacDonald malaria model,[3] Yorke and Hethcote's model of gonorrhea,[4] Angela McLean's model for measles vaccination in tropical countries,[5] Anderson and May's model for measles vaccination in UK, Anderson and Trewhella's model for wildlife reservoirs of bovine tuberculosis,[6] Smith and Grenfell's and Smith's models for controlling gastrointestinal nematode infections in ruminants,[7] Medley, Guatt and Bundys' models for controlling soil-borne nematode infections of humans[8] and Robert's model of cestode infections of humans and domestic animals. In agriculture, a model constructed by Anderson and Levins showed that the most important factor in preventing the spread of a virus in bean plants is preventing the arrival of the white fly (see paper by Pamela Anderson and F. J. Morales in this volume, pp. 181–194), as opposed to reducing its abundance once it has arrived. For the purpose of exploring interventions against the spread of Lyme disease, Sandberg, Awerbuch and Spielman constructed a model and showed that reduction of deer in a particular site wouldn't eliminate Lyme disease. Massive killing of deer to below a certain threshold would be required to achieve this goal.

In the course of the conference, several modeling problems were posed which belong on our research agenda:

1. The social science group raised the question of the incorporation of risk and social factors in modeling. The difficulties are obvious. We do not have equations for: people's behavior, the relation between the frequency of a threat to health and the perception of that threat, the structure of power as it impinges on the dynamics of institutional decision making, or the production of knowledge. Therefore the most common kind of modeling, which attempts to describe the processes of concern by systems of precisely specified simultaneous equations, is not available. However, more qualitative modeling approaches might be a first step (see paper by Tamara Awerbuch in this volume, pp. 232–241).

2. What is the effect of nutrient enrichment or overfishing on the relative abundance of the edible and the inedible (and sometimes toxic) plankton species? Here the numerical computation of solutions to differential equations and the qualitative analysis of the networks of interactions in the marine ecosystems are available methods.

3. Stephen Morse asked if already stressed ecosystems, which have been partly degraded by run-off, would be more vulnerable to the climatological anomalies that are part of the normal environmental fluctuation. This can be viewed as a problem in sensitivity analysis applied to models of large marine

[a] For other references please see paper by Tamara Awerbuch "Evolution of mathematical models of epidemics" and paper by Gary Smith "Characteristics of the host-parasite interactions that promote parasite persistence" in this section.

ecosystems. The technical side of the sensitivity analysis is less problematic than the decisions as to what indicators of ecosystem health to use.

4. What is the effect of an alternative reservoir or host on the prevalence of vectored infectious disease? It can have opposite effects, increasing the vector population but reducing the fraction of the vector population that transmits infection to people. Therefore the outcome has to be modeled with more detail before a conclusion can be reached.

5. The recent outbreak of a hantavirus disease in the southwestern United States (at Four Corners) has been linked to short-term weather conditions affecting rodent food resources against a background of regional ecological change associated with "development." Short-term modeling has estimated that the basic reproductive rate for the epidemic (see chapter by Gary Smith) is between 1 and 2. This means that a small perturbation in the mouse population may be enough to control the infection in humans. Therefore the CDC recommended clearing of the areas around homes to reduce the local carrying capacity of the environment for mice. Since mouse population density is a component of the reproductive rate of the disease, this may be sufficient to protect the human population. We are still in need of a concerted effort to link already extensive knowledge of rodent population dynamics with their parasites in multi-species models.

RECOMMENDATIONS

Mathematical modeling should be incorporated into the research agendas for the preparation for new and resurgent diseases. This work would include:

1. The continued development of the compartment type models for specific diseases that take into account their special features and allow quantitative conclusions.

2. Qualitative models are needed to understand the dynamics of multi-species interactions in aquatic and terrestrial ecosystems subject to perturbation.

3. Models of the within-host dynamics of infection and response are needed in order to understand the parameters of population level dynamics.

4. Models of vulnerability, behavior, and intervention are needed to make epidemiology a truly biosocial science.

5. Models of pathogen evolution are needed to take into account the special features of genetic change and symbiosis in microorganisms.

6. Finally, research is needed to develop new mathematical approaches designed for the new epidemiology in which greater complexity is combined with less precise specification.

Mathematical models require knowledge of the diseases in order to be relevant. There is a current need for a comprehensive database integrating pathosystem information of human, veterinary, and plant pathosystems.

REFERENCES

1. Ross, R. 1911. The Prevention of Malaria, 2nd edition. London: John Murray.
2. Ross, R. 1916. An application of the theory of probabilities to the study of *a priori* pathometry, Part I. Proc. R. Soc., Ser. A **92:** 204–230.
3. MacDonald, A. 1957. The Epidemiology and Control of Malaria. London: Oxford University Press.
4. Yorke, J. A., H. W. Hethcote & A. Nold. 1978. Dynamics and control of the transmission of gonorrhea. Sex. Transm. Dis. **5:** 51–56.
5. McLean, A. R. & R. M. Anderson. 1988. Measles in developing countries. Part I. Epidemiological parameters and patterns. Epidemiol. Infect. **100:** 111–133.
6. Anderson, R. M. & W. Trewhella. 1985. Population dynamics of the badger (*Meles meles*) and the epidemiology of bovine tuberculosis (*Myobacterium bovis*). Phil. Trans. R. Soc., London, B **310:** 327–381.
7. Smith, G. & B. T. Grenfell. 1990. Population biology of pseudorabies in swine. Am. J. Vet. Res. **51:** 148–155.
8. Medley, G. F., H. L. Guatt & D. A. P. Bundy. 1993. A quantitative framework for evaluation of the effect of community treatment on the morbidity due to ascariasis. Parasitology **106:** 211–221.

Integrating a Social Sciences Perspective into an Approach to New Disease

Introduction—Social Sciences Section

The emergence of new disease cannot be understood fully without understanding its social dimensions. Perceptions of disease, of what constitutes disease risk for both individuals and groups, of what is considered biologically abnormal, and what is considered an appropriate response to "disease," are culturally and socially mediated. Recognition of disease depends on perception of threat or identification of a deviation from the natural order, the expected course of events. Social factors not only shape patterns of risk but also influence how individuals, communities, and societies take action when confronted by a threat.

The papers that follow explore some of the ways social processes shape pathways of infection and disease. Social processes define the basis of public understanding of risk, causation, and the nature and capacity of response to disease. In many ways, exposure, the distribution and intensity of risk, and the framing of response are determined by socioeconomic and political conditions. Such forces as oppression, discrimination, historical memory, and notions of community will influence public attitudes and ultimately health-related behaviors.

The exploration of these social issues will be best served by the development of an integrated agenda for theory and empirical inquiry. Studies of disease emergence should incorporate insights of both the biological and the social sciences—including perspectives from economics, politics, anthropology as well as the behavioral sciences. These papers begin to map the social terrain on which new diseases emerge.

Emerging Epidemic Diseases

Anthropological Perspectives

JOHANNES SOMMERFELD

Harvard Institute for International Development
1 Eliot Street
Cambridge, Massachusetts 02138

Epidemics, whether induced by new or well-known infectious agents, are not exclusively biological occurrences. To a large extent they involve people's representations and behaviors: people whose behaviors change the ecology of an existing host-agent relationship; people afflicted by a disease or by its stigma; people at risk and people protecting themselves; journalists and other professional groups whose reports and attitudes fashion public opinion; and scientists whose conceptual frameworks, hypotheses, and public health recommendations contribute to making an epidemic also a social and cultural process. In this paper I will discuss the role of social and cultural factors in the evolution of infectious disease epidemics. These factors refer to collective behaviors and representations as they are, to a large extent, shaped by society and culture. It is argued that behavioral patterns and representations are important factors in the emergence and spread of epidemic disease. Their discussion here aims at broadening the biomedical focus on pathogens and vector-host relationships as the ultimate and sole causes of infectious disease epidemics by including social and cultural factors that facilitate the spread of disease in human populations.

This paper reviews social science literature on epidemics so as to familiarize non-social scientists with its source. First, I will briefly describe and outline developments within the biocultural approach to medical anthropology pertaining, specifically, to emergence factors of new diseases. Second, I will review the literature on cultural and social reactions to epidemics during the evolution and containment of epidemics. Third, I will discuss the public health implications of a framework that takes into consideration the cultural and social aspects of an epidemic process.

Two major conceptual approaches within the health-related social sciences are preoccupied with human disease and offer empirical or theoretical material to the study of epidemics. Bio-social and bio-cultural approaches study disease from the perspective of human ecology and focus on cultural and social emergence factors in epidemics. Cultural anthropological, ethnomedical, and historical work contributes more to the understanding of how epidemics are interpreted by human populations and how humans behave when confronting epidemic disease.

BIOCULTURAL RESEARCH AND EMERGENCE FACTORS

Biocultural anthropology investigates the link between biological, social, behavioral, and cultural factors in studies of human disease.[1] The focus of biocultural anthropology has traditionally been on cultural and social adaptation of human populations in a particular ecological setting[2] and how culture, behavior, and society influence the transmission of infectious agents to hosts.[3-5] It has also been documented how epidemics emerge in societies when adaptive mechanisms deteriorate, particularly as a consequence of political subjugation,[6] economic development,[7] culture contact, social change and acculturation,[8,9] and the alteration of a population's ecological setting (cf. ref. 10).

Macrosociological behavioral phenomena such as population movements or the alteration of the environment have been shown to contribute to the emergence of new or resurgent epidemics. Population movements encompass mass migratory phenomena of various underlying reasons (e.g., famine, war, economic breakdown, political unrest), as well as international travel or trade. A new series of viruses reached human populations because of massive alterations of the environment. Deforestation, for example, has largely contributed to the epidemic occurrence of Kyasanur Forest disease.[10] Ecological degradation has also contributed to the epidemic emergence of Lassa, Marburg, Ebola and many other viruses.[11] Urbanization with its ecological consequences has led to outbreaks of dengue fever, particularly in cities of developing countries.[12] Microlevel behavioral factors contributing to the emergence of epidemic infectious disease include feasting patterns, dietary practices, hygiene, sexual behavior, and the handling of animals, which all influence in one way or another individual risk of exposure to disease.

Prospective research within the bio-cultural approach has recently been added to traditionally more retrospective research designs. Scientists are now beginning to document how economic activities as well as social and cultural change affect the bio-cultural adaptation of populations to their natural habitat and how this subsequently leads to the emergence of new diseases. Medical anthropologist Carol Jenkins, for instance, in a collaborative project involving virologists and entomologists, has set up a prospective case-control study involving four villages in the highlands of Papua New Guinea. Her team investigates the impact of large scale logging on the health of villagers by systematically documenting economic, social, and cultural change as well as existing and emerging infectious agents in humans and animals.[13] A further challenge to future biocultural research will be to critically contextualize biocultural data with a political-economic perspective taking into consideration large-scale societal, political, and economic ramifications of health and medical care.[14] The emergence of epidemic disease will then be investigated not only in its micro-societal and ecological context but also in the context of macro-societal forces that contribute to the living conditions of the affected population and to the political economy of health and health care in the respective society as well.

PATTERNS OF REACTIONS TO EPIDEMIC DISEASE

A large body of literature from an historical and socio-cultural perspective has documented social and cultural repercussions of epidemics in time and space. Examples include, the impact of the AIDS epidemic on social institutions in the United States,[15] the role of epidemics in the political subjugation and conquest of societies,[6] the evocation of collective fears and representations,[16] and, historically, the use of epidemics in controlling the sick and often powerless as well as the healthy in order to redefine intra-societal power relations.[17] A major focus of comparative work has been to describe universal as well as society-specific patterns of reactions to epidemics. McGrath,[18] in reviewing worldwide ethnographic evidence from the Human Relations Area File (HRAF), a cross-cultural data base at Yale University, suggests six historically common behavioral patterns of social responses to epidemics: 1) flight or migration from the epicenters of the epidemic; 2) development of therapeutic as well as preventive measures that are commonly not the norm (*e.g.*, ceremonies, quarantine); 3) blaming and scapegoating individuals or institutions; 4) resignation or acceptance of the disease; 5) ostracism of sick individuals and those at risk; and 6) intragroup conflict. However, a certain society as it is shaped by cultural, political, and economic forces, may exhibit society-specific reactions to epidemics. Fox,[19] for example, in an historical analysis of responses to epidemics in the United States since the 18th century, reports prototypical reactions to epidemic disease that include: 1) an underestimation of the severity of the problem; 2) fear and anxiety; 3) flight, denial, and scapegoating of carriers, particularly foreigners, and 4) business-civic coalitions in controlling the shape of public health interventions.

Cultural anthropologists who are confronted with epidemics during their fieldwork in a community have provided a number of in-depth ethnographic case-reports about collective reactions to epidemics (*e.g.*, refs. 10, 20, and 21; *cf.* ref. 22). Most of these accounts focus on how people's belief systems influence health-care behavior. In the face of an epidemic, human populations interpret epidemic disease within the framework of pre-existing culture-specific representations. Nichter[10] has documented how an outbreak of Kyasanur Forest disease in southwest India was interpreted in terms of moral transgression against local patron deities and how this interpretation further influenced the health-seeking behavior of the affected population. Nichter's case study also suggests that certain biological characteristics of the epidemic, in his case the specific loci of the epidemic and the signs and symptoms of the disease, are reinterpreted within cultural theories pertaining, more specifically, to health, the nosology and etiology of disease, the nature of healing, and more generally, to misfortune, life, and death. Folk etiologic and nosologic representations of this kind can shape group behavioral responses in the face of a spreading epidemic. Nichter, for instance, showed how villagers preferred private practitioners and disregarded hospital facilities set up specifically for Kyasanur Forest disease patients.

Illness representations are generally not uniform and stable but rather are in flux during the course of an epidemic. In fact, multiple explanations can co-exist and new categorizations can emerge, especially for imported epidemic infections. Even widely shared models, for instance attributing certain diseases to deities, can change over time or adapt to a particular epidemic situation. Mariamman, a pan-Indian Goddess traditionally associated with smallpox, became linked with other sicknesses of the poor such as tuberculosis, after the eradication of smallpox.[23] She also became associated, at one point during the 1984 epidemic, with the appearance of Kyasanur Forest disease in southwest India.[10]

Biomedical terms such as malaria are often popularized and then incorporated into the pre-existing medical system without further elaboration of their conceptual implications (*e.g.*, mode of transmission, risk factors, prevention).[24] Widely shared cultural models are usually the outcome of a societal process where consensus is reached over time.[21] It is also possible that populations already have a specific illness model for a re-emerging epidemic and that they describe these symptoms to health care practitioners. Sign and symptom recognition or knowledge of an infectious agent, however, rarely implies exclusive compliance with public health measures. Coreil,[20] in her account of an anthrax epidemic in Haiti, showed that health-seeking behavior of anthrax patients implied concurrent usage of traditional therapeutic approaches, an observation also made in China during a cholera epidemic.[25]

Ideas and behavioral patterns can be transmitted from person to person just like infectious agents. Epidemics are, in fact, recognized as such and interpreted by humans, a phenomenon that can be studied within the framework of an "epidemiology of representations."[26] Public reactions to epidemics often involve the triggering of specific associations that pertain to the larger society's belief system. Consider, for example, the idea of AIDS as a "gay plague" or the representation of the hantavirus epidemic as a "Navajo flu." Paralleling the biologic epidemic, these representations may become "epidemic" themselves and can affect an unexpectedly large number of minds in a short period of time. The course of the AIDS epidemic suggests that emerging epidemics can produce social and cultural repercussions on a larger societal and even global level. Social and cultural epidemics of this kind (*cf.* refs. 27 and 28) can spread quickly and with strong "social virulence," which may have enormous economic consequences for the affected population. Consider, for example, the identification of Haiti in 1982 with the HIV virus which cost its economy millions of dollars in tourism revenues and hundreds of jobs due to the exodus of investors.[29]

Other representations become endemic in a population. For example, the belief that the "common cold" is caused by exposure to cold temperature, although a relic of humoral medicine, is an endemically held representation. The AIDS epidemic provides a prime example of how representations become endemic on a macro-societal level. Although there are national and regional differences in ideological reactions to AIDS, prototypical patterns include scapegoating, stigmatization, accusation, metaphorization, and collective preventive, and curative representations.[27,28,30-32]

Worldwide medical ethnographic material documents the existence of lay or folk sectors within a given health care system where folk nosologic as well as etiologic notions—often contradicting biomedical assumptions—provide meaning to the sick person, his or her social network, and health-care behavior.[33] These notions often reflect the social location of people who hold them, *e.g.* the poor, the marginalized. Their divergence from biomedical explanatory models also needs to be seen in the context of societal class relations.

Cultural assumptions and models of disease causality and prevention are important to know because they can influence a population's reaction to epidemic disease. Evidently the severity of the response depends to a large extent on how the afflicted perceive their risks. Risk perception, on the other hand, changes with a person's perceived amount of control over an exposure.[34] It is equally important to note that popular notions of risk differ in many cases from scientific usages of the concept, a discrepancy of languages of risk that often uncovers ideological and class-related perspectives.[35]

In some cases, collectively held beliefs conflicting with biomedical knowledge have been shown to propagate an epidemic and to jeopardize public health measures. Examples range from the rejection or unawareness of the infectious agent and the underlying germ theory in a cholera epidemic in China[25] to the rejection of the efficacy of immunizations due to religious and moral convictions during a diphtheria epidemic in a religious sect in Colorado.[36] It has recently been stated that an entire continent (Africa) "underreacts" to the HIV-pandemic because the majority of its inhabitants is "not fully convinced that biomedical determinism is the only force operating in the world." [37]

It is important to recall at this point that academic or scientific epidemiology may be paralleled by a lay or popular epidemiology. This may involve the use and reinterpretation of epidemiologic findings for socio-political purposes, such as in the case of AIDS activism, or the incorporation of epidemiologic knowledge into larger belief systems, as in the case of the interpretation of the hantavirus epidemic by Navajo healers who saw it within the framework of their larger socio-cosmological theories.

Epidemics thus need to be considered as social processes that are socioculturally and epidemiologically constructed.[38,39] Societal institutions as different as healer groups, scientific disciplines, or public media are important catalysts in the production of popular attitudes and reactions to an epidemic process. They can produce or reproduce early or preliminary epidemiologic findings and create strong public representations. An editorial recently published in the *Lancet* provocatively asked whether "epidemiologists cause epidemics." [40]

Epidemics are not simply reflected by social and cultural systems on the micro- as well as on the macro-level; social and cultural repercussions can also positively and negatively impact the biological process of an epidemic. Panic, flight and migration from the foci of the epidemic may either break the chain of transmission or accelerate its transmission. McGrath[18,31] and Wallace,[41] have argued that social disruption resulting from social responses to an epidemic can in fact increase the biological impact of epidemics. Wallace,[41] for instance, described and modeled the effects of social disintegration, defined as the breakdown of social control and coping mechanisms, as an important co-factor in accelerating the spread of AIDS in New York City minority neighborhoods.

PUBLIC HEALTH IMPLICATIONS

The extent of cultural and social reactions to a new disease depends on a number of factors: the virulence and pathogenicity of the agent; the pathway of transmission; the disease manifestations; and its repercussions on cultural and societal mores. However, public health interventions in an epidemic may have little success when, as in the case of emerging dengue fever epidemics in Honduras: i) awareness and concern of a population vis-a-vis an epidemic is low and needs to be increased; ii) knowledge about the vector and its lifecycle is limited;[12] or iii) the disease is not considered life-threatening and its symptoms are not viewed as signs of severe sickness. Communities can even have conflicting ideas about the causes and the most appropriate prevention of the disease and therefore fail to comply with established programs to contain an epidemic. Behavioral change is more likely to occur when members of the affected population are aware of the infectious agent, its route of transmission, and behavioral risk factors.[4] Dissemination of etiologic knowledge alone is not necessarily followed by behavior change, particularly when risky behavior is co-determined by socio-economic, socio-political, or cultural factors. Public health interventions, especially health education, need to be based on group priorities and risk perceptions. They need to take into account local belief systems and practices in their social and cultural as well as economic contexts. Health communication measures, beyond simply disseminating biomedical knowledge, also need to inform target populations at risk of how behavior change is feasible within existing social, economic and cultural constraints.

There is an increasing interest in more interdisciplinarity and methodological "triangulation" between epidemiologists, virologists, and social scientists in infectious disease research.[42–44] During the investigation phase of an epidemic, a combination of rapid epidemiologic and social science assessments (cf. ref. 45) would strengthen the effort. Why not back up epidemiologic surveillance with a "surveillance" of cultural, behavioral and social repercussions? Social and cultural processes involved in an epidemic can be explored through non-numerical, qualitative techniques including less structured exploratory research methods, such as open-ended key-informant interviews, structured observations at the household level, or more formalized rapid ethnographic assessment techniques. Social scientists can then help elucidate what might motivate the affected population to change risk behavior and sustain behavioral patterns needed to contain the epidemic. During the investigation phase of an epidemic particularly in non-Western settings, it is important to understand epidemic-related community beliefs that are of potential conflict with biomedical knowledge. More in-depth, long-term ethnographic research will be needed to contextualize these belief patterns in the larger framework of the respective society and to develop viable community-based prevention approaches. Biocultural research in geographic areas undergoing rapid ecological and demographic changes can prove useful in constructing early warning systems with regard to prevention and containment efforts of impending infectious disease epidemics.

On a more theoretical level, epidemics need to be conceptualized as both biologic and social occurrences. There are recent theoretical efforts within anthropology to conceptualize human health and disease beyond the conventional epidemiological model of host-pathogen-environment interactions. These important advances look at disease and health as products of "mutually interacting organic, inorganic and cultural environments." [46] Beyond these attempts to integrate within disciplines there is, as Rosenfield[47] has persuasively argued, a strong need for an analytic framework that transcends contemporary disciplinary borders and bridges the social and the biomedical perspectives in applied health research. Research on new diseases would benefit from developing stronger transdisciplinary linkages between the biomedical and social sciences and their various subdisciplines.

ACKNOWLEDGEMENTS

I am grateful to James Trostle, Richard A. Cash, and Janet McGrath for their encouraging and useful comments on earlier drafts of this paper.

REFERENCES

1. McElroy, A. 1990. Biocultural models in studies of human health and adaptation. Med. Anthropol. Quart. 4(3): 243–265.
2. Alland, A. 1969. Ecology and adaptation to parasitic diseases. In Environment and Cultural Behavior. A. P. Vayda, Ed. New York: Natural History Press.
3. Dunn, F. L. 1984. Social determinants in tropical disease. In Tropical and Geographical Medicine. K. S. Warren & A. A. F. Mahmoud, Eds. New York: McGraw Hill.
4. Brown, P. J. & M. C. Inhorn. 1990. Disease, ecology, and human behavior. In Medical Anthropology. Contemporary Theory and Method. T. M. Johnson & C. F. Sargent, Eds. New York: Praeger.
5. Inhorn, M. C. & P. J. Brown. 1990. The anthropology of infectious disease. Ann. Rev. Anthropol. 19: 89–117.
6. McNeill, W. H. 1976. Plagues and Peoples. Garden City, NY: Doubleday.
7. Hughes, C. & J. Hunter 1970. Disease and development in Africa. Soc. Sci. & Med. 3: 443–493.
8. Wirsing, R. 1985. The health of traditional societies and the effects of acculturation. Current Anthropol. 26(3): 303–322.
9. Jenkins, C. et al. 1989. Culture change and epidemiological patterns among the Hagahai, Papua New Guinea. Human Ecol. 17(1): 27–57.
10. Nichter, M. 1987. Kyasanur forest disease: An ethnography of a disease of development. Med. Anthropol. Quart. 1(4): 406–423.
11. Preston, R. 1992. Crisis in the hot zone. The New Yorker, 26 October: 58–78.
12. Kendall, C. et al. 1991. Urbanization, dengue, and the health transition: Anthropological contributions to international health. Med. Anthropol. Quart. 5(3): 257–267.
13. Gibbons, A. 1993. Where are 'new' diseases born? Science 261 (6 August): 680–681.
14. Leatherman, T. L., A. H. Goodman & R. B. Thomas. 1993. On seeking common

ground between medical ecology and critical medical anthropology. Med. Anthropol. Quart. 7(2):202–207.

15. JONSEN, A. R. & J. STRYKER, Eds. 1993. The Social Impact of AIDS in the United States. Washington, DC: National Academy Press.

16. GILMAN, S. 1988. Disease and Representation: From Madness to AIDS. Ithaca, NY: Cornell University Press.

17. FRANKENBERG, R. 1992. The other who is also the same. The relevance of epidemics in space and time for prevention of HIV infection. Int. J. Health Serv. 22(1): 73–88.

18. McGRATH, J. W. 1991. Biological impact of social disruption resulting from epidemic disease. Am. J. Phys. Anthrop. 84(4): 407–419.

19. FOX, D. M. 1989. The history of responses to epidemic disease in the United States since the 18th century. Mount Sinai J. Med. 56(3): 223–229.

20. COREIL, J. 1980. Traditional and Western responses to an anthrax epidemic in rural Haiti. Med. Anthropol. 4(1): 79–105.

21. FARMER, P. 1990. Sending sickness: Sorcery, politics, and changing concepts of AIDS in rural Haiti. Med. Anthropol. Quart. 4(1): 6–27.

22. IMPERATO, P. J. 1974. Cholera in Mali and popular reactions to its first appearance. J. Trop. Med. Hyg. 77(12): 290–296.

23. EGNOR, M. 1982. The changed mother, or what the smallpox goddess did when there was no more smallpox. Contr. Asian Stud. 18: 26–45.

24. COIMBRA, C. E. 1988. Human factors in the epidemiology of malaria in the Brazilian Amazon. Hum. Org. 47(3): 254–259.

25. HSU, F. L. 1955. A cholera epidemic in a Chinese town. In Health, Culture, and Community. B. Paul, Ed. New York: Russell Sage Foundation.

26. SPERBER, D. 1985. Anthropology and psychology: Towards an epidemiology of representations. Man 20(1): 73–89.

27. EARICKSON, R. J. 1990. International behavioral responses to a health hazard: AIDS. Soc. Sci. & Med. 31(9): 951–962.

28. HEREK, G. M. & E. K. GLUNT 1988. An epidemic of stigma – public reactions to AIDS. Am. Psychol. 43: 886–891.

29. FARMER, P. 1992. Aids and Accusation: Haiti and the Geography of Blame. Berkeley, CA: University of California Press.

30. AGGLETON, P., G. HART & T. DAVIS. 1991. AIDS—Social Representations, Social Practices. Sussex: Palmer Press.

31. McGRATH, J. W. 1992. The biological impact of social responses to the AIDS epidemic. Med. Anthropol. 15(1): 63–79.

32. FORD, N. & S. KOETSAWANG. 1991. The socio-cultural context of the transmission of HIV in Thailand. Soc. Sci. Med. 33(4): 405–414.

33. KLEINMAN, A. 1978. International health care planning from an ethnomedical perspective: Critique and recommendations for change. Med. Anthropol. 2: 71–94.

34. FOEGE, W. H. 1988. Plagues: Perceptions of risk and social responses. Soc. Res. 33(5): 331–342.

35. HAYES, M. V. 1992. On the epistemology of risk: Language, logic and social science. Soc. Sci. & Med. 35(4): 401–407.

36. PRINCETON, J. C. 1988. A diphtheria epidemic in a religious sect: An anthropological assessment of a public health intervention. Med. Anthropol. Quart. 2(1): 75–79.

37. CALDWELL, J. C., I. O. ORUBULOYE & P. CALDWELL. 1992. Underreaction to AIDS in sub-Saharan Africa. Soc. Sci. & Med. 34(11): 1169–1182.

38. INGSTAD, B. 1990. The cultural construction of AIDS and its consequences for prevention in Botswana. Med. Anthropol. Quart. 4(1): 28–40.

39. OPPENHEIMER, G. M. 1988. In the eye of the storm: The epidemiological construction of AIDS. In AIDS: The Burdens of History. E. Fee & D. M. Fox, Eds. Berkeley, Los Angeles, London: University of California Press.

40. LANCET 1993. Editorial: Do epidemiologists cause epidemics? Lancet 341 (April 17) 993–994.

41. WALLACE, R. 1993. Social disintegration and the spread of AIDS. Soc. Sci. & Med. 37(7): 887–896.

42. JANES, C. R. *et al.*, Eds. 1988. Anthropology and Epidemiology. Dordrecht: D. Reidel.
43. HOLLAND, C. V. 1989. Man and his parasites: Integration of biomedical and social approaches to transmission and control. Soc. Sci. & Med. **29**(3): 403–411.
44. ANKRAH, E. M. 1989. AIDS: Methodological problems in studying its prevention and spread. Soc. Sci. & Med. **29**(3): 265–276.
45. MANDERSON, L. & P. AABY. 1992. An epidemic in the field? Rapid assessment procedures and health research. Soc. Sci. & Med. **35**(7): 839–850.
46. ARMELAGOS, G. J., T. LEATHERMAN, M. RYAN & L. SIBLEY. 1992. Biocultural synthesis in medical anthropology. Med. Anthropol. **14**: 35–52.
47. ROSENFIELD, P. 1992. The potential of transdisciplinary research for sustaining and extending linkages between the health and social sciences. Soc. Sci. & Med. **35**(11): 1343–1357.

Health Transitions and Complex Systems

A Challenge to Prediction?[a]

CRISTINA DE A. POSSAS[b]

Department of Population and International Health
Harvard School of Public Health
665 Huntington Avenue
Boston, Massachusetts 02115

MARILIA B. MARQUES[c]

Oswaldo Cruz Foundation
Av. Brasil 4036 Sala 715
Manguinhos 21040-361
Rio de Janeiro, Brazil

INTRODUCTION

This paper discusses to what extent the emergence and global dissemination of new and resurgent infectious diseases such as AIDS, cholera, malaria and tuberculosis, is contributing to the complexity of health profiles and how this may affect the predictability of dominant health-transition approaches. These approaches have been supported by demographic assumptions on possible long-term health consequences of population aging, based mainly on mortality indicators. The crucial technological and financial implications of non-infectious chronic and degenerative diseases affecting a growing older population, have been their main focus.

However, despite being, as shown by Olshansky *et al.*[1,d] a major health-transition trend in the contemporary world, population aging does not necessarily lead to an exclusive tendency towards these non-infectious diseases. To the contrary, other important demographic and non-demographic dimensions of the health transition should also be considered.

On one hand, the main processes influencing the contemporary demographic dynamics—population aging, population growth, population mobil-

[a] We thank Dr. Richard Levins, Harvard Working Group on New and Resurgent Diseases, Harvard School of Public Health, for his insightful comments. We also thank the Oswaldo Cruz Foundation and the National Research Council in Brazil (CNPq) for the financial support.

[b] Former Takemi Fellow, Harvard School of Public Health. Member of the New and Resurgent Diseases Group. Currently Professor, National School of Public Health, Oswaldo Cruz Foundation, Rua Leopoldo Bulhoes 1480-3.andar sala 326, Manguinhos-Rio de Janeiro, RJ21040, Brazil.

[c] Visiting Fellow, Takemi Program, Harvard School of Public Health. Coordinator, Nucleus for Science and Technology Studies, Oswaldo Cruz Foundation, Rio de Janeiro, Brazil.

[d] Olshansky *et al.*[1] recently suggested that population aging tends to surpass population growth as the major policy issue, affecting both developed and developing countries.

ity and population differentiation—are undergoing important and decisive changes, which interact in complex ways with new and resurgent infectious diseases. Diseases closely related to population mobility and poverty, such as AIDS and cholera, provide good examples of the impact of these changes.

On the other hand, it should be considered that the appearance of these infectious diseases does not seem to be a restricted or cyclical phenomenon. To the contrary, they have persisted and surpassed national frontiers, increasingly affecting developing and also, unexpectedly, developed countries. Diverse global changes in marine and terrestrial ecosystems[2–4] are increasingly being related to their emergence and dissemination, although some hypotheses are still controversial. Drug and pesticide resistance, environmental change, behavioral change, migration and poverty, among others, have provided a fertile field for their rapid spread. Social and political trends affecting most countries such as the declining power of the working class vis-à-vis corporations have been the foundation of many of these changes and should be carefully examined.[e]

Although more information is necessary on the impact of these global ecosystem changes on the health conditions of populations, there is enough reasonable evidence suggesting that they are contributing worldwide to the emergence of new and resurgent infectious diseases.[4] The overlap of these emerging diseases with other infectious and non-infectious diseases is leading to increasingly complex health profiles.[6]

There are also indications that, although infectious and non-infectious diseases affect diverse social groups, their overlap tends to concentrate on the poor. As shown by Briscoe,[7] on the basis of data from Brazil, and as illustrated by Possas,[6] the poorest segments of the population are often more likely to be exposed to a broader range of risks and thus to diverse disease patterns.[f]

The inadequacy of traditional health transition approaches[g] to confront this complexity is our primary focus. Following insights from former publications,[4,9] we try here to anticipate, in a long-term perspective, some crucial conceptual, methodological and policy issues that should be considered in the discussion of an alternative framework.

We suggest that a comprehensive transdisciplinary approach, incorporating the contributions of the scientific study of complexity, based on the recent

[e] A good analysis of these social and political processes in the contemporary world can be found in Offe.[5]

[f] Our definition of "disease pattern" is the one adopted by Possas.[8] "Disease patterns" are defined as structures expressing the concentration of diverse **risk conditions** for disease, in populations exposed to each one of these conditions. Patterns of "co-prevalence" of infectious and non-infectious diseases refers to specific structures of risk conditions when these diverse diseases are associated. In our approach, **"disease patterns"** should **not** be identified with **"health profile,"** defined by Possas as the distribution of incidence of diverse diseases over the same population.

[g] These approaches, which we will discuss later, are designated as "traditional" with the meaning that they have been persisted as references for several decades and are now incorporated as "common sense" in public health.

advances of ecology, evolutionary theory, social and information sciences, can provide important elements to the formulation of a new health transition framework.

THE EPIDEMIOLOGICAL RATIONALE

Social and health policies in the contemporary world often respond to market and political demands and have not been, in most cases, oriented by a strict epidemiological rationale.[b] Nevertheless, recently international agencies and policy-makers in developed and developing countries have become increasingly interested in the design of new strategies to anticipate health-transition trends.

Two major issues account for this motivation. First, the escalating political and financial pressures on social welfare and health care from an aging population; and second, the emergence and rapid dissemination of new and resurgent infectious diseases, also increasingly affecting costs.

Both issues need further analysis. The first, related to the increase in the proportion of deaths from chronic and degenerative diseases as populations get older, has often been explained as the "natural" ill-health outcome of senescence, resulting from cumulative effects of diverse risk factors.

Murray et al.,[10] arguing against this widely held belief, maintain, in a recent World Bank book[11] that adult mortality rates from these non-infectious diseases decline simultaneously with the overall mortality rate decline. However, as Possas[9] has shown previously, they decline much less in the older age groups, particularly those above 60 years of age. This has important policy implications which should be considered, especially in some newly industrialized developing countries, where life expectancy is increasing and infectious diseases still dominate.

The second issue is the rise of new and resurgent infectious diseases, such as AIDS, cholera, tuberculosis, and malaria. Their increasing incidence and prevalence in different regions of the globe suggest that, despite significant declines in mortality related to them, infection and parasitism are a crucial and often underappreciated force in the health transition dynamics.

Dominant epidemiologic explanations, focusing on the consequences of population aging, have resulted in some demographically based typologies, designed to locate countries in diverse health-transition stages.[i] These typologies can be misleading, if possible long-term health consequences of social and environmental trends leading to new and resurgent infectious diseases, are minimized. Demographically based typologies can only be

---

[b] An additional observation here is that "policy" formulation and implementation are the result of political processes involving diverse contradictory interests. Therefore, data and theory are instruments, but not determinants of health outcomes.

[i] The health-transition stages conceived by Omran illustrate these typologies well.

useful to approach health transition if their strict demographic dimension is acknowledged.

HEALTH TRANSITION: APPROACHING COMPLEXITY

Health Transition as a Descriptive Concept

An important contribution of Caldwell et al.[13] was the introduction of a comprehensive approach to the concept of health transition as defined in a collaborative project between the Rockefeller Foundation and the Health Transition Centre at the Australian National University, which focuses on the social, cultural and behavioral determinants of health.

This approach provides important elements for understanding demographic and health-transition relations in the contemporary world and certainly contributed to a new perspective on the original formulations of Omran[12] and Lerner.[14]

Nevertheless, more extensive discussions on the conditions, nature and patterns of health and demographic transitions are needed.

Following Tabah's[15] definition of the demographic transition,[16] we propose that health transition should be understood as a descriptive concept which pictures a process rather than a theory or law.

Our viewpoint contrasts with dominant developmental approaches to health transition, which often forge theories or laws trying to identify abstract and universal health transition trends.

Their main limitation is trying to generalize, according to their teleological[j] (or finalistic) definitions of the health transition from a relatively recent phenomenon in human evolution occurring in a period only in the last two centuries.

Despite extraordinary gains in life expectancy, decline in mortality for infectious diseases and relative increase in mortality for non-infectious diseases, the evolution in these indicators should not be identified as a permanent long-term trend, whose steps would necessarily follow the stages of socio-economic development, in an unilineal sequence.

Health Transition and Socio-economic Development: The Impasse of Convergence Theories

The concept of transition has its origin in the Latin word transitio which means "change or passage from one stage to another."

Concerning the demographic transition, it has been described as a continu-

---

[j] As defined by Nagel,[17] "A system is teleological if it has a mechanism which enables it to maintain a specific property despite environmental change."

ous process evolving from high mortality and fertility regimes to low mortality and fertility regimes, when the transition would be "completed." [k]

In a similar approach, dominant health-transition theories have defined this ordered progression as the outcome of socio-economic development. Health-transition trends are related to different socio-economic development stages, which may express an influence of evolutionary approaches to economic development, such as the one formulated by Rostow.[19]

These health-transition theories have found support in the shift of the proportion of deaths in the last two centuries of industrialization and urbanization in most industrialized and newly industrialized societies. As shown by Bell,[20] during this period these countries moved from an "underdeveloped" stage marked by high mortality from infectious and reproductive diseases and high fertility rates, to a "developed" one dominated by low mortality and concentrated on non-infectious chronic and degenerative diseases and accidents, with high life expectancy and low fertility rates.

These assumptions of regularity and ordered progression have extended to epidemiology concepts and arguments supported by the convergence theories in demography, which assume that developed and developing countries tend in the long term to converge gradually to similar demographic and health profiles.

These utopic convergence assumptions have been challenged by the complex and uneven processes underlying economic development and health transition in different societies. Certainly, a present day "developing" country is not like the present "developed one" a century ago.

The emergence of new diseases like AIDS and other infectious diseases apparently introduces, particularly in advanced societies, an unexpected deviation in this assumed regular and ordered trajectory.

Thus, we propose that two distinct processes should be considered in the comprehension of health transition trends: the first is the secular tendency of improvement of health levels which are related to overall improvements (certainly not for everyone!) in general life conditions associated with socio-economic development; the other are episodes of outbreaks of a disease in specific societies or risk populational groups.

To what extent and in which direction this last process will affect the secular trend is presently unpredictable.

Demarcating the Boundaries: Demographic and Health Transitions

We believe, unlike Cleland,[21] that clearer boundaries between issues of the demographic transition and issues of the health transition are necessary. Despite important dynamic interactions between demographic and health

---

[k] An analysis of this process in mortality transition can be found in Palloni.[18]

transitions,[1] this last concept refers to a broader and apparently more complex range of processes.

We view the demographic transition as particular epidemiological processes—mortality and fertility—within the health transition.

A comprehensive health-transition framework should integrate and demarcate three dimensions: mortality transition, morbidity transition, and reproductive transition (for the concept of reproductive transition, see Palloni[22]).

Two major issues should be considered here: the first refers to a necessary distinction between the different roles of the reproductive transition in demographic and health transitions, differentiating health consequences of reproduction from the demographic issues of reproduction.

Curiously, Cleland[21] provides a good argument for this distinction, assuming that "in study of the health transition, reproduction is of importance only insofar as it presents a particular set of health problems and consequences and only insofar as the determinants of reproductive behaviour and health behaviour are common."

The other refers to the need for a clearer conceptual distinction between morbidity and mortality transitions. Despite the widely acknowledged limitations of self-perceived as well as physician-attributed morbidity data,[10] which contribute to the restriction of epidemiological analysis to mortality indicators, this distinction between morbidity and mortality is possible at the conceptual level (diseases such as blindness or leprosy provide good examples of elements of morbidity independent from mortality).

At the theoretical level, this differentiation was proposed in the 1970s in

---

[1] Where there is an initial demographic transition toward an older population, the number of small children **per household** diminishes. This reduces exposure within the household, so that where within-family transmission is important (*e.g.*, measles, pinworms, tuberculosis), demographic change alters transmission rates. The conceptual distinction between demographic and epidemiological change should not, of course, obscure their dynamic interactions. As suggested by Levins in a personal communication, an example can illustrate these interactions:

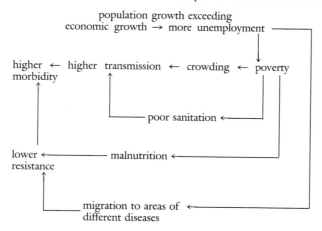

Brazil by Arouca[23] in his critical approach to the concept of "natural history of diseases." Incorporating philosophical and epistemological contributions to medicine from Canguilhem[24] and Foucault,[25] he provides enough reasonable evidence against the notion of a continuous and steady progression from initial symptoms of disease to death.

This critical approach brings important insights to the current debate on the relative role of morbidity and mortality in health transitions. It supports our argument that morbidity and mortality transitions, despite being strongly related, seem to refer to qualitatively different phenomena, requiring therefore diverse approaches.[m]

Mortality and Morbidity Transitions: Diverse Phenomena

Morbidity cannot be inferred from mortality. Despite the important increase in life expectancy worldwide, related to the decline of fertility and mortality as countries develop, there is not sufficient evidence—even in developed countries—that related morbidity indicators have declined following the same trend expressed for mortality rates.

In this aspect, our approach differs from the one of Murray et al.[10] Despite recognizing that mortality rates express in different ways a portion of the burden of illness, they conclude with the observation that "many, although not all, major causes of morbidity also cause mortality and, therefore, are captured in good quality mortality data."

Instead, our argument here is that morbidity cannot be captured in good quality mortality data, even if some determinants of morbidity also lead to mortality. To the contrary, we suggest that mortality and morbidity transitions should rather be viewed as distinct, although related, processes in health transitions, which respond to the interaction of complex and diverse causal and non-causal relations.

Our conclusion is that no linear causality link between morbidity and mortality rates should be assumed. Although they constitute powerful instruments to measure health trends, these rates refer to specific quantitative indicators which are limited in their capacity to express the diverse and complex social processes operating in health transitions.

Therefore, developing alternative methodologies combining qualitative and quantitative approaches to health transitions, rather than trying to extract universal laws from numerical indicators, is the appropriate scientific procedure to explain their dynamics in the current stage of knowledge.

Health Transitions and Complex Systems

Diverse approaches and definitions for "complex system" have been developed internationally and pervade the contemporary scientific debate on complexity.

---

[m] An argument to support this differentiation is: if age-specific morbidity and related mortality remain unchanged, then there is a "health transition" that reflects only a change in age structure.

An overview of diverse definitions for "system" since Bertalanffy (1956) can be found in Baker.[26] He shows that, in spite of their diverse theoretical affiliations, authors seem to agree in essence that "a system is a set of units or elements that are actively interrelated and that operate in some sense as a bounded unit." He stresses that what is new, as Ackoff (in Baker[26]) has pointed out, is "the tendency to study systems as an entity."

He also identified, in contrast with increasing specialization of knowledge, a renewed quest for a "general systems theory," that is a "body of organized theoretical constructs which can be employed to discuss the general relationships of the empirical world" and "bridge the gaps among disciplines." [26]

Recently, new challenges have emerged from important developments in the applications of general system theory to living systems and in the study of ecological complexity. The notion of "complex system" emerged from diverse new scientific perspectives and has generated distinct frameworks and models.[27-31] However, it is interesting to note that more than two decades later, Cowan[30] would define "complex system" in a definition similar to the one identified by Baker for 'system': "Complex systems consist of many relatively independent parts that are highly interconnected and interactive."

A crucial methodological problem for biological sciences and for public health is the difficulty of translating emerging biological arguments into values for the parameters of diverse abstract models. Taylor[32] has accurately identified these methodological constraints. He provides important insights to the discussion, contrasting "morphological" approaches to complex systems, developed by mathematical ecologists, who focus on particular mathematical systems or sampling from universes of permitted parameters combinations for such systems, with "developmental" approaches to complexity, focused on the construction and turnover of those systems, which require "reworking theory to embrace the particular and the contingent of local and historical circumstances."

A new non-morphological approach to health transition complexity (or "developmental," as suggested by Taylor) will demand a long-term transdisciplinary effort, addressing a broad range of theoretical, computational and empirical problems.

This approach requires taking into account that the health profiles of populations do not necessarily evolve as a simple response to socio-economic stages, but unfold in intricate social economic, demographic and cultural processes, which demarcate specific conditions of exposure and vulnerability of populations to risks in various ecosystems.

Whitehead[33] contributes to this new historical and social perspective. He says: "Many natural systems—from animal populations to the weather or the level of rivers—are complex systems where apparently distinct forces interact with each other, and where what happens in the past is very important for what is going to happen in the future. Clearly this could also apply to complex social systems, including financial markets, international crises, and regime transitions."

In this new perspective, modeling can provide important tools. Models that respect complexity can improve simulations for alternative health transition scenarios, assuming diverse initial conditions for exposure and vulnerability to risk factors.

There is some reasonable evidence suggesting that slight changes in the initial positions of populations across conditions of vulnerability (age, sex, occupation, *etc.*) and exposure to risks (chemicals, new infectious agents, *etc.*), in diverse ecosystems, can lead to very different trends in the evolution of health profiles. This was illustrated previously in a population-based model developed by Possas,[6] which incorporates data from Brazil, where it is suggested that it is possible to identify the impact of slight changes in these initial conditions on specific health profiles of human populations.

A common objection is that these models often require support from sophisticated computerized mathematical procedures but usually lack adequate input from quality mortality and morbidity data, which limits their output. However, lack of accurate information on the universe population should not be an obstacle for health-transition models. Qualitative approaches and simulation strategies addressing complexity can help to minimize these constraints.[n]

CONCLUSION

Health profiles of populations have evolved globally towards complex patterns of co-prevalence of infectious and non-infectious diseases, which result from diverse interactions of a broad range of risk factors, most of them not yet fully understood.[o] [6,20,38,39]

New and resurgent infectious diseases are obviously challenging the predictability of prevailing health-transition models. However, although complex systems are sometimes thought to be highly unpredictable, unpredictability should not be assumed as a necessary feature of complexity. Owing to a large number of variables and connectivity, stability issues and other conditions affecting complex systems need to be demonstrated.

We have warned here of the risks of overestimating health care needs of an aging population at the expense of confronting new and resurgent infectious

---

[n] Alternative statistical tools to overcome under-reporting of epidemiological information, as the one proposed for infant mortality in Brazil by Landmann,[34] or, as suggested by Possas,[6] risk tables projecting estimates for the health profile of populations, might help to overcome these data restrictions to approach health transition complexity.

[o] Speth and others from the World Resource Institute (see Waldrop,[28] 1992) argue that global sustainability is possible only if human society undergoes at least six fundamental transitions within a few decades: **demographic, technological, economic, social, institutional** and **informational** transitions. The study of complex systems is critical to meet the challenges posed by these diverse transitions (Gell-Mann, in Waldrop[28]). However, we would add to their list a new missing component: "A **health transition** to a world where the ability to identify, anticipate and minimize exposure of populations to behavioral and environmental risks bridges the gap between the health status of developed and developing nations and within nations."

diseases.[p] This policy option may have important detrimental consequences, such as 1) rapid dissemination of global epidemics; 2) increasing political demands for health care; 3) spiraling health care costs, resulting from the overlap of infectious and non-infectious diseases on health profiles; and 4) inadequacy of existing surveillance systems and health care structures to face this new reality.

We agree with Callahan,[35,36] who shows that most of the health needs of the elderly often lead to long-term and technology-intensive care, although in most cases they cannot yet be adequately met in the current stage of medical development.

This debate is clearly permeated by an equity issue: since infectious diseases tend to concentrate on the poor, who live in conditions favoring a lower life expectancy, a shift of emphasis to the diseases of the aged might contribute to a minimization of policy strategies focusing on the health problems of the poor. This can contribute (besides leading to unacceptable social discrimination) to an aggravation of global epidemics affecting all social strata.

Of course, trading-off the health of the young versus the old is a false problem. Many diseases of the elderly are laid down in youth.[q] Thus, the main policy issue is instead how to build a healthful society for everyone.

Conferring a new status on the so far peripheral public health programs and on biomedical research and development aimed at infectious diseases emerges therefore as a priority strategy and a main challenge in the contemporary world.[40]

This will require important long-term investments at both national and international levels, including support to transdisciplinary approaches to health, design of innovative epidemiological methods to approach complexity, implementation of international monitoring networks, and development of strategies to define and respond to health policy priorities.

However, this approach should not be limited to the public health domain. Non-public health approaches to health can be decisive in confronting this challenge, reducing the vulnerability of populations to risks. Social and political issues such as equity, structure of the labor market, land use, environmental protection and education, among others, should also be incorporated into this new framework.

---

[p] This is also a risk for developing countries. Gwatkin[37] has correctly suggested that a health strategy focusing on chronic diseases among adults and the elderly might be considerably more relevant for regions with low mortality levels than for high-mortality regions. However, even in low-mortality regions, given the social heterogeneity and increasing poverty in many developed countries, this strategy might be carefully discussed, since it might underestimate the dissemination of important infectious diseases. The same reasoning is valid, for opposite reasons, for high mortality societies, where non-infectious diseases are increasingly affecting more influential upper social groups and those who are occupationally exposed.

[q] Many examples, such as plaque formation in the arteries of children, illustrate this argument.

REFERENCES

1. OLSHANSKY, S. J., B. A. CARNES & C. K. CASSEL. 1993. The aging of human species. Sci. Am. April: 46–52.
2. ANDERSON, D. M. 1989. Toxic Algal Blooms and Red Tides: A Global Perspective. *In* Red Tides: Biology, Environmental Science and Toxicology. T. Okaichi, D. Anderson & T. Nemoto, Eds. Elsevier Science Publishing Co.
3. SHOPE, R. 1991. Global climate change and infectious diseases. Environ. Health Perspect. 96: 171–174.
4. LEVINS, R., C. A. POSSAS, T. AWERBUCH, U. BRINKMANN, I. ECKARDT, P. EPSTEIN, N. MAKHOUL, C. PUCCIA, A. SPIELMAN & M. WILSON. 1993. Preparing for New Infectious Diseases. Harvard Working Group on New and Resurgent Diseases. Department of Population and International Health, Harvard School of Public Health, Working Paper n. 8.
5. OFFE, C. 1985. Disorganized Capitalism. Cambridge, MA: MIT Press.
6. POSSAS, C. A. 1992. Sociological Approach to Epidemiological Analysis: A Tool for Developing Countries. Takemi Research Paper, Harvard School of Public Health, Boston.
7. BRISCOE, J. 1990. Brazil: The New Challenge of Adult Health. (A World Bank country study). Washington, DC: The World Bank.
8. POSSAS, C. A. 1989. Epidemiologia e Sociedade: Heterogeneidade Estrutural e Saúde no Brasil. São Paulo: HUCITEC. [Epidemiology and Society: Structural Heterogeneity and Health in Brazil].
9. POSSAS, C. A. 1993. A dimensão saúde da transicão demográfica: Uma discussão conceitual. *In* Proceedings IV Conferencia Latino-Americana de Población: La Transición Demográfica en América Latina y el Caribe. México City. [Health dimension of the demographic transition: a conceptual discussion].
10. MURRAY, C. J. L., G. YANG & X. QIAO. 1992. Adult mortality: Levels, patterns and causes. *In* The Health of Adults in the Developing World. G. A. Feachem *et al.,* Eds. New York: Oxford University Press.
11. FEACHEM, G. A. *et al.,* Eds. 1992. The Health of Adults in the Developing World (a World Bank Book). New York: Oxford University Press.
12. OMRAN, A. R. 1971. The epidemiological transition: A theory of the epidemiology of population change. Milbank Mem. Fund Quart. 49: 509–538.
13. CALDWELL, J. C. 1989. Introductory thoughts on health transition. *In* What We Know about Health Transition: The Cultural, Social and Behavioural Determinants of Health. J. Caldwell, S. Findley, G. Santow, W. Cosford, J. Braid & D. Broers-Freeman, Eds. The Proceedings of a International Workshop, Canberra, Vol. I.
14. LERNER, M. 1973. Modernization and health: A model of the health transition. Paper presented to the Annual Meeting of the American Public Health Association, San Francisco, CA.
15. TABAH, L. 1989. De una transición demográfica a otra. Boletin de Población de las Naciones Unidas 28: 1–16. [From one demographic transition to another].
16. CHACKIEL, J. & J. MARTINEZ. 1993. Transición demográfica en América Latina y El Caribe desde 1950. *In* Proceedings IV Conferencia Latino-Americana de Población: La Transición Demográfica en América Latina y el Caribe. México City. [Demographic Transition in Latin American and the Caribbean since 1950].
17. NAGEL, E. 1979. Teleology revisited and other essays in the philosophy and history of science. New York: Columbia University Press.
18. PALLONI, A. 1989a. The meaning of health transition. *In* What We Know about Health Transition: The Cultural, Social and Behavioural Determinants of Health. J. C. Caldwell, S. Findley, G. Santow, W. Cosford, J. Braid and D. Broers-Freeman, Eds. The Proceedings of an International Workshop. Canberra, Vol. I.
19. ROSTOW, W. W. 1960. The Stages of Economic Growth: A Non-Communist Manifesto. New York: Cambridge University Press.
20. BELL, D. 1993. Some implications of the health transition for policy and research. *In*

Health and Social Change: An International Perspective. L. Chen, A. Kleinman & N. Ware, Eds. Cambridge, MA: Harvard School of Public Health.

21. CLELAND, J. 1989. The idea of the health transition. *In* What We Know about Health Transition: The Cultural, Social, and Behavioural Determinants of Health. J. C. Caldwell, S. Findley, G. Santow, W. Cosford, J. Braid & D. Broers, Eds. The Proceedings of an International Workshop, Canberra, Vol. I.

22. PALLONI, A. 1989b. Methodological problems in the study of the health transition. *In* What We Know about Health Transition: The Cultural, Social, and Behavioural Determinants of Health. J. C. Caldwell, S. Findley, G. Santow, W. Cosford, J. Braid & D. Broers, Eds. The Proceedings of an International Workshop, Canberra, Vol. I.

23. AROUCA, A. S. 1975. O dilema preventivista: Contribuição para a compreensão e crítica da medicina preventiva. PhD. Thesis, Medical School of the State University of Campinas, UNICAMP, São Paulo. [The preventivist dilemma: Contribution toward understanding and critical approach to preventive medicine].

24. CANGUILHEM, G. 1978. On the Normal and the Pathological. Author's thesis, Strasbourg 1943, with 3 additional essays. Dordrecht, Holland; Boston: D. Reidel Pub. Co. c1978.

25. FOUCAULT, M. 1978. Preface 1978 edition of Canguilhem's 1943 thesis. See reference 24.

26. BAKER, F. 1970. General systems theory, research and medical care. *In* Systems and Medical Care. A. Sheldon, F. Baker & C. P. McLaughlin. Cambridge, MA: Massachusetts Institute of Technology Press.

27. LEVINS, R. & R. LEWONTIN. 1985. The Dialectical Biologist. Cambridge, MA: Harvard University Press.

28. WALDROP, M. M. 1992. Complexity: The Emerging Science at the Edge of Order and Chaos. New York: Simon & Schuster.

29. LEWIN, R. 1992. Complexity: Science on the Edge of Chaos. New York: Macmillan Pub. Co.; Toronto: Maxwell Macmillan.

30. COWAN, G. A. 1993. Interview. *In* Adapting to Complexity, R. Ruthen. Sci. Am. Jan: 130–140.

31. NICOLIS, G. & I. PRIGOGINE. 1989. Exploring Complexity: An Introduction. New York: W.H. Freeman and Company.

32. TAYLOR, P. J. 1985. Construction and Turnover of Multispecies Communities: A Critique of Approaches to Ecological Complexity. Thesis, Department of Organismic and Evolutionary Biology, Harvard University, Cambridge, MA.

33. WHITEHEAD, L. 1993. On reform of the state and regulation of the market. World Dev. 21(n. 8): 1371–1393.

34. LANDMANN, C. S. 1993. Estimativas da mortalidade infantil como função da distribuição etária dos óbitos registrados: Proposta de um procedimento. PhD. thesis, National School of Public Health, Oswaldo Cruz Foundation, Rio de Janeiro, RJ. [Estimate of infant mortality as function of age distribution of registered deaths].

35. CALLAHAN, D. 1987. Setting Limits: Medical Goals in an Aging Society. New York: Simon and Schuster.

36. CALLAHAN, D. 1990. What Kind of Life: The Limits of Medical Progress. New York: Simon and Schuster.

37. GWATKIN, D. R. 1993. Distributional implications of alternative strategic responses to the demographic-epidemiological transition—an initial inquiry. *In* The Epidemiological Transition: Policy and Planning Implications for Developing Countries. J. N. Gribble & S. H. Preston, Eds. Washington, DC: National Academy Press.

38. BOBADILLA, J. L. & C. A. POSSAS. 1993. Health policy issues in three Latin American countries: Implications of the epidemiological transition. *In* The Epidemiological Transition: Policy and Planning Implications for Developing Countries. J. N. Gribble & S. H. Preston, Eds. Washington DC: National Academy Press.

39. FRENK, J., J. L. BOBADILLA, C. STERN, T. FREJKA & R. LOZANO. 1991. Elements for a theory of the health transition. Health Transition Rev. 1: 21–38.

40. MARQUES, M. B. 1989. A Reforma Sanitária Brasileira e a Política Científica e Tecnológica Necessária. Série Política de Saúde n. 8. Rio de Janeiro, Fiocruz, NEP. [The Brazilian Health Reform and Necessary Science and Technology Policy].

Disease, Population and Virulence

Thoughts about Measles Mortality

MICHEL GARENNE,[a,c] JOHN GLASSER,[b] AND
RICHARD LEVINS[a]

[a]Department of Population and International Health
Harvard School of Public Health
665 Huntington Avenue
Boston, Massachusetts 02115

[b]National Immunization Program
Centers for Disease Control
Mail-stop E-61
1600 Clifton Road
Atlanta, Georgia 30333

INTRODUCTION

Over the last 120 years or so, most of the world has experienced a dramatic decline in mortality, often called the "epidemiological transition" or the "health transition," which began with a decline in mortality due to infectious and parasitic diseases.[1] The mortality decline is usually attributed to successful public health policies, to improved nutrition, and to better living conditions. However, this is still a matter of intense debate in the literature. Mortality from many common infectious diseases is now so low in developed countries that one forgets how lethal they were in the previous century. This is the case for instance for measles, one of the main killers of children in the past. This change occurred very rapidly in the span of human history, within 2 to 3 generations. However, emerging infectious diseases, such as AIDS, remind us how lethal infections can be, despite good nutritional status, modern medicine, and high standards of living.

Measles is one of the most studied infectious diseases and was a major threat in the recent past. It surfaces again and again in the literature together with plague, cholera, smallpox and a few others. It has stimulated the imagination of writers and is even mentioned in one of Charlie Chaplin's movies. A recent epidemic in a religious community of Philadelphia (1990) reminded us how lethal this disease can be even in wealthy, well-nourished communities, when proper preventive and curative care are not provided.[2] Measles is an "old disease" for the human population. It was identified in the 10th century by Rhazes, a Persian physician and possibly in the 7th century by a Hebrew

[c] Author to whom correspondence should be addressed at the Harvard School of Public Health, Room 1208; Tel.: (617)-432-0418; Fax: (617)-432-2181; E-Mail: MGARENNE @HSPH.HARVARD.EDU.

physician, Al Yehudi.[3] Measles has therefore been prevalent for at least 30 human generations, and maybe many more. Measles is a disease of high density populations, requiring large groups of 500,000 to 1,000,000 people to sustain itself.[4] It may therefore not have existed prior to the Neolithic period.

Recent issues in the literature on infectious diseases, many of them presented in this volume, deal with emerging diseases and their lethality. In this paper, we review what we have learned from the past with respect to measles mortality. We review what we observe when a disease such as measles appears in a virgin population and what we are discovering concerning the dynamics of measles transmission as a risk factor for measles mortality. This review is not meant to be exhaustive, but presents a few arguments for the debate on new diseases.

THE DISEASE

Measles is caused by a virus, first isolated by Enders in 1954.[5] The measles virus is a spherical, single stranded RNA virus, member of the genus *Morbillivirus*, in the family of *Paramyxoviridiae*. The virus is transmitted by aerosols produced by the cough, during the first few days of clinical infection. The disease is very contagious, and it infects virtually everybody who has not been vaccinated, generally during the first 10 to 15 years of life. The infection is almost always clinically apparent and easy to recognize. It occurs usually once in a lifetime, although second infections rarely have been documented.

The case fatality rate (probability of dying when infected) can be high, up to 25% for infants in developing countries. However, the case fatality rate decreases dramatically with age, at least up to 15 years. In the worst mortality situations, measles can be responsible for the premature deaths of about 5% of all newborn children. Death occurs within 3 to 4 weeks of the first clinical manifestation of measles and is usually caused by a secondary infection, such as pneumonia, bronchiolitis, laryngitis (croup), diarrhea, *etc.* Death sometimes results from the viremia *per se.* Measles can also provoke a severe malnutrition and can be responsible for delayed mortality. It can also cause a persistent infection, leading to a rare disease, subacute sclerosing panencephalitis (SSPE).

DEFINITION OF VIRULENCE

A key factor in understanding the mortality from a disease is the virulence of the germ. One would like to define case fatality as the product of the virulence of the disease and the level of immunity of the host. However, virulence is difficult to define and is not independent from the immunity of the host. In animal populations, the virulence of a germ is more standardized, because experimentation is possible. In well-controlled animal populations, the virulence of a germ is defined by its lethality for a given inoculum. The mortality usually increases dramatically with the inoculum, the "lethal dose 50" (LD_{50}) being defined as the number of organisms required to kill 50% of challenged experimental animals.[6] This ambiguity in the concept of virulence makes it almost impossible to distinguish from mortality in human populations, in which the immunity of the host seems to play the most important role. In fact, the pathophysiologic process requires various microbial products, the virulence factors. They include the factors for overcoming anatomic barriers, factors for avoiding and disrupting humoral defenses and factors directed at phagocytic cells.

The measles virus is assumed to have stayed relatively constant over the years. Although it now has a low lethality in developed countries, it still can cause major damage as shown in the Philadelphia epidemic and among immunosuppressed people, such as AIDS patients.[7]

ADAPTATION

Adaptation of the host and the pathogen is another often cited mechanism for determining mortality. The classical example is that of Myxomatosis, a viral infection of rabbits. This virus has some similarities with the measles virus and its case study may be relevant for measles. Myxomatosis is caused by a virus, common among Brazilian rabbits, among which it is rarely lethal. However, the disease was found to be almost always lethal among European laboratory rabbits, which had not been previously exposed to the disease. It was later introduced to control previously introduced rabbits that had become pests in Australia. When spread into this wild rabbit population, it had a lethality of 99%. However, within a few years, both the virus and rabbit evolved. Within two years the virus became less lethal, even among laboratory animals (about 80% lethality). Within 15 years (about 30 generations), a new rabbit population equilibrium was reached, with about 20% susceptible.[8] How this experiment applies to human diseases is unclear. Germs can probably evolve as rapidly among human populations as they do among rabbits. However, human populations reproduce more slowly than rabbits, and 30 generations represent about 1000 years for humans, a totally different time scale!

Adaptation of the germ seems to be determined by its reproductive success. Ewald has recently made a series of observations relating the virulence of a germ to its transmission pattern.[9] The parasite evolves depending on the mode of transmission and the survival of the host. If death of the host is detrimental to its reproduction, the parasite will tend to evolve towards less virulent forms. If death does not matter or is advantageous, the parasite will become more virulent. A clear example has been recently given by analyzing several species of fig wasps that are infected by nematodes.[10] In the species where only one wasp lays eggs in the fig, the nematodes depended totally on the survival of this single host for their reproductive success and were virtually harmless. In other species where more hosts are found, the nematodes were pathogenic, and virulence increased with the number of potential hosts.

In the case of measles, there does not seem to be any obvious advantage of the disease to be more or less lethal. In fact, the virus is transmitted during the prodromal phase, that is before the index case is severely sick, and survival of the index case is unlikely to affect the reproductive success of the virus. Therefore, changes in mortality would be a secondary consequence of evolution for successful reproduction and transmission during the first days after infection. For instance, a slower rate of reproduction might extend the asymptomatic stage and increase transmission, or successful infection may involve the ability to suppress the immune system, increasing later virulence. Or, concentration of the virus in the respiratory tract may enhance transmission, but reduce the rash. Symptoms may evolve in ways that do not obviously fit along a virulence axis.

VIRGIN POPULATIONS

An old disease can become a new disease when it arrives in a virgin population. Perhaps the most striking example of this is the case of measles and smallpox in the new world. The Indian population of the New World came about 15,000 years before Columbus and seems not to have been exposed to these deadly diseases prior to the arrival of Europeans. These two diseases seem to have been responsible for the death of about 90% of the Indian population within less than a century. Francis Black recently re-analyzed this extreme mortality from diseases that were causing the death of only a few percent of the European population at the same time.[11] His hypothesis is based on the lower genetic diversity of the Indian population.

Black argues that a virus grown in one host is preadapted to a genetically like host and thereby gains virulence by passage between two such hosts. This seems to be a plausible explanation for the measles virus. The measles virus replicates with "low fidelity," changing even while infecting a single host. Some immunogenic sequences change during replication. The host histocompatibility (MHC) antigens present a restricted set of viral peptides and the immune response selects against viruses with these peptide sequences. When they pass to a new host, they meet new MHC genes and different peptides. When the virus encounters a similar host, it is "preadapted," and therefore likely to be more lethal. The lethality of a disease in a population is likely to be a function of its genetic diversity. There is evidence that the Indian population has a lower genetic diversity than other human groups. This could explain why measles could kill such a high proportion of people (90%), whereas it killed at most 5% of the populations of Africa and Europe in the past.

DYNAMICS OF EPIDEMICS

Another important observation is that of Anderson and May concerning the coevolution of hosts and parasites.[12] The authors note that "low virulence is generally associated with effective immunological or non-specific responses that tend to suppress pathogen replication with a concomitant reduction in transmissibility." There are a few observations showing that measles mortality varies within the same population according to the dynamics of the epidemics.

At the level of the population, a few observations suggest that the dynamics of the epidemics has also an impact on case fatality. For instance, Picken noted that the case fatality rates for measles were lower in rural areas than in urban areas of Scotland at the turn of the century.[13] There was a monotonic relationship between population density and case fatality rates, the areas with the highest densities having the highest case fatality rates. The author also noted a relationship with the size of the household, and observed that measles was more lethal among soldiers (living in crowded situations) than in the general population of the same age. In Senegal, epidemics with the highest lethality also had the highest secondary attack rate.

A similar phenomenon has been reported in Senegal at the household level. Garenne *et al.* studied the dynamics of measles transmission within the large Sereer compounds, where up to 20 measles cases could occur in the same outbreak.[14] There was a very strong effect of the generation of measles cases within the compound, that is the second generation in the household had much higher mortality than the first (the index cases), the third generation higher mortality than the second *etc.* The case fatality was roughly multiplied by two at each generation, and was 16 times higher in the fifth generation as compared to the first generation. This could be explained either by a cumulative "dose effect" (the generations being more and more sick and transmitting higher doses of viruses) or by a genetic adaptation effect (the virus becoming more and more adapted to the genetic background of family).

DISCUSSION

There are many other examples of similar ecological regularities with other diseases. For instance, Ewald argues that when outbreaks of pathogenic E. coli in hospitals last less than a week, few deaths occur, whereas higher case fatality rates are noted when they last longer.[9]

Historical records also show us how deadly "new diseases" can be. When the plague came in Europe in 1348, it killed almost half of the population within a few years. It took about 100 years to reach the population level of 1347. Malaria was killing similarly high proportions of European settlers in Africa prior to the widespread use of quinine. Recent projections of the demographic impact of AIDS in Africa show that under the current pattern of transmission and lethality, the HIV virus might cause the premature death of about half the population within a few decades. Therefore, it is of the utmost importance to identify the direction of evolution of the virus during the present pandemic.

REFERENCES

1. PRESTON, S. H. 1976. Mortality Patterns in National Population. New York: Academic Press.
2. ROGERS, D. V., J. S. GINDLER, W. L. ATKINSON & L. E. MARKOWITZ. 1993. High attack rates and case fatality during a measles outbreak in groups with religious exemption to vaccination. Ped. Infect. Dis. J. **12**: 288–292.
3. PREBLUD, S. R. & S. L. KATZ. 1988. Measles vaccine. *In* Vaccines. S. A. Plotkin & E. A. Mortimer, Eds.: 182–222. Philadelphia: W.B. Saunders Co.
4. ANDERSON, R. M. & R. M. MAY. 1991. Infectious Diseases of Humans: Dynamics and Control. Oxford: Oxford University Press.
5. ENDERS, J. F. & T. C. PEEBLES. 1954. Propagation in tissue cultures of cytopathogenic agents from patients with measles. Proc. Soc. Exp. Biol. Med. **86**: 277–286.
6. HEWLETT, E. L. 1990. Toxins and other virulence factors. *In* Principles and Practice of Infectious Diseases. G. L. Mandell, R. G. Douglas & J. E. Bennett, Eds.: 2–9. Third edition. New York: Churchill Livingstone.
7. KAPLAN, L. J., R. S. DAUM, M. SMARON & C. A. McCARTHY. 1992. Severe measles in immunocompromised patients. J. Am. Med. Assoc. **267**: 1237–1241.
8. MACFARLANE, B. & D. O. WHITE. 1972. Natural history of infectious disease. Cambridge: Cambridge University Press. Fourth Edition.
9. EWALD, P. W. 1993. The evolution of virulence. Sci. Am. April: 86–93.
10. HERRE, E. A. 1993. Population structure and the evolution of virulence in nematode parasites of fig wasps. Science **259**: 1442–1455.
11. BLACK, F. 1992. Why did they die? Science **258**: 1739–1740.
12. ANDERSON, R. M. & R. M. MAY. 1982. Coevolution of hosts and parasites. Parasitology **85**: 411–426.
13. PICKEN, R. M. F. 1992. The epidemiology of measles in a rural and residential area. Lancet **339**: 1349–1353.
14. GARENNE, M. & P. AABY. 1990. Pattern of exposure and measles mortality in Senegal. J. Infect. Dis. **161**: 1088–1094.

Economic Development and Tropical Disease[a]

UWE K. BRINKMANN

Department of Population and International Health
Epidemiology, Tropical Public Health
Harvard School of Public Health
665 Huntington Avenue
Boston, Massachusetts 02115

INTRODUCTION

Development stands for an improved quality of life through gains in health, education, living standards, and higher income. Development is based on economic growth or so it is perceived since development is found to be more advanced where greater economic development has occurred. The common creed is, that those countries that have not "developed" yet will do so in the future, or are doing so now.

In the "developed" industrialized countries of Europe, North America and Austral-Asia infectious diseases have disappeared even before antibiotics and vaccines have been available. With the expectation that the same will happen in the "developing" countries, infectious diseases, and with them all tropical diseases, are regarded as a thing of the past, merely lingering on, an "unfinished agenda."[1,2] Unfortunately, reality does not agree with this optimistic view of global and continuous progress. Endemic parasitic diseases still affect more people than any other condition. Malaria has made a comeback in many countries where it was thought to have disappeared. Tuberculosis is once again a serious threat to public health, even in "developed" countries. A wholly new infection, AIDS, has emerged and developed into a global epidemic, seemingly out of nowhere. Yet all indicators of development: GDP per capita, average life expectancy at birth, and per capita income have been rising in almost all countries, including the "developing" countries over the past decades.[3] Why did economic growth not lead to the expected development in terms of health? How do tropical diseases and economic development relate to each other? The present article explores the interaction of development and disease in those countries that struggle to develop, and which are close enough to the equator to be called tropical.

---

[a] This is a revised version of a paper published in the Public Health Magazine of Bayer, A. G. and is reprinted with permission. Dr. Uwe Brinkmann died suddenly in June 1993 while on a site visit in Brazil.

303

TROPICAL DISEASES AND THE ENVIRONMENT

Tropical parasitic diseases result from the infection with mono- or multicellular microorganisms. They differ from bacterial and viral agents in an important aspect. The human host is not able to develop protective immunity. The human immune system will only prevent severe illness and will limit the number of parasites below a maximum number that varies individually. This immunity has to be acquired through episodes of illness or prolonged infection. It is of relatively short duration and requires reinfection to be maintained.

The agents of tropical disease take unique advantage of the environment. Many employ insect vectors to emerge from the host, for transportation, and to enter the next host. The vector will protect the parasite with its body while providing nutrients from its body and an environment inside its body in which the parasite can multiply at the same time. The mouth parts of vectors are specialized tools for the penetration of the host's surface. Without them the parasite would be trapped inside the host's body and would be unable to get into the host. Even if infectious agents like schistosomes have maintained some ability in some of their stages to live freely, they expose themselves only for very brief periods of their life cycle to the dangers of the environment. They enter abundant intermediate hosts. Inside them they remain as long as the intermediate host lives. They constantly multiply within that host and free-living stages continuously emerge from it, ready to enter any available definitive host immediately. Because of these peculiarities of their life cycle, tropical parasite populations exhibit a remarkable degree of temporal stability. They tend to be robust to perturbation either from seasonal changes in climate or the introduction of control measures.[4]

All tropical diseases are linked to water for their transmission. Insect vectors breed in or close to water. Most of them cannot survive in extremely arid conditions. If the transmission between hosts does not involve vectors, it occurs in water or at least it requires humid conditions.

ECONOMIC GROWTH AND THE ENVIRONMENT

The most important factor of economic growth in the Northern Hemisphere, industrialization, has not played the same role in the predominantly agrarian developing countries of the south. The generation of hydroelectric power, the exploitation of minerals, and the intensification of agriculture occupy important places. All these factors interfere also to a large degree with the environment and with human ecology.

The construction of hydroelectric dams has created large artificial lakes. These lakes have covered forests and cultivated land. The people who inhabited the land formerly were displaced and forced to migrate elsewhere. At the same time these schemes have attracted large numbers of people to work on the construction of the dam and related installations. Most dams were located in remote areas and their construction took several years. Labor forces consisted mainly of unskilled workers. Almost all developing countries have a surplus of unskilled labor. If workers are housed cheaply, this saves on construction expenses and labor disputes are unlikely. After the construction of dams, the lakes provide opportunities for fishermen. The water of the lake or that of the regulated rivers downstream can be used to create irrigation schemes. Again, this will draw migrants in search for land and jobs.

The most direct way to intensify agriculture is to use more water. This will overcome the limitations imposed by drier periods of the year and allow extension of the period of cultivation to the entire year. Many parts of the world possess fertile soil that only needs water to allow the growth of plants. Globally, 15% of all cultivated areas are irrigated. They produce more than 40% of the agricultural output. Every year the irrigated areas expand by 1.5%.[5]

Other means to increase agricultural production are to expand cultivation into virgin tropical forests or wetlands, to introduce special plants bred for high yield, to prevent loss of production from pests, or to provide fertilizer.

Socially, agriculture oriented to contribute to economic growth is fundamentally different from traditional subsistence farming. It requires sophisticated technology to maintain irrigation and specialized knowledge to handle pesticides and machinery. Economic skills are needed to plan investment, to service loans, and to observe markets. Most farmers have never been trained to cope with the challenges of intensive agriculture. In the transition from subsistence to cash crop agriculture many farmers lose their land and become migrant workers. As long as there are uncultivated areas, some of them will try to resettle in more and more marginal situations, encroaching on tropical forests, mountain slopes too steep for machines, and poor soils. This then leads to the destruction of forest reserves, erosion, and desertification as a result of soil depletion. Poor and landless migrants will be especially attracted by promises of hidden treasures. They will endure hardship and will flock in large numbers to remote jungles accepting improbable prospects to mine gold or gems. Women will cast aside traditional values to become prostitutes as this appears to be their only hope to gain riches without possessing particular skills or knowledge.

TROPICAL DISEASES AND ECONOMIC GROWTH

Economic growth can favor the transmission of tropical diseases indirectly via its impact on the environment. The environment may be more favorable for insect vectors, intermediate hosts of parasites and animal reservoirs. The human host can become more vulnerable as a result of malnutrition which will be a part of poverty. Poverty is often a byproduct of economic growth when development leads to a polarization of society and when mechanisms for a social redistribution of goods are insufficient. Human migration as another byproduct of economic growth exposes humans to local varieties of infectious agents against which they possess only partial or no acquired immunity.

The spillways of hydroelectric dams may provide breeding places for the simulium vectors of onchocerciasis.[6] Artificial lakes, reservoirs, irrigation systems are colonized by aquatic and amphibious snails that can act as the intermediate hosts of schistosomiasis. This infection has always been endemic in Mali (West Africa). However, its prevalence exceeds 50% in all areas with intensified irrigated agriculture. It is found to be below 20% in all other parts of the country, even if water is abundant.[7] The prevalence of schistosomiasis rose significantly after the introduction of irrigation in Africa, South America, and Asia.[5,6,8] When irrigation was used to expand the cultivation of rice in Zanzibar, it turned out that the paddy fields provided excellent breeding grounds for malaria vectors.[9] Irrigation generally enhances the transmission of malaria, schistosomiasis, filariasis, and arboviruses like Japanese encephalitis.[6]

The introduction of fish farming in small artificial ponds in the rice fields of Northeast Thailand provided both intermediate hosts of opisthorchiasis: aquatic snails and fish. Formerly an insignificant infection maintained largely by civet cats, it presently affects 50% of the population of 17 million and is linked to the highest incidence of cholangiocarcinoma anywhere in the world.

The use of pesticides in intensive agriculture kills more than the pests; often large numbers of non-target organisms are eliminated at the same time. Since they lack food, predators of insects are likely to disappear as well. Malaria vectors that have become resistant as a result of earlier attempts at eradication using residual insecticides will find an ideal ecological niche in such situations. Their explosive multiplication has led to malaria epidemics.[10]

The extension of agricultural cultivation into virgin tropical forests may mean the invasion of existing zoonotic transmission cycles. The elimination of the original animal host like the giant sloth in the Amazon Region of Brazil may make humans become the alternative definitive host of leishmaniasis.[10]

When partially or non-immune groups of migrants are exposed to an infectious agent, they will suffer more severe morbidity. Illness will also not be restricted to children but will occur among adults. This effect is often aggravated because migrants are usually poor and uneducated. They will live under poor sanitary conditions and will neither possess the means nor will they know how to avoid exposure. Outbreaks of tropical diseases like malaria may occur during exhausting journeys as well as when migrants settle in unfamiliar environments.[11]

When the Brazilian Amazon Region was opened through the construction of the Transamazon highway in the 1970s, and when landless migrants started to establish small farms in the area, the previous decline of malaria was reversed.[12] In Arba Minch, Ethiopia, the incidence of malaria doubled over the span of two years and adult morbidity increased by 10% as a result of the immigration of non-immunes to a development project.[13] In an area of stable malaria in Somalia an outbreak of malaria occurred with 22 times more infections than usual after new settlers had moved into an agricultural project in the South.[14] The prospect of finding gold has lured thousands into the Brazilian Amazon. Malaria epidemics are frequent among the miners. The hope to become rich through finding rubies or sapphires in the jungles along the Thai-Cambodian border has drawn a constant stream of non-immunes from the poor provinces of Thailand. Their incorrect use of antimalarials for prophylaxis has led to the emergence of drug resistance and its spread. Their presence has kept malaria transmission alive despite all efforts of one of the best malaria control programs.

In some cases the relation between economic growth, agriculture, and tropical diseases is even more complex. An outbreak of malaria occurred when the cultivation of coffee was introduced to an area of stable malaria in southern Thailand in 1986. Normally coffee plantations are not good breeding grounds for the Anopheline vectors of malaria. The disease was endemic in the area and adults possessed a sufficient degree of acquired immunity. In this case forest had to be cleared. The work was done by indigenous workers and migrants who had come from other parts of Thailand. The ecological change had provided excellent breeding for a different malaria vector (*Anopheles minimus*). The indigenous workers had acted as asymptomatic carriers of the parasite. Poor housing conditions for the workers had increased their exposure.[15] In another part of Thailand, malaria had disappeared when forest was replaced by cassava plantations. However, in the 1980s when its market value dropped, cassava was replaced by rubber plantations and orchards and malaria re-invaded the area.[11] FIGURE 1 shows how intensive agriculture is linked to the increase of tropical diseases.

Economic growth may indirectly lead to an increase of tropical diseases. It is certainly necessary to control, prevent, and cure them. The observation[8] that schistosomiasis prevalence had dramatically increased after small dams were constructed in a region of Mali led to the creation of a national control program. This was sponsored over more than ten years by a foreign donor. Concentrated efforts led to chemotherapeutic mass treatment of more than

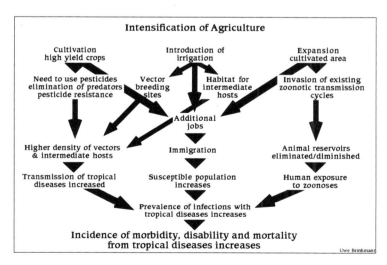

FIGURE 1. Intensive agriculture is an important factor of economic growth in many developing countries. The flow chart links intensive agriculture to the increase in the incidence of disease resulting from the infection with agents of tropical diseases.

75,000 persons and a substantial reduction of schistosomiasis prevalence in the most affected parts of the country.[16] In Kenya the relation between economic development and malaria prevalence has been studied.[17] It was observed that malaria prevalence had no impact on production as long as social structures and relationships insured against production losses. Significantly high levels of income enabled the community to bring down malaria morbidity and mortality through improved health care. Changing the construction of dams and irrigation systems may make it more difficult for vectors and intermediate hosts of parasites to breed.[18] Provisions can be made to give access to water to the population without exposing them to the transmission of schistosomiasis.[19] Expert systems have been designed to forecast the potential vector-borne disease problems in irrigation systems.[20] Multi-objective planning and resource allocation models have been developed to identify a most effective sequence of disease control and development programs that might serve as frameworks for a development that optimizes economic growth yet strives for better health at the same time.[21] FIGURE 2 also leads from intensive agriculture as an element of economic growth to tropical disease. This time however, it shows how development may help to prevent morbidity, disability and mortality.

Over time the strategies to achieve development have changed. Rapid industrialization as well as import substitution have been given up. The World Development Report for 1991[3] recommends the investment into the "human" capital through education and the development of skills. The World Develop-

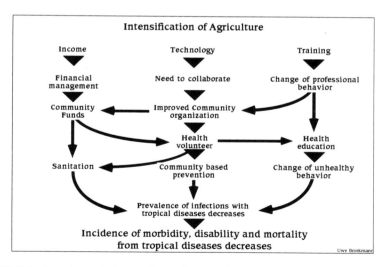

FIGURE 2. Intensive agriculture will contribute to development and create higher incomes. The flow chart links intensive agricultural production to the development of public health and the prevention of tropical infections. This combined with improved curative services will diminish morbidity, disability and mortality resulting from tropical disease.

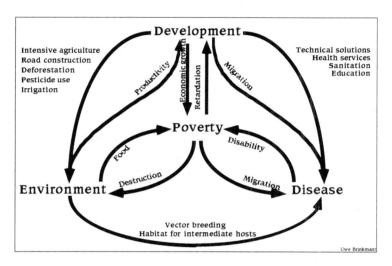

FIGURE 3. Economic growth has ecological side effects that may increase the transmission and severity of tropical diseases. It may also help communities to cope better with threats to health resulting from tropical infectious agents.

ment Report for 1992[22] admits that economic growth is associated with severe degradation of the natural world. It recognizes that though economic growth is essential for development, it is a highly imperfect proxy for it. The people who suffer from the side effects of economic growth are often different from those who benefit from it. FIGURE 3 combines the two roles of economic development with regard to tropical diseases. At its center is poverty. Presently, more than one fifth of all humans, 1.1 billion persons, live in absolute poverty.[22] The conditions under which these people live and their desperate struggle to improve their lot often causes more disease, including tropical disease, as was shown above. The unequal access to resources and the decrease in the quantity and quality of renewable resources is the cause of political and ethnic conflict in developing countries.[23] Yet wealth is not the solution to poverty. The life expectancy of residents of Harlem, New York is lower than those of much poorer populations, *e.g.*, of Bangladesh. The difference is a better social organization and education.[24] Is it possible to answer the question about the relationship between economic development and tropical diseases? Nicolis and Prigogine[25] have developed the mathematics of complex interactions in elementary physics. Applying it to human society they wrote: . . . "A basic question that can be raised is whether, under those circumstances, the overall evolution is capable of leading to some kind of global optimum, or, on the contrary, whether each human system constitutes a unique realization of a complex stochastic process whose rules can in no way be designed in advance."[25] A little further in the same text they assume that the latter is probably right.

SUMMARY

Development stands for an improved quality of life through gains in
health, education, living standards, and higher income. Development is based
on economic growth. Although all indicators of development: GDP per
capita, average life expectancy at birth, and per capita income have been rising
in almost all countries, including the "developing" countries over the past
decades, economic growth did not lead to the expected disappearance of
infectious diseases. Economic growth is associated with severe degradation
of the natural world. Though economic growth is essential for development,
it is a highly imperfect proxy for it. The people who suffer from the adverse
effects of economic growth are often different from those who benefit from
it. Economic development shows two faces with regard to tropical diseases:
it is essential for their prevention and cure and it contributes to their transmission and severity through its impact on the environment. The pivotal point
is poverty. If economic growth leads to improved education and social organization, even adverse effects can be mastered by the community.

REFERENCES

1. COMMISSION ON HEALTH RESEARCH FOR DEVELOPMENT. 1990. Health Research, Essential Link to Equity in Development. Oxford: Oxford University Press.
2. JAMISON, D. T. & W. H. MOSELY. 1991. Disease control priorities in developing countries: Health policy responses to epidemiological change. Am. J. Pub. Health **81:** 15–22.
3. WORLD BANK. 1991. The challenge of development. *In* World Development Report 1991. Washington, DC: Oxford University Press, pp. 1–51.
4. ANDERSON, R. M. & R. M. MAY. 1982. Population dynamics of human helminth infections: Control by chemotherapy. Nature **297:** 557–563.
5. BERGQUIST, N. R., M-G. CHEN & K. E. MOTT. 1988. Schistosomiasis in the context of rice production systems in developing countries. *In* Vector-borne Disease Control in Humans through Rice Agroecosystem Management.: 143–151. International Rice Research Institute, WHO/FAO/UNEP.
6. BRADLEY, D. J. 1977. The health implications of irrigation schemes and man-made lakes in tropical environments. *In* Water Wastes and Health in Hot Climates. R. Feachem, M. McGarry & D. Mara, Eds.: 18–29. Chichester, UK: John Wiley & Sons.
7. HUNTER, J. M., L. REY & D. SCOTT. 1982. Man-made lakes and man-made diseases. Soc. Sci. Med. **16:** 1127–1145.
8. BRINKMANN, U. K., R. KORTE & B. SCHMIDT-EHRY. 1988. The distribution and spread of schistosomiasis in relation to water resources development in Mali. Trop. Med. Parasitol. **39:** 182–185.
9. KHATIBU, A. I. Irrigation development and malaria incidence in Zanzibar. *In* Malaria and Development in Africa. Washington, DC: American Association for the Advancement of Science Sub-Saharan Africa Program, pp. 121–126.
10. COOPER-WEIL, D. E., A. P. ALICBUSAN, J. F. WILSON, M. R. REICH & D. J. BRADLEY. 1990. The impact of development policies on health. Geneva: World Health Organization.
11. KONDRASHIN, A. V., R. K. JUNG & J. AKIYAMA. 1991. Ecological aspects of forest malaria in Southeast Asia. *In* Forest Malaria in Southeast Asia. V. P. Sharma and A. V. Kondrashin, Eds. New Delhi: World Health Organization.
12. SAWYER, D. R. & D. O. SAWYER. 1992. The malaria transition and the role of social science research. *In* Advancing Health in Developing Countries: The Role of Social Research. L. C. Chen, A. Kleinman & N. C. Ware, Eds.: 105–122. New York: Auburn House.

13. NEGA, A. Population migration and malaria transmission in Ethiopia. *In* Malaria and Development in Africa. Washington, DC: American Association for the Advancement of Science Sub-Saharan Africa Program, pp. 181–189.

14. WARSAME, W. Impact of population movements on malaria transmission in Ethiopia. *In* Malaria and Development in Africa. Washington, DC: American Association for the Advancement of Science Sub-Saharan Africa Program, pp. 217–221.

15. SARAVUDH SUVANNADABBA. 1991. Deforestation for agriculture and its impact on malaria in southern Thailand. *In* Forest Malaria in Southeast Asia. V. P. Sharma & A. V. Kondrashin, Eds.: 221–226. New Delhi: World Health Organization.

16. BRINKMANN, U. K., C. WERLER, M. TRAORE & R. KORTE. 1988. The National Schistosomiasis Control programme in Mali, objectives, organization, results. Trop. Med. Parasitol. **39:** 157–161.

17. MWABU, G. M. Economic development and malaria prevalence. *In* Malaria and Development in Africa. Washington, DC: American Association for the Advancement of Science Sub-Saharan Africa Program, pp. 167–180.

18. PIKE, E. G. 1987. Engineering against Schistosomiasis/Bilharzia, Guidelines toward Control of the Disease. London: Macmillan Publishers.

19. BRINKMANN, A. & R. STEINGRUBER. 1986. Possible modifications in the construction of small dams to prevent the spread of schistosomiasis. Trop. Med. Parasitol. **37:** 199–201.

20. BIRLEY, M. H. 1989. Forecasting potential vector borne disease problems on irrigation schemes. *In* Demography and Vector-borne Diseases. M. W. Service, Ed.: 255–270. Boca Raton, FL: CRC Press Inc.

21. PARKER, B. R. 1983. A program selection/resource allocation model for control of malaria and related parasitic diseases. Computers and Operations Res. **10:** 357–389.

22. WORLD BANK. 1992. Development and environment. *In* World Development Report 1992. Washington, DC: Oxford University Press, pp. 1–206.

23. HOMER-DIXON, T. F., J. H. BOUTWELL & G. W. RATHJENS. 1993. Environmental change and violent conflict. Sci. Am. February (1993): 38–45.

24. SEN, A. 1993. The economics of life and death. Sci. Am. May (1993): 40-47.

25. NICOLIS, G. & I. PRIGOGINE. 1989. Exploring Complexity. New York: W.H. Freeman and Company.

Human Movements and Behavioral Factors in the Emergence of Diseases

Commentary

LAURIE GARRETT

Newsday/*Science Section*
235 Pinelawn Road
Melville, New York 11747

We seem to live in a period of unprecedented human movement, human interaction, and a sheer increase in the numbers of *Homo sapiens* on the planet (FIG. 1). It is expected that the world's population will reach 6 billion by the year 2000. Population growth is correlated with a dramatic increase in human density (FIG. 2). Human density is unevenly distributed. Concentration occurs mostly in large and growing urban centers and is produced by the migration of people from rural areas into the cities (TABLE 1). Thus, the increase in human density leads to a dramatic growth of urban centers.

The city of Boston, for example, underwent a radical change in its urbanization pattern between 1830 and 1850. Prior to 1830 it was much safer to be a resident of Boston than a resident of England, particularly London. The life expectancy as a resident of Boston was much higher than anywhere in England at the time. That shifted in 1850 because of a huge stream of people moving to Boston, primarily due to immigration, and to an escalation in sheer population density.[1]

In Asia we have seen a serious urbanization shift in the second half of this century. In 1955 there were about 270 million urbanites in all of Asia. By 1985 this number reached 750 million people living in urban centers. The World Bank predicts that 1.3 billion Asians will live in urban centers by the year 2000. Urban centers will be transformed into giant megacities (defined as exceeding 10 million people in population) as a result of this human movement and birth-driven population growth. In 1950 we had only 2 megacities—New York and London (TABLE 2). Today, 10 megacities exist around the globe and by the year 2000 it is projected that there will be 24 of such giant cities, according to World Bank, UNDP and WHO projections.

This dramatic urbanization process is located mostly in the Americas and East and South Asia (TABLE 2). Many urban services considered essential to health may be deficient in these growing megacities. Such deficits in urban and health services will not be limited to megacities in developing countries. For instance, the expansion and urbanization of Tokyo has been so radical and so fast that only 40% of the population of Tokyo has sewage services that are linked to sewage process treatments before the waste makes its way into the sea. This is notable, given that Japan is arguably one of the 2 or 3 wealthiest countries in the world.

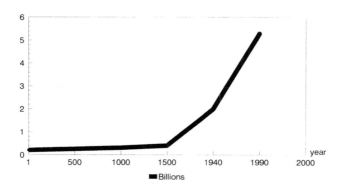

FIGURE 1. Population growth.

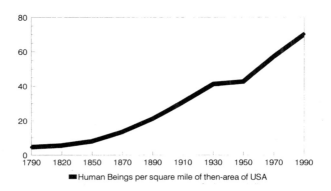

FIGURE 2. Population density, United States.

TABLE 1. Population in Urban and Rural Areas in the United States, Africa, and the World

	Date	% Urban	% Rural
United States	1910	45.6	54.4
	1950	59.6	40.4
	1990	75.2	24.8
Africa	1970	34.0	66.0
(UN projection)	2010	50.0	50.0
World	1900	14.0	86.0
(World Bank projection)	2010	50.0	50.0

TABLE 2. Megacities (Metropolitan Populations Exceeding 10 Million)

1950 (2)	New York, London
1980 (10)	*Americas:* Buenos Aires, Rio de Janeiro, São Paulo, Mexico City, Los Angeles, New York
	East Asia: Beijing, Shanghai, Tokyo
	Europe: London
2000 (24)	*Africa:* Cairo
	Americas: Buenos Aires, Rio de Janeiro, São Paulo, Mexico City, Los Angeles, New York
	East Asia: Beijing, Shanghai, Osaka-Kobe, Tokyo-Yokohama
	South Asia: Dacca, Bombay, Calcutta, Delhi, Madras, Jakarta, Baghdad, Teheran, Karachi, Bangkok, Manila, Istanbul
	Europe: Paris (London drops off the list)

With regard to housing conditions in many of these rapidly expanding cities, WHO and UNDP estimated that in 1985 there were 100 million homeless adults and 100 million abandoned children living in urban areas worldwide. In 1981, 40% of the residents of Nairobi were classified as living in housing that was so substandard that it was not officially mapped.

As part of the urbanization process, people from rural areas bring their rural diseases into the urban centers and start the process of urbanization of rural diseases. This process has been well documented for leishmaniasis and Chagas disease. Contamination of the blood supplies with *Trypanosoma cruzi* (the cause of Chagas disease) has become a very serious problem in some parts of Latin America. In Buenos Aires 6% of the blood supply was contaminated in 1985. In some other urban centers in Argentina contamination rates reached 20%, in Brazilia 15%, and in Santa Cruz, Bolivia, up to 63% of the blood supply was contaminated.

Urbanization is not the only process of human movement which is correlated with the emergence of infectious diseases. The ongoing movement of refugees around the globe, caused by political and economic crises, should be of immediate concern. At present, it is very difficult to obtain accurate numbers of refugees. Between 1980 to 1989 the annual numbers of refugees increased by 75%, reaching an estimated 15,093,900 refugees in 1989, according to the International Organization on Migration. Today, the amount of refugee movement in the world is certainly beyond this figure. The fall of the Berlin Wall, followed by the destabilization of national boundaries and the nationalistic warfare in many parts of the world, have made it difficult for international organizations to track the refugee movements. They estimated that the amount of refugee movement has at least doubled since 1989.[2]

Air traffic is another means of human movement that is of importance for the emergence and transmission of infectious diseases. FIGURES 3 and 4 show that air traffic, domestic and international, is increasing steadily. An end to this steady increase is not expected. Airplanes have become a routine form of travel, used by some people much the same way as trains and buses. Thus, our planet is shrinking into a global village as humans find that there are fewer and fewer places considered too exotic or distant.

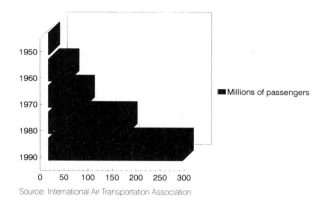

FIGURE 3. Air traffic—international.

On board the aircraft, either in the bodies of passengers or in the luggage and cargo, many kinds of pathogens easily cross national and geographic boundaries. Further, because of changes in the air-circulation systems of aircrafts, the potential for transmission of infectious diseases has increased. According to the Centers for Disease Control, in the last 6 years there have been reports of more than 25 outbreaks of enteric diseases related to food consumption on the aircraft or from infected personnel serving the food to passengers. Among these diseases are shigellosis, cholera, typhoid fever, salmonellosis, and staphylococcal food poisoning.

In addition to the transmission of enteric disease, tuberculosis transmission associated with air flights has been reported. One case involved an infected flight attendant with active tuberculosis. Twenty-three flight crew

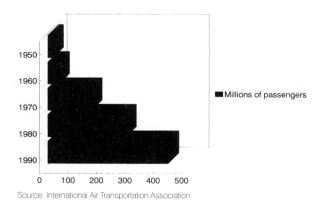

FIGURE 4. Air traffic—domestic.

TABLE 3. Reported Cases of Sexually Transmitted Diseases, 1992

Disease	Reported Cases, 1992 (millions)
Trichomonas	120
Chlamydia	50
HPV	30
Gonorrhea	25
Herpes simplex	20
Syphilis	3.5
Chancroid	2
HIV (1992 only)	1.5

Source: World Health Organization.

members on international flights on which she flew tested positive for tuberculous infection, according to CDC. So far, no passengers have been documented to have been TB-infected by this flight attendant.

In 1979 there was an influenza outbreak on board a Boeing 747 aircraft. 72% of the passengers and crew members were infected.

Airlines are reducing fresh air circulation in order to save jet fuel. When jet fuel costs increased drastically more than a decade ago, carriers began looking for ways to reduce their operating costs. Recirculating the air was less expensive than bringing in outside air, which has to be pressurized and brought to the proper temperature. As a result, new aircrafts have been redesigned. Prior to 1980, before the redesign of circulation units, the entire air of the plane was replaced by fresh air every 3 minutes. The air in planes today is either never replaced with fresh air or, if it is so, it takes about 30 minutes to recirculate the entire air space of the cabin, according to airline testimony last year before Congress.

The human movements described above—urbanization, development of megacities, refugee movement, and air travel—are related to the recent increase in sexually transmitted diseases (STDs). The reported cases of sexually transmitted diseases are increasing worldwide (TABLES 3 and 4). In the United States there have been special problems with reporting and documenting selected STDs.

TABLE 4. Reported Cases of Syphilis, Hepatitis B and Gonorrhea in the United States from 1940 to 1990

Year	Syphilis (all stages)	Hepatitis B	Gonorrhea
1940	472,900	not reported	175,841
1950	217,558	not reported	286,746
1960	122,538	not reported	258,933
1970	91,382	not reported	600,072
1980	68,832	19,015	1,004,029
1985	75,000	26,600	911,000
1990	134,000	21,100	690,000

TABLE 5. Institutionalization, USA

	1980	1990
Prisons/Jails	329,821	774,375
Shelters	not reported	190,406
Military	671,000	589,700
Dorms	1,994,000	1,953,558
Nursing Homes	1,426,000	1,772,032

The reported cases of syphilis over the last 30 years reveals an interesting trend (TABLE 4). For over 25 years the disease declined. This decline reversed and cases of syphilis reached a high point in 1990. Between 1985 and 1990 the incidence rates for syphilis rose from 11.45 to 20.10 per 100,000 population.[3]

In case of gonorrhea, the incidence rate started to decrease in the 1980s. This decrease might have been caused by the introduction of condom programs and sex education in connection with the emergence and spread of HIV infections. Unfortunately, in some high risk communities, such as young gay men and sexually active African Americans, gonorrhea incidences are now rising, as are HIV rates.

The increase of sexually transmitted diseases is closely related to the enormous increase in population density caused by urbanization.

Urbanization cannot be understood only as a demographic process. It is accompanied by changes in value systems between the generations. The traditional rural moral standards change as new generations move into the urban centers. In many developing countries, the rapid social transitions with the corresponding changes in value systems have taken place under the influence of standards of the so-called developed world. Among the many new values adopted, altered sexual behavior will place these populations at greater risk for acquiring STDs.

Finally, two more processes should be mentioned which are correlated with the emergence of infectious diseases.

First, there has been a marked increase in institutionalization in certain populations in the United States (TABLE 5). The most dramatic increase is seen in prisons and jails. The reason for this increase are federal and state

TABLE 6. Medical Device Implants, USA, 1988

Type	Number (thousands)
Artificial joints	1,625
Fixation devices	4,890
Ear vent tubes	1,494
Breast implants	544
Shunt or catheter	321
Heart valve	279
Pacemaker	460

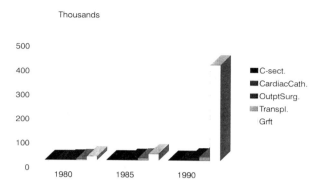

FIGURE 5. Surgical procedures, USA.

changes in drug enforcement laws, mandating incarceration for possession and sale of small amounts of illegal substances. The result was more street arrests and a larger number of people rotated through the jails. The major increase of institutionalized people in prisons and jails happened between 1980 and 1990 and resulted from an increase in drug-related arrests, according to the U.S. Department of Justice.

Hospital practice and medical practice present risk for the emergence of some infectious diseases. Procedures that involve putting foreign objects or tissues into a human body have increased radically (TABLE 6 and FIG. 5). For the first time, a number of procedures were performed placing animal tissue, such as baboon livers or hearts, into human bodies. No agency has seriously asked what kinds of microorganisms might be transplanted along with a baboon liver and what the consequences of such contaminated transplants might be. This is particularly important, given that the recipients of transplants are severely immunosuppressed. Such procedures might provide new niches for viruses to cross inter-species barriers.

REFERENCES

1. ROSENKRANTZ, B. 1993. Personal communication.
2. LEDERBERG, J., R. E. SHORE & S. C. OAKS, JR. Eds. 1992. Emerging Infections: Microbial Threats to Health in the United States. Institute of Medicine. Washington, DC: National Academy Press.
3. CDC. 1992. Summary of notifable diseases, United States, 1992. Morbidity and Mortality Weekly Report 1992. **41**(55): 68.

New Diseases

The Human Factor

LINCOLN C. CHEN

Department of Population and International Health
Harvard School of Public Health
665 Huntington Avenue
Boston, Massachusetts 02115

That the emergence of new diseases can be shaped by human forces is well demonstrated in history, for example the devastation of New World populations during the period of European exploration. There is every reason to believe that the contemporary world movements of people and goods, as well as changing human behavior, will play an even more important role in the emergence and transmission of new disease into the future. The human factor may be called "anthropogenesis," or caused by humankind.

Anthropogenesis may be considered in two ways: the first concerns changes in the number, composition, and distribution of people, while the second is what people actually do—called rather loosely human activity, human behavior, or health behavior. FIGURE 1 shows these two components of anthropogenesis. Under the demographic component, there are three parameters of concern—the size, composition, and distribution of human populations. These demographic dimensions are entirely determined by three simple demographic variables—the birth, death, and migration rates.

World population size today is about 5.5 billion, having tripled from 1.7 billion at the beginning of this century. With rates of growth having peaked in the mid-1970s, world population is growing at about 2 percent annually. World population will certainly cross the threshold of 6.0 billion by the turn of the century. Depending upon projections, world population size may eventually reach anywhere from about 8 to 20 billion people by the end of the next century. Such growth is unprecedented in human history. It is also highly imbalanced. Of the 90 million new additions each year, over 90% are in the so-called developing regions of the world. The most rapidly growing region is sub-Saharan Africa, followed by the Middle-East. Because of its very large base population, Asia's increases are very large in absolute numbers. Lower growth rates are to be found in Latin America. Most industrialized societies have attained replacement level fertility, and growth, if any, is confined mostly to immigration.

Changing numbers is being accompanied by changing age and gender composition of the population. Declining fertility and improved longevity are leading to increasingly more adults and elderly people in populations. An elderly age profile characterizes much of the industrialized world, with developing countries also demonstrating the same shifts, although less markedly. Poorly understood are the implications of such age composition shifts for the immunological profile of entire populations, not of individuals.

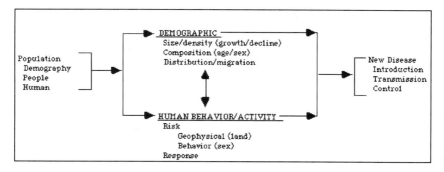

FIGURE 1. New Diseases: Anthropogenesis.

Finally, the geographic distribution of human populations is shifting also very rapidly, owing both to differential population growth and migration. Indeed, some have noted that the most dramatic demographic phenomenon of our times is in distribution rather than in numbers. Whereas the world population was predominantly rural and dispersed at the beginning of this century, we will be living in an urbanized world by the next century. Urbanization is accelerating to a level where about half of the world's people will be living in cities by about the year 2010. Twenty of the world's largest cities, most of them in developing countries, will have populations exceeding 10 million. Internationally migration may also be important but its magnitude is minuscule in comparison to rural-urban shifts.

Under human behavior in relation to health, a loosely used term, we can consider two overlapping yet distinctive dimensions. First is "human activity" which can be defined as actions related to people's production, consumption, and other activities for managing their social and physical environment for generating their quality of life. These human activities are not primarily "health-seeking" or health-directed, although they may have important health implications. A second type of human behavior is directly related to health. High-risk personal "health behavior" is illustrated by changing sexual practices and intravenous drug abuse, and health-seeking behavior in the utilization of preventive and therapeutic health services. This distinction between human activity and health behavior has been made because each relates to different determinants, although both can generate significant health consequences. These distinctions in human behavioral health risks are made because while the latter has direct consequences for health risk, the former has indirect effects. For example, with modern technology humans today have the capacity to drastically alter our geophysical environment—witness recent concerns over global warming due to carbon dioxide production. These geophysical changes can affect health in many ways. Along a parallel track, certain population subgroups may pursue high-risk health behavior, resulting in very direct health consequences.

TABLE 1. Demographic Causes of Emergence

	Population Intrusion	Urbanization	Air Travel
Bacteria			
Borrelia (Lyme)	x		
Viruses			
Dengue		x	x
Filovirus			x
Hantavirus	x		
HIV-1		x	x
Lassa		x	
Ross River	x		
Yellow fever		x	x
Protozoa			
Giardia			x
Malaria		x	x
Strongyloides			x

Source: IOM report, 1992

The relationship of demographic and human behavioral anthropogenesis with new diseases can assume several dimensions in terms of the introduction of new diseases, their dissemination or transmission, and of course ultimately their control or decline. If these human factors are juxtaposed with the recent list of new diseases from the Institute of Medicine (IOM) report,[1] TABLE 1 is produced listing the demographic causes of disease emergence according to bacteria, viruses, and protozoa. The demographic factors considered by the IOM report are population intrusion, urbanization, and air travel. These in turn have been linked to some specific pathogens. Noteworthy is the fact that, as shown in the IOM report, most of the pathogens associated with these demographic factors are viral, rather than bacterial or protozoan. Interestingly, cholera is not listed (perhaps because the focus of the report is on diseases that threaten the United States), although several other water-borne infections, like giardia, are listed.

Because human movement appears to play such an important role in anthropogenesis, TABLE 2 was designed to present some speculative relationships between migration and disease emergence. Migration in TABLE 2 is classified according to historical, national, and international categories. These, in turn, are associated with certain socioeconomic correlates and implications for disease emergence and transmission.

The movement of people has occurred throughout human history. Cyclic movements were common among hunter-gatherer societies and nomadic populations. Many of these movements were seasonal, following resource bases for livelihoods. Because population densities and inter-group contact were low, these movements were unlikely to be associated with significant human-to-human disease transmission. Another more dramatic historical movement was the period of European exploration of new worlds. These movements for exploration, conquest and settlement brought Europeans into

TABLE 2. New Diseases and Migration

Migration Typology	Sociodemographic Correlates	Disease Implications
Historical		
Cyclic	Hunter-gatherer	Low density
	Seasonal, nomadic	Low contact
Exploratory	Conquest, settlement	Smallpox, measles
National		
Labor	Seasonal employment	Malaria (Thailand)
Rural-urban	Urbanization	Dengue (Latin America)
Forced	Displaced	
International		
Labor	Economic	Tuberculosis
Forced	Refugees	Malaria (Cambodia)
Air travel	Commercial	HIV, STD
	Recreational	
	Social	
Sea/land		

contact with populations previously unexposed to many human pathogens. The decimation of indigenous populations due to smallpox and measles has been well documented in the history of the Americas.[2]

Today, intra-national migration streams are extremely frequent but poorly documented. Seasonal and intermittent rural-urban and rural-rural movements are driven in part by the search for economic opportunity—jobs in cities, farms. In his study of the development of drug-resistant malaria in Thailand, Uwe Brinkmann was attempting to document how intra-national movement of Thai labor to gem mines could be associated with indiscriminate antimalarial drug use and the consequent development and transmission of drug-resistant malaria in Southeast Asia. Perhaps the largest movements of residents within countries, taking place in virtually all countries around the world, has been rural-urban, resulting in massive urbanization. Illustrative health problems associated with the density and growth of urban populations, without corresponding water, sanitation, and other amenities, are the recent explosive outbreaks of dengue fever, for example in Mexico and other areas of Latin America. Finally, a neglected dimension of intra-national movement is "displaced peoples," forced to flee their homes by political crisis, conflict, and war. It is estimated that there are over 20 million displaced persons in the world today due to these crises, as in ex-Yugoslavia and in many countries of Africa.

International migration would seem to play a predominant role in global disease transmission. The long-term and steady movement of labor from economically disadvantaged to more prosperous countries is an on-going process. Disease transmission is not common with these migration streams, although tuberculosis may be an example of an infectious disease that could be transmitted by such migratory streams. The world today has about 18 million international refugees, defined as people forced to flee their homes across international boundaries because of political and economic crises. Refugees are classified only for political purposes; people forced to move internationally owing to natural calamities such as environmental catastrophes, earthquakes, and cyclones are not officially classified as refugees. Considerable attention has been focused on the last category of international movement, that is air travel, because of its volume, the rapidity of movement, and our inability to screen and control disease transmission. International air travel today numbers over 500 million international crossings annually for commercial, recreational, and social purposes. HIV and sexually transmitted diseases are among those diseases facilitated by this mode of migration. There have been reports that disease transmission via respiratory routes could be accelerated by recent airline policies to restrict the volume of fresh recycled air within newer aircraft.

One final note about international movements may be made. While people may be the primary carriers of concern, trade of goods can also act as a carrier for disease transmission. "Diseases do not need visas," a participant at the workshop underscored. The recent cholera outbreak in Peru that has subsequently spread to many countries in Latin America has been postulated to be due to the discharge of ballast water from Asian tankers delivering goods to Latin America. This transmission pattern, if true, did not involve human-to-human contact, but rather the movement of pathogens associated with their ecologic niche.

Let me close with three key questions. 1) Are we dealing with an unprecedented human situation in terms of demography and behavior? The answer, I believe, is yes, profoundly so. Our species has never before experienced the sheer scale of the movement and velocity of growth we currently have. 2) Second, what can we look forward to in a future world where national barriers of all types are being dismantled rapidly? We have already virtually unrestricted international movement of money and finance, information and knowledge, science and technology, and increasingly goods and services. These movements are perhaps one of the hallmarks of our century. Can we keep people within political boundaries while we have unrestricted movement of all of these other factors of production and consumption? I submit that it would be very difficult to do so; thus, international migration will surely play a key role in new diseases in the future. 3) Finally, given these movements, can we expect to see again the type of massive population destruction that McNeill[3] described for the age of world exploration? Will some populations be wiped out as unexpected new diseases are introduced into previously non-exposed populations? Such is a possibility, of course; indeed, some considered HIV/AIDS as one such possible candidate. But, it is equally possible that such rapid and complete movement of people around the world would generate over time endemicity of disease, rather than epidemics, leading to low-grade but chronic disease prevalence in world populations with increasingly a previously exposed and immunized population. This scenario would be far more likely with diseases that we already know about; whether these global demographic and human dynamics would introduce a new Andromeda strain that could threaten us as a species remains unknown.

REFERENCES

1. LEDERBERG J, R. E. SHOPE & S. C. OAKS, JR., Eds. 1992. Emerging Infections: Microbial Threats to Health in the United States. Institute of Medicine. Washington, DC: National Academy Press.
2. CROSBY, A. W., JR. 1972. The Columbian Exchange. Westport, CT: Greenwood Press.
3. McNEILL, W. H. 1976. Plagues and Peoples. New York: Anchor Press/Doubleday.

Theoretical and Social Approaches: Discussion

Part A. The Biosocial Nature of Disease Emergence

RICHARD LEVINS: I would like to comment on the question of the biosocial nature of disease. I think we have to consider several different meanings.

First, if we would write an equation for an epidemic it would involve the parameters of transmission, development of symptoms, recovery, acquisition and loss of immunity. All of these seem to be medical parameters. But, when we unpack any of the parameters they become social, as the probability of transmission depends on who is where in an area of an outbreak and the success of a transmission depends on the vulnerability of the host. The recovery rate will depend on the access people have to medical care. I'm not sure, what exactly would influence the duration of immunity.

Second, the perception of the disease process is a truly social phenomenon. Whether something is regarded as acceptable or unacceptable depends, historically, on who does the regarding and for whom. For example, during the heyday of the plantation sugar economy in the Caribbean a 10 year life expectancy for a slave on a sugar plantation was essentially good health. Health interventions by the owner of the plantation were required only to extend the life expectancy to that point. Obviously, the slaves did not agree with this limitation in their life expectancy and therefore developed their own alternative health system. The result was a dual health system with different perceptions and different methods of curing.

The third major aspect refers to the question of patterns of knowledge and ignorance about a disease. Such patterns depend on the way in which the health profession is organized internally, its relation to other disciplines, how the health profession is connected to the society as a whole, and who is recruited to the health professions.

Our knowledge about a disease depends essentially on who owns the production of knowledge and therefore what kinds of problems get priority or will be ignored.

Finally, the structure and the amount of intervention we design to control a disease outbreak depends strongly when an intervention becomes desirable. Sometimes we have to face a rather bizarre situation, where we have to prove that a disease is costing money before we can convince somebody to do anything about it.

In conclusion, when we talk in a general way about the biosocial nature of disease we have to differentiate and examine each of the different aspects, I mentioned above. It is just too simple to say that there are social factors and biological factors. Rather, we should assume that each entity in the

325

interaction is inextricably both—social and biological—and has to be understood from both perspectives.

PAUL EPSTEIN: I would like to extend the host/environment/pathogen model and offer another model for this discussion.

If we expand "environment" and include the climate system, further, substitute ecosystems for the host and substitute "indicator" species for agents, we can then derive health outcomes.[a] The health or integrity of an ecosystem is related to the diversity within it, its stability, the productivity, the yields and to the vulnerability to stresses, especially to the invasion of organisms. A simplified agricultural system, for example, is vulnerable to invasion. A simplified deforested system is vulnerable to stresses such as flooding, as in Bangladesh and Honduras. The interaction between stresses and the ecosystem result in changes in indicator species. Some responses may occur relatively rapidly. The abundance of insects and rodents on land and algae in coastal systems, are prime examples. Changes in indicator species are directly related to health outcomes: Algae and biotoxins produce damage in fish and shellfish; algae are correlated with cholera outbreaks; insect pests damage plants and might have harmful effects on humans; and rodents carry viruses (hantavirus) and bacteria (plague). Adaptation is one response or intervention, and involves social, biological and behavioral factors. Behavioral factors can be as simple as the following examples: putting hats on to protect from ozone depletion or using lime juice for water and seafood disinfection (a good method, saving forests from being used to boil water).

Surveillance is another response, which is mostly aimed at outcomes. Surveillance could be expanded to include indicator species, which means to monitor (and then manage) insects and algal populations.

For ecosystem management (secondary prevention) we must, for instance, reduce deforestation, not straighten out rivers. Primary prevention in the global system involves policies on fossil fuel use and forestry.

These elements make up an integrated assessment. Adaptation, surveillance, primary and secondary prevention are social and behavioral factors which determine disease emergence and ecosystem health.

How does this framework translate into practical programs for surveillance and management?

We have discussed algae as a vector for cholera and also the emergence of "O139 Bengal," a new variant of cholera. O139 Bengal has the potential to spread directly (through "neighborhood" dispersion) or indirectly (through "hierarchical" dispersion) in ballast in ships, for instance, to Australia, Indonesia and to Africa.

We have further the opportunity to monitor multiple parameters under the rubric of large marine ecosystems (LME) described by Kenneth Sherman (watersheds, fishing policies, plankton, temperature, currents, etc.).[b] Remote

[a] See also Epstein on ecosystem health in the Conceptual Framework Section (pp. 423–435).
[b] See paper by Kenneth Sherman "Coastal ecosystem health: A global perspective" in this volume (pp. 24–43).

sensing to follow algal (phytoplankton) blooms will play an important part. We will be able to examine algae and copepods for biotoxins and for cholera.

In this way we can integrate health monitoring into an ongoing system driven by UNCED (UN Conference on Environmental and Development, Rio de Janeiro, June 1992) and the environmental movement, to monitor ecosystems and meteorological conditions.

LAURIE GARRETT: I have to note that your model has no human beings in it. Where are they in the causality of disease?

EPSTEIN: Humans are one of the species.

GARRETT: So we're part of environment?

EPSTEIN: We are primary drivers of as well as responders to environmental changes through participation in biological processes and through behavioral, social, economic and political processes. As one of the species, we are now changing the environment at a greater rate than any other species has, that we are aware of. We are also threatening to exhaust resources and overwhelm other species. We are definitely part of the ecosystems and the global system.

PAMELA ANDERSON: What we need is a biosociological construct. I was noticing, that we are still breaking down along disciplinary lines. The question remains, what kind of proposals have we to develop such a biosociological construct?

HARVEY FINEBERG: One question for Pamela: What steps do you think we should take either as a group or more generally in order to foster the kind of genuine interdisciplinary exchange that is behind the comment you made?

ANDERSON: I would like to see some of the ideas debated across disciplinary lines. How do we make it happen that social scientists and physicians, despite their specialization, really discuss some of the issues raised in the discussions of this workshop concerning the emergence of new diseases?

The first step is to believe the findings from other disciplines. The second step would be to select examples—case-in point diseases—and exercise the research in a transdisciplinary framework.

GARRETT: I think that we are most comfortable with the research about the emergence of new microbes. We can observe and analyze the biological processes in the laboratory or in the field. It becomes less comfortable for us to explore the human behavior related to the emergence and reemergence of diseases.

Why do people participate in behaviors that put them and other people at risk? It's very difficult to remove judgmental aspects from the research about human behavior and health. If we analyze modes of transmission of pathogens through human-to-human contact we will face ethical and moral questions related to human rights and the historical violation of human rights in a society.

This research demands understanding of the cultural, political and social determinants of people's behavior, thus the incorporation of social and anthropological research.

EPSTEIN: Poverty and inequities are strongly related to increased vulnerability of populations, for instance through increased exposures to toxins. Poverty and inequality are also driving factors of environmental change.

People sell drugs, sell their bodies, sell their organs; sell everything they can because of poverty and inequities. Inequities and poverty drive them to cut down forests. These factors are directly linked to health and to increasing ecosystem vulnerability.

FINEBERG: This is a very intriguing point, especially in relation to the different ways in which we have used the idea of the "human factor" in our sessions today. In the first sessions on water-borne and vector-borne diseases the influence of human action was predominantly constructed in terms of either commercial activity or the changes the human population produced in the environment. The discussions in the small working groups seemed to convey a larger sense of the social construct of illness and the understanding of disease. In these discussions human-to-human attitude, interaction, and relationship were addressed and not only the interactions of humans to environment or humans to disease vectors.

Part B. Population Movements and Infectious Diseases

TAMARA AWERBUCH: I like Dr. Chen's table on population movements very much.[a] I may add to the aspect of national migration, the movement from urban to rural areas. An example is the movement of people from the cities in Brazil to rural areas. Mostly, they move to the Amazon in order to create new agricultural land by destroying the forests. By doing so, the settlers create new habitats for mosquitoes. They will get infected with malaria because, coming from urban areas, they are not immune to malaria. This disease becomes endemic in the Brazilian Amazon.

To study all components of population movements, population growth, and the interactions between vectors, pathogens and hosts, we should apply mathematical modeling.

PAMELA ANDERSON: In plant sciences we are confronted with the problem of movement of seeds. Eighteen percent of the identified and characterized plant viruses are vertically transmitted.[b] Pathogens are transmitted through the seeds. Further research might even show that 1/3 of all plant viruses are transmitted vertically.

The boundaries of quarantine become particularly important to prevent such vertical transmission of plant pathogens through seed movement. We know at least 10 groups of viruses for which seed transmission is important. In analyzing the seed movements in relation to the spread of plant diseases we might be able to identify patterns of mobility or movement.

---

[a] See also commentary by Lincoln Chen in this section (pp. 319–324).
[b] For the definition of "vertical transmission," please see the glossary.

Reflecting on the discussion about surveillance, I think we have focused the arguments on surveillance of static populations. In my opinion, we have to connect these models of surveillance with our knowledge about mobile populations. In plant science the seeds represent mobile populations. We should, in addition to the existing surveillance concepts, develop a surveillance system for mobile populations.

Such a surveillance system should be based on identified patterns of movement, including the movements of people.

ROBERT SHOPE: I want to add an example of the long-range transport of infectious disease vectors. This work was done by Robert Sellers at Pier Bright, England.[1]
He made basically two observations.

In the framework of a study about blue tongue disease in animals on Cyprus, they identified the species of culicoides as the vector of blue tongue disease. Cyprus is the natural habitat of this culicoides species. At the same time they conducted parallel studies about this disease in England. They could capture specimens of culicoides in England too. Surprisingly, these specimens belonged to the same species they found on Cyprus. The conclusion was, that the England specimen had been carried with the wind from Cyprus to England.

The other example I want to mention is related to the African horse sickness. Seller could trace the disease from sub-Saharan Africa to the Middle East. He concluded that this disease distribution is correlated with the directions of the winds. The African horse sickness is also a culicoides-transmitted disease.

Both examples seem to indicate that the movements of the infectious disease vectors contribute largely to the distribution and spread of the disease.

RICHARD LEVINS: I want to add three points to the discussion.

First, the experience has shown that most introductions of species, including parasites, into new areas are unsuccessful. The species fail to establish themselves in the new eco-niche. Nevertheless, there are circumstances in which species could establish themselves in new areas fabulously well. To explain these successful introductions we have a theory of the ecology of invasions which was first developed by Elton.[2] Further, it would be possible to overwork the existing biogeographic theory for the specific context of the introduction of parasites into new areas.

My second comment is related to changes in the human population. It seems to me that we picture population movements as something that happens independently from us, as another kind of climate change. After the change took place and after we identified it, we try to respond to the problem.

I would suggest that we develop either invited or uninvited health impact statements in relation to the population movements in the world. With such health impact statements we could analyze critically the various programs for development—both the large-scale programs focusing on development schemes of a whole country and the more localized ones, like the development of hydroelectric projects that involve changing the ecology and demography of a particular region. The goal of such evaluations is to calculate the impact of development programs or changes in human populations on health in a country or a region *prior* to the environmental changes these events produce.[c]

For example, in regard to the Brazilian Amazon we discussed the relationship between deforestation and the resurgence of malaria in this region. I'm really concerned with an ethical problem, that we take measurements that would facilitate the conquest of the Amazon without regard to the concerns of the people who live there.

My third problem is that we, as the "intervenors" (of health or development programs), are parts of the system. When we talk about the dynamics of these changes, the behavior of ministries of health and governments become important. One aspect in this regard is social memory. How long does it take before either a government or a ministry of health decides that the problem is solved? This decision would include closing down the laboratory and spending money somewhere else. The duration of memory, either in a general population or among the health community, is a parameter of social dynamics which has to be analyzed at the same scale as the rate of natural selection or the rate of spread of a pathogen.

Looking at human behavior includes looking at the behavior of the communities of people who are trying to deal with health. Bureaucratic inertia is a component of this behavior.

LINCOLN CHEN: You have to remember that the whole concept of migration is definitional. In other words, did I migrate from Boston to come to this meeting?

We can get very different migration rates depending on where we would draw boundaries for migrating populations and, most important, for what purposes we would draw such boundaries. The statistics about population movements will show what we defined to be a movement or migration. The defined boundaries that we impose will influence the ways of dealing with population movements and their causes, like urbanization or refugee movement. I don't think that national boundaries are inappropriate. Our public systems have to be organized by administrative and political units which include, at one level, nations. The existence of nations or national boundaries cannot replace the need to think globally about the movement of diseases.

CRISTINA DE A. POSSAS: In this workshop we discussed only population growth and population mobility as elements of population dynamic. I would like to add two other important elements of population dynamic—population aging and population differentiation. Both processes should be discussed in their relationship to new and resurgent disease.

Population differentiation includes social differentiation, changes in the structure of the labor market, and changes in the political organization of the labor force. Population differentiation is correlated with poverty and, as discussed by Laurie Garrett, poverty strongly affects the emergence of infectious disease.

---

[c] See also paper by Uwe Brinkmann on economic development and tropical diseases in this volume (pp. 303–311).

CHEN: I would like to summarize this discussion.

In this session we discussed issues related to the disciplines: demography (population studies), anthropology (human behavior), and infectious disease epidemiology (the design of a framework for disease transmission and the interaction between people and new diseases). We focused the discussion on human behavior and human-to-human interactions, including sex behavior and infectious disease. Further we reflected on the question of social and economic change, especially the globalization of our societies and economics. It seems that there is only the global unit which provides the basis to deal with the changes and movements of human species, no matter what boundaries we draw on our maps.

In this context I am reminded of a book by Jacques Attali called *Millennium*.[3] In this book Attali looks into the next century. He describes a nomadic person as an individual unit with an individual number, who owns his or her computer and portable phone to participate in the global economy and society. In the next century, there will be another type of nomadic person which Jacques Attali does not describe in his book. This other nomad will not own a computer or a modem or a telephone. He or she will be a refugee, on the move into cities to struggle for survival. Both types of nomads will change disease emergence essentially. Thank you very much.

REFERENCES

1. SELLERS, R. F. 1992. Weather, Culicoides, and the distribution and spread of blue tongue and African horse sickness virus. *In* Blue Tongue, African Horse Sickness and Related Orbiviruses. T. E. Walton & B. I. Osburn, Eds.: 284–290. Boca Raton, FL: CRC Press.
2. ELTON, C. S. 1958. The ecology of invasions by animals and plants. London: Chapman and Hall.
3. ATTALI, J. 1992. Millennium. Winners and Losers in the Coming World Order. New York: Random House, Inc. Translated from the French by L. Conners and H. Gardels.

Part C. Human Movements and the Spread of Infectious Diseases

LEONARDO MATA: One of the present population movements that concerns us greatly in Costa Rica is tourism. For example, every year one million people travel to Spain as tourists. The proportion of tourists in comparison to the local population sums up to 1 tourist to 40 natives, more or less.

In small islands or nations like Barbados, Costa Rica, or Hawaii, this proportion is shifted considerably. In Costa Rica, for example, with a total population of about 3 million people, every year about 600,000 tourists visit the country. Tourism is an important figure for the national economy of Costa Rica.

The stream of tourists, seeking sunshine and relaxation, has an enormous impact on the lifestyle of the native population in Costa Rica. In this regard, sexually transmitted diseases, especially AIDS, became a very sensitive issue for the tourism industry and, of course, for health officials of the country.

Further, the highest cumulative incidence rates of AIDS in the world are not in Africa, but in the Caribbean. In the Bahamas and French Guinea, there are as many as 3,000 to 4,000 cases of HIV-infected persons per million.

LAURIE GARRETT: I mentioned that there are 100 million abandoned children living in the urban centers worldwide. For most of those children, there is only one way to earn their living—sex trade. "Sexploitation" is increasing globally and is strongly related to urbanization. An increasing number of people move to poor urban centers and they will find almost no resources for living. Sex trade becomes the only way they can earn their living. On the other hand, sex tourism continues to attract every year millions of tourists.

We could look at the streets of New York and we would find prostitutes who work there. These prostitutes are infected with several different agents. Almost 50% of them are HIV infected.

In my opinion, sexually transmitted diseases have the highest probability of crossing national boundaries very rapidly.

If we map the routes of global heroin and cocaine trade and further, if we map the international centers of sex tourism and "sexploitation" in the world, we would find overlapping areas with the centers of HIV incidence, centers of hepatitis B, and other STDs.

STEPHEN MORSE: There have been talks about eroticizing safe sex and providing alternative ways for professional sex workers to earn their livelihood. These efforts have moved very slowly. I think, this indicates how important it is, today, to organize appropriate social interventions and to motivate people to accomplish these interventions.

Despite the years of warning that AIDS would become a pandemic in Asia, there was a great deal of denial that prevented actions to stop the penetration of HIV into Asia. Regarding the factor—movement of people into cities—there is another aspect to consider. In some parts of the world, for instance in India, young men will move into the cities for work and leave their families behind. While in the cities, they may seek prostitutes, professional sex workers.

Then, these people, after having made money in the city, may return to their families in the rural areas and they will bring AIDS to these communities. This demographic pattern may feed epidemics in far off places.

RICHARD CASH: The notion of national boundaries and borders inhibits our thinking and our ability to deal with infectious diseases. Take the examples of sexually transmitted diseases. There is a tendency that one country blames another one for the introduction and spread of STDs. When syphilis was introduced into Europe, the French called it the "English Disease" and the English, of course, blamed it on someone else.

The spread of AIDS among commercial sex workers (CSWs) in Thailand was first blamed on international tourists. In fact, most of those using CSWs are Thai men. By focusing on people from "outside" countries, like tourists, health officials might ignore the risk factors within their own country.

The movement of people is not stopped by national borders, even when policy and behavior are significantly different between countries. China, for example, has had a rigorous program for years, aimed at controlling the spread of STDs. The closing of brothels, education of prostitutes, mass treatment, and a conservative policy have contributed to reduce STDs significantly. As borders open, and behaviors change, however, it is expected that STDs will increase in China during the next few years.

There should be a way that we can focus more on the movement of disease, without lines on the map. It might help to view the spread of diseases from satellite photographs rather than from a geopolitical perspective.

GARRETT: I agree with everything Richard said. But, I am not so visionary. It is hard for me to look ahead and to picture a time when public health would be considered important enough, universally, that government planners would be willing to ignore borders for the sake of public health. Such perspective does not exist now, and it takes a powerful imagination to picture it for the future.

GARY SMITH: National boundaries are important, in my understanding, because they represent actual barriers for movements. We have talked about the extent of movements across boundaries. We should as well consider the role of national boundaries in inhibiting population movements. Regarding my own field of research, national boundaries are shown to be inhibitory to animal movements. In my opinion, it is not especially visionary to think of a system where those national boundaries can be broken down, at least in terms of population movement. The European Community, for example, has done exactly this—they broke down the national boundaries to a certain extent. There is some concern about the consequences that increased travel and trade would have on the spread of human as well as animal diseases in Europe. Both aspects have to be explored—the fact that small national boundaries do inhibit movement, and on the other hand, that it is not totally visionary to think of a global organization that abandons national boundaries.

Vulnerability and the Distribution of Exposures

Concept Paper

Infectious diseases are caused not by pathogens alone but by the exposure of vulnerable populations or individuals to pathogens. Therefore reducing vulnerability and exposure is a major aspect of preparation for new disease threats, along with prediction, detection with rapid response and prevention in a long-term coherent strategy.

Vulnerability is the measure of harmful impact resulting from a given negative input or stressor on individuals or populations. It is therefore the inverse of tolerance or resistance. Vulnerability to emerging diseases is simultaneously social and biological, mediated by factors such as depressed immune response, reduced generalized host defenses, limited social support, increased social disruption, poor economic status, and exposure to pollutants, toxins and infectious agents. Each of these may increase vulnerability and reduce tolerance through an impact that is both biological and social. Indeed, the social/biological dichotomy in epidemiology is false and ultimately misleading. We define the domain of concern as intrinsically biosocial.

Vulnerabilities and exposures are unequally distributed across societal and national boundaries. All the categories of class, race, gender and ethnicity which differentiate privileges and oppressions also affect vulnerability. Toxic waste dumping in the United States, for example, has been concentrated in African American and Native American communities; person-to-person transmission of pathogens is related to population density by way of the frequency of "contact," while contact itself is defined by the mode of transmission. Many vector-borne and water-borne diseases are concentrated in poor third world communities. Finally, the research effort has been uneven, producing a pattern of knowledge and ignorance determined by the priorities of those allocating research resources.

We can analyze the vulnerabilities of individuals or populations (groups of people sharing common social, economic or demographic characteristics) by examining the probabilities of events along a causal sequence of conditional probabilities: the probability of exposure to an infectious agent, the probability of transmission to a host if there is exposure, the probability of infection if the agent is transmitted, the probability of disease if infection occurs, and the probability of partial or complete recovery or death following disease. These links may be subdivided more finely. Some of the same factors, such as the state of the immune system or access to health care, intervene at several stages in the sequence. All these events may vary among individuals and populations.

Public health workers distinguish between the risk status of people and the interventions they receive (including clinical therapy). Risk status captures aspects of people's lives that influence the exposure and its consequences.

The access to and efficacy of treatment may also vary: the more vulnerable groups often receive less efficacious treatment, increasing the rate at which infection leads to disease and death.

The first question then is, what measures can we take to reduce vulnerability and exposure? These fall into the general category of "horizontal resistance" in which a broad generic program is used to reduce exposure and vulnerability prior to the appearance of new diseases. These include measures to reduce exposure to pathogens and vectors such as limiting deforestation, careful design of irrigation systems, controlled disposal of used rubber tires, and provision of sewer services in the expanding cities; reduction of nutrient runoff and erosion into fresh water and marine habitats; sex education and the means for applying that education. Other measures affect transmission, such as the provision of less crowded housing, use of mosquito nets; improvement of vitamin A nutrition and the reduction of air pollution in the community and workplace to maintain the integrity of the respiratory tract epithelium. Some measures are directed at strengthening elements of the immune system and improving access to medical care. In all these cases vulnerability can be reduced without precise prediction of specific diseases since these interventions offer protection or improve outcomes for a wide range of possible epidemiological threats. Some of these measures involve expansions of traditional public health activities while others fall outside the sphere of the health professions but are no less necessary to health.

Social inequity is an important condition underlying vulnerability. Exploited and stressed individuals and populations are at greater risk of emerging and resurgent diseases. In addition, because they cannot avoid exposure to unsafe conditions in their social or physical environment at home or at work or play, they are often constrained by their circumstances into unwanted and unsafe choices and offered limited access to therapeutic interventions. Thus vulnerability must be seen as a system property whose locus is the social structure even where that structure is expressed through individuals and individual behaviors.

A strategy to reduce vulnerability should be included in all economic and technological development programs. The health impacts of development should be examined on different spatial and time scales as they affect the pattern of local moment to moment conditions but also the broad societal changes operating over decades.

Detection, Surveillance, and Response to Emerging Diseases

Introduction

Substantial erosion has occurred of the traditional resources needed to address detection, surveillance and response to infectious diseases. These include a loss of well-trained professionals, as well as redirection of traditional infrastructures which have historically formed the foundation of those important services. This erosion is not limited to a single stratum of the public health infrastructure, but rather involves losses at all levels: hospital, state and regional laboratories, universities, national and international centers. Technical advances have, in many cases, improved our ability to identify specific pathogens or their genetic fingerprints, but these advances have been at the expense of more traditional procedures. The result has too often been an increased reliance on "kits" for diagnostic procedures, with a resulting loss of the skills necessary for traditional isolation or cultures of pathogens. Likewise, the molecular revolution has been accompanied by a dramatic reduction in training opportunities in basic laboratory-oriented courses in microbiology and parasitology, for example. Thus, we are faced with diminished human resources to face the challenge of detection, surveillance, and response to emerging diseases.

In general, the technical tools necessary to detect emerging diseases are available; however, they are not appropriately distributed or widely used. Key infrastructural resources to support critical detection efforts, such as serum and tissue banks and repositories for strains of microbes, are generally lacking. Strengthening of detection and surveillance capabilities at the local, state, and federal level is needed. Novel approaches to detection and surveillance are needed, with establishment of partnerships of public health professionals with health care providers, professional organizations, and universities. Expanded opportunities for input of information are needed. For example, the lay public is often an excellent source of first alert of outbreaks, as well as a potential mobilizing force for acquisition of funding for response activities. Current examples include the recent *E. coli* O157:H7 outbreak of hemolytic-uremic syndrome, recognition and response to Lyme disease, and marine environmental issues. Perhaps directed public involvement efforts should be explored, such as telephone call-in lines manned by local public health facilities, to provide detection and surveillance information, especially for milder diseases that would not necessarily require hospitalization. Public education efforts might also contribute to this effort, as by television programs of popular themes that include a health component. "How to be a hero" was suggested, with the example of the critical observations of a single individual which led to recognition of the *E. coli* outbreak, resulting in the prevention of several thousand cases.

Surveillance is likewise threatened by eroding infrastructures and loss of key personnel. Accurate surveillance information is required, however, to form the basis for any quantitative evaluation of interventions and cost-effectiveness analysis. Fortunately, some kinds of surveillance can be conducted rather inexpensively, and this may be a component of larger, research-oriented projects. To be fully successful, however, surveillance should be conducted on a global scale, since we have often seen that events in one part of the world may quickly have consequences in another. Surveillance, at least on a national scale, should be the responsibility of the government. Unfortunately, funding for surveillance programs is difficult to obtain, even for government agencies, and is virtually impossible for the typical university researcher. To overcome this, sustainable partnerships have been formed between government, universities, and even private industry, to link both surveillance and research with shared objectives of interest to all parties.

An argument can be made that response efforts have been hurt by the concept of "eradication" (*i.e.*, smallpox) or "elimination," rather than the often more appropriate response of "control and containment" (as needed, for example, for cholera). Likewise, statistical measurements of mortality alone may not accurately reflect the burden of morbidity, and the two should not be confused.

Surveillance entails knowing what to measure. In the case of new and emergent diseases, knowing what to observe may be obscure. One way to identify key observations comes by understanding the network of interactions of pathogens, hosts, vectors, and the ecology of these organisms. A surveillance system will not measure everything, hence tools are required to decide on early-warning indicators.

Models are one tool that can aid surveillance. Not all kinds of models will be helpful; models used for surveillance should be general, omitting precision. Because these are for emergent diseases, the models should sacrifice some realism in the sense that they entertain unconventional assumptions (*e.g.*, a non-O1 *Vibrio* can produce cholera).

Models cannot be made for every possible new disease or pathogen. Criteria need to be developed that identify most probable disease candidates. One procedure to develop criteria would begin with the list of diseases and pathogens developed in the Institute of Medicine report. This could be refined by looking at the set of assumptions that produced that list.

Another procedure to identify disease candidates would derive from deductions from actual events. One criterion might suggest a search for diseases normally absent when coupled to unusual or abnormal ecological or biological or physical conditions that seem likely to persist. The experience with the hantavirus of New Mexico associated with the unusually high rodent population makes this criterion a likely candidate. It also suggests other rodent-borne diseases should be examined.

Another criterion comes from the aberrant reports or outliers that cannot be explained. The detection of non-O1 vibrios in the midst of a pandemic of diarrheal disease with cholera-like symptoms, signals the need to develop models that can consider outlandish reports as possible. The models would be aids to suggest what would be the patterns of disease that a non-O1 vibrio would present compared to an O1 vibrio. There are no guarantees that sufficient biological knowledge would have been available to have made such a model prove useful. It would be worthwhile for major health organizations, like the CDC and WHO, to have modeling groups specifically attached to surveillance units.

Indirect (Unanticipated) Effects of
Intervention

Public health interventions have in many cases had unanticipated, indirect effects. These "surprise events" have been both positive and negative. Measles vaccine has benefits that would not have been apparent if surveillance had measured only cases of measles. Conversely, recent studies showed vaccination of infants with high titer measles vaccine (Edmondston-Zagreb strain) at a young age led to increased mortality, most apparent in girls. Thus our definition of disease needs to include total long-term disease burden and may need to extend beyond the primary disease that is the target of intervention.

Malaria control efforts may have short-term benefits following use of insecticide, but in a longer time frame may lead to rebound in malaria with the emergence of mosquito resistance. In other settings, spraying efforts to reduce mosquitoes met with human social resistance as the insecticides eliminated wasps that were predatory to bedbugs or caterpillars, resulting in increased human bedbug infestation or collapsed roofs due to caterpillar destruction. Pesticide spraying may kill the targeted species, but also claim untargeted animals, such as cats, allowing for a surge in pathogen-carrying rodent populations.

These examples illustrate several principles:

1. Any disease or public health intervention must be pursued with careful consideration of its full impact. Planners of projects aimed at microbial or vector suppression on a large scale must recognize that later cessation or diminution of efforts may produce a microbial or vector rebound effect that exceeds original levels, resulting in iatrogenic emergence.
2. Consideration of any intervention should follow a multidisciplinary approach that encompasses the social, behavioral, cultural, policy/governmental, biological, ecological and medical aspects of the proposed intervention at the planning stage.
3. Unintended secondary impacts of interventions may not be apparent until months or years following their execution. This underscores the need for long-term monitoring of populations and ecologies following interventions.
4. Some indirect impacts of interventions could have been anticipated had the planned actions been approached with proper skepticism and analysis. But that may not always be the case. This highlights the potential benefit of involving persons from a range of disciplines to extend the scope of understanding possible indirect consequences.
5. Time frames for concern and activity are different for curative physicians vs. public-health advocates.

6. Mathematical models can be used to alert researchers to outcomes that might not have been anticipated. An example comes from models of rabies in wildlife which suggest that vaccination levels insufficient to eradicate the virus actually increase the absolute density of rabid animals.

Global Surveillance for Recognition and Response to Emerging Diseases

JAMES W. LEDUC AND EUGENE TIKHOMIROV

Division of Communicable Diseases
World Health Organization
20, Avenue Appia
Geneva, Switzerland CH-1211

The World Health Organization (WHO) is attempting to exercise its leadership and coordinating roles by creating a global surveillance program for recognition and response to emerging diseases. This program will be proactive in nature, broad in scope, and truly international in perspective. It will be horizontal in that it holds the potential to address viral and bacterial pathogens, as well as zoonoses. Parenthetically, the program will also have the capability to recognize biological warfare events, an area of increasing international concern. The stimulus for this program is the current pandemic of HIV and AIDS, but it is based on the realization that pathogens mutate, develop resistance, and are continually challenging the human population. Concurrent with this are changes that place humans at greater risk of infectious disease, such as urban over-crowding, global warming, and changing social values.

The program will target activities at the country level by making maximum use of existing WHO Collaborating Centers located throughout the world. The objective of the program will be recognition of new, emerging, or re-emerging diseases, and drug-resistant microorganisms. The routine reporting of all infectious diseases is neither practicable nor sustainable, and will not be the goal of this program. Recognition of unusual disease occurrences, coupled with an appropriate response mechanism, is however, an attainable goal which we hope will be achieved through this program.

The focus of the program is to enhance laboratory capabilities so that local reference centers are prepared to rapidly recognize novel outbreaks as they occur, and to complement this effort with a stronger intervention capacity at the WHO headquarters level, so that prompt, coordinated action can be taken in conjunction with the Regional Offices. In addition, the program will strengthen local capabilities to systematically monitor bacterial resistance to antimicrobials. Widespread installation of WHONET, a computer-based program will facilitate the management of antibiotic susceptibility test results. Training components will build local human resources in outbreak investigation, laboratory studies, and surveillance. Research opportunities in epidemiology, microbiology, disease prevention and control, and health systems development will evolve from the program as better definitions of both common pathogens and emerging diseases are realized.

During the past decade, numerous emerging and re-emerging infectious diseases have been recognized. In addition to HIV and AIDS, dengue hemor-rhagic fever dramatically invaded the Americas, causing a massive outbreak in Cuba in 1981, which severely challenged the national health care facilities.[1] More recently, dengue hemorrhagic fever has been documented in Brazil and Venezuela. It threatens other Latin American nations, as well as Asian and Pacific countries, including Australia, where dengue transmission was recently recorded in northeastern parts of the country for the first time in decades.[2–4] Pandemic cholera reappeared in South America in 1991 after that region was cholera-free for many years,[5] and a new cholera strain, *V. cholerae* O139, which appears to elude the protective immunity of persons previously infected with other strains of cholera, emerged in 1993 in the Indian subcontinent.[6] In Russia, diphtheria has made a dramatic resurgence in 1991 to 1993,[7] and in Africa, epidemic yellow fever was recognized for the first time ever in Kenya.[8] Rift Valley fever virus, an important pathogen of both domestic animals and humans, was documented in Egypt in 1993, the first time since the devastating outbreak of 1977–1978, when thousands of animals and hundreds of humans were infected.[9] Elsewhere in Africa, Lassa fever continues to cause epidemics, including nosocomial outbreaks with fatalities in doctors and nurses, in much of West Africa. And in the United States, a highly fatal form of hantavirus infection, a rodent-borne zoonosis, was recognized for the first time in 1993.[10] This disease, with a clinical presentation of acute pneumonitis leading to death in from 50 to 75% of those affected, is perhaps the best example of both a dramatic new disease, and of how well-prepared laboratory and field investigations can be quickly mobilized to define and combat an emerging infectious disease problem.

Emerging infections are not, however, limited to the appearance of dra-matic epidemics of new diseases. Common bacterial pathogens regularly de-velop resistance to antimicrobial agents.[11] After each new antibiotic has be-come widely used, it tends to lose its effectiveness as resistance develops. Many strains of gonococci, for example, became resistant to sulfonamides, then later to penicillin. Most strains of staphylococci became resistant to penicillin, then to methicillin, and recently to fluoroquinolones.[12] Strains of shigella became resistant to tetracycline, ampicillin, and then trimethoprim.[13] Pseudomonas strains have quickly become resistant to many new drugs, and a quarter of the clinical isolates of *Haemophilus influenzae* are resistant to ampicillin. Other gram-negative bacilli have become resistant to nearly all of the available antibiotics, including new broad spectrum antibiotics such as cephalosporins. Such resistance is a hazardous and costly problem in devel-oped countries, but in the developing world, where routine susceptibility testing and costly new antibiotics are not readily available, it is increasingly life-threatening.

A comprehensive program for surveillance of antimicrobial resistance, which is adaptable to all member states, is an appropriate goal for WHO. A pilot study towards this goal was conducted between 1987 and 1992, and led to the development of WHONET, a computer program for microbiology laboratories to facilitate the management of antibiotic susceptibility test results from routine clinical isolates.[14] Analytical programs utilizing these data aid local hospitals in understanding the epidemiology of antimicrobial resistance, assist in the development of rational antibiotic prescription practices, and help infection control programs. WHONET may be used in isolation on a personal computer, or in conjunction with larger computing resources. By 1994, WHONET was in use in over 100 hospitals, institutes and laboratories in 26 countries, primarily in the Americas, the Western Pacific and in Europe.

We hope to complete revision of a new edition of WHONET (WHONET 3), evaluate it in limited field tests, and expand the network of national microbiology laboratories which use WHONET. This will make available at the local level a resource to aid in the selection of appropriate antibiotics, identify local resistance patterns, and assist in quality control programs. Where needed, we will also provide limited assistance in establishing local antibiotic screening capabilities. The network will also allow ongoing surveillance of antimicrobial resistance, not only at the local level, but also regionally and globally.

OBJECTIVES

Development Objectives for Global Surveillance of Infectious Diseases

Critical elements of the surveillance and response system include a network of reference centers that assist national services in disease diagnosis and investigation, which has access to potentially significant or novel clinical observations, as well as to the patients or animals affected. These centers need the capability to conduct preliminary epidemiological investigations in close collaboration with national services following recognition of novel events. The centers will also assist countries with laboratory-based diagnostics to differentiate common illnesses from new syndromes or introductions. The centers will require a communications capability so that information may be rapidly and reliably relayed to WHO and other centers that may share an interest in their findings. An option for informal communications must exist, so that preliminary information can be shared as observations are made and investigations begun, before formal announcement of a problem is made. WHO will in turn need to coordinate appropriate responses to recognized events, which will include providing assistance in field investigations and problem definition, coordinating confirmation of laboratory results, organizing consultations of experts to decide upon the most effective intervention strategies, and then implementing those specific interventions to identified problems. Targets for surveillance will include both human and animal pathogens.

By the end of 1995, we hope to have accomplished the following objectives.

A. Have in place a dynamic, interactive, global network of Collaborating Centers able to rapidly recognize, investigate, report outbreaks of infectious diseases, and differentiate "normal" from "new," emerging, or re-emerging infections.

B. Organize a system whereby critical laboratory reagents, equipment and technologies are rapidly institutionalized into the routine capabilities of each Collaborating Center.

C. Create an ongoing training program for both technicians and professionals whereby new skills are introduced into the national laboratories and Collaborating Centers.

D. Expand existing global response capacity within WHO to assist in investigation and control of recognized outbreaks. Included would be close coordination with programs such as the Expanded Program on Immunizations, the Special Program for Research and Training in Tropical Diseases, the Control of Tropical Diseases Program, and other programs where effective preventive interventions are stressed.

E. Foster frequent, easy, inexpensive, informal communications between Centers and with WHO and other interested organizations. This could take the form of expanded E-mail communications, or perhaps inexpensive satellite communications for remote locations.

Development Objectives for Monitoring Bacterial Resistance to Antimicrobial Agents

The original WHONET program and documentation is now in its second revision, and a third edition is under development. Initial efforts in our plans to monitor antimicrobial resistance will focus on completion of WHONET 3, evaluation of the program under field conditions, and modification of it to meet local needs. Following the quality control test, we will collect and analyze the results, then hold a workshop to evaluate the trial, standardize the methods used, determine the geographic localities where additional sites are required, and define means of information exchange. When we have refined the WHONET program, expansion to the widest possible number of users should be appropriate, and we will attempt to increase the number of participating laboratories, establish a network of national, regional, and international reference laboratories, and maintain a global surveillance system through continued quality control, technical assistance, and information exchange.

We hope to complete the following efforts by the end of 1995.

A. Establish a network of regional and national reference laboratories to ensure continuous information on antimicrobial resistance from representative geographic areas worldwide. These laboratories would identify global trends in resistance, and offer a mechanism for early detection of new resistance patterns.

B. Offer specific interventions based on the data accumulated from A above. These might include offering guidance in the development and use of new antibiotics, and recommending ways of preserving the efficacy of older ones; comparison of antibiotic practices and determination of the most efficient and cost-effective usages; detection and potentially prevention of the international spread of resistant plasmids or strains; and offering global warnings on the emergence of resistant strains.

Through the efforts described here, we hope to strengthen national capacities in disease surveillance and control, thereby building health infrastructure, while helping to promote research capabilities by improving disease problem definition and assisting in training and corrective interventions.

REFERENCES

1. GUZMAN, M. G., G. P. KOURI, J. BRAVO, M. CALUNGA, M. SOLER, S. VAZQUEZ & C. VENEREO. 1984. Dengue haemorrhagic fever in Cuba. I. Serological confirmation of clinical diagnosis. Trans. R. Soc. Trop. Med. Hyg. **78**: 235–238.
2. PAN AMERICAN HEALTH ORGANIZATION. 1992. Dengue and dengue haemorrhagic fever in the Americas: An overview of the problem. Epidemiol. Bull. **13** (Special Edition): 1–2.
3. WHO. Dengue and dengue haemorrhagic fever, Venezuela. WER **68**: 316–317.
4. STREATFIELD, R., D. SINCLAIR, G. BIELBY, J. SHERIDAN, M. PEARCE & D. PHILLIPS. Dengue serotype 2 epidemic, Townsville, 1992–93. Communicable Dis. Intell. **17**: 330–332.
5. WHO. 1991. Cholera. WER **66**: 55–56; 61–63; 65–70.
6. ALBERT, M. J., A. K. SIDDIQUE, M. S. ISLAM, A. S. G. FARUQUE, M. ANSARUZZAMAN, S. M. FARUQUE, & R. B. SACK. 1993. Large outbreak of clinical cholera due to Vibrio cholerae non-O1 in Bangladesh. Lancet **341**: 704.
7. CDC. 1993. Diphtheria outbreak—Russian Federation, 1990–1993. MMWR **42**: 840–847.
8. WHO. 1993. Yellow fever, Kenya. WER **68**: 159–160.
9. WHO. 1993. Rift Valley fever, Egypt. WER **68**: 300–301.
10. CDC. 1993. Update: Hantavirus pulmonary syndrome—United States, 1993. MMWR **42**: 816–820.
11. O'BRIEN, T. F. & MEMBERS OF TASK FORCE 2. 1987. Resistance of bacteria to antibacterial agents: Report of Task Force 2. Rev. Infect. Dis. **9** (Suppl. 3): S244–S260.
12. MURRAY, B. E. 1991. New aspects of antimicrobial resistance and the resulting therapeutic dilemmas. J. Infect. Dis. **163**: 1185–1194.
13. TAUXE, R. V., N. D. PUHR, J. G. WELLS, N. HARGRETT-BEAN & P. A. BLAKE. 1990. Antimicrobial resistance of *Shigella* isolates in the USA: The importance of international travelers. J. Infect. Dis. **162**: 1107–1111.
14. O'BRIEN, T. F. & J. M. STELLING. 1994. A computer program (WHONET) that files and analyzes all information on each isolate at each center improves multicenter surveillance of resistance to antimicrobial agents. Abstract book, 6th International Congress for Infectious Diseases, Abstract 1321, p. 404.

Emerging Infectious Diseases in the United States

Improved Surveillance, a Requisite for Prevention

RALPH T. BRYAN,[a] ROBERT W. PINNER, AND
RUTH L. BERKELMAN

Office of the Director
National Center for Infectious Diseases
Centers for Disease Control and Prevention
Atlanta, Georgia 30333

INTRODUCTION

Once expected to be eliminated as a significant public health problem, infectious diseases remain the leading cause of death worldwide and a leading cause of illness and death in the United States.[1] As society, technology, and the environment change, pathogens can evolve or spread, altering the spectrum of infectious diseases. Emerging infections are those diseases whose incidence has increased within the past two decades or whose incidence threatens to increase in the near future.[2] Many factors or combinations of factors can contribute to disease emergence (TABLE 1). Newly emergent infectious diseases may result from the evolution of existing organisms; known diseases may spread to new geographic areas or new human populations; or previously unrecognized infections may appear in humans living or working in changing ecologic conditions that increase their exposure to insect vectors, animal reservoirs, or environmental sources of novel pathogens. Diseases may re-emerge owing to the development of antimicrobial resistance in existing agents (*e.g.*, gonorrhea, malaria, pneumococcal disease) or breakdowns in public health measures for previously controlled infections (*e.g.*, cholera, tuberculosis, measles).

Numerous examples demonstrate that emerging infectious diseases are a global problem (TABLE 2). In the United States, toxic shock syndrome and Lyme disease illustrate how new technology or products (super absorbent tampons) and changing ecology and human demographics (reforestation, increased deer populations, suburban migration), respectively, can foster the emergence of new microbial threats.[3,4] Other societal changes, such as our expanding use of child care facilities, have contributed to the emergence of infectious diseases that threaten children and staff in child care centers as well as other household members in infected children's

[a] *Present address:* IHS-HQW, Epidemiology Branch, 5300 Homestead Dr. N.E., Albuquerque, NM 87110; Fax (505) 837-4181.

TABLE 1. Factors in Emergence[a]

Categories	Specific Examples
Societal events	Economic impoverishment; war and civil conflict; population migration
Health care	New medical devices; organ or tissue transplantation; drugs causing immunosuppression; widespread use of antibiotics
Food production	Globalization of food supplies; changes in food processing and packaging
Human behavior	Sexual behavior; drug use; travel; diet; outdoor recreation; use of child care facilities
Environmental changes	Deforestation/reforestation; changes in water ecosystems; flood/drought; famine; global warming
Public health infrastructure	Curtailment or reduction in prevention programs; inadequate communicable disease surveillance and diagnostic capacity; lack of trained personnel (epidemiologists, laboratory scientists, vector and rodent control specialists)
Microbial adaptation and change	Changes in virulence and toxin production; development of drug resistance; microbes as cofactors in chronic diseases

[a] Adapted from reference 2.

homes. Recent examples of child care-related infectious disease threats include *Escherichia coli* O157:H7, shigellosis, giardiasis, cryptosporidiosis, hepatitis A virus, and rotavirus.[5]

RECOGNIZING THE PROBLEM

Emerging infections such as acquired immunodeficiency syndrome (AIDS), Lyme disease, or hantavirus pulmonary syndrome and reemerging infections such as tuberculosis (TB) or cholera vividly illustrate that we remain highly vulnerable to the microorganisms with which we share our environ-

TABLE 2. Examples of Emerging Infectious Diseases, 1993

Inside United States
- *E. coli* O157:H7
- Cryptosporidiosis
- Coccidioidomycosis
- Multidrug-resistant pneumococcal disease
- Vancomycin-resistant enterococcal infections
- Influenza A/Beijing/32/39
- Hantavirus infections

Outside United States
- Cholera in Latin America
- Yellow fever in Kenya
- *Vibrio cholerae* O139 in Asia
- *E. coli* O157:H7 in South Africa and Swaziland
- Rift Valley fever in Egypt
- Multidrug-resistant *Shigella dysenteriae* in Burundi
- Dengue in Costa Rica and Panama
- Diphtheria in Russia

ment. Although many serious infectious diseases are preventable, current approaches to health care make effective control difficult.

Timely recognition of emerging infections requires early warning systems to detect new threats to health before they develop into public health crises. Prompt detection of these new threats depends on careful monitoring by modern surveillance systems and a thorough understanding of trends in incidence and distribution of known infectious agents. Better domestic and international surveillance systems to monitor these trends and detect emerging and reemerging infectious diseases are needed.

Surveillance of selected infectious diseases in the United States is based on state laws and regulations that require reporting of these diseases to health departments, generally by physicians or laboratories, to direct prevention and control programs. This notifiable disease system depends heavily upon voluntary collaboration between the Centers for Disease Control and Prevention (CDC) and state and local health departments, as well as those who report cases. However, reporting is generally incomplete, in part because of inadequate resources. Results from a recent survey by the Council of State and Territorial Epidemiologists (CSTE) further illustrate the inadequacy of existing infectious disease surveillance by documenting the limited number of professional positions dedicated to infectious disease surveillance in most states. For example, in 12 of the 50 states surveyed, no professional position is dedicated to surveillance of food-borne and water-borne diseases.[6] Also, no federal resources are provided to state and local health departments to support the national notifiable disease system in contrast to categorical disease programs such as those targeting AIDS, TB, certain cancers, and lead poisoning. In addition, the ability of state public health laboratories to support surveillance and control of infectious diseases has diminished, and health department services, such as insect vector and rodent control programs, have been dismantled in many states.

As highlighted in three recent reports by committees of medical and public health experts convened by the National Academy of Science's Institute of Medicine (IOM), the ability of the U.S. public health system and our health professionals to deal with emerging infectious disease problems is in jeopardy.[2,7,8] The earliest of these reports, published in 1987, "The U.S. Capacity to Address Tropical Infectious Disease Problems,"[7] documented our poor state of readiness to recognize, treat, or control infectious disease threats emanating from the tropics—regions which have yielded microbial threats such as cholera, Lassa fever, chloroquine-resistant malaria, and penicillin-resistant gonorrhea. The second report, "The Future of Public Health," published in 1988, concluded that the U.S. public health system is in disarray and emphasized that the U.S. approach to public health has too often been crisis-driven or reactive, a costly approach that limits the application of cost-saving preventive strategies.[8] The third IOM report, "Emerging Infections, Microbial Threats to Health in the United States," published in 1992, highlighted the ongoing threat to domestic and global health from emerging infectious diseases.[2]

TABLE 3. *Addressing Emerging Disease Threats: A Prevention Strategy for the United States,* Summary of Goals

Goal I	**Surveillance**
	Detect, promptly investigate, and monitor emerging pathogens, the diseases they cause, and the factors influencing their emergence.
Goal II	**Applied Research**
	Integrate laboratory science and epidemiology to optimize public health practice.
Goal III	**Prevention and Control**
	Enhance communication of public health information about emerging diseases and ensure prompt implementation of prevention strategies.
Goal IV	**Infrastructure**
	Strengthen local, state, and federal public health infrastructure to support surveillance and implement prevention and control programs.

In collaboration with other federal agencies, state and local health departments, international organizations, academic institutions, and professional societies, CDC has developed a prevention strategy containing four goals that emphasize a multidisciplinary approach to the recognition and prevention of emerging infections (TABLE 3).[b]

The following discussion focuses on Goal I of this strategy and will highlight five important elements of improved surveillance for emerging infections: 1) strengthening the national notifiable disease system, 2) establishing sentinel surveillance networks, 3) establishing population-based emerging infections epidemiology and prevention centers, 4) developing a system for enhanced global surveillance, and 5) applying new tools and novel approaches to surveillance.

APPROACHING THE PROBLEM—IMPROVED SURVEILLANCE

To provide the vigilance and rapid response capability required to better detect, contain, and prevent emerging infectious diseases, improved surveillance systems must be developed. Surveillance serves several purposes: it permits disease patterns to be characterized by time, place, and person; detects epidemics; suggests hypotheses for epidemiologic investigation; evaluates prevention and control programs; projects future health care needs; and helps lower health care expenditures by facilitating earlier implementation of intervention strategies.[9,10] A well-functioning surveillance system is the most effective way to maintain vigilance for and ensure timely response to emerging infectious diseases. Because the ability to detect what is new or emerging depends on the capacity to know and track the routine, surveillance with appropriate laboratory support can function as an early warning system for emerging infections.

[b] The CDC plan is entitled *"Addressing Emerging Infectious Disease Threats: A Prevention Strategy for the United States."* Copies may be obtained by writing to the National Center for Infectious Diseases, office of Program Resources-EP, Mailstop C-14, Centers for Disease Control and Prevention, Atlanta, GA 30333.

Many elements are required for effective surveillance. Information originates with someone in a hospital, laboratory, or clinic who detects a case, records it, and transmits the data needed for public health action to a local or state health department. Data from laboratories, hospital clinical records, or sources of vital statistics are often insufficient, and direct communication with patients or their health care providers may be required. At its origin, surveillance of infectious diseases must be thorough, and data must be recorded accurately and transmitted promptly. At each level of data collection, the quality of the information must be evaluated, and information from many sources must be combined and transmitted to the next level.

Data received through surveillance must be analyzed correctly, synthesized clearly, and disseminated effectively. The timeliness of this process is crucial to its efficacy. Each link in the surveillance chain must function well for the system to work. Most importantly, information gained through surveillance must lead to action by the public health system that includes investigating outbreaks, designing and implementing interventions, and evaluating the effectiveness of new or existing interventions. To accomplish effective infectious disease surveillance, the United States needs a national system that integrates laboratory and epidemiologic data. With effective surveillance, early identification of emerging infectious disease threats is more likely because problems can be recognized at any of several levels—at local or state health departments or at CDC, where national surveillance data are compiled and analyzed.

Modern society presents numerous challenges to surveillance. For example, assessing the health of under-served or transient populations, such as migrant workers, the homeless, or inner-city minorities, is difficult, but is extremely important because such populations are often most vulnerable to emerging infectious diseases. By targeting vulnerable populations for surveillance, opportunities for improved health care delivery and earlier recognition and containment of emerging infectious disease threats are enhanced. Likewise, infectious diseases that emerge abroad and threaten other nations through travel, immigration, and commerce challenge existing surveillance capabilities.

Strengthening National Notifiable Diseases Surveillance

The nation's notifiable disease surveillance system forms the foundation for our ability to know and track the routine. Certain infectious diseases—such as multidrug-resistant (MDR) TB, meningococcal meningitis, and botulism—warrant prompt detection of all cases because they cause substantial morbidity and mortality, require specific public health interventions, or may signal a potential outbreak. State public health authorities, other infectious disease experts, and CDC should reexamine currently reportable diseases, establish criteria for making a disease reportable, and explore ways to enhance rapid reporting of cases from clinical laboratories and health care practitioners. States must also examine the need to develop statutory requirements that clinical laboratories submit isolates of designated organisms of public health importance to the state laboratory. National infectious diseases surveillance must be flexible enough to include newer problems, such as *E. coli* O157:H7-associated hemolytic uremic syndrome (HUS), hantavirus pulmonary syndrome, or multidrug resistance in common pathogens (*e.g.*, pneumococcus, *M. tuberculosis*).

Enhanced surveillance for important food-borne and water-borne diseases, for example, is needed, including the addition of important emerging infections such as *E. coli* O157:H7 to the national notifiable disease system. Infectious agents continue to contaminate food sources and food-borne outbreaks of emerging infections are no longer isolated events involving only limited numbers of people. Evidence for these trends includes recent outbreaks of salmonellosis associated with the consumption of dairy products (domestic cheese, eggs); shigellosis associated with commercial airline food; and contamination of powdered milk products and infant formula with *Salmonella*.[11-17] In addition, in early 1993, hamburgers contaminated with *E. coli* O157:H7 and served at a fast-food restaurant chain caused a multistate outbreak of severe hemorrhagic colitis and hemolytic uremic syndrome, resulting in the deaths of at least four children.[18,19]

Water-borne outbreaks due to emerging pathogens may also be on the rise. In the spring of 1993, a municipal water supply contaminated with the intestinal parasite *Cryptosporidium* caused the largest recognized outbreak of water-borne illness in the history of the United States. An estimated 403,000 persons in Milwaukee, Wisconsin, developed prolonged diarrhea, and approximately 4,400 required hospitalization. (Personal communication: Jeffrey P. Davis, M.D., Communicable Disease Epidemiologist, Wisconsin, December 1993.)

In most areas of the United States, existing surveillance systems are inadequate to rapidly recognize outbreaks such as those caused by *E. coli* O157:H7 and *Cryptosporidium*. It is likely that improved surveillance and early recognition of these problems would prevent significant numbers of new infections through rapid investigation and institution of appropriate preventive interventions such as recalling hamburger contaminated with *E. coli* O157:H7 and issuing boil water advisories to interrupt transmission of *Cryptosporidium*. In addition, accurate disease surveillance can measure the effectiveness of regulations to ensure safe food and water.

National surveillance requires adequate infrastructure, including well-trained personnel within state health departments and local communities in addition to efficient and secure communications among CDC, state and local health departments, public and private laboratories, and health care providers. To establish a system that can effectively meet the threat of emerging infectious diseases, ties between these groups must be strengthened.

Establishing Sentinel Surveillance Networks

The use of sentinel events to enhance surveillance is an effective public health tool that has proven useful in the monitoring of many diseases. Sentinel networks, linking groups of participating individuals or organizations to a central data receiving and processing center, have been particularly helpful in monitoring specific infections or designated classes of infections. Examples of such networks currently in use at CDC are the National Nosocomial Infection Surveillance (NNIS) system,[20] the National Respiratory and Enteric Virus Surveillance System (NREVSS), the Pediatric and Adult/Adolescent Spectrum of Human Immunodeficiency Virus (HIV) Disease Projects, and the domestic influenza surveillance network.

Expanded use of the sentinel network concept will improve our ability to detect and monitor emerging infections. With the cooperation of state and local health departments, CDC has proposed to establish a series of electronically linked Sentinel Surveillance Networks, organized according to information source, that will use novel and traditional data sources to compile information important to the assessment of emerging infections (TABLE 4).

Clinician or laboratory-based networks provide a mechanism for rapid interaction/consultation among members when unusual syndromes (*e.g.*, unexplained adult respiratory distress syndrome, idiopathic CD4 lymphocytopenia, or eosinophilia-myalgia syndrome) or laboratory isolates are detected. Networks of selected physicians' groups may also provide early warning of newly emerging syndromes of uncertain but probable infectious origin such as febrile diarrheal illnesses, meningitis and encephalitis, or hemorrhagic fevers. Such networks may also allow a more effective means for monitoring occupationally acquired infections in hospital and laboratory personnel. Other networks could focus on the emergence of drug-resistant pathogens (*e.g.*, clinical microbiology laboratories). Special consideration should also be given to the formation of veterinary networks to monitor established zoonotic diseases (*e.g.*, brucellosis, salmonellosis, cryptosporidiosis) or the increasing incidence of animal infections with zoonotic potential (*e.g.*, bovine tuberculosis, bovine spongiform encephalopathy).

Establishing Population-based Emerging Infections Programs

To complement and support local, regional, and national surveillance and research efforts, CDC has recently proposed that a network of population-

TABLE 4. Examples of Potential Participants in Sentinel Surveillance Networks

- Blood Banks
- Clinical Microbiology Laboratories
- Emergency Rooms
- Family Practitioners
- Gynecologists
- Infectious Disease Specialists
- Internists
- Medical Examiners
- Pediatricians
- Travel and Tropical Medicine Clinics

based Emerging Infections Programs be established. The proposed programs will be developed through cooperative agreements with health departments and will be strategically located in sites across the country that offer access to various population groups. CDC will work with state and local health departments to establish these programs, building upon existing capacities and partnerships whenever possible. In turn, state health departments may choose to work with local academic institutions and other governmental or private-sector organizations to carry out program projects. The programs' purpose will be to forge strong links with local medical and public health personnel, and community representatives in order to establish continuous sources for population-based data as a foundation for conducting a variety of surveillance, epidemiologic, and prevention research projects relevant to emerging infections. These programs will also provide excellent opportunities for training public health professionals through cooperative arrangements between health departments, academic centers, and joint CDC/National Institutes of Health (NIH) training programs in infectious disease epidemiology.

In addition to providing population-based information, these programs will interact with special populations including the rural and inner-city poor; under-served women and children; the homeless; and immigrant or refugee groups. Other special population groups may also benefit from the proposed programs' activities. For example, an increasing percentage of our population is elderly or immunosuppressed, and a growing number of persons are immunosuppressed because of HIV infection, organ transplantation, or cancer chemotherapy. These population groups are at increased risk for emerging and drug-resistant infections, and their medical management is complex and costly. Specifically, these groups are highly susceptible to opportunistic infections, and an ever-expanding array of such infections is being seen in patients with AIDS and other forms of immunosuppression.[21]

Although their presence may facilitate the reporting of new infections or rare syndromes recognized by health professionals in the area, these programs are not expected to significantly improve our ability to actually detect previously unknown or unrecognized infectious diseases. Rather, they are designed to assess the public health impact of emerging infections and to evaluate methods for their prevention and control.

These population-based programs will provide a powerful tool for integrating information from many different places and sources, and about different emerging diseases. At the same time, national trends can be evaluated by combining information from the same project conducted at several programs across the country. Programs will maintain the necessary flexibility to accommodate changes in specific projects as the need for information changes. Some projects will be conducted at all programs, while others might be carried out in only a few (TABLE 5).

Priority activities will include:

1) Conducting active population-based surveillance projects to obtain detailed information about selected diseases for which adequate infor-

TABLE 5. Potential Projects and Locations for Emerging Infections Programs in the United States

POTENTIAL PROGRAM LOCATIONS	Food-borne Disease Surveillance and Prevention (*e.g.*, *E. coli* O15:H7)	Opportunistic Infections in HIV-infected Inner City Populations (*e.g.*, MDR TB)	Drug Resistance in Nursing Homes and Child Care Facilities (*e.g.*, MDR Pneumococcal Disease)	Febrile and Diarrheal Illness in Migrant Farm Workers (*e.g.*, Malaria, Typhoid)	Unexplained Deaths of Possible Infectious Etiology in Young Adults (*e.g.*, ARDS)	Etiologic Agents in Community-Acquired Pneumonia (*e.g.*, *Mycoplasma*)
Northeast	X	X			X	
Mid-Atlantic	X	X			X	X
Southeast	X	X	X		X	
South	X	X		X	X	X
Midwest	X		X	X	X	
Southwest	X		X		X	X
West	X	X	X	X	X	
Northwest	X		X	X	X	X
U.S. Pacific Isles	X				X	X
U.S. Caribbean Isles	X	X			X	X

mation is currently unavailable, such as multidrug-resistant pneumococci and various food-borne infectious diseases.

2) Conducting special projects such as evaluating new diagnostic tests for Lyme disease; assessing illnesses that are often not specifically diagnosed but whose trends and etiologic information are important (*e.g.*, diarrhea, community-acquired pneumonia); and investigating the relationships between infections and chronic diseases (*e.g.*, hantavirus infections and hypertensive end-stage renal disease, hepatitis C and chronic liver disease).[22,23]

3) Conducting behavioral surveillance projects designed to assess trends in behaviors that either increase or decrease risk for infectious disease (*e.g.*, trends in food preparation and consumption practices, sexual behavior, travel, or exposure to animals).

4) Examining infectious diseases in the context of populations at risk, recognizing that the incidence of many emerging diseases will be highest among under-served populations and the immunosuppressed.

5) Implementing and evaluating pilot prevention and intervention projects for emerging infectious diseases that focus on safe food preparation in the home, handwashing in child care settings, appropriate use of antibiotics in clinical settings and in the community, and personal protection devices for clinical and laboratory personnel potentially exposed to infectious agents.

6) Providing technical assistance; epidemiologic, behavioral science, and laboratory expertise; and training to other agencies, institutions, or organizations in a Program's area when needed, such as during the investigation of outbreaks.

Developing Enhanced Global Surveillance for Emerging Infections

Although infectious disease threats often emerge in regions remote from the United States, they are readily transported here.[24–32] However, practical mechanisms for the early detection of such threats, such as international infectious disease surveillance systems, are rudimentary. Cholera provides an excellent example of the need for sound international surveillance capability. Cholera has recently returned to the Western Hemisphere in epidemic proportions after almost a century's absence (FIG. 1). Through October 1993, at least 900,000 cases of infection were detected and over 8,000 persons died. Although cholera initially reemerged in Peru, the disease has occurred throughout Latin America, and cases have been imported into the United States where more cases occurred in 1992 than in any other year since national cholera surveillance began in 1962.[15,25] Moreover, the *Vibrio cholerae* O1 strain responsible for cholera in Central and South America has been isolated from oysters and oyster-eating fish captured in oyster beds along U.S. Gulf Coast waters.[26]

More recently (1993), a newly described toxigenic strain of *Vibrio cholerae*, *V. cholerae* O139, has emerged in southern Asia where it is causing epidemic

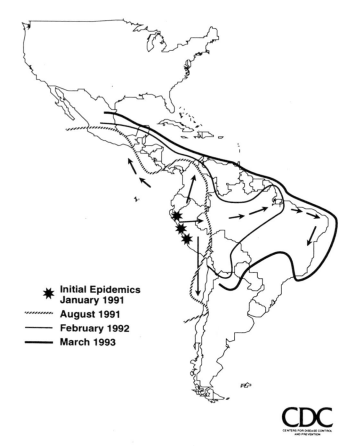

FIGURE 1. Spread of epidemic cholera—Latin America, 1991–1993.

cholera-like illness and has largely replaced *V. cholerae* O1 strains in many areas. Standard diagnostic tests for cholera are inadequate for this new strain, and neither currently formulated vaccines nor prior infection with *V. cholerae* O1 is protective. This new form of cholera is spreading, and an imported case has already occurred in a U.S. traveler returning from India.[27]

Effective approaches to surveillance on an international scale should include early detection capability and the capacity—national, regional, or international—to generate public health responses.[32] However, public health infrastructure and infectious disease expertise vary widely from country to country. Even in industrialized nations, a more timely and effective information exchange about emerging infectious disease problems is clearly needed.[33,34] For many developing countries, where this task will be the most difficult, established infrastructures, such as those in place for polio and

Guinea worm eradication efforts, and existing resources, such as those available from ministries of health, the World Health Organization (WHO), Institut Pasteur, the International Clinical Epidemiology Network (IN-CLEN), the U.S. Agency for International Development (USAID), the U.S. Department of Defense (DOD), NIH and CDC regional facilities or field stations, universities, and many other nongovernmental organizations, may be useful in efforts to improve international cooperation in detecting and evaluating emerging infectious disease threats.

Through enhancement and linkage of existing centers and networks, CDC has proposed that a global consortium of epidemiology and biomedical research centers be established to promote the detection, monitoring, and investigation of emerging infections. These centers would emphasize the integration of epidemiology and laboratory science. The consortium would be established in close cooperation with local ministries of health and operate under the direction of an international steering committee with representatives from CDC and other appropriate federal and international agencies or organizations. A central office for coordinating operations of the consortium, possibly at WHO, will be established. Initial steps would include review of the current and potential capabilities of various existing research facilities and surveillance systems, such as the WHO-sponsored arbovirus and hemorrhagic fever surveillance networks. Areas of expertise that are critical to meeting consortium goals of improved detection, monitoring, and investigation of emerging infections include epidemiology, clinical medicine (accompanied by ready access to patients and appropriate health care facilities), and laboratory sciences, particularly diagnostic microbiology. Expertise in related disciplines such as field ecology (*e.g.*, mammalogy, entomology) and behavioral sciences will also be important. To minimize startup costs and avoid lengthy delays, the highest priority for initial inclusion in the consortium would be given to facilities that currently maintain expertise in several of these disciplines (see TABLE 6).

The consortium members would assist their host countries by providing training and support to local and regional scientists and public health officials, aiding outbreak investigations in the region, and assisting with the formulation of public health policies. Laboratory and epidemiology back-up would be available from CDC and other collaborating organizations.

Applying New Tools and Novel Approaches to Surveillance

Infectious disease surveillance—both U.S. and global—should utilize modern computing and communications technologies to transform data into usable information quickly and effectively. Accurate, efficient data transfer with rapid notification of key partners and constituents is critical to effectively addressing emerging infectious disease threats. The systematic evaluation of new and innovative tools for the collection and analysis of epidemiologic data will enhance the speed with which technological, mathematical, and statistical advances are brought into use in efforts to better understand emerg-

TABLE 6. Examples of Potential Members of a Global Consortium of
Epidemiology/Biomedical Research Programs/Centers

Existing Networks
  • CDC Field Epidemiology Training Programs (FETPs)
  • PAHO Polio Eradication Surveillance System
  • International Clinical Epidemiology Network (INCLEN)
  • International Office of Epizootics (OIE) Worldwide Information System
  • WHO Arbovirus and Hemorrhagic Fever Collaborating Centers
  • WHO Global Influenza Surveillance Network
Existing Research Facilities
  • Caribbean Epidemiology Centre (CAREC), Trinidad
  • CDC, National Center for Infectious Diseases Field Stations
  •   (Cote d'Ivoire, Guatemala, Puerto Rico, Kenya, Sierra Leone, Thailand)
  • Department of Defense, U.S. Army and Naval Medical Facilities
  •   (Brazil, Egypt, Indonesia, Kenya, Peru, Philippines, Thailand)
  • Food and Agriculture Organization of the United Nations (FAO) Reference Centers
       (Argentina, Brazil, Colombia, Czech Republic, France, Germany, Hungary, Kenya,
       Panama, Senegal, Spain, Sri Lanka, Thailand, UK, Uruguay, USA)
  • French Scientific Research Institute (ORSTOM) (*e.g.,* Central African Republic,
       Congo, Cote d'Ivoire, Guinea, Senegal)
  • Instituto de Nutricion para Centro America y Panama (INCAP), Guatemala
  • International Center for Diarrheal Disease Research, Bangladesh (ICDDR,B)
  • NIH, National Institute of Allergy and Infectious Diseases Supported Projects
       (Brazil, Colombia, Israel, Mali, Mexico, Philippines, Sudan, Uganda, Venezuela,
       Zimbabwe)
  • Pasteur Institutes
       (*e.g.,* Algeria, Central African Republic, French Guiana, Iran, Madagascar, Morocco,
       New Caledonia, Senegal, Vietnam)

ing infections. Included in this process will be the appropriate evaluation and
utilization of:

1) **Secure networks for the transmission of sensitive information.**
   Such networks are essential components of effective surveillance systems and should be designed to interface easily with national and
   international communications infrastructures for information dissemination and networking (*e.g.,* BITNET, INTERNET) being developed
   through the proposed High Performance Computing and High Speed
   Networking Applications Act of 1993.
2) **Automatic and direct reporting from physicians' offices, hospitals,
   and private and public laboratories.**
   Comprehensive health insurance and universal access to health care
   will facilitate this process and improve surveillance. Reporting would
   be received by state health departments as soon as cases are suspected
   or identified.
3) **Computer-based patient record technology.**
   Participation by public health professionals in the development of this
   capability is important to ensure that these systems are compatible
   with automated public health surveillance systems while maintaining
   patient confidentiality.

4) **Plans to integrate existing and planned information systems.**
INTERNET can provide the physical framework for improved information exchange and the establishment of "information superhighways" for public health. Existing national surveillance systems should be modified to use common standards and protocols, ensuring that data are stored in compatible formats and retrievable via easy-to-use interfaces.

5) **Geographic information systems (GISs) and satellite imagery.**
GISs allow geographically oriented information about disease distribution to be visually and analytically linked to images of the environment. These images and data can include satellite-generated images, housing or other location data obtained from hand-held Global Positioning Systems (accurate to less than a meter), digitized street maps, and census data. This technology may be particularly useful in monitoring environmental changes that could affect the emergence of infectious diseases.[35,36]

6) **New statistical and mathematical modeling methods.**
New methodology for analyzing time-space clustering, GIS data, and data from longitudinal studies needs critical assessment for potential applications to the problems of emerging infections. Newer mathematical models can be used in both hypothesis-generating and confirmatory analyses, and may provide excellent opportunities for anticipating or forecasting changes in the incidence or distribution of important emerging or reemerging infectious diseases such as rabies.[37]

CONCLUSION

This article has emphasized the surveillance elements in CDC's plan, *Addressing Emerging Infectious Disease Threats: A Prevention Strategy for the United States* (TABLE 3). With this plan as a guide, implementation of these approaches to surveillance, based on public health priorities and resource availability, should provide a solid foundation for broader efforts to prevent emerging infectious diseases in this country.[38]

SUMMARY

Emerging infectious diseases such as prolonged diarrheal illness due to water-borne *Cryptosporidium*, hemorrhagic colitis and renal failure from food-borne *E. coli* O157:H7, and rodent-borne hantavirus pulmonary syndrome as well as reemerging infections such as tuberculosis, pertussis, and cholera vividly illustrate that we remain highly vulnerable to the microorganisms with which we share our environment. Prompt detection of new and resurgent infectious disease threats depends on careful monitoring by modern surveillance systems. This article focuses on five important elements of improved surveillance for emerging infections: 1) strengthening the national notifiable disease system, 2) establishing sentinel surveillance networks, 3) establishing population-based emerging infections programs, 4) developing a system for enhanced global surveillance, and 5) applying new tools and novel approaches to surveillance.

ACKNOWLEDGMENTS

Several sections of this paper represent the collaborative efforts of many individuals. The authors wish to express gratitude to those persons from CDC and elsewhere who contributed to, and critically reviewed, this paper. We are particularly indebted to Judith R. Aguilar, Robert P. Gaynes, Allen W. Hightower, James M. Hughes, and C. J. Peters for their invaluable input.

REFERENCES

1. WHO. 1992. Global Health Situations and Projections, Estimates 1992. Geneva.
2. INSTITUTE OF MEDICINE. 1992. Emerging Infections: Microbial Threats to Health in the United States. National Academy Press, Washington, D.C.
3. DAVIS, J. P., P. J. CHESNEY, P. J. WAND, et al. 1980. Toxic-shock syndrome: Epidemiologic features, recurrence, risk factors, and prevention. N. Engl. J. Med. **303**: 1429–1435.
4. CDC. 1993. Lyme disease—United States, 1991–1992. MMWR **42**: 345–348.
5. THACKER, S. B., D. G. ADDISS, R. A. GOODMAN, B. R. HOLLOWAY & H. C. SPENCER. 1992. Infectious diseases and injuries in child day care: Opportunities for healthier children. JAMA **268**: 1720–1726.
6. OSTERHOLM, M. 1993. Council of State and Territorial Epidemiologists Survey on Surveillance. Personal Communication. Minnesota Department of Health.
7. INSTITUTE OF MEDICINE. 1987. The U.S. Capacity to Address Tropical Infectious Disease Problems. National Academy Press. Washington, D.C.
8. INSTITUTE OF MEDICINE. 1988. The Future of Public Health. National Academy Press. Washington, D.C.
9. HENDERSON, D. A. 1976b. Surveillance of smallpox. Intl. J. Epidemiol. **5**: 19–28.
10. BERKELMAN, R. L. & J. W. BUEHLER. 1991. Surveillance. In Holland N. H., R. Detels, G. Knox, Eds. Oxford Textbook of Public Health, 2nd edit., Vol. 2: Methods of Public Health. New York: Oxford University Press. p. 161.
11. WOOD, C. W., K. L. MacDONALD & M. T. OSTERHOLM. 1992. Campylobacter enteritis outbreaks associated with drinking raw milk during youth activities: A 10-year review of outbreaks in the United States. JAMA **268**: 3228–3230.
12. HEDBERG, C. W., J. A. KORLATH, J. Y. D'AOUST, et al. 1992. A multistate outbreak of Salmonella javiana and Salmonella oranienburg infections due to consumption of contaminated cheese. JAMA **268**: 3203–3207.
13. HEDBERG, C. W., M. J. DAVID, K. E. WHITE, et al. 1993. Role of egg consumption in sporadic Salmonella enteritidis and Salmonella typhimurium infections in Minnesota. J. Infect. Dis. **167**: 107–111.
14. HEDBERG, C. W., W. S. LEVINE, K. E. WHITE, et al. 1992. An international foodborne outbreak of shigellosis associated with a commercial airline. JAMA **268**: 3208–3212.
15. CDC. 1992. Cholera associated with an international airline flight. MMWR **41**: 134–135.
16. DuPONT, H. L. 1992. How safe is the food we eat? (Editorial). JAMA **268**: 3240.
17. CDC. Salmonella serotype Tennessee in powdered milk products and infant formula—Canada and the United States, 1993. MMWR **42**(26): 516–517.
18. CDC. Preliminary report. 1993. Foodborne outbreak of Escherichia coli O157:H7 infections from hamburgers—western United States. MMWR **42**(4): 85–86.

19. CDC. Update. 1992–1993. Multistate outbreak of *Escherichia coli* O157:H7 infections from hamburgers—western United States. MMWR **42**(14): 258–263.
20. GAYNES, R. P., S. BANERJEE, G. EMORI, *et al.* 1991. The Nosocomial Infections Surveillance (NNIS) System: Plans for the 1990s and beyond. Am. J. Med. 116S–120S.
21. GRADON, J. D., J. G. TIMPONE & S. M. SCHNITTMAN. 1992. Emergence of unusual opportunistic pathogens in AIDS: A review. Clin. Infect. Dis. **15**: 134–157.
22. ALTER, M. J., H. S. MARGOLIS, K. KRAWCZYNSKI, *et al.* 1992. The natural history of community-acquired hepatitis C in the United States. N. Engl. J. Med. **321**: 1899–1905.
23. GLASS, G. E., A. J. WATSON, J. W. LEDUC, *et al.* 1993. Infection with a ratborne hantavirus in U.S. residents is consistently associated with hypertensive renal disease. J. Infect. Dis. **167**: 614–620.
24. LEDERBERG, J. 1988. Medical science, infectious disease, and the unity of humankind. JAMA **260**: 684–685.
25. CDC. 1992. Update: Cholera—western hemisphere. MMWR **42**(5): 89–91.
26. CDC. 1993. Isolation of *Vibrio cholerae* O1 from oysters—Mobile Bay, 1991–1992. MMWR **42**(5): 91–93.
27. CDC. 1993. Imported cholera associated with a newly described toxigenic *Vibrio cholerae* O139 strain—California, 1993. MMWR **42**(26): 501–503.
28. MALDONADO, Y. A., B. L. NAHLEN, R. R. ROBERTO, *et al.* 1990. Transmission of *Plasmodium vivax* malaria in San Diego County, California, 1986. Am. J. Trop. Med. Hyg. **42**: 3–9.
29. CDC. 1993. Malaria in Montagnard refugees—North Carolina, 1992. MMWR **42**: 180–183.
30. GELLERT, G. A., A. K. NEUMANN & R. S. GORDON. 1989. The obsolescence of distinct domestic and international health sectors. J. Pub. Health Pol. **10**: 421–424.
31. HENDERSON, D. A. 1992. Strategies for the twenty-first century, control or eradication? In: Walker D., Ed. Global Infectious Diseases: Prevention, Control, and Eradication. Springer-Verlag. 227–234. Vienna.
32. HENDERSON, D. A. 1993. Surveillance systems and intergovernmental cooperation. *In* Emerging Viruses. S. S. Morse, Ed.: 283–289. New York: Oxford University Press.
33. BARTLETT, C. & N. GILL. 1993. International surveillance of disease. Communicable disease control after Maastricht: Germs and solidarity. Lancet **341**: 997–998.
34. DESENCLOS, J. C., H. BIJKERK & J. HUISMAN. 1993. Variations in national infectious diseases surveillance in Europe. Lancet **341**: 1003–1006.
35. ROGERS, D. J. & B. G. WILLIAMS. 1993. Monitoring trypanosomiasis in space and time. Parasitology 106:S77–S99.
36. EPSTEIN, P. R., D. J. ROGERS & R. SLOOF. 1993. Satellite imaging and vector-borne disease. Lancet **341**: 1404–1406.
37. COYNE, M. J., G. SMITH & F. E. McALLISTER. 1989. Mathematic model for the population biology of rabies in the mid-Atlantic states. Am. J. Vet. Res. **50**: 2148–2154.
38. BERKELMAN, R. L., R. T. BRYAN, M. T. OSTERHOLM, J. W. LEDUC & J. M. HUGHES. 1994. Infectious disease surveillance: A crumbling foundation. Science **264**: 368–370.

Pneumonia in the United States

Shifting Perceptions of Causality

MARY E. WILSON

Mount Auburn Hospital
330 Mount Auburn Street
Cambridge, Massachusetts 02238
and
Department of Population and International Health
Harvard School of Public Health
665 Huntington Avenue
Boston, Massachusetts 02115

The clinical syndrome of pneumonia in the United States over the past few decades illustrates the myriad events that have changed what microbes are associated with the disease and our perceptions of cause. In midcentury most pneumonias were thought to be caused by several bacteria, with the pneumococcus being most frequent, and viruses, usually unidentified.

Over the past four decades, we have come to recognize a growing number of specific viral and non-viral pathogens, as well as chemical agents, that cause pneumonia in humans. In 1961 Chanock et al.[1] used immunofluorescence to demonstrate that an agent, previously known as the Eaton agent, was found in the majority of non-bacterial pneumonias in military recruits. The following year the organism was successfully grown on agar and identified as a mycoplasma (*Mycoplasma pneumoniae*). This organism is now recognized as a common cause of pneumonia, especially in young adults. Progress in scientific technology allowed identification of an agent that helped to explain what was observed epidemiologically.

An outbreak of pneumonia at a hotel in Philadelphia, the site of the 1976 American Legion convention, precipitated intense investigation. A total of 221 persons developed pneumonia and 34 died. Not until many months later was a bacterium recovered from autopsy lung specimens. The bacterium, later named *Legionella pneumophila*, had never previously been known to cause human disease.[2] Studies since have shown that legionella was not new. It was implicated retrospectively in an epidemic that led to 15 deaths in 1965 in a psychiatric hospital in Washington, D.C. (stored serum was tested.) The organism had not been identified earlier because it does not grow on the usual culture media used in microbiology laboratories and is not visible when sputum is examined with Gram's stain, a commonly performed test for bacteria. Since the Philadelphia outbreak, good diagnostic tests have been developed to allow recognition of this pathogen, a widely distributed organism in the

362

environment and an important cause of community-acquired and nosocomial pneumonia. In this example, an intense focus of resources on a highly
visible population led to studies that went beyond conventional techniques
to identify an organism that had gone unnoticed. Water handling systems,
air conditioners and water cooling tanks, which allow dispersal of the
organisms, and a growing population of immunocompromised patients at
heightened risk may contribute to an increase in the number of infections
in recent decades.

Chlamydia pneumoniae (or TWAR, after the first two isolates TW-183
and AR-39) was recognized as a major cause of pneumonia after several
outbreaks of pneumonia swept northern Europe in the 1980s.[3] Now
recognized to have a worldwide distribution and to infect persons of all
ages, this organism explains yet more of the cases of pneumonia that in
past years probably would have been attributed to an unknown virus.
Epidemiologic events prompted intensified investigation; scientific expertise
that derived from work done on trachoma and genital chlamydiae helped
inform research in this area.

In the early 1980s, *Pneumocystis carinii*, a fungal organism long known
to cause severe pneumonia in leukemic patients and other compromised
hosts, was found in a number of young men who did not have any of
the known risk factors for pneumocystis pneumonia. Over the next few
years thousands of cases occurred, later found to be associated with the
immune suppression caused by the human immunodeficiency virus. Clinical
features of the infection in these patients differed in important respects
from disease described as typical in the textbooks. The appearance of a
rapidly growing and uniquely vulnerable population redefined the frequency
and expected manifestations of this infection.

In 1989 a number of patients sought medical care for an illness that
frequently included cough and shortness of breath along with fevers,
myalgias, and arthralgias. Prominent eosinophilia was found on laboratory testing. About 90% had pulmonary infiltrates on chest x-rays. In
some patients the disease was progressive and fatal. By mid-1990 more
than 1500 cases and 27 deaths had been identified. The disorder was
called eosinophilia-myalgia syndrome (EMS) after its distinctive clinical
features. Early epidemiologic studies associated EMS with the ingestion
of L-tryptophan, typically taken as a nutritional supplement to treat insomnia
and depression. Moreover, epidemiologic studies linked disease to exposure
to L-tryptophan made by a single manufacturer. Spectral and chemical
analyses of the suspect tryptophan demonstrated distinctive findings,
suggesting the presence of contaminants in certain lots of tryptophan that
could trigger the disorder.[4] Of note is the structural similarity between
one of the contaminants, 3-(phenylamino)alanine, and the 3-(phenylamino)
1,2-propanediol impurity found the rapeseed oil implicated in causing a
similar syndrome in Spain several years also.[5] EMS, with symptoms that
suggested a possible infectious disease, was associated with a chemical
contaminant ingested in a drug available without prescription in the
United States. Epidemiologic studies implicated L-tryptophan; sophisti-

cated chemical techniques were necessary to identify potential chemical causes.

In June 1993 a cluster of cases of pulmonary disease with rapid progression and high mortality occurred in the southwestern United States. A virus not previously associated with pulmonary disease in the United States was found and identified as a hantavirus, one of a group of viruses known to cause a disease in Asia and Europe, commonly described as hemorrhagic fever and renal syndrome.[6] Although the hantavirus-associated disease in the United States was initially thought to be restricted to one geographic focus, now that diagnostic tools have been developed, disease has been identified in at least 16 states. Several events may have contributed to the initial cluster of cases and its recognition: climatic events that supported an expanded rodent population, heightened awareness in an area anticipating cases of plague, and deaths in previously robust young persons. (This outbreak is discussed in detail in the paper by S. Morse in this volume.) The wide range of symptoms caused by agents in the same virus group shows that similar organisms do not necessarily cause similar diseases, and that the relation between taxonomic and clinical distance is an area awaiting exploration.

The CDC and NIH have estimated that in the United States between 50,000 and 150,000 persons die each year from unexplained respiratory disease. How many other as yet unrecognized pathogens and perhaps environmental toxins are participating? The above examples reflect a sample of the kinds of events that are shaping apprehension of the pathogens found in one clinical syndrome and the way we identify them. They also show that the presence of potential pathogens in the environment may be insufficient to lead to human disease. Changes in the human host, amplification of the microbe because of shifts in climate, technology, behavior, or other events may allow disease to manifest. The recent upsurge in coccidioidomycosis shows the interaction of several, seemingly unrelated events, in contributing to an increase in reported cases (see insert).

The experience with pneumonia illustrates that there may be a hierarchy of diagnostic difficulty and resources needed for recognition and identification of organisms in the laboratory. Social, environmental, and technological events influence frequency of disease and timing of recognition. Climatic events may lead to expansion of frequency and of geographic distribution. Organisms readily seen and grown in clinical laboratories will usually be recognized, if they appear in populations with access to laboratory evaluation. However, the media and reagents in clinical laboratories are selected to identify that which we know can cause disease and expect to find. This means that we are unlikely to identify something we are not looking for unless it closely resembles something we know. Thus we may characterize drug-resistant forms of common bacteria but are less likely to pick up an unusual or different organism. The media and culture techniques used in microbiology laboratories support the growth of only a small fraction of microbes in our environment. The epidemiologic circumstances often provide the clues that push investigators to go beyond their usual testing.

COCCIDIOIDOMYCOSIS

The spores of the soil-associated fungus *Coccidioides immitis*, when airborne, can be inhaled by humans leading to pulmonary infection and, in some instances, dissemination to other organs. Its appearance in humans generally coincides with the geographic areas where soil and climatic conditions permit its survival in soil.[6] Weather patterns can influence its spread. For example, in 1977, high velocity winds in the southern extreme of the San Joaquin Valley in California carried aloft soil containing arthroconidia of the fungus and dispersed it over an area encompassing approximately 87,00 km^2, an area the size of the state of Maine. This resulted in epidemic infection outside of the usual endemic area.[7] In the early 1990s the number of cases reported in California increased dramatically (*e.g.*, from an annual average of 428 cases during 1981–1990 to more than 4000 cases annually in 1992 and 1993).[8] Factors identified as potentially associated with the marked increases included weather conditions (heavy rains following a prolonged drought), activities that disturb the soil and facilitate spread (*e.g.*, disruption of soil with the 1993 earthquake in southern California was followed by an increase in the cases of acute coccidioidomycosis in the affected region), and a growing population of vulnerable persons (*e.g.*, non-immunes moving into the area, increasing numbers of persons immuno-compromised by HIV, chemotherapy, and various diseases).

REFERENCES

1. CHANOCK, R. M., L. HAYFLICK & M. F. BARILE. 1962. Growth on artificial medium of an agent associated with atypical pneumonia and its identification as a PPLO. Proc. Natl. Acad. Sci. USA **48:** 41.
2. FRASER, D. W., T. TSAI, W. ORENSTEIN, *et al.* 1977. Legionnaires' disease: Description of an epidemic of pneumonia. New Engl. J. Med. **297:** 1183–1197.
3. GRAYSTON, J. T., C-C. KUO, S-P. WANG, *et al.* 1986. A new *Chlamydia psittaci* strain, TWAR, isolated in acute respiratory tract infections. New Engl. J. Med. **315:** 161–168.
4. PHILEN, R. M., R. H. HILL, W. F. FLANDERS, *et al.* 1993. Tryptophan contaminants associated with eosinophilia-myalgia syndrome. Am. J. Epidemiol. **138:** 154–159.
5. MAYENO, A. N., E. A. BELONGIA, F. LIN, S. K. LUNDY & G. J. GLEICH. 1992. 3-(Phenylamino)alanine, a novel aniline-derived amino acid associated with the eosinophilia-myalgia syndrome: A link to the toxic oil syndrome? Mayo Clin. Proc. **67:** 1134–1139.
6. WILSON, M. E. 1991. A World Guide to Infections: Diseases, Distribution, Diagnosis. New York: Oxford University Press.
7. FLYNN, N. M., P. D. HOEPRICH, M. M. KAWACHI, K. K. LEE, R. M. LAWRENCE, E. GOLDSTEIN, G. W. JORDAN, R. S. KUNDARGI & G. A. WONG. 1979. An unusual outbreak of windborne coccidioidomycosis. New Engl. J. Med. **301:** 358–361.
8. CDC. 1994. Update: Coccidioidomycosis—California, 1991–1993. Morbidity and Mortality Weekly Report **443:** 421–423.

Diagnosis of New and Resurgent Diseases

Contributions from Longitudinal Community Health Research

JOHN B. WYON[a]

Department of Population and International Health
Harvard School of Public Health
665 Huntington Avenue
Boston, Massachusetts 02115

INTRODUCTION

This paper introduces the principles of longitudinal community health research (LCHR) through a brief history of its origins. We then explore some LCHR projects to illustrate how it can help us approach new and resurgent diseases.

John Gordon, a bacteriologist, physician, and epidemiologist, had an experience in 1934 which set him on the path of Longitudinal Community Health Research (LCHR). He was then Director of Field Studies for The Rockefeller Foundation in Iesi, Romania. He was determined to document an epidemic of scarlet fever from the first to the last case; he therefore designed and conducted a long-term study of every child in the community of Iesi where he predicted a scarlet fever epidemic would arise. This involved visiting every child twice a week to swab their throats to detect the first, subsequent and last cases. The epidemic did come and he did document it.

During the second world war Gordon was Chief of Preventive Medicine for all U.S. forces in Europe, and later in East Asia. The communities he now studied were military and civilian population units. Military records gave him accurate numerators and denominators for measuring the changing severity and frequencies of many medical and health issues. He knew that, given basic longitudinal, community-based data, he could be master of the frequencies of disease outbreaks. In the context of LCHR this mastery gave him a powerful and subtle tool to investigate immediate and underlying determinants of the frequencies and severity of the diseases he pursued.

In the late 1940s Gordon set out to conduct a scientific field test of the capacity of birth control methods to change the birth rate of some selected rural communities in a developing country. He knew that the community-based field methods he had developed in Romania would be appropriate to poor, largely illiterate rural Indian communities. The birth control message

[a] *Address for correspondence:* 143 Fairway Road, Chestnut Hill, MA 02167-1847.

and materials would be delivered door to door by monthly home visits. He wanted to be sure that the birth control was available when couples were ready.

But he had a second focus in mind. He recognized that the same monthly visits would provide the opportunity to collect prospective data with which it would be possible to measure accurately death, birth and migration rates, and to learn in detail many of the local determinants of these rates. As a check on the prospective records of population dynamics he planned annual censuses of the communities after the initial census. The study was conducted in villages of the Punjab, India. Headquarters were in the small town of Khanna. The field work lasted from 1953 to 1960, and a further six months in 1969;[1] from 1984 to 1988 Dr. Monica Das Gupta conducted her own follow-up study in the same villages.[2]

RECOGNITION OF A NEW OR RESURGENT DISEASE

Several criteria for recognizing a disease as "new" were listed in a table presented in an article published by members of the Harvard Working Group on New and Resurgent Diseases.[3] As I read the table on page 55 of this report by Levins et al., five out of the ten listed criteria for recognition refer to increased perception of severity; four refer to changes in frequency in time or space; and one refers to a property of the pathogen. Thus I would conclude that changing severity and frequencies of suspected new diseases provide major identifying characteristics of new or resurgent infectious diseases for their recognition. Identification of etiologic agents is also, of course, an important component of the recognition.

After recognition and diagnosis of the determinants of individual cases, and of their severity and frequencies, comes the need to prevent or cure the disease. Studies of the frequency and severity of cases, particularly of deaths from these diseases, provide invaluable data for the identification of important preventable determinants underlying the immediate cause of an infective disease, its severity and its frequency. Such studies can reveal what kinds of people are at greater risk of suffering a disease. Besides providing data to exploit the standard epidemiologic classes of time, place and person, LCHR can supply in addition rich data for cohort and life table studies.

CONNECTIONS AMONG DISEASE DETECTION, DIAGNOSIS AND CONTROL

Modern nations appoint public health or medical practitioners to be responsible for detecting and controlling disease problems in the country and its subdivisions.

Practitioners face the challenge that after detecting a new or resurgent disease they must then seek to comprehend (diagnose) its immediate causation, and the underlying causes or determinants of its frequency and severity in the population for whom they are responsible. The effective design, management and evaluation of feasible control programs depend on the success of these efforts. Criteria for evaluating control programs are to be conceived particularly in terms of declines in the frequency and severity of the disease. Rigorous evaluations of programs intended to control the disease help to clarify the diagnosis.

With very few exceptions, such as natural disasters, epidemics and pandemics have multiple causes and determinants. The short-term goals of disease control are to limit deaths, serious disease, and their sequelae. Long-term goals are to limit the further spread of the disease, and if possible to eliminate the disease from the region for which the practitioner is responsible. Achieving these goals entails setting up surveillance procedures to ensure that future epidemics are detected as early as possible.

Societies want to get as much protection from serious or distressing disease as they can. The prime task of the responsible public health practitioners is therefore to provide concepts and data by which the society can consider and decide on priorities and by which to judge what control operations are feasible. The practitioners must be able to ask and answer the question: In this population, what are the most frequent, serious, preventable or treatable pathologies?

A health information system is therefore a prime requirement for these practitioners. In this paper I explore how the longitudinal community approach to health issues contributes to a health information system.

RESURGENT DISEASES IN INDIA

A brief history of the discovery of some infectious diseases in India provides a backdrop to the LCHR practiced in Gordon's Khanna Study. Today we are well aware that among poor populations diarrheas and pneumonias account for a major proportion of all deaths in the first two years of life. This was not recognized until recently.

From 1896 to 1945: The Last Classical Largely Uncontrolled Quarantinable Epidemics in India

For centuries largely illiterate registrars in Indian villages have been keeping records of births, deaths, and other events. FIGURE 1[4] indicates that from 1896 to 1945 they recorded fever as the cause of about 50 percent of deaths. According to these records the classical quarantinable diseases of cholera, smallpox and plague together accounted for about 15 percent of deaths. Dysentery and diarrhea accounted for less than 5 percent, respiratory diseases about 5 percent, and other causes 20 to 25 percent.

FIGURE 2[4] indicates that during these 50 years only one or two percent of recorded deaths were ascribed to smallpox, and the frequencies of deaths from plague and cholera epidemics were subject to wide swings. Although smallpox, cholera, and plague are highly recognizable, especially during an

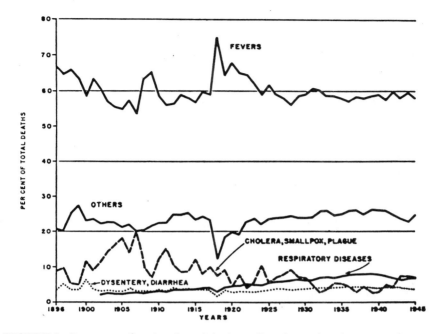

FIGURE 1. Percentage of total registered deaths attributed to each major group of causes, British India: 1896 to 1945. Source: Davis.[4]

epidemic, the percentage of annual deaths ascribed to any one of these diseases never exceeded 14 percent.

In the early decades of this century the village registrars did recognize diarrhea, as distinct from epidemic cholera, and pneumonia as important causes of death, but in small proportions. Those who analyzed the reports of the village registrars gave no tabulations by age or sex for those years.

1958, Ten Years Post-Independence, and 13 Years Post-Second World War

In the mid-1930s The Rockefeller Foundation established in India five rural primary health units near major cities. The Singur Health Unit near Calcutta was one of these. In 1957 the directors of the Singur Health Unit conducted a general health survey of the population they served. Data were collected from 5352 out of the 118,000 persons in the area.[6] The survey included retrospective questions on deaths. The 99 deaths they recorded at all ages suggested a death rate in the first year of life of 65/1000, and in the next four years of 28/1000. These are believable rates, but they carry a large standard error. Based on the ratios of the first year compared to the 1–5 year death rates now being recorded the ratio of 65 to 28 indicates a relatively

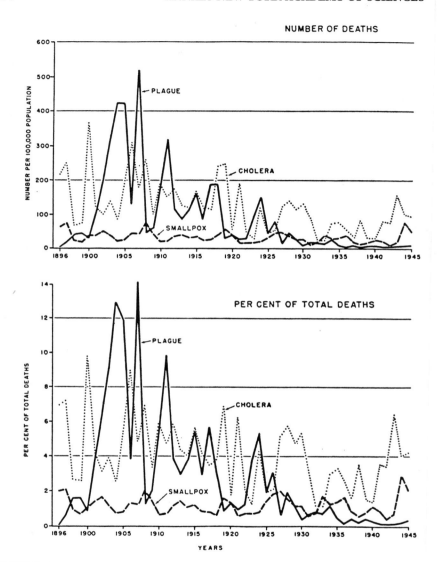

FIGURE 2. Registered deaths from plague, smallpox and cholera per 100.000 population, and per 100 deaths: British India, 1896–1945. Source: Davis.[4]

high death rate in the second year of life, and therefore almost certainly a high death rate in later months of the first year of life.

However, these rates were based on few recorded deaths. With five deaths in the first year of life, and two in the second year diarrhea appeared to be the leading cause of death in the first five years of life. Pneumonia, asphyxia and tetanus each contributed two or three deaths. These findings stimulated no comment from the investigators. To them the death rates of early childhood were quite moderate, and they expected the causes of death they found.

1952 to 1969, Results from the Khanna Study

Study Design and Field Method

The Khanna Study[1] was was based on the principles of LCHR by collecting prospective data at home visits within whole defined rural communities. Two geographically separated groups of villages provided sites for the prospective measurement of birth rates for four years in test populations of 8000 people (with birth control offered each month to every married couple) and control populations of 4000 persons (no birth control). The project was conducted in the Punjab, India.

The key features of field work relevant to the frequency and severity of diseases were: 1) the populations of whole villages served as the primary units of observation, and 2) monthly home visits made possible accurate prospective observations on sicknesses, deaths, other vital and reproductive events and birth control practices. The key features of data analysis were to exploit the prospective records of person-time exposed to the possibility of disease and death, cohort analyses and applications of the life table method.[7]

The field method for this study was based on direct field interviews conducted by a Punjabi staff of men and women living in the village assigned to them. Five special studies were developed: medical diagnosis of all deaths; medical care of fatal cases; obstetric practices; sicknesses and child feeding among children born during the span of the project; and the epidemiology of unintentional traumatic injuries and deaths in the scientific control villages. The system of recording data allowed for cross-reference of events, such as births or deaths, among the various study records.

High Death Rates in the Second Year of Life

According to the data given in FIGURE 3 the first year death rate in the Khanna villages, 1956 through 1959, was ten times that in the United States in 1951; but the second year death rate in the Khanna villages was 30 times the U.S. rate. This startling finding later turned out to be commonplace in poor communities.[8] Until findings from the Khanna Study were published, age-specific death rates of children were usually given only as infant mortality, deaths per 1000 live-births, and as deaths per 1000 population aged 1 to 5 years.

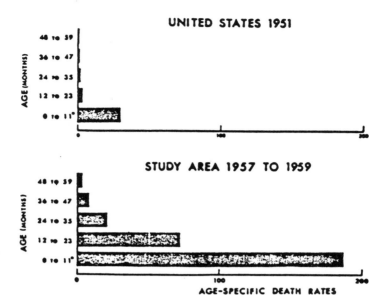

FIGURE 3. Annual death rates of preschool children by single years of age, villages of the Khanna Study area 1957 to 1959, and of the United States, 1951. Source: Wyon and Gordon,[1] Figure 87.

FIGURE 4 illustrates the value of using person-years of experience as the denominator for examining death rates at age intervals of a few months. It documents that the death rate fell off sharply after the first month of life, but then returned to significant levels for the 12 months from 6–18 months of age; in this case particularly among females. The 6–18 or 6–24 month period of high mortality has now been reported frequently elsewhere. The excess female mortality is characteristic chiefly of highly male-dominated cultures.

Medical Diagnosis of Causes of Death

By visiting every family every month, and through other sources of information, the Khanna Study staff have confidence that they detected virtually every death among residents in the study villages within one week of the event. A physician visited the family promptly and took a medical history of the fatal illness. In many cases a physician had seen the sick person before death. Occasionally other medical reports were available.

TABLE 1 shows that acute diarrheal disease was far the most frequent diagnosis of cause of death at all ages, followed by pneumonia and tuberculosis. The deaths from diarrhea, pneumonia and tetanus turned out to be dominantly from young children. Measles just made the first ten causes of

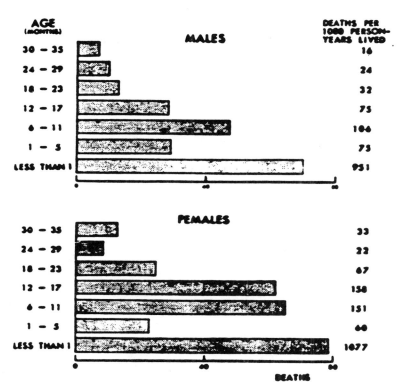

FIGURE 4. Estimated deaths of children from 1000 live-births, and death rates, by sex, 1955 to 1959, selected Khanna Study villages, life-table analysis. Source: Wyon and Gordon,[1] Figure 90.

TABLE 1. The First Ten Causes of Death, as Determined by Individual Case Study—Test and Control A Villages, January 1957 to December 1959

Cause of Death[a]	Number of Deaths	Deaths per 100,000 Population per Year
Acute diarrheal disease	68	187.2
Pneumonia	44	121.1
Tuberculosis	40	110.2
Tetanus	33	90.8
Heart disease	29	79.8
Birth injuries	29	79.8
Cancer	28	77.1
Typhoid fever	26	71.6
Accidents	23	63.3
Measles	18	49.5

[a] SOURCE: Wyon and Gordon,[1] Table 17.

death, and was confined to young children. Deaths from unintentional traumatic injuries were also among the first ten causes of death.

Tetanus of the Newborn

Tetanus killed 30 out of every 1000 live born children in the first 8 to 10 days of life, but it was almost unknown to the local medical profession and at the two teaching hospitals in the city of Ludhiana only 25 miles away with good transportation available. This established tetanus of the newborn as a newly recognized or resurgent, highly fatal, frequent disease in the Punjab, and in other parts of India. The infection appears to be related chiefly to contamination by animal dung during the cutting and dressing of the umbilical cord. Immunization of mothers against tetanus before or during pregnancy effectively prevents tetanus of the newly born.

Deaths Grouped by Potential for Prevention and by Age

During the three calendar years 1957 to 1959 the study staff detected 651 deaths in the 11 villages—12,000 people. We used these data to address the question: In these communities what are the most frequent, preventable causes of death?

With the goal of prevention in mind we distinguished four categories of causes of deaths attributed to preventable infections, and frequently concomitant preventable malnutrition. These groups were 1) tuberculosis, 2) diseases preventable by immunization, 3) infections complicated by serious malnutrition, and 4) fecal-borne diseases without serious malnutrition; these are diarrheas of persons over five years old. Detailed diagnoses of causes of death are given in Wyon and Gordon.[1]

Under the heading of **Selected Infections with Malnutrition** FIGURE 5[1] indicates that in their first year of life about 70 per 1000 of the children less than one year old died from enteric and respiratory infections complicated by severe malnutrition. The death rate from these causes in the second year of life was almost 40 per 1000. FIGURE 6[5] shows that in Guatemala the peak incidence of cases of diarrheal disease was 0.8 cases per child per *month* in the age group 18–23 months. Even if the diarrhea rate at these ages is much higher in Guatemala than in India, we can start to recognize the huge burden of infections in the first two years of life among these poor people; the extraordinarily high mortality from these "simple" infections becomes much more credible. Yet the rate of "loose bowels" and coughs and colds among children at these ages from our own personal and family experience at these ages is perhaps one third to one quarter of the rate in Guatemala. But our children are not so intensely exposed to virulent enteric and respiratory organisms as those near Khanna and in Guatemala, and the nutritional state of our children is much better; therefore, the severity of these attacks is much less. During the ages of children aged 0–35 months in Guatemala almost 90

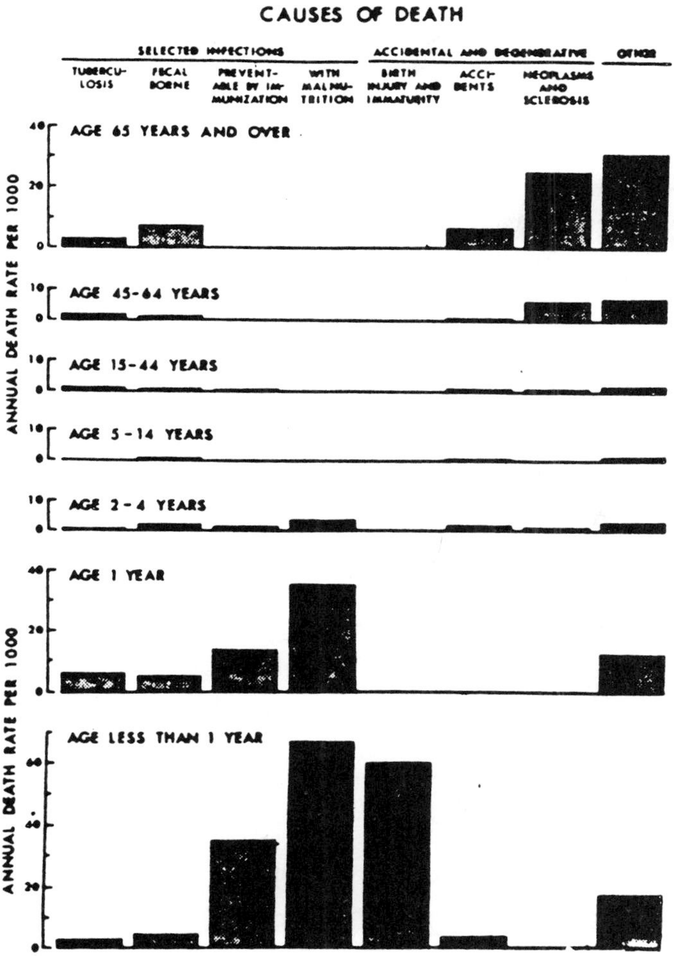

FIGURE 5. Death rates per 1000 persons per year, by causes of death grouped according to possible preventive techniques, and by age. Source: Wyon and Gordon,[1] Figure 94.

out of 100 person-months of experience were marked by a case of diarrhea; 30 percent by upper respiratory disease, and 27 percent had lower respiratory disease; whereas only 10 percent had one of the "infectious diseases of child-hood" (chicken pox, measles etc.).[8]

It is important to note that the physicians at Khanna made no diagnoses of deaths due to malnutrition as such. We did not conduct anthropometric measurements to determine nutritional status. In the early 1950s those techniques were still being worked out as a field method.

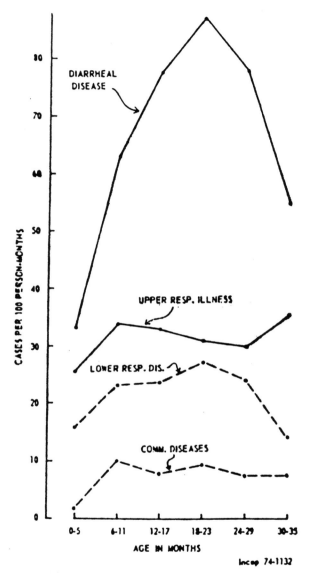

FIGURE 6. Incidents of common infectious diseases among children in the first few years of life, by age in months, Guatemala. Source: Mata,[5] Chapter 12, adapted from Table 12.3. See also Figure 12.3a.

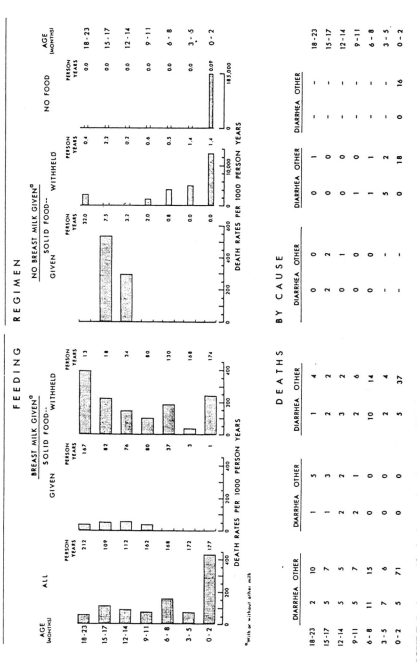

FIGURE 7. Age specific death rates by trimesters of life from birth to two years of age, deaths and causes of death, by feeding regimen, selected villages of the Khanna Study. The data result from monthly observations of 779 children. Each month each child was determined to be receiving breast milk, with or without solid food; no breast milk with or without solid food; or no food at all. Causes of death are given as from diarrhea or from other causes. Source: Wyon and Gordon,[1] Figure 92.

Returning to FIGURE 5,[1] three other categories of causes of death among the children living near Khanna were those ascribed to: 1) birth injury and immaturity, 2) injury, and 3) neoplasms and sclerosis. The remainder are given as other.

Each of the eight categories of grouped cause-specific death rates in FIG-URE 5 is subdivided by age, starting with the first year; the second year, and the third to fifth years of life (years 2–4), then by spans of 10, 20, 30, and 20 years of age until we arrive at 65 years and over.

Conclusions from Figures 4, 5, and 6

The categories of deaths preventable with relatively well-established technologies are dramatically concentrated in the first two years of life. The data in FIGURES 4,[1] 6,[8] and 7[1] presented here still further identify the crucial age span of 6 to 18 months of age when a high proportion of deaths can be prevented using simple techniques. This was a major discovery in the 1950s of newly recognized categories of preventable deaths. FIGURE 7 provides strong evidence from the Khanna Study that breast fed children from ages 6 to 24 months of age who were receiving solid food were only one third or less likely to die than children of the same ages not receiving solid food to supplement their mother's breast milk. No other field study has yet reported these observations.

The capacity of the staff of primary health care systems to identify specific children in defined communities at high risk of dying from these preventable diseases is another important part of the diagnosis.[9] This capacity arises from their systematic home visiting. Longitudinal community health practititioners can, through the data they collect in the course of their daily practice, fill in the gaps left by approaches through clinics and through rallies organized by mobile staff units visiting at agreed locations and times. This practical application of the principles of LCHR is now being put to practical test in a few primary health care programs in Bolivia and elsewhere.[10]

APPLICATIONS OF LCHR TO CONTROL NEW AND RESURGENT INFECTIOUS DISEASES

Primary Health Care in Bolivia

In 1979 Dr. Henry Perry of North Carolina set out to develop a primary health care service to cover a population of about 250,000 persons in the Andes Mountains of Bolivia.[10] John Wyon agreed to contribute ideas towards

---

FIGURE 8. Deaths by age in months, three primary health care programs in Bolivia. **a:** Carabuco (high Andes—13,000 feet above sea level); **b:** Mallco Rancho (Andes valleys—8000 feet); **c:** Montero (tropics—600 ft). Source: Perry and Sandavold.[9]

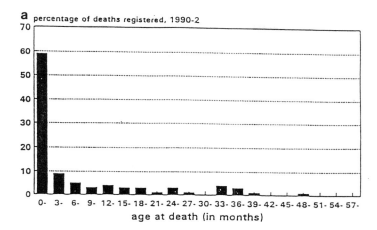

a percentage of deaths registered, 1990-2

age at death (in months)

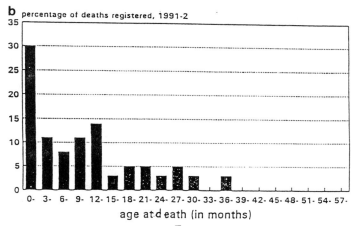

b percentage of deaths registered, 1991-2

age at·d eath (in months)

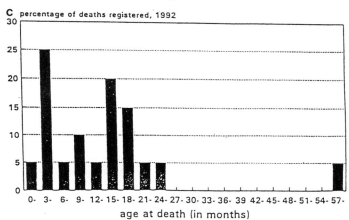

c percentage of deaths registered, 1992

age at death (in months)

this effort on field and analytic methods derived from The Khanna Study in India and elsewhere. The program is known as Andean Rural Health Care (ARHC).

The decision to evaluate the project in terms of declining death rates led to the adoption of the LCHR approach used at Khanna. The challenge was to measure local rates of sickness and death, and their determinants, in the context of an on-going primary health care project.

The staff developed what they now call their Census-Based, Impact-Oriented approach. Over the past decade the field staff have developed programs in three highly distinct ecologic zones at 13,000, 8000, and 600 feet above sea level, and with important cultural differences. The programs are based on routine periodic contact with every person in the communities.[9,10] Efficient health information systems have been developed appropriate to each locality. The staff ask themselves the question: "in these communities what are the most frequent, serious, preventable or treatable problems and what are the determinants of these problems?" They answer their question by analyzing the data they collect from the communities they serve to measure the community-based rates of sickness, death, *etc.*

FIGURE 8 displays the distribution of deaths by month of age in the first two years of life from the three primary health care sites in Bolivia. The marked differences in the distributions of deaths clearly indicate that high priority attention is indicated at different ages in the three ecologic regions.

The staff at each location have more work to do to achieve a clearer understanding of the most frequent, serious, preventable problems affecting their communities, and the determinants of these problems. But they have the tools with which to pursue these inquiries. They can measure severity and frequencies of specific syndromes. In a word, the staffs of these primary health care programs are able to diagnose re-emerging infectious diseases in their defined communities and to recognize new diseases.

SUMMARY AND CONCLUSIONS

Concepts

In my understanding, new and resurgent diseases are either new to the medical professions, or reflect expressions of diseases already known to health agencies, but now appearing with increased severity, frequency or extent (geographic or social).

Aspects of Diagnosis

We may recognize some or all of:

1. cases as sporadic events, or as epidemics or endemics of the disease;
2. changes in the severity, frequency, or geographic or social location of cases within communities or populations;

3. the multifactorial determinants of the disease, its frequency, and its manifestations, such as clinical features, vectors of infections, factors promoting or diminishing frequencies and distributions of cases by age or sex among individuals, families or communities, and how any or all of these may point towards causation, and therefore to possible control;
4. physical, biological and social determinants of changes in severity, frequency and location, with emphasis on preventable or curable determinants;
5. applications of the above insights to determine critical features of disease control programs—their design, management and evaluation, relevant to demonstrated high priority specific diseases affecting specific communities.

Longitudinal Community Health Research and Practice

1. LCHR increases our capacity to recognize and measure the features of severity, frequency and distributions of cases, epidemic or endemic disease, and to recognize some of the determinants of these features,
2. LCHR is based on a) defining appropriate communities, b) defining and detecting, prospectively, cases and vital events within those communities, and c) obtaining continuous records of denominator populations of the defined communities so that changes in morbidity and mortality rates can be measured accurately.

In general terms LCHR can fill in accurately many gaps left by conventional clinical and vital records, and by conventional surveys, in the available information on disease incidence and prevalence, on the vital events of births, deaths and migrations and on the populations at risk of disease and vital events.

REFERENCES

1. WYON, J. B. & J. E. GORDON. 1971. The Khanna Study: Population Problems in the Rural Punjab. Cambridge, MA: Harvard University Press.
2. DAS GUPTA, M. 1987. Selective discrimination against female children in rural Punjab, India. Popul. Dev. Rev. **13:** 77–.
3. LEVINS, R. et al. 1994. The Emergence of New Diseases. Am. Scientist. **84:** 52–60.
4. DAVIS, K. 1951. The Population of India and Pakistan. Princeton, NJ: Princeton University Press.
5. MATA, L. 1978. Children of Santa Maria Cauque. Cambridge, MA: Massachusetts Institute of Technology Press.
6. SEAL, S. C., K. C. PATNAIK, P. C. SEN & L. M. BHATTARCHARJI, et al. 1959. Report of the Resurvey of Singur Health Unit Area: 1957–58. All India Institute of Hygiene and Public Health, Calcutta.
7. POTTER, R. G., J. B. WYON, M. PARKER & J. E. GORDON. 1965. Applications of field studies to research on the physiology of human reproduction: Lactation and its effects on birth intervals in eleven Punjab villages, India. In Public Health and Population Change. M. C. Sheps & J. C. Ridley, Eds.: 377–399. Pittsburgh, PA: University of Pittsburgh Press

8. GORDON, J. E., J. B. WYON & W. ASCOLI. 1967. The second year death rate in developing countries. Am. J. Med. Sci. **254:** 357–380
9. PERRY, H. & I. SANDAVOLD. 1993. Routine systematic home visitation as a strategy for improving access to services and program effectiveness: Lessons from Bolivia and the U.S. *In* Global Learning for Health. R. Morgan & R. Raus, Eds.: 175–185. Washington, DC: National Council for International Health.
10. PERRY, H. 1989. The Census-based Impact-Oriented Approach and its Application by Andean Rural Health Care in Bolivia, South America. Available from Andean Rural Health Care: Lake Junaluska, NC.
11. SILVA, K. T. 1987. Final Report on the Sarvodaya Malaria Control Research Project, Anuradhapura District, Sri Lanka. Moratuwa, Sri Lanka: Sarvodaya Movement.

Surveillance: Discussion

Part A. The Possibilities and Limitations of Surveillance

ANDREW SPIELMAN: I would like to argue in terms of a dual approach to monitoring. One focus should be laid on the optimization of a routinized system of surveillance. Another approach should emphasize exactly the other way. New diseases are inherently novel. There will be aspects to new diseases that are unpredictable, inherently unpredictable. New diseases or aspects of the emergence of new diseases will possibly escape a monitoring routine.

Most of the discussions this morning have been based on establishing a routine system. I would like to suggest that we also place a certain amount of emphasis and money on developing research capacities for those academics who are working on anticipating the unusual. If we could have, in parallel with the routine surveillance system, a system of grant or contract awards for research to cope with the unpredictable of disease emergence, we could have a large payoff by a relatively small investment.

ROBERT TESH: I want to question the whole notion of a surveillance system. In particular, I want to question the usefulness of surveillance for those areas where it is very likely that new diseases will emerge, for example in parts of Africa where people are coming in contact with areas that they have not come into contact with before.

I really question the possibility of developing a routine surveillance system given the limitations of the scientific community in these areas. I think, what we are really asking for is a type of awareness. For example, people working at the mission hospital in Zaire should be able to look out for unusual circumstances that might support the emergence of a new disease. In my understanding, surveillance by its very nature is looking for things that are already known or described. Surveillance in the common sense does not focus on looking for new things, circumstances, alterations in environments and populations.

The question remains: Are we looking for an awareness for the unusual in relation to the emergence of new diseases, or are we looking for the kind of surveillance that we traditionally think about? I would like your response to that.

RALPH BRYAN: I think we are talking about a combination thereof. My comments were focused on surveillance in the United States. Jim LeDuc may be a better person to ask about concepts for international surveillance and international sensible networks in relation to that criticism. I think Ruth pointed out that it is important to have a system in place where people can communicate about unusual events or observations.

IRINA ECKARDT: I would like to support Dr. Tesh's criticism. The belief in collecting more data by using the latest technology, like remote sensing or modern computer technology, is a basic element in traditional surveillance strategies. I am strongly convinced that even with the help of modern technologies we will not break through the barrier to anticipate and predict disease emergence in the different parts of the world. To overcome this barrier requires new thinking, a critical reflection on the preconditions of theories and models in the medical sciences, and a strongly transdisciplinary organization of research.

I would like to repeat Pamela's comment that it is important to develop a framework before the field research starts. We have to think about the basic elements in our models before we design our field research and before we collect data. The model itself should not be static, but dynamic. It has to be open to changes and corrections. Changes might be necessary in relation to the new knowledge we gain from the field, for example anthropological data about the people living in the areas of our research, comments from other research projects, or changes in the political or social structure of the country we are working in.

An interactive process of modeling and data collection would make both modes of surveillance—the "routine system" and the "awareness system" (to look out for the unusual and to report it)—possible. I am not arguing that we should give up the possibilities that modern technologies, especially remote sensing, provide to improve surveillance. I would rather support Andy's suggestion to develop both—the routine system and the system for developing our abilities to look for the unusual.

At the same moment it is very important to develop simple communication procedures, in accordance with the specific level of economic development in a specific country. (The people working in the mission hospital in Zaire might not have computers with a modem to report the unusual event via e-mail to WHO or CDC.) These communication procedures should contain a kind of check-list of what is necessary to do and to report in case of a new epidemic. The check-list should be designed in a way that it survives the rotation of different national and international projects in a specific country. It should be both—adjusted to the native modes of communication in a country and designed to provide the fundamental information about an epidemic. To seek the simplest and most reliable communication structure requires again anthropological and sociological research.

RUTH BERKELMAN: That is a very good point. I want to add something. When we talked about a global consortium Bob Shope and many people have been involved in, we talked about three key elements for detection of new disease. 1) You have to have access to the clinical population. 2) You need some basic laboratory support. 3) You have to have some epidemiologic expertise, so that you would know what to do when you are confronted with a new disease and how to categorize it. Not the data *per se* are important to detection but having people in the field that have access to those three key elements. Generally these people in the field are conducting research. They are not just out there waiting for something to happen. On the other hand, when you look at systems where people are in touch, for example with the health departments in the United States, they have some routine systems they use. They can call the health department when something unusual happens.

In the case of the hantavirus outbreak in New Mexico, a kind of awareness was present because people were very worried about plague that year. They had been in contact and because a single epidemiologist in an Indian Health Service reported his observation that plague was right in the area, the outbreak of the hantavirus could be detected relatively fast. In this case, the communication between the different Health Services, CDC and the local population proved to be a major part in the detection and identification of this epidemic.

I agree that data collection describes past events, not future events. But it is important to have a kind of routine system, including the collection and report of epidemiological data. It is as important as the routine system to have people in the field who are trained to look out for the unusual and report it.

ROBERT SHOPE: I would like to make a suggestion for Ralph's system of research on emerging infections and for a surveillance system. Usually you would ask in a laboratory what diseases they are diagnosing there. I think, it might be even more valuable to ask what diseases they are not diagnosing. In other words, in how many cases of encephalitis for which they have stored sera was it not possible to make a diagnosis? Furthermore, it should be possible to collect those undiagnosed sera in some sort of serum bank or long-term storage. Comparisons between these sera and newly identified and diagnosed or undiagnosed ones would be possible.

I think such a serum bank would have been useful to you for a study of the acute respiratory disease syndrome in New Mexico and other locations in the United States. Obviously there had been some cases scattered throughout the United States. If you had a systematic collection of acute respiratory syndrome cases, including some sort of materials like sera, you could have gone back to those in the case of the Four Corners outbreak.[a]

TESH: I want to follow up on something that Bob Shope said. Some of you had asked if there were certain sequences or antigenic characteristics that would allow us to identify a pathogen. For those of you who are not virologists I want to explain this. Among the viruses there are families and certain serogroups. Many of them have antigenic characteristics or genetic sequences in common and among them some are pathogens and some are not. We don't know why one virus is a pathogen and why another virus is not. Perhaps one virus that is now not a pathogen will become a pathogen under different circumstances and environmental conditions. It would be a little simplistic to take a virus and to predict that this virus will or will not become a pathogen. In fact, for most viruses even if we know that they are pathogenic, we can hardly identify which viruses are more pathogenic or which are less. We really don't know the processes that make a virus pathogenic.

SHOPE: I think that two things are important. First, we have to develop clinical surveillance. The other important component is finding the protoplasm and documenting the biodiversity by isolating and collecting viruses.

---

[a] For detailed discussion about the hantavirus outbreak in the United States, see "Hantaviruses and the Hantavirus Outbreak in the United States" and "Disease in Evolution: Hantavirus," in this volume (pp. 199–207 and 208–224, respectively).

DONALD ROBERTS: Bob, would you have had the yellow fever vaccine if there had been no surveillance in Africa?

SHOPE: The answer is no. We would not have had the vaccine. Yellow fever very definitely was a disease that was occurring in the United States until roughly 1900. This disease was a problem of our own, and it could be again a problem for the United States.

RITA COLWELL: I think it is important to give the following comment. Data and virus strains have gone into the CDC. There is the problem, in my opinion, that the information system has not been interactive. I really enjoyed hearing Dr. Bryan's talk and that you are interested in connecting the CDC system with physicians and laboratories. It is important to make the system truly interactive. If you can develop such an interactive system, you would have a great research opportunity.

BRYAN: One basic factor of good surveillance is good feedback. If we are going to establish a good surveillance system, we have to have that interactivity you're talking about.

COLWELL: I would like to reemphasize a point that was made earlier by another speaker. Usually, there are very valuable investigators doing research projects in the field who may not know the epidemiology, but who may be able to observe and analyze the events that contribute to an epidemic. A major point is that cooperation and collaborative work with such research teams is very effective. I think that in the past some CDC teams have not been so interested in partnerships during an investigation of an outbreak or epidemic. At least, some people in the field got that impression.

RICHARD LEVINS: I would like to discuss long-term prediction in addition to surveillance. There is the need to have a data base which will allow us to ask the kinds of questions that ecologists would ask almost routinely. For instance, questions such as: What is the host range of viruses of a particular group as against the host range of bacteria or fungi? Is it true that the physiological similarity of lungs across mammals means that there would be more shared pathogens of lungs than of guts? Do viruses have any climatic restrictions other than those imposed by their vector? There are many hypotheses which come out of ecology. For example: Is it true for reservoir populations as it is true for plants that the greater population size the greater the number of species of parasites that inhibit it?

In order to be able to recognize whether a particular virus is more likely to be pathogenic, we would have to have a data base in which a systematic position of viruses and their hosts can be established. Such a data base should be broadly accessible. The design of the data base could be compared with the process of development of the Human Relations Area File that was set up at Yale by anthropologists. Originally they had just a few ideas, geometric figures or images on their collected pottery. Over the years they have added tolerance and more information into the data base.

In relation to the recognition and identification of new and resurgent diseases it would be a great help to have a systematic place where people can interrogate the data bank. What are the systematic properties? How many diseases are there in bears compared to diseases in mice? This general compendium is needed in order to be able to answer many questions that we're asking now, even if this is always going to be restricted by uneven searching and the quality of the data.

BRYAN: One thing we have proposed in a larger document related to emerging infections in the United States is the creation of a national infectious disease data base that is accessible to people doing research in public health and infectious diseases.

PAMELA ANDERSON. One problem, also for the design of an infectious disease data base, is to define "new" in relation to infectious diseases. The Harvard Working Group on New Diseases defined new in a very broad sense. A disease can also be new to an area, and it is often called a "threatening disease." There are papers on "threatening diseases" in Africa, for example.

We are teaching our students to identify vectors which we don't have yet in Central America because we know that if those vectors appear, a specific pathogen is very likely to appear as well. This "new" pathogen might have the potential to wipe out our banana industry or our soybean industry.

To teach the students about vectors and pathogens that are currently not in area and to teach them an awareness, to look out for such unusual vectors and pathogens, is another kind of surveillance. Actually, it is very cheap because it is incorporated into the educational system.

When we are talking about expanding the surveillance system, we should not forget that there is a whole army of ecologists working in the field, already doing, for example, rodent research. A large amount of our theory in public health and epidemiology is derived from basic population studies in ecology. If we would be able to coordinate the research in ecology or even zoology, we could get a lot of data from such networks. To establish such a network is, again, not very expensive.

Part B. Institutions and Surveillance

LAURIE GARRETT: I want to add the following facts to the discussion. Because of a new drug policy, every year hundreds of thousands of people circulate through the jails in the United States. Typically, they stay in the jails for less then 7 days. During that time they undergo several diagnostic procedures, including screening tests for tuberculosis and HIV infection. The results of these routine tests show that the poor populations in inner cities or urban areas who rotate in and out of the jail are at very high risk for infection with new or resurgent diseases. In these populations the rate of intravenous drug use and the rate of STDs is very high. The development of a routine surveillance system for these populations, in connection with jail physicians, is an important element in a national surveillance strategy for the United States.

RUTH BERKELMAN: I want to add something to Laurie's comment. Actually, a number of HIV surveys are conducted throughout the country, not only in prisons, but also in STD clinics, drug treatment facilities, shelters for the homeless or in homeless persons. These surveys are also used to screen for other pathogens, like the HTLV-1 and HTLV-2.

GARRETT: My reason for mentioning jails as a place of study is because of the difficulties inherent in studying other populations, such as the homeless and persons attending clinics for STDs or intravenous drug use. These populations may be highly recalcitrant and even violent. In contrast, persons in jails theoretically have no weapons and their identities can be verified. Persons can be followed and seen again in six months or a year. It seems to me that a great opportunity is being missed.

RALPH BRYAN: In jails you have a captive audience. It's a window of opportunity for surveillance. I think we should further develop a surveillance network for other forms of institutionalization, like nursing homes or even child-care facilities.

Nosocomial Amplifiers of Microbial Emergence

LAURIE GARRETT

Newsday/*Science Section*
235 Pinelawn Road
Melville, New York 11747

Morse has described a two-step process for the emergence or reemergence of microbial disease: the "viral trafficking" of microbes from one species or locale to another, followed by dissemination of the introduced microbe.[1] I suggest an intermediate step may be necessary, particularly for microbes not readily transmitted by respiratory contact or through highly mobile vectors: amplification. If neither the host nor the vector frequently changes locales, it is unlikely that a localized outbreak will graduate to epidemic status within the immediate local human population. Indeed, a microbe may occasionally circulate through the human population, unnoticed, for generations until an amplification event raises its presence to outbreak or epidemic status.

Amplification, then, might be defined as any process which markedly increases microbial population, from a modest or virtually invisible homeostatic host relationship to one of significantly greater host infection rates and microbial transmission.

Several factors—environmental and social—might serve as amplifiers, including the routine presence and exposure to unprocessed human waste (for enteric microbes), extreme high density housing (for respiratory microbes), widespread intravenous drug abuse (for blood-borne microbes), and local population ratios on the order of 3 : 1 or more of men to women (for sexually transmitted agents).

The post-World War II history of emergence indicates that medical facilities (hospitals, missionary outposts, dispensaries, and clinics) can readily serve as amplifiers.

Nosocomial transmission does not, in and of itself, constitute amplification, as most incidents of microbial passage from human to human via medical equipment, fellow patients, procedures, or personnel do not result in a significant expansion in microbial population, or in the epidemiological range of susceptible hosts. A medical facility (inpatient or outpatient) constitutes an ecology of concentrated microbes infectious to humans spanning the gamut of potential pathogens, modes of transmission, and parasitic compatibility with *Homo sapiens*. Humans enter the facility from the larger environment, in which the pathogenic microbes often exist in a more dilute or isolated relationship to the hosts. Following treatment (which may or may not be successful), the humans return to the larger environment.

In the facility's ecology many potential hosts are temporarily or permanently compromised immunologically, have particularly vulnerable portals of

389

microbial entry (wounds, suture sites, skin dressing, pneumonitis) and interact intimately with a variety of pieces of equipment, apparatuses, and personnel. The opportunities for nosocomial transmission of microbes are multitudinous. Less numerous are chances for amplification, resulting in expansion of the epidemiologic host range of the microbe, the microbe's movement from the facility into the larger human environment, or significant spread within the facility.

For some microbes it can be argued that medical establishments of one kind or another are the primary amplifiers of their presence among human hosts.

Every known outbreak of Ebola (caused by the Ebola filovirus) has resulted from amplification in a medical setting. Antibody-positive individuals can be found throughout Africa,[2] yet only three significant outbreaks of the disease have ever come to world attention. The first recognized outbreak of the disease occurred in Yambuku, Zaire in the winter of 1976, its precise origin never clarified. The index case of the outbreak, however, was a man who sought care at the Yambuku missionary hospital. Every case thereafter could be traced either to the hospital or to relatives of individuals who had attended clinics or been hospitalized for other reasons prior to developing Ebola hemorrhagic disease.[3] Investigation by a World Health Organization team revealed that the primary sources of transmission were the five syringes used by missionary personnel for all injections performed by the facility: some 300–600 injections per day.

Clearly, the practice of reusing five syringes on all patients amplified what began as a remote occurrence of a not-readily-transmissible disease.

Similarly, the 1976 and 1979 Ebola outbreaks in southern Sudan revolved around extremely impoverished, under-supplied medical facilities. Though it appears that both outbreaks began with cases in a cotton factory in N'zara,[3] the epidemics only occurred when the index cases were amplified in medical facilities. The toll among medical personnel, fellow-patients, and relatives was severe.[4]

Although there clearly is an endemic sylvatic pattern to Lassa fever, dramatic outbreaks in 1969, 1970, 1972, 1974, 1989, 1992, and 1993 in West Africa all resulted from medical facility-based transmission.[5] Again, sporadic cases resulting from rodent exposures (*Mastomys natalensis*) that undoubtedly occur frequently in West Africa were amplified radically through human blood-to-blood or continuous respiratory exposure during medical procedures, the sharing of food and water by co-warded patients, locating Lassa cases upwind of maternity patients, reuse of medical syringes, and a tracheotomy performed on a Lassa victim.[6–11]

The origin of the 1976 swine flu in the United States has never been explained, nor has its apparent extremely limited spread within the Fort Dix military base during the winter of that year. A total of 155 GIs on the base ultimately tested antibody positive against the Shope swine antigen; thirteen developed influenza as a result; one died. The diseased individuals were members of different regiments which had no contact over the epidemic's course. Intraregimental spread, or transmission within barracks, was not a significant problem. A sergeant who performed mouth-to-mouth resuscitation in an attempt to revive the recruit who died of influenza did not, himself, become infected.[12]

Army investigators found two sites that were visited by all those who contracted swine influenza: the central intake area where GIs and recruits were processed following the Christmas holidays, and the medical dispensary. Because the individual soldiers who became ill initially passed through the processing center on several different days, the investigators were unable to identify a shared mode of transmission at that site. All the primary cases visited the fort's medical dispensary, however, for reasons other than influenza prior to developing flu, and could have been exposed at those times through a variety of means. It is therefore possible that the Fort Dix dispensary served as a swine flu amplifier in 1976, expanding a probably single zoonotic infection into a local outbreak.

Although the Legionnaires' disease bacterium can be transmitted to humans by a number of means involving moist air exposure, hospitals have clearly been sites of amplification on several occasions. Contaminated air conditioning systems and wound exposure to nonsterile water have been major culprits.[13–19]

Outbreaks of multidrug-resistant bacteria and mycobacteria have frequently arisen from medical facilities, with index case infections amplified many times over through inadequate staff hygiene,[20–22] syringe or device reuse,[23,24] device packaging,[25] air recirculation through hospital wards,[26–29] septic catheters or IV lines,[30–32] septic surgical procedures, often involving implants of various medical devices, limbs, or joints,[33–36] respiratory assistance equipment,[37,38] and inadequate protection of personnel in pathology labs.

A Florida outpatient clinic where HIV-positive men received inhaled pentamidine for *Pneumocystis carinii* prophylaxis was the setting for an epidemic of multidrug-resistant tuberculosis.[39]

Similarly, co-housing HIV-positive patients on wards with individuals suffering active TB has resulted in epidemics of both drug susceptible and multidrug-resistant tuberculosis in several places worldwide over the last five years.[26–29]

The spread of methicillin-resistant *Staphylococcus aureus* (MRSA) within hospital facilities is now such a pervasive and serious problem in the United States that some hospital wards must periodically be shut down, potentially contaminated materials destroyed, the facility heavily treated with disinfectant, and, only then, reopened.[40,41] Such radical steps for elimination of sites of hospital amplification of MRSA are particularly necessary for burn wards, where severely immunosuppressed patients with large, exposed skin surface areas are particularly vulnerable.

Multiple outbreaks of influenza A have been documented in medical institutions and other closed populations. Amantadine-resistant strains have emerged and spread in nursing home residences when the anti-viral agent amantadine was used prophylactically to control outbreaks.[42]

Not all nosocomial infections result in disease amplification; most cases remain individualized. Amplification results when one of two events occur:

the microbes' advantage becomes great enough to allow expansion from the medical setting to patients' relatives and external society, or, the overall burden of incidents over time in medical facilities leads to a cumulative increase in societal levels of infection.

Most of the cases described above are indicative of the first mode of nosocomial amplification.

Examples of the second—widespread sporadic entries into the community with secondary spread and persistence—might include hepatitis B,[43–47] vancomycin-resistant enterococci,[48,49] respiratory syncytial virus,[52] MRSA (methicillin-resistant *Staphylococcus aureus*),[40,51,52] multi-resistant *S. pneumoniae* and *Staphylococcus epidermidis*,[40] fluoroquinolone-resistant *Serratia* and *P. aeruginosa*, aminoglycoside-resistant agents (streptococci, pseudomonas, enterococci, enterobacteriaceae).[40]

There is clear evidence that antibiotic-resistant bacteria often first emerge in livestock due to widespread use of the drugs in the poultry, dairy, and beef industries. Zoonotic events occur among livestock handlers and meat and dairy consumers. But widespread human infection with the new strains often follows hospital amplification.[53]

If Lassa, Ebola, and hepatitis B can be readily amplified in a medical setting, it is reasonable to assume any bloodborne, emergent organism may—or, in fact, does—take advantage of similar amplification settings. Among the organisms one might expect to see exploiting medical settings or medical interventions for emergence amplifications are: acyclovir-resistant herpes simplex and zoster,[54] gancyclovir- and foscarnet-resistant cytomegalovirus, HTLV-1, HTLV-II, multidrug-resistant malaria, the gamut of hemorrhagic fever viruses, and an untold number of organisms not yet identified.

Medical interventions have clearly been at the crux of numerous—perhaps most—drug-resistant bacterial outbreaks, and it can be safely predicted that the range of both the organism species possessing genes that confer resistance, and the spectrum of drugs to which any given species is resistant will increase through medical amplification.

"In our hospitals, where antibiotic consumption continues to increase, the nosocomial flora consists of many resistant bacteria," Gentry writes.[52] "And infections acquired in the nosocomial setting are now far more severe than their community-acquired counterparts."

As for respiratory-transmitted organisms, measles and tuberculosis have clearly demonstrated the continuing, often lethal, role of the medical amplification setting. Few hospitals anywhere in the world that were constructed after World War II were designed to anticipate airborne contagion. Indeed, contemporary hospital design in wealthy nations may serve as a more efficient amplification ecology than its developing world counterparts because energy efficiency and criminal (or psychiatric) security provisions virtually eliminate individualized patient ventilation or air control. Though such hospitals may have a handful of designated positive-pressure or air-isolated rooms, the bulk of all patients breathe the same, recirculated, potentially microbe-laden air.

Nosocomial amplification can best be distinguished from iatrogenesis in that no policy or medical practice appears to be singularly responsible for these events. Indeed, it is the routine of medicine, its very mundaneness, that lays at the root of the problem. Nosocomial amplification occurs even when health providers try to do their jobs day in and day out, using available resources as well as they can. Adherence to CDC Universal Precautions is not always possible, even when providers at all tiers of a facility are conscientious.

It may, therefore, be the case that medical facilities—particularly inpatient—are ideal settings for surveillance and monitoring of microbial emergence, as they appear to represent critical sites for amplification. It would seem judicious to investigate means whereby providers might better recognize novel diseases or microbes and rapidly report such discoveries to an established surveillance network. At this time such routine reportage is haphazard in wealthy countries and virtually nonexistent in developing countries.

It may well be impossible to anticipate and prevent initial microbial emergence—Morse's "viral trafficking" or microbial cross-species movement. But amplification may be quite amenable to mitigation, particularly in medical settings where, presumably, the collective enterprise is motivated to prevent human disease.

REFERENCES

1. MORSE, S. S. 1993. Examining the origins of emerging viruses. *In* Emerging Viruses. S. S. Morse, Ed. Chapter 2. New York: Oxford University Press.
2. PAIX, M. A., J. D. POVEDA, D. MALVY, et al. 1988. A sero-epidemiological study of hemorrhagic fever viruses in an urban population of Cameroon. Bull. Soc. Pathol. Exot. et de ses Filiales 81: 679–682; BOIRO, I., N. N. LOMONOSSOV, V. A. SOTSINSKI, et al. 1987. Clinico-epidemiologic and laboratory research on hemorrhagic fevers in Guinea. Bull. Soc. Pathol. Exot. et de ses Filiales 80: 607–612; VAN DER WAALS, F. W., K. L. POMEROY, J. GOUDSMIT, et al. 1986. Hemorrhagic fever virus infections in an isolated rainforest area of central Liberia. Trop. Geograph. Med. 38: 209–214.
3. PATTYN, S. R. 1978. Ebola virus haemorrhagic fever: Proceedings of an International Colloquium on Ebola Virus Infection and Other Haemorrhagic Fevers held in Antwerp, Belgium, 6–8 December, 1977. Amsterdam: Elsevier/North-Holland Biomedical Press.
4. BARON, R. C., J. B. McCORMICK & O. A. ZUBEIR. 1983. Ebola virus disease in southern Sudan: Hospital dissemination and intrafamilial spread. Bull. WHO 61: 997–1003.
5. ROLLIN, P., L. WILSON, J. CHILDS, et al. 1993. Lassa fever epidemic in Plateau State, Nigeria—1993. Presentation to the Annual Meeting of the American Society for Tropical Medicine and Hygiene, Atlanta, October 1993.
6. CAREY, D. E., et al. 1972. Lassa Fever—Epidemiological Aspects of the 1970 Epidemic Jos, Nigeria. Trans. R. Soc. Trop. Med. Hyg. 66: 402–408.
7. FRAME, J. D. 1975. Surveillance of Lassa fever in missionaries stationed in West Africa. Bull. WHO 52: 593–598.
8. FRASER, D. W., et al. 1974. Lassa fever in the eastern province of Sierra Leone, 1969–1972. I. Epidemiology studies. Am. J. Trop. Med. Hyg. 23: 1131–1139.
9. FISHER-HOCH, S. P., O. TOMORI, G. I. PEREZ-ORONOZ, et al. Transmission of lethal viruses through routine parenteral drug administration. Personal communication, unpublished, 1993.
10. MERTENS, P. E., et al. 1973. Clinical presentation of Lassa fever cases during the hospital epidemic at Zorzor, Liberia, March–April 1972. Am. J. Trop. Med. Hyg. 22: 780–784.
11. TROUP, J. M., et al. 1970. An outbreak of Lassa fever on the Jos Plateau, Nigeria, in January–February, 1970. Am. J. Trop. Med. Hyg. 19: 695–696.
12. TOP, H. F., JR. & P. K. RUSSELL. 1977. Swine influenza A at Fort Dix, New Jersey (January–February 1976). IV. Summary and Speculation. J. Infect. Dis. 136: S376–S380.

13. LATTIMER, G. L. & R. A. ORMSBEE. 1981. Legionnaires' disease. New York: Marcel Dekker, Inc.
14. KAUFMAN, A. F., J. E. MCDADE, C. M. PATTON, et al. 1981. Pontiac fever: Isolation of the etiologic agent (*Legionella pneumophila*) and demonstration of its mode of transmission. Am. J. Epidemiol. **114:** 337–347.
15. FOY, H. M., P. S. HAYES, M. K. COONEY, et al. 1979. Legionnaires' disease in a prepaid medical-care group in Seattle 1963–75. Lancet (April 7): 767–770.
16. SARAVOLATZ, L., L. ARKING, B. WENTWORTH & E. QUINN. 1979. Prevalance of antibody to the Legionnaires' disease bacterium in hospital employees. Ann. Intern. Med. **90:** 601–603.
17. HELMS, C. M., M. MASSANARI, R. P. WENZEL, et al. 1988. Legionnaires' disease associated with a hospital water system. J. Am. Med. Assoc. **259:** 2423–2426.
18. NAHAPETIAN, K., O. CHALLEMEL, D. BEVRTIN, et al. 1991. The intracellular multiplication of *Legionella pneumophila* in protozoa from hospital plumbing systems. Res. Microbiol. **142:** 677–685.
19. ALARY, M. & J. R. JOLY. 1992. Factors contributing to the contamination of hospital water distribution systems by Legionellae. J. Infect. Dis. **165:** 565–569.
20. KISLAK, J. W., T. C. EICKHOFF & M. FINLAND. 1969. Hospital-acquired infections and antibiotic usage in the Boston City Hospital—January 1964. New Engl. J. Med. **271:** 834–835.
21. SCHLABERG, D. R. 1981. Evolution of antimicrobial resistance and nosocomial infection. Am. J. Med. **70:** 445.
22. WEINSTEIN, R. A. & S. A. KABINS. 1981. Antimicrobial resistance. Am. J. Med. **70:** 449.
23. LIVORNESE, L. L., S. DIAS, C. SAMEL, et al. 1992. Hospital-acquired infection with vancomycin-resistant *Enterococcus faecium* transmitted by electronic thermometers. Ann. Intern. Med. **117:** 112–116.
24. HALEY, R. W., D. H. CULVER, W. M. MORGAN, et al. 1985. Increasing recognition of infectious diseases in U.S. hospitals through increased use of diagnostic tests, 1970–76. Am. J. Epidemiol. **121:** 168–181.
25. ANONYMOUS. 1971. How the septicemia trail led to the IV bottle cap. Hosp. Pract. 35–45, 151–154.
26. BLOCK, A. B., P. T. DAVIDSON, et al. 1991. Tuberculosis in patients with the Human Immunodeficiency Virus infection. New Engl. J. Med. **324:** 1644–1650.
27. PEARSON, M. L., J. A. JEREB, T. R. FRIEDEN, et al. 1992. Nosocomial transmission of multidrug-resistant *Mycobacterium tuberculosis*. Ann. Intern. Med. **117:** 191–196.
28. EDLIN, B. R., J. I. TOKARS, M. H. GRIECO, et al. 1992. An outbreak of multidrug-resistant tuberculosis among hospitalized patients with the acquired immunodeficiency syndrome. New Engl. J. Med. **326:** 1514–1521.
29. DOOLEY, S., B. EDLIN, M. PEARSON, et al. 1992. Multidrug resistant nosocomial tuberculosis outbreaks in HIV-infected persons. Presentation to the VIII International Conference on AIDS, Amsterdam, 1992.
30. RAAD, I., W. COSTERTON, I. V. SABHARWA, et al. 1993. Ultrastructural analysis of indwelling vascular catheters: A quantitative relationship between luminal colonization and duration of placement. J. Infect. Dis. **168:** 400–407.
31. PALLARES, R., M. C. PUJOL, C. PENA, et al. 1993. Cephalosporins as risk factors for nosocomial *Enterococcus faecalis* bacteremia. Arch. Intern. Med. **153:** 1581–1586.
32. STAMM, W. E. 1981. Nosocomial infections: Etiologic changes, therapeutic challenges. Hosp. Pract. (August): 75–88.
33. NATIONAL NOSOCOMIAL INFECTIONS SURVEILLANCE SYSTEM. 1991. Nosocomial infections rates for interhospital comparison: Limitations and possible solutions. Infect. Control Hosp. Epidemiol. **112:** 609–621.
34. OLSON, M., M. O'CONNOR & M. D. SCHWARTZ. 1984. Surgical wound infections: A 5-year prospective study of 20,193 wounds at the Minneapolis VA Medical Center. Ann. Surg. **199:** 253–259.
35. CRUISE, P. J. E. 1981. Wound infection surveillance. Rev. Infect. Dis. **3:** 734–737.
36. HALEY, R. W., D. H. CULVER, W. M. MORGAN, et al. 1985. Identifying patients at high risk of surgical wound infection. Am. J. Epidemiol. **121:** 206–215.

37. STINE, T. M., A. A. HARRIS, S. LEVIN, et al. 1987. A pseudo-epidemic due to atypical mycobacteria in a hospital water supply. JAMA **258:** 809–811.
38. HARKNESS, G. A., D. W. BENTLEY & K. J. BOGHMANN. 1990. Risk factors for nosocomial pneumonia in the elderly. Am. J. Med. **89:** 457–463.
39. FISCHL, M. A., R. B. UTTAMCHANDANI, G. L. DAIKOS, et al. 1992. An outbreak of tuberculosis caused by multiple-drug-resistant tubercle bacilli among patients with HIV infection. Ann. Intern. Med. **117:** 177–183.
40. NEU, H. C. 1992. The crisis in antibiotic resistance. Science **257:** 1064–1073.
41. JARVIS, B. Personal communication, Centers for Disease Control, 1993.
42. MAST, E. E., H. W. HARMON, S. GRAVENSTEIN, et al. 1991. Emergence and possible transmission of amantadine-resistant viruses during nursing home outbreaks of influenza A (H_3N_2). Am. J. Epidemiol. **134:** 988–997.
43. CENTERS FOR DISEASE CONTROL. 1990. Summary of the Agency for Toxic Substances and Disease Registry Report to Congress. Morbidity and Mortality Weekly Report **39:** 822–824.
44. HU, D. J., M. A. KANE & D. L. HEYMANN. 1991. Transmission of HIV, hepatitis B virus and other bloodborne pathogens in health care settings: A review of risk factors and guidelines for protection. Bull. WHO **69:** 623–630.
45. THOMAS, D. L., S. H. FACTOR, G. D. KELEN, et al. 1993. Viral hepatitis in health care personnel at the Johns Hopkins Hospital. Arch. Intern. Med. **153:** 1705–1712.
46. KENT, G. P., J. BRONDUM, R. A. KEENLYSIDE, et al. 1988. A large outbreak of acupuncture-associated hepatitis B. Am. J. Epidemiol. **127:** 591–598.
47. SHAW, F. E., C. L. BARRETT, R. HAMM, et al. 1986. Lethal outbreak of Hepatitis B in a dental practice. JAMA **255:** 3261–3264.
48. CENTERS FOR DISEASE CONTROL. 1993. Nosocomial enterococci resistant to vancomycin—United States, 1988–1993. Morbidity and Mortality Weekly Report **42:** 597.
49. FRIEDEN, T. R., S. S. MUNSIFF, D. E. LOW, et al. 1993. Emergence of vancomycin-resistant enterococci in New York City. Lancet **342:** 76–79.
50. LECLAIR, J. M., J. FREEMAN, B. F. SULLIVAN, et al. 1987. Prevention of nosocomial respiratory syncytial virus infections through compliance with glove and gown isolation precautions. New Engl. J. Med. **317:** 329–334.
51. COHEN, M. L. 1992. Epidemiology of drug resistance: Implications for a post-antimicrobial era. Science **257:** 1050–1055.
52. GENTRY, L. O. 1991. Bacterial resistance. Orthop. Clin. North Am. **22:** 379–388.
53. PEREZ-TRALLERO, E., M. URBIETA, C. L. LOPATEGUI, et al. 1993. Antibiotics in veterinary medicine and public health. Lancet **342:** 1371–1372; ENDTZ, H. P., G. J. RUIJS, B. VANKLINGEREN, et al. 1991. Quinolone resistance in *Campylobacter* isolated from man and poultry following introduction of fluoroquinolones in veterinary medicine. J. Antimicrob. Chemother. **27:** 199–208.
54. The NIAID reported the first such case on December 9, 1993 in an individual with recurrent genital herpes.

The Environment, Remote Sensing, and Malaria Control

DONALD R. ROBERTS

Department of Preventive Medicine/Biometrics
Uniformed Services University of the Health Sciences
Bethesda, Maryland 20814

MARIO H. RODRIGUEZ

Director, Center for Malaria Research
Tapachula, Mexico

INTRODUCTION

There is increasing interest in environmental protection to conserve ecological processes, preserve genetic diversity and sustain use of natural ecosystems. In public health, concern for the environment focuses on contributions of the environment to emergence of diseases, including the arthropod-borne diseases. In the case of environmental protection, the goal is to prevent human intrusions and modifications of natural environments for the primary purpose of living resource conservation. In efforts to protect public health, the primary goal should be to prevent human intrusion and modification of pristine environments in order to protect human populations from extensions of pathogens from natural foci[a] of disease.[1] In each case, protection of the natural environment is emphasized. The International Council of Scientific Unions and the International Geosphere-Biosphere Program emphasize the need for global data and information systems to address environmental and conservation concerns.[2] Among health professionals, the need is also recognized for global monitoring and information systems on environmental issues and emerging diseases.[3,4]

Improved communications and space-science technologies, such as remote sensing, offer hope of new, more holistic approaches to surveying, monitoring and controlling the arthropod-borne diseases. The promise of these technologies has surfaced at a time when global and national efforts at vector and disease control are faltering, for example *Aedes aegypti* and malaria, respectively.

REMOTE SENSING TECHNOLOGY

Remotely sensed data of various types and of various scales can be used to elucidate and predict the temporal and spatial distributions of disease

---

[a] Natural foci of disease are environments, undisturbed by human activities, where vectors, pathogens and recipients of infection (vertebrate hosts) reside.

vectors. Low resolution data (*e.g.*, US National Oceanic and Atmospheric Administration satellite data) have been used to plot normalized difference vegetation indexes (NDVIs) indicative of where or when vectors of Rift Valley fever or African trypanosomiasis might occur[5,6] (see FIG. 14 in REMOTE SENSING SECTION). Such low resolution data are useful for general studies of broad zones or regions. Higher resolution data from Landsat or SPOT satellites can be used to study the temporal and spatial distributions of disease vectors in association with small earth surface features, rice fields, villages, rivers, *etc.*[7–9] (see FIG. 13 in REMOTE SENSING SECTION). Work with high resolution data can take advantage of increasingly specific knowledge of the vector-environmental associations. In other words, information on how different surface features will impact the local presence and abundance of the vector species can be used in interpretations of satellite data. Consequently, background studies on the relationships of the environment to disease-vector-host associations are needed for appropriate use of remote sensing technology.

Background studies should be designed to detect, identify and analyze the environmental determinants of disease vectors in the real world; define the scale for detecting, identifying and analyzing environmental determinants with satellite data; and finally, validate analyses of satellite data with *in situ* (ground truth) data (FIG. 1). The results of these studies can be used to

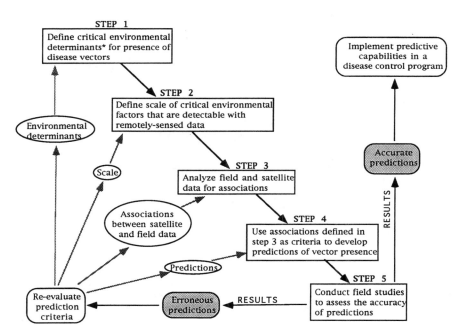

FIGURE 1. A paradigm of required studies leading to applications of remote sensing data to predict the spatial distributions of disease vectors. * Indicates earth surface features, *e.g.*, rivers, ponds, pastures, forest edge that influence the presence and abundance of disease vectors.

prepare and execute regional schemes of disease and vector control, predict future events, and plan and develop projects for preventing disease risks. The background studies' data are derived from field studies, and should be amenable to computer manipulation. For many other categories of background data, remote sensing is the only cost-effective means of acquiring data to study, monitor, and hopefully, contain or mitigate existing and emerging vector and disease problems.

Arthropod-borne diseases in particular are strongly associated with certain environmental conditions. Indeed, the principal environmental conditions, such as temperature and rainfall, regulate the geographical and seasonal distribution of many arthropod-borne diseases. Recognition of the interactions between humans, disease vectors and the environment date back far into the history of infectious disease research. The relationships were formalized in Pavlovsky's research in Russia and his writings on landscape epidemiology.[1] Pavlovsky noted that arthropod-borne disease exists when there are specific climate, vegetation, soil, and favorable microclimate in the places where vectors, donors and recipients of infection take shelter. Furthermore, he noted that disease circulation takes place only when the environmental conditions are favorable. Examples of diseases that are regulated by environmental conditions include leishmaniasis, African trypanosomiasis, malaria and others.

REMOTE SENSING TECHNOLOGY AND MALARIA CONTROL

Today malaria continues to be the leading cause of morbidity and mortality in humans throughout the tropics, with an estimated 270 million people affected. Despite efforts to eradicate the disease, it has made a dramatic resurgence within the last 20 years. Furthermore, morbidity and mortality from malaria are at almost unprecedented levels.[10]

Application of remote sensing to study and assist in the control of malaria and other arthropod-borne diseases is the subject of a National Aeronautics and Space Administration (NASA)-sponsored study.[11] The NASA project[b] is designed to demonstrate the use of remote sensing technologies to develop predictive models of malaria vector abundance on a local to regional scale.

Human malaria is an anthroponosis, as such it is only found in association with human populations. It is not an emerging disease or a disease associated with natural foci, as defined by Pavlovsky.[1] Indeed, malaria foci only occur when humans, vectors and the malaria parasites occur together. However,

---

[b] Participants in the NASA-sponsored project include the following individuals and organizations: Louisa Beck, Sheri Whitney and Mike Spanner, NASA Ames Research Center, Moffett Field, California; Eliska Reimankova and Robert Washino, University of California, Davis, CA; Mario H. Rodriguez, Americo Rodriguez and Juan Hernandez, Centro de Investigacion de Paludismo, Tapachula, Mexico; Jack Paris, California State University, Fresno, CA; Carl Hacker, School of Public Health, University of Texas in Houston; LLeweLLyn J. Legters, Donald Roberts and Sylvie Manguin, Uniformed Services University of the Health Sciences, Bethesda, MD.

since malaria is transmitted by *Anopheles* mosquitoes, human malaria is associated with natural environments to the same extent that the mosquito vectors are associated with natural environments.

The NASA project was conducted in three phases and we are currently in phase III. The first phase was conducted on population abundance of *Anopheles freeborni* in rice fields of the Central Valley of California. The first phase of work tested the concept that remote sensing and ground surveillance data incorporated into a geographic information system (GIS) could be used to predict the temporal and spatial occurrences of *A. freeborni* larval populations. In brief, we found that early developing rice fields (defined by remotely sensed data) in closest proximity to livestock pastures produced greater densities of larvae than more slowly developing fields located further from pastures. The remote sensing reflectance data and GIS measurements of rice field-distances from pastures were adequate to predict nearly 90% of the high-producing fields almost 2 months before peak densities of *Anopheles* larvae.[7]

Phase II was conducted in the state of Chiapas, Mexico in collaboration with the Centro De Investigaciones de Paludismo in Tapachula. The general approach for Phase II studies has been described previously.[12] The first priority for Phase II studies was to improve understanding of the biology of the primary malaria vector species *A. albimanus,* on the Coastal Plain. Initial research was directed at defining the relationships of *A. albimanus* larval abundance with a variety of environmental variables. The relationships of the dominant aquatic plants with the presence and abundance of larvae were particularly germane to our research interests. In phase II research, habitats were defined by dominant plants; habitats were then clumped (by use of cluster analysis) into habitat-types. Habitat-types were then used to characterize the larger vegetation units. The vegetation units, unlike habitats and habitat-types, were generally discernible with remotely sensed data. A habitat was defined as a body of water with a dominant vegetation, for example *Eichhornia*. The habitat-types were defined strictly on botanical and limnological parameters. Analysis of variance was employed to investigate relationships among habitat-types and the density of larvae. These studies showed that selected growth forms of plants contributed positively, neutrally, or negatively to the presence and abundance of *A. albimanus* larvae. Finally, the larger vegetation units, which were detectable with remotely sensed data, were characterized with certain mixes of habitat-types and larval densities.[13-16]

In conducting current phase II research, a GIS was developed that includes digitized map attribute data, geolocated and classified remotely sensed data, and field surveillance data. A standardized program of surveillance with UV-updraft light traps and ground verification of breeding sites surrounding villages was used to obtain the *in situ* data. The satellite data are used to identify villages and classify vegetation units surrounding villages. Relying on previously defined associations of vegetation units with *A. albimanus* larval abundance, remotely sensed data were used to define the associations of vegetation units and individual villages with high or low densities of *A. albimanus* mosquitoes.[8]

TABLE 1. Studies Conducted on the Uses of Remote Sensing to Predict the Spatial Distribution of *Anopheles* Mosquitoes in California, Mexico and Belize

Studies	California	Mexico	Belize
Step 1: Define environmental determinants		X	X
Step 2: Define scale		X	X
Step 3: Define associations between remote sensing and field data	X	X	
Step 4: Develop predictions about spatial distribution of vectors		In process	X
Step 5: Assess accuracy of predictions		In process	X

Source: Wood *et al.*,[7] Beck *et al.*,[8] and Roberts *et al.*[9]

In a separate program of research,[e] remote sensing and cartographic data were employed to predict localities of high and low malaria vector densities during the dry season along the Hummingbird Highway in Belize (see color FIG. 13). Predictions were based on environmental criteria derived from two years of field studies. Predictions were developed by remote sensing specialists with no previous experience in Belize and no field data. The criteria for predictions related to presence of waterways, elevation, amount of forest between houses and selected waterways, and presence of humans. Once predictions were developed, field surveys were conducted in April and May, 1993 to verify presence and abundance of vectors. This blind test was the first time that remotely sensed data have been used to develop highly accurate prospective predictions about the spatial distributions of malaria vectors.[9] Although the SPOT multispectral satellite data employed in this test were from 1990, still the data interpretations relating to ground cover and sites of houses and human activities were generally accurate. While single houses with thatch roofs could not be detected, there were other characters indicative of human activities, and thus presence of humans.

Studies in California, Mexico and Belize differed in terms of approaches as defined by the paradigm in FIGURE 1 (TABLE 1). Field work conducted by Dr. Robert K. Washino on *A. freeborni* in California precluded the need for preliminary field studies (step 1). Additionally, the determination of scale for integrating remote sensing and field data (step 2) was fixed by size of the sampling unit, *i.e.*, rice field. Studies were performed to define associations between spectral and *in situ* data;[7] but no tests of predictions were performed (steps 4 and 5). In Mexico, extensive field studies (step 1) were conducted to define associations of *A. albimanus* with environmental determinants.[13-16] These studies were followed by a detailed study of associations between remotely sensed and *in situ* data (step 3).[8] Based on the latter study, predic-

[e] Eliska Reimankova, University of California, Davis, CA; Jack Paris, California State University, Fresno, CA; LLeweLLyn J. Legters, Donald Roberts and Sylvie Manguin, Uniformed Services University of the Health Sciences, Bethesda, MD; Jorge Polanco, Ministry of Health, Belize City, Belize.

tions of vector abundance in different villages will soon be developed (step 4) and tested with field data (step 5). For studies in Belize, extensive field studies (step 1) were conducted to define associations of *A. pseudopunctipennis* populations with environmental determinants.[15,17] Specific environmental determinants that were detectable with multispectral satellite data were identified. Since we were very confident of the predictive power of these environmental determinants for presence of *A. pseudopunctipennis* mosquitoes, no study of associations between remotely sensed and *in situ* data (step 3) was conducted. Consequently we were able to skip step 3 and complete steps 4 and 5 by developing predictions and testing the predictions with field survey data.

SUMMARY

Results of studies in California, Mexico and Belize demonstrate the value of remote sensing technology for studying vector-borne diseases. These studies have also shown that it is necessary to fully define the environmental factors associated with the presence of vectors and disease transmission, and to be able to detect these environmental factors with image data. These studies, and other published reports,[5,6] are demonstrating many potential uses of remotely sensed data in managing and targeting vector and disease control measures.

REFERENCES

1. PAVLOVSKY, E. N. 1960. Natural Nidality of Transmissible Diseases with Special Reference to the Landscape Epidemiology of Zooanthroponoses. Frederick K. Plous, Jr., translator and Norman D. Levine, editor. Urbana and London: University of Illinois Press (1966). 261 pp.
2. BARRETT, E. C. & L. F. CURTIS. 1992. Introduction to Environmental Remote Sensing. New York: Chapman and Hall. 426 pp.
3. LEGTERS, L. J., L. H. BRINK & E. T. TAKAFUJI. 1993. Are we prepared for a viral epidemic emergency? *In* Emerging Viruses: 269–282. S. S. Morse, Ed. New York: Oxford University Press.
4. HENDERSON, D. A. 1993. Surveillance systems and intergovernmental cooperation. *In* Emerging Viruses. S. S. Morse, Ed.: 283–289. New York: Oxford University Press.
5. LINTHICUM, K. J., C. L. BAILEY, F. G. DAVIES & C. J. TUCKER. 1987. Detection of Rift Valley fever viral activity in Kenya by satellite remote sensing imagery. Science **235:** 1656–1659.
6. ROGERS, D. J. & S. E. RANDOLPH. 1991. Mortality rates and population density of tsetse flies correlated with satellite imagery. Nature **351:** 739–741.
7. WOOD, B., R. WASHINO, L. BECK, K. HIBBARD, M. PITCAIRN, D. ROBERTS, E. REJMANKOVA, J. PARIS, C. HACKER, J. SALUTE, P. SEBESTA & L. LEGTERS. 1991. Distinguishing high and low anopheline-producing rice fields using remote sensing and GIS technologies. Prev. Vet. Med. **11:** 277–288.
8. BECK, L. R., M. H. RODRIGUEZ, S. W. DISTER, A. D. RODRIGUEZ, E. REJMANKOVA, A. ULLOA, R. A. MEZA, D. R. ROBERTS, J. F. PARIS, M. A. SPANNER, R. K. WASHINO, C. HACKER & L. J. LEGTERS. 1993. Remote sensing as a landscape epidemiological tool to identify villages at high risk for malaria transmission. Am. J. Trop. Med. Hyg. In press.
9. ROBERTS, D. R., J. F. PARIS, S. MANGUIN, R. E. HARBACH, R. WOODRUFF, E.

REJMANKOVA, J. POLANCO, B. WULLSCHLEGER & L. J. LEGTERS. Predictions of malaria vector distributions in Belize based on multispectral satellite data. Am. J. Trop. Med. Hyg. Submitted.

10. INSTITUTE OF MEDICINE. 1991. Malaria. Obstacles and Opportunities. S. Oaks, Jr., V. Mitchell, G. Pearson & C. Carpenter, Eds. Washington, D.C.: National Academy Press. 309 pp.

11. AMES RESEARCH CENTER. 1988. A Project Plan for Vector-Borne Disease Predictive Modeling (Project Di-Mod). Moffett Field, CA: Ames Research Center.

12. ROBERTS, D., M. RODRIGUEZ, E. REJMANKOVA, K. POPE, H. SAVAGE, A. RODRIGUEZ-RAMIREZ, B. WOOD, J. SALUTE & L. LEGTERS. 1991. Overview of field studies for the application of remote sensing to the study of malaria transmission in Tapachula, Mexico. Prev. Vet. Med. **11:** 269–275.

13. SAVAGE, H., E. REJMANKOVA, J. ARREDONDO-JIMENEZ, D. ROBERTS & M. RODRIGUEZ. 1990. Limnological and botanical characterization of larval habitats of two primary malaria vectors, *Anopheles albimanus* and *Anopheles pseudopunctipennis,* in coastal areas of Chiapas state, Mexico. J. Am. Mosquito Control Assoc. **6:** 612–620.

14. REJMANKOVA, E., H. SAVAGE, M. REJMANEK, J. ARREDONDO-JIMENEZ & D. ROBERTS. 1991. Multivariate analysis of relationships between habitats, environmental factors and occurrence of anopheline mosquito larvae *Anopheles albimanus* and *A. pseudopunctipennis* in southern Chiapas, Mexico. J. Appl. Ecol. **28:** 827–841.

15. REJMANKOVA, E., H. SAVAGE, M. RODRIGUEZ, D. ROBERTS & M. REJMANEK. 1992. Aquatic vegetation as a basis for classification of *Anopheles albimanus* Weidemann (Diptera : Culicidae) larval habitats. Envir. Entomol. **21**(3): 598–603.

16. RODRIGUEZ, A., M. RODRIGUEZ, J. HERNANDEZ, R. MEZA, E. REJMANKOVA, H. SAVAGE, D. ROBERTS, K. POPE & L. LEGTERS. 1993. Dynamics of population densities and vegetation associations of *Anopheles albimanus* larvae in a coastal area of southern Chiapas, Mexico. J. Am. Mosquito Control Assoc. **9**(1): 46–57.

17. REJMANKOVA, E., D. ROBERTS, R. HARBACH, J. PECOR, E. PEYTON, S. MANGUIN, R. KREIG, J. POLANCO & L. LEGTERS. 1993. Environmental and regional determinants of *Anopheles* (Diptera: Culicidae) larval distribution in Belize, Central America. Environ. Ent. **22**(5): 978–992.

Part C. Surveillance and Funding

LINCOLN CHEN: I think probably the biggest challenge for detection and surveillance is cost. Everything we have said during this workshop has a price tag. The remaining questions are: How do you prioritize? What do you do at what cost to give you the highest returns? It is necessary, in my opinion, to discuss all the suggestions made during the workshop in relation to cost and cost effectiveness.

I want to add that, as someone who worked in the population-based longitudinal surveillance system, I don't think that we ever picked up any new diseases from a routine system. The workers in the surveillance system were not sensitized to look for something unusual. They were routinized, indeed.

ROBERT SHOPE: We have some experience in trying to raise money to carry out certain activities such as serum banks and long-term surveillance. Lincoln is correct that one has to put a price tag on everything we are doing. I would say it more practically. You have to find somebody who will give you the money to do the research you have planned. The solution that we figured out after several failures is to design a research program, which somebody wants to support along with surveillance. Surveillance could be a component of that research. Under such circumstances I think that it is practical to go out and obtain money.

I can give you an example. The army in Thailand has been doing a hepatitis A vaccine trial. They followed a cohort of 40,000 Thai children for a period of at least 2 years, maybe longer. In addition, as a component of the hepatitis A vaccine trial, they have done a general disease survey. In other words, they did case finding among the 40,000 Thai children. They took acute and convalescent sera from each child who missed 3 or more days of school and kept the records of the results of the survey. They are now able to go back and to identify other disease incidence rates in cases where the school absence was not caused by hepatitis A. For instance, they have identified the incidence of dengue fever in that population. I think there are similar opportunities in the United States and overseas where such a set-up could be used.

PAUL EPSTEIN: Keeping in mind what Lincoln charged us with, cost effectiveness, one of the three areas that Ralph presented for monitoring emerging diseases was strengthening general surveillance of simple sentinel populations. I think Laurie's suggestion on prison populations is excellent. The third area you listed was sentinel areas or critical strategic sites. I would like to explore that for a moment. We know that indicator species are being followed by some "group." For example, rodents are being followed by ecologists that health epidemiologists are not necessarily in touch with. Critical regions are also being followed by environmentalists using remote sensing and GIS (geographic information system) work. In the Amazon, for example, satellite images indicate extensive road building in Amazonia. While the area is "only" 7% deforested, the ecological effects of fragmentation and "edge effects" add another 15%, in terms of the impact on diversity. This is an area where malaria is blossoming.

DONALD ROBERTS: I would like to comment on the remote sensing activity that can fit into this discussion. One of the obstacles that we have encountered in the attempt to use remote sensing and GIS in public health has been the belief that this technology is a very expensive toy. I would like to emphasize that remote sensing is really not that expensive. Within the program of research we carried out in Belize, the minor cost factor was the remote sensing work. The field research was, in terms of a limited budget, very expensive. You could actually buy a very sophisticated software package that would run on a 486 computer for $3,000. A remote sensing image from the spot satellite system (a single scene of 60 × 60 kilometers) would cost $1,500.

The cost question should be discussed more in relation to the usefulness of this technology in public health research and the possible applications that should be made of the technology.

Basic Elements in a Conceptual Framework for New and Resurgent Disease

Introduction—Conceptual Framework Section[a]

RICHARD LEVINS

Department of Population and International Health
Harvard School of Public Health
665 Huntington Avenue
Boston, Massachusetts 02115

During the workshop we could recognize an imbalance between the contributions from the social sciences and the natural sciences. This imbalance was never really resolved. In the plenary sessions and the workshop discussions we made several steps towards a coherent approach to epidemiology, but we could not achieve the basic elements for an unified approach to disease. Such unified approach to disease would be built on the basis of transdisciplinary research.

We recognized the importance of integrating social and biological aspects of the disease process in our discussions, and we identified key areas and problems in relation to an approach to new diseases where such integration is still missing. Especially the research on the "human factor" of diseases emergence requires strong interactions and collaboration between different disciplines of science, crossing the boundaries between social sciences and natural and medical sciences.

One reason for the difficulty we had during the workshop establishing an integrated approach to disease is related to a lack of clarity about the definition of a conceptual framework for this approach. The comments regarding an integrated conceptual framework for disease emergence were expressed on different levels of abstraction, reflecting either different processes in the evolution of new and resurgent diseases or different levels of understanding and modeling of disease evolution.

In the following I will identify some basic prerequisites for a conceptual framework. The elements of a conceptual framework include:

- a statement of the problem,
- the goals,
- the objects of study,

---

[a] This introduction is based on written contributions to the issue of a conceptual framework for the research on new diseases which were submitted by the participants of the workshop.

- the subject of the study, and
- the means of the study.

The statement of the problem should start off with rejecting the model of an epidemiological transition. The model of an epidemiological transition supports the belief in a secular decrease in infectious disease to their complete replacement by other medical problems. Contrary to this belief, we would characterize the present period in a different way. We are living in a period of extremely large scale changes in society, the physical environment, populations, pathogens, knowledge, and also in the resources socially made available for coping with these problems. Therefore, we are living in a period in which increased encounters with both familiar and unfamiliar diseases are very likely to occur.

The second element of a conceptual framework is our goals. The obvious, immediate goal is reducing infection. But, focusing on infection is not enough. We are more directly concerned with disease and reduction of infection is a surrogate for reduction of disease. We want to reduce the vulnerability of populations and we want to reduce our own uncertainty about future disease emergence. This is a permanent activity. Finally, it should be our goal to seek for understanding of the process of coping with disease, the areas of our own competence and blindness and the obstacles we face in trying to deepen that understanding.

The third element of a conceptual framework is choosing the objects of study. Again, we could identify some immediate objects of interest. These immediately given objects of interest might be particular infections or particular diseases. Studies of the pathogen, of classes of pathogens, and of hosts, both human and non-human, have to be added to the list of objects of interest in a conceptual framework to confront the emergence of disease. In addition to these objects we have to move to the study of qualities or processes, like vulnerability, evolution, population range, the expansion and contraction of populations and our own activity.

The fourth element in a conceptual framework is the subject of the study. Who is behind the discussion of recommendations, the design of intervention strategies, or the distribution of money for medical or anthropological research?

I think, we realize now, that health is too serious a matter to be left to the medical professions and the public health professions alone. At this workshop we came together from a variety of different disciplines and we could recognize the process of the formation of a new health community. This health community will bring medical, veterinary, and plant pathologists, evolutionists, ecologists and social scientists, climatologists and marine biologists together to face a commonly perceived threat—endemic infectious diseases. An important part of that process is to establish language correlation, by defining terms that would be used very differently in our different spheres of expertise.

The fifth element is a discussion of means, including concept clarification, and the development of theoretical premises for an approach to infectious disease emergence. We recognize that teaching, preparing people to carry out surveillance or development programs is crucial. We can not simply decide we will look for pathogens without considering who will do the looking. How can we be sure to have a good chance of finding pathogens and recognizing them?

In the face of our own ignorance in dealing with the unknown I think we need a mixed strategy. After we have made our best guess as to what needs to be done, we have also to consider what might happen if we are wrong in our guess and our decision. Prior to the realization of health programs we should think about alternatives. What else might be helpful to cope with a problem, with a disease outbreak?

We need a mixed strategy that combines levels, disciplines and approaches, short term and long term, and theoretical, experimental and observational ways of exploring.

Challenging Complexity

Conceptual Issues in an Approach to New Disease

IRINA ECKARDT[a]

Museum of Comparative Zoology
Harvard University
26 Oxford St.
Cambridge, Massachusetts 02138

and

Department of Population and International Health
Harvard School of Public Health
665 Huntington Ave.
Boston, Massachusetts 02115

Patricia Rosenfield discussed in her paper "The potential of transdisciplinary research for sustaining and extending linkages between the health and social sciences" the importance of the formation of conceptual frameworks in the design of transdisciplinary projects:

> Representatives of different disciplines are encouraged to transcend their separate conceptual, theoretical, and methodological orientations in order to develop a shared approach to the research, building on a common conceptual framework.[1]

A "common conceptual framework" is based on the definition and analysis of research problems in the development of new approaches. These new approaches should "represent the historical and present-day reality in which health problems are situated" [1] more closely.

Without any doubt, the project to explore the evolution of new and resurgent disease aims at the development of a new conceptual framework within health sciences. In constructing such a framework clarification has to be achieved in regard to the following points:

- structure of the framework,
- disciplines of science which will contribute to research and modeling,
- theoretical and epistemological premises which have to be defined, and
- possible connections between theoretical research, practical or applied research, and modeling.

The design of a new conceptual framework for the research on "disease in evolution" is an integrative part of ongoing research. In the process of exploring the complex evolution of new and resurgent disease theoretical and episte-

---

[a] Address correspondence to Dr. Eckardt at Falkenberger Ch.132(0502), Berlin D-13057 Germany.

mological questions will arise simultaneously and new premises will be formulated. The important aspect is to ask such questions and, by doing so, to confront the limitations of our current understanding, our current systems of terms, and our methods to model disease emergence.

I will define some theoretical premises for the project on the evolution of new and resurgent disease in this paper. But first, I should clarify the difference between a conceptual framework (the term used by Patricia Rosenfield) and a theoretical framework (see discussion on integrated epidemiology, Part B in this section). This differentiation marks and separates different levels of abstraction and generalization in the present enterprise to understand complex evolutionary processes, like the evolution of new disease.[2]

The development of new theoretical frameworks in science requires fundamental changes in science policy, science methodology, and science sociology. Theoretical frameworks are changing as they confront the limits of present scientific techniques, methods and theories.

The growing influence of evolutionary thinking in several scientific disciplines, including the humanities, characterizes the development of a new theoretical framework in this century. The framework of evolutionary thinking has not only been applied in the majority of biological disciplines,[3] but also in physics,[4] ecology,[5] sociology,[6] and other scientific fields.[7] Different single theories and concepts describing and identifying different evolutionary processes in nature, societies, and artificial life[b] have been developed within this framework. Thus, a new theoretical framework is not based on one "true" theory exclusively, but originates in the process of theory formations. Theory formations consist of concepts and theories which have been developed relatively simultaneously. Such theory formations cover a wide range of disciplines in science and lead to the design of new subfields.[9]

In the terms of philosophy of science, the construction of new theoretical frameworks marks **paradigm changes in science.**[10] The completion of paradigm changes can be recognized only in retrospection.

The current, intensive research on complex processes in nature, society and artificial life, for example, might result in the construction of a new theoretical framework for future research.[11] The framework of evolutionary thinking would then be incorporated in this new framework.

In the development of new conceptual frameworks the focus is laid on the definition and identification of **selected** research problems and the development of new approaches in order to solve these problems. For example, the models of disease emergence which have been developed according to our present understanding, the concepts which have been constructed on the basis of such models, and the different efforts to develop new methodological and theoretical premises (see for instance the paper on cellular automata by

---

[b] Artificial life in this context describes a new form of reality which cannot be understood as a simple reflection and model of processes and structures in nature.[8]

Kiszewski and Spielman, pp. 249–259 in this volume) will contribute to a theory on the evolution of new and resurgent disease. And, as different researchers are working on this problem, it is very likely that different, alternative and complementary, theories and concepts on disease evolution will emerge.

Conceptual frameworks are essential elements in the development of theoretical frameworks. Changes in theoretical frameworks will influence the essential norms of thinking and modeling in a given period of the development of science. As a result, a new theoretical framework will change the value systems by which scientific truth is defined. The development of conceptual frameworks will influence our knowledge and understanding of a **specific** scientific problem, like the emergence of new disease, and in a more **general** way the existing theoretical frameworks, like the framework of evolutionary thinking.[12]

The following discussion contributes to the design of a conceptual framework for understanding the complex evolution of new and resurgent infectious disease. Despite all modern and advanced technologies, drugs, pesticides, health surveillance systems, and the various international activities of different health organizations, it is currently not possible to predict and anticipate the emergence and virulence of new pathogens. The health sciences are still limited to reacting only after new epidemics occurred.

Thus, the research problem on which our efforts are focused can be identified with the question: Why have the health sciences been caught by surprise with new or reemerging disease until today? And further: What are the major theoretical, conceptual, and methodological problems which have to be solved in order to develop techniques, models, and information networks to surpass the boundaries of our current understanding of the emergence of new infectious disease? The most important assumption in exploring this research problem—that the emergence of new and known infectious disease is a **complex evolutionary process in which several natural and social processes are interacting**—implies not only several demands for the development of an adequate research strategy, but identifies the theoretical framework within which this new concept will arise—the framework of evolutionary thinking.

Looking back in the history of health sciences, specialization has been a characteristic feature, determining the course of disease prevention, surveillance and cure. Specialization of health sciences has been accompanied by the dominance of a bio-medical conceptual framework for all health-related problems.

The following features are implied in the bio-medical conceptual framework:

- the focus on causal explanations and the development of different concepts of causality—unidirectional causes, the differentiation between contributing and component causes and necessary and sufficient causes, and webs of causes;[13]

- the separation of internal from external causes of diseases—pathogens which are invading bodies and causing diseases; and
- the differentiation of different organ systems according to their exposure to infections.

The development of microbiology and genetics, the improvement of known technologies, and the introduction of new ones, led to the belief that with the steady progress of health sciences the burden of infectious disease in humans would be erased from this planet.

If we were able to identify pathogens with the help of modern technologies and microbiology, and if we were able to map their genetic compositions, we would know our "enemies" and we could control them.

If we were able to treat people with powerful drugs, like antibiotics, and if we were able to fight disease vectors with pesticides and other chemicals we could make the world a better place and prevent great pandemics.

And then came Lassa fever (1969), Ebola hemorrhagic fevers (1976), and several severe cholera epidemics.

Poverty has been correlated with the burden of infectious disease for as long as we have records of great pandemics.[14] Nevertheless, the belief in the power of modern health sciences was accompanied by the belief in progressive economic development, which would provide opportunities for better sanitation systems, better nutrition, better education, and better health care, even in third world countries. Pandemics would decrease with the increase in the world's wealth.

And than came AIDS (1981)

Drastic changes in existing patterns of social relations among and within nations, breakdowns of societies, and population migration have been determinants of outbreaks of infectious diseases in all parts of the world. Moreover, the destruction of our natural environment supports the emergence of new pathogens and the contact between humans and pathogens.

And before AIDS came Lyme disease (1975) and Legionnaire's disease (1978), and afterwards came cyanobacteria-like bodies causing diarrhea (1990),[e] and hantavirus pulmonary syndrome (1993).

Obviously, there has been a discrepancy between the expectations and beliefs and the real ongoing processes of emergence and reemergence of infectious disease in all parts of the world. The knowledge and data available on the history and evolution of infectious disease in plants,[16] animals and humans[17] has not been used to bring the conceptual framework closer to the reality of infectious disease emergence. The collected data and facts about epidemics and pandemics provide a basis for the development of a systematic

---

[e] What were initially described as "cyanobacteria-like bodies" have now been identified as cyclospora.[15]

approach to new and resurgent disease. Further, the development of new models of complex evolutionary processes and the theoretical premises of these models enable us to combine the systematic approach with an evolutionary basis. Mainly owing to the specialization of health sciences and the traditional bio-medical framework this development of a **systematic (evolutionary) approach** has been delayed in health sciences.

Frederick Murphy summarized in his paper "New, emerging and reemerging infectious diseases" most of these diseases reported during the last decades. Referring only to two "case-in-point" examples Murphy described, the limitations of the common framework in health sciences can be shown. Legionellosis was first identified in the 1976 outbreak in Philadelphia. As in all other cases of new or reemerging diseases the search for the responsible virus or, in this case bacteria, began. The results were very surprising:

> As efforts were made to sanitize such water sources, it was found that the Legionella bacteria live and grow inside free-living protozoa [such as the harmless protozoa used in high school biology laboratories]. This would have been but a curiosity, except for the fact that when inside its protozoan host the bacteria are very resistant to chlorine—the chlorine used to treat water never contacts the bacteria.[18,d] (p. 33)

Murphy further draws the conclusion that we are facing a complex environment which is somehow related with the emergence of disease. Research activities should be focused on this relationship, on the "mysterious econiches" [18] (p. 14) in which pathogens are evolving. In the second example quoted from Murphy's paper we see again surprising facts concerning the emergence of new and known disease.

> In 1990 cyanobacteria, that is blue-green algae, were found to be the cause of diarrhea in some patients who had recently traveled to tropical countries and in some patients with AIDS.[18] (p. 34)

The surprising fact was that cyanobacteria-like bodies[e] had been considered as completely harmless microorganisms living in peaceful coexistence with humans. What processes transformed this peaceful coexistence into a harmful relationship for humans?

There is no evidence so far that the organism itself has been evolutionary transformed. Its prevalence might be, nevertheless, correlated with ecological changes, especially in the marine ecosystems. The increase of underserved and immunosuppressed populations[f] with greater vulnerability to infection and the development of new techniques to diagnose the infection (which previously may have been lost in the background of undiagnosed diarrhea infections) led to the identification of cyclospora as a human pathogen.

---

[d] Only very high concentrations of chlorine can kill legionella. Contaminated water supplies are still treated with chlorine in order to eliminate bacteria, like legionella.
[e] "Cyanobacterium-like bodies" have now been identified as cyclospora.[15]
[f] See also the paper by Bryan et al., "Emerging Infectious Diseases in the United States: Improved Surveillance, a Requisite for Prevention," in this volume (pp. 346–361).

Hence, besides ecological and biological (genetic) processes which alter microorganisms and transform them into pathogens, social, cultural, behavioral as well as political (the fact that there is an increasing part of the world's population with only very limited health care) processes determine changes in the complex web of interactions which shape the evolution of new and resurgent disease.

Both "case-in-point" diseases, quoted from Murphy's paper, exemplify limitations of our current ability to identify and recognize pathogens and vectors of new infectious disease. Our knowledge of ecosystems and the social factors which contribute to disease emergence is still quite limited. Ecosystems, new diseases, and social systems are surely related in complex ways. Because of this complexity it is assumed that disease emergence is predictable only in a very limited way.

This assumption—that disease emergence is complex with only limited predictability—contains in my opinion a dangerous oversimplification of the picture. The notion of surprise might have been exchanged for the idea that things are complex, too complex to be predictable. Hence, we are not surprised anymore, because we know, generally, that disease evolution is an ongoing, complex process in which new diseases will emerge and known diseases will reemerge.

The design of an international surveillance system has been identified as a necessary task within the development of a sufficient prevention strategy.[8] A worldwide surveillance system or network would include, for instance, outposts of specialists, training programs to educate the staff in hospitals and clinics, information networks using satellite technology, and communication networks between industrialized and third world countries. Such a system would reduce the impact of epidemics. It might shorten the time which is needed to identify a new disease. But, we know, that our prevention strategies and interventions will necessarily be limited because disease emergence is a complex phenomenon. So, we are not surprised anymore, when our national and international surveillance systems fail in predicting an outbreak of a new disease or a known disease in new environments.

It seems that there is still a research problem to solve, besides the development of better surveillance systems, better preventive strategies, and better drugs and chemicals to control disease pathogens and vectors:

Is it possible to understand and reconstruct the complex processes involved in disease emergence in a way that would allow us to predict and to anticipate new and reemerging disease?

First, some words about the definition of complex and complexity. It is widely accepted to equate the terms complex and complicated. Systems, processes and phenomena which are very complicated, and for that reason difficult to understand, are characterized as complex.[19] This conflation is, in my opinion, problematic.

---

[8] See Bryan et al., pp. 346–361.

Complicated and simple are descriptions which have been influenced by the level of development of technology and science during the history of humankind. Likewise, these descriptions are essentially dependent on the access the observer or investigator had to the knowledge of the time and the major theoretical and religious systems. Referring again to the example of legionellosis, the legionella bacteria developed an incredible adaptation enabling them to live and grow inside free-living protozoa. To develop such an adaptation, complex interactions between these two species within an existing ecosystem were necessary.

Shall we describe these interactions and the adaptation the bacteria developed as complicated? Or, are we rather confronted with a simple, but very efficient mechanism for this microorganism to construct the environment according to its needs?

In co-evolution, the feedback of the products of natural selection on the course of selection undermines unidirectional evolutionary inference. Thus, the descriptions "complicated" and "simple" are not very useful for understanding the complex interactions between pathogens, other microorganisms, disease vectors and the pathogen's hosts.

Instead of dissecting reality into opposing features, an analysis of complex phenomena starts with the identification of the large number of variables involved in the case, and continues with the search for the *interactions* of these variables.[20] The emergence of Legionnaire's disease was not only determined by the co-evolution of the legionella bacteria and protozoa but also by human technology, human behavior, and the vulnerability of the human host.

The variability of conditions caused by, for example, the introduction of new technologies, the destruction of our natural environment and changes in human behavior, is itself an environmental feature to which species have to adapt. Thus, such technologies like pipes with debris, which provide a niche for protozoa and legionella, cooling towers, vegetable-misting devices, and fountains might have contributed to the emergence of Legionnaire's disease.

If we include environmental, social, and behavioral factors, the increase in an immunosuppressed population, the perspective of the pathogen, and interventions by health organizations and ministries of health in our conceptual framework, we will end up with a very large number of interacting variables. The struggle to understand this system of interacting variables and processes defines the challenge of understanding complexity.

The reconstruction of a system of interacting variables involved in disease emergence in models and theory, demands essentially transdisciplinary cooperation, because the knowledge about different variables emerges from different scientific disciplines. For example, contributions from marine ecologists, microbiologists, epidemiologist, engineers, and social scientists were necessary to understand the emergence of Legionnaire's disease.

Specialists from different disciplines can add important knowledge on the behavior of complex living systems, to help us understand the evolution of new or known pathogens. Evolutionary ecology, for example, contributes the concept that inputs percolate through the system and the impacts may occur far from the entry of forces or substances into the system. Thus, responses to external influences and disturbances are mostly not unidirectional. Ecosystems are not poised in equilibrium but rather are dynamic and constantly changing.[21]

Moreover, if we assume that all parameters of an epidemic are bio-social, the incorporation of social sciences[h] is substantial for understanding disease emergence. Comparative studies between plant, animal and human diseases and ecosystems might allow the recognition of common patterns of infectious disease emergence.

Pattern recognition means, in this context, identification and understanding of general, recurring connections of interacting variables and processes involved in disease emergence and interventions against disease. Patterns may occur as structural as well as functional connections of interactions between processes and variables. Patterns and their evolution in natural, artificial or social systems are modes in which complexity exists. Thus, it is possible to identify pattern recognition as one keystone in understanding complex systems.

Not all variables involved in the emergence of new and known infectious disease are measurable. The measurements might be incorrect because variables changed after they had been measured. The method of statistical data analysis is therefore limited. Mathematical equations may lack the level of specificity which would be necessary to reflect the complexity of the processes and interactions involved in disease emergence. With these methods we can only reconstruct parts of the whole phenomenon. The development of such epistemological "tools" like pattern recognition, causal analysis, and statistical and mathematical modeling will be determined by changes in the existing theoretical and conceptual frameworks.

In the following I identify some patterns of changes in natural and social environments which favor emergence of new disease. The identification, understanding, and modeling of these patterns indicate the scope of the conceptual framework on the evolution of new and resurgent disease.

Ecological Patterns

The ongoing climate changes, global warming, the enlargement of the ozone hole, the further pollution of the earth's water reservoirs, and the

---

[h] "Social sciences" is used in this paper in a very broad and general sense. I do not intend to reduce social sciences to behavioral sciences. Anthropology, for example, plays an increasing role in understanding the cultural factors and determinants involved in disease emergence.

creation of historically new environments, like toxic dumps, agriculture which relies on monocultures, and biofilms, are processes which result in devastating changes within existing ecosystems. The emergence of new disease and the upsurges of "old" disease can be identified as one result of the change of natural environments in all parts of the world.[i]

Social Patterns

Migration due to dramatic social changes, wars, economic collapse of societies, and the existing wealth differences between the industrialized world and the third world, and within countries, influence the exposure of non-immune populations to infectious diseases. AIDS, medical treatments that cause suppression of the immune system, *etc.*, contribute to an increase in the vulnerability of the human host to infectious diseases. Modern travel by airplane opens up immense possibilities for pathogens and disease vectors to overcome geographical barriers just by using the human system of transportation.[j]

Biological Patterns

The biological processes of mutagenesis and natural selection are present in natural ecosystems. The destruction of our natural environment as well as increasing in population movement might act as new selection pressures resulting in increasing plasticity of known viral and bacterial strains.

For example, the extensive use of pesticides and other chemicals against disease vectors and pathogens changes the natural relationships between predator and prey. The destruction of natural enemies opens up new niches for the very animals and microorganisms we targeted to kill. Vectors and pathogens were pushed into selection processes favoring the survival of resistant strains and populations.[k]

The identification of these patterns involved in disease emergence and reemergence supports the notion that we are living in an interconnected world, in which ecological and social processes affect all nations and all societies on this planet. And if ecological and social processes determine disease evolution, the emergence of new infectious disease and the reemergence of known disease will affect as well all nations and all societies without regard to their developmental and economic status.

The challenge to understand the complexity of this interconnected world marks the substantial change of the current theoretical framework.[22] The

[i] See paper by Paul Epstein on "Ecosystem Vulnerability" (pp. 423–435) for case-in-point diseases.

[j] See paper by Uwe Brinkmann on "Economic Development and Tropical Diseases" (pp. 303–311). In addition, the commentaries and discussion parts in the Social Sciences Section in this volume are focused on the identification of social patterns of disease emergence.

[k] See paper by Richard Levins (pp. 260–270) on "Natural Selection in Pathogens" for examples.

efforts to develop a new conceptual framework to understand complex disease evolution will contribute to the development of this new theoretical framework and introduce changes in the traditional bio-medical framework of health sciences.

REFERENCES

1. ROSENFIELD, P. 1992. The potential of transdisciplinary research for sustaining and extending linkages between the health and social sciences. Soc. Sci. Med. **35**(No. 11): 1351.
2. SCHAFFNER, K. F. 1993. Discovery and Explanation in Biology and Medicine. Chicago: The University of Chicago Press.
3. MAYR, E. 1982. The Growth of Biological Thought. Diversity, Evolution and Inheritance. Cambridge, MA, London: The Belknap Press of Harvard University Press.
4. EIGEN, R. & R. WINKLER. 1993. Laws of the Game. How the Principles of Nature Govern Chance. Princeton, NJ: Princeton University Press. (translation from German)
5. CODY, M. L. & J. M. DIAMOND, Eds. 1975. Ecology and Evolution of Communities. Cambridge, MA, London: The Belknap Press of Harvard University Press.
6. LUHMANN, N. 1984. Soziale Systeme. Frankfurt am Main: Suhrkamp.
7. LEKSON, S. H., T. C. WINDES, J. R. STEIN & W. J. JUSTICE. 1988. The Chaco Canyon Community. Sci. Am. **259**: 100–109.
8. LANGTON, CH. G., Ed. 1989. Artificial Life. Santa Fe Institute Studies in the Sciences of Complexity, Proceedings, Vol. 6. Redwood City, CA: Addison Wesley.
9. GELL-MANN, M. 1988. The concept of the institute. In Emerging Syntheses in Science. D. Pines, Ed. Redwood City, CA: Addison-Wesley.
10. KUHN, T. S. 1962. The Structure of Scientific Revolutions. Chicago, London: The University of Chicago Press; 1977. The Essential Tension. Chicago and London: The University of Chicago Press. pp. 293–320.
11. LEWIN, R. 1992. Complexity: Life at the Edge of Chaos. New York: Macmillan Pub. Co.
12. CASTI, J. L. 1994. The cognitive revolution? Idealistic Studies **28**: 19–38.
13. AHLBOM, A. 1984. Criteria of causal association in epidemiology. In Health, Disease, and Causal Explanation in Medicine. L. Nordenfelt & B. I. B. Lindahl, Eds.: 93–98. Dordrecht. Boston. Lancaster: D. Reidel, Kluwer: FAGOT, A. M. 1984. About causation in medicine: some shortcomings of a probabilistic account of causal explanations. *ibid*, pp. 101–126.
14. EPSTEIN, P. R. 1992. Commentary—Pestilence and Poverty—historical transitions and the great pandemics. Am. J. Prev. Med. **8**: 263.
15. ORTEGA, Y. R., CH. R. STERLING, R. H. GILMAN, V. A. CAMA & F. DIAZ. 1993. Cyclospora species—a new protozoan pathogen of humans. New Engl. J. Med. **328**(18): 1308–1312; BENDALL, R. P., S. LUCAS, A. MOODY, G. TOVAY & P. L. CHIODINI. 1993. Diarrhoea associated with cyanobacterium-like bodies: A new coccidian enteritis of man. Lancet **341**: 590–592.
16. ANDERSON, P. K. 1991. Epidemiology of insect transmitted plant pathogens. Dissertation in the Department of Population and International Health, Harvard School of Public Health.
17. WILSON, M. E. 1991. A World Guide to Infections. New York: Oxford University Press.
18. MURPHY, F. A. 1992. New, emerging and reemerging infectious diseases. Unpublished manuscript.
19. ARTHUR, B. W. 1993. Why do things become more complex? Sci. Am. May: 144.
20. BECHTEL, W. & R. C. RICHARDSON. 1993. Discovering Complexity; Decomposition and Localization as Strategies in Scientific Research. Princeton, NJ: Princeton University Press.
21. LEVINS, R. 1993 Personal communication.
22. KELLERT, S. H. 1993. In the Wake of Chaos: Unpredictable Order in Dynamical Systems. Chicago: The University of Chicago Press; KAUFFMAN, S. A. 1992. The Origins of Order: Self-organization and Selection in Evolution. Oxford, New York: Oxford University Press; NICHOLIS, G. & I. PRIGOGINE. 1989. Exploring Complexity. New York: W. H. Freeman.

Developing Paradigms to Anticipate Emerging Diseases

Transmission Cycles and a Search for Pattern[a]

MARK L. WILSON

Department of Epidemiology and Public Health
Yale University School of Medicine
60 College Street
New Haven, Connecticut 06520-8034

Predicting the emergence of diseases constitutes a critical challenge for future research. Although new diseases continue to be recognized, characterized and compared, we lack an approach for systematically employing such knowledge to guide future action. How can we develop systems for analyzing existing ecological, epidemiological and social change in a manner that will sharpen surveillance? What common characteristics of new diseases might be exploited in efforts designed to improve detection and prevention? Are there properties or processes of recognized emerging diseases that might be used to forecast when and where other such new diseases will appear, or whom they might affect?

This essay suggests a method for classifying transmission cycles of recently emergent infections in order to identify common ecological and epidemiological patterns that might be used to anticipate similar future events. By comparing emergent diseases according to their transmission characteristics, factors that maintain the corresponding pathogens in nature become the objects of study. The goal, then, is to identify mechanisms by which previously uninfected organisms or regions become vulnerable to infection. In particular, this approach is designed to identify components of transmission that are particularly susceptible to environmental change generated by human activities.

The events that promote disease emergence are considered in terms of a) movement of people or of the infectious agents themselves and b) particular kinds of human behavior that may increase the likelihood of transmission. Disease emergence may, thereby, occur as a result of increased local incidence, geographic distribution or severity of symptoms.

CHARACTERIZING TRANSMISSION

Diseases may be classified on the basis of the kinds of hosts that are naturally infected by the pathogen and their usual mechanism of transmission.

[a] Supported by a grant from the MacArthur Foundation (9008073 Health).

418

Anthroponotic diseases include those in which people are the sole natural hosts for the pathogen, and zoonotic diseases those including human infection by a pathogen that is naturally maintained in non-human hosts, generally vertebrate animals (TABLE 1). Directly transmitted infections pass through close physical contact between hosts, including aerosol or venereal contact; and indirectly transmitted infections pass by means of another host, such as by the bite of a vector arthropod. Diseases generally can be classified unambiguously by these criteria. Certain zoonotic infections such as monkey-pox and Lassa fever, however, can become anthroponotic for brief periods of time. The goal, then, is to classify diseases in a manner that provides a framework for comparing characteristics that may be linked to emergence.

The following discussion employs this schema to classify the likely means by which exotic pathogens might be introduced into new sites, or by which preexisting pathogens are likely to emerge owing to changes in human behavior (TABLE 1). A hierarchy of complexity that identifies factors or events necessary for disease emergence becomes evident. This process permits development of general, robust principles for transmission systems that help predict emergence. The likelihood that a pathogen will be imported, for example, may be examined on the basis of the changes in the number of factors in the transmission system. The equation could include a weighting function that quantifies the importance of each step or factor that would interact with its probability. Such an approach also may permit comparisons of diseases that have recently emerged, and the development of testable hypotheses of characteristics that predispose certain diseases to continue to emerge. For example, does environmental change promote the emergence of vector-borne zoonoses? Are directly transmitted anthroponoses more likely to appear when human migration or population density increases? Answers to questions such as these may be sought either by a systematic examination of available data describing past events, or by a more theoretical approach that models interactions that represent processes which lead to change. In practice, a mixed strategy that employs both approaches probably will be most productive.

Ultimately, predictions concerning new diseases can be formulated. Although it seems unrealistic to expect precision as to the time and place of emergence, analysis of the general features of emerging diseases should assist future inquiry and may suggest sites in which surveillance should be particu-

TABLE 1. Effect of the System of Transmission and of Human Behavior on the Transport of Pathogens into New Sites

System of Transmission	Number of Factors	Pathogen Movement or Behavior
Anthroponotic		
Direct	Few	Human, Vehicle
Indirect	Some	Human, Vector, Vehicle
Zoonotic		
Direct	Some	Reservoir, Human, Vehicle
Indirect	Many	Vector, Reservoir, Human, Vehicle

larly vigilant. In this manner, prediction can be seen as enhancing our awareness of new disease patterns, as well as increasing the likelihood of recognizing a new disease as soon as it appears.

HUMAN MIGRATION AND PATHOGEN TRANSPORT

Pathogens may appear in new sites through three or more processes, including: a) transfer of infectious agents into new sites, b) introduction of competent reservoirs and vectors, or c) changes in demographic or immune status of human populations. Does the mode of transmission affect the likelihood of importation? Examples exist for each of the categories,[1] suggesting that movement of people or pathogens can lead to emergence of diseases of different types (TABLE 2). However, diseases transmitted by certain pathways should be more prone to transport and establishment, hence more likely to emerge. For example, directly transmitted anthroponoses such as measles and rubella require only the introduction of the pathogen into a previously unaffected region for disease to emerge.

Although diverse modes of importation may be available to pathogens with particularly complex transmission cycles, the conditions required for their maintenance may be highly constrained. For example, for malaria to become established following introduction by a parasitemic human, competent, human-biting anopheline mosquitoes must already exist in the region. Indeed, transport of infections in vectors would seem less likely than in people. Other zoonoses such as schistosomiasis will become established only if the required intermediate hosts are present. The highly involved cycles of indirectly transmitted zoonoses such as Rift Valley fever typically require a variety of competent vertebrate hosts and particular vector species for the virus to be introduced. Although seasonal variations may permit transient outbreaks, emergence of vector-borne zoonoses that leads to endemicity may be infrequent. A framework such as this permits analysis of when and where exotic agents are likely to form stable introductions.

TABLE 2. Examples of Diseases That Have Recently Emerged Owing to Human and Animal Movement or Transport of Inanimate Material, Grouped According to the Kind of Transmission System

System of Transmission	Transport of Pathogen in	Disease	Type or Means of Transport or Movement
Anthroponotic			
Direct	Human	Measles	Travel
	Vehicle	Cholera	Ship ballast
Indirect	Human	Malaria	Immigration into deforested sites
	Human	Dengue	Inter-island travel
Zoonotic			
Direct	Vertebrate	Rabies	Infected raccoons to hunt
Indirect	Vertebrate	Rift Valley fever	Infected sheep into Egypt

TABLE 3. Examples of Diseases That Have Emerged Owing to Human Behavioral Interactions with the Environment; Diseases are Grouped According to their Natural System of Transmission

System of Transmission	Object of Change	Disease or Pathogen	Behavior or Environmental Change
Anthroponotic			
Direct	Humans	HIV/AIDS	Sexual activity
	Material	Hepatitis B	Sharing of needles
Indirect	Humans	Filariasis	Poor drainage of water
	Vector	Yellow fever	Stored water, containers
Zoonotic			
Direct	Vertebrate	Venezuelan hemorrhagic fever	Agriculture/food preparation
	Material	Giardiasis	Camping, untreated water
Indirect	Vertebrate	Lyme disease	Increased habitat for host
	Vector	Japanese encephalitis	Pig culture and drainage

HUMAN BEHAVIOR AND ENVIRONMENTAL CHANGE

The emergence of a second group of diseases can be ascribed largely to human behaviors that have altered the environment, or to the manner in which environment change affects certain ecological cycles (TABLE 3). As before, diseases are grouped according to their natural system of transmission. Similar questions also can be asked: Do certain human behaviors more often lead to the emergence of diseases that have particular types of transmission? Can these characteristics of transmission be used to identify categories of human-environment interactions that increase the risk that a new disease will appear?

Numerous examples of emerging diseases associated with behavioral changes are available for most categories of transmission (TABLE 3). In general, pathogens having complicated transmission cycles seem to emerge in response to changes in human behavior or environmental change as readily as do those that develop more simply. People generally become exposed to novel zoonoses or anthroponoses as a result of altered patterns of human activity, and this may occur whether the cycle is simple or complex. The advent of readily available hypodermic needles and technological advances such as organ transplantation and blood transfusion have created alternative pathways for the emergence of novel anthroponoses.

FUTURE EFFORTS

Although one system has been proposed here as a framework for organizing emerging diseases and searching for pattern, other such systematic approaches also could be useful. For example, by classifying agents according to the immune response they invoke in people, specifically whether protection is partial or complete, life-long or short-lived, other criteria for comparing diseases may prove instructive. Perhaps introduced pathogens that typically induce full, life-long protection against reinfection are less likely to generate disease emergence than ones whose immunogenicity is more variable. Diseases may also be analyzed by comparing the host specificity of the pathogen, asking how many kinds of host organisms it can parasitize. Disease agents whose host range is very narrow may be less likely to emerge than those which can propagate in a wide variety of hosts or survive in a hostile environment.

An analytical approach is required if we are to fully exploit the extensive and diverse information on emerging diseases that is accumulating. A systematic and thorough cataloging and comparison of pathogens and their characteristics could help identify types of agents that share common features that predispose to emergence. Multiple features may increase these probabilities exponentially. Such information may facilitate establishment of categories of agents that are associated with particular conditions, thereby guiding surveillance. Although it is unlikely that we will ever be able to predict the emergence of a particular disease at a precise time and place, analysis of the general features of emerging diseases should assist future inquiry, and should focus attention on human activities that create public health threats.

REFERENCE

1. LEDERBERG, J., R. E. SHOPE & S. C. OAKS, JR., EDS. 1992. Emerging Infections, Microbial Threats to Health in the United States. Washington, DC: National Academy Press.

Framework for an Integrated Assessment of Health, Climate Change, and Ecosystem Vulnerability

PAUL R. EPSTEIN[a]

Harvard Medical School
The Cambridge Hospital
1493 Cambridge Street
Cambridge, Massachusetts 02139

INTRODUCTION

Periods of ecological change may be associated with extinctions of some species and the emergence of new ones—in particular, pests and pathogens. An altered balance of species combined with a stressful environment may increase the selection of opportunistic and toxin-producing organisms, and contribute to the redistribution of vectors and animal reservoirs of disease. This paper presents a framework for an integrated assessment of climate change and ecosystem vulnerability using biological indicator species for detection. It has six components: 1) The Climate System, 2) Ecosystems, 3) The Social System, 4) Indicators, 5) Outcomes, and 6) Responses (see FIG. 1). Those familiar with the health paradigm of causality will see one analogous to the environment, two, the host and three, the agent.

Insects are especially sensitive biological indicators in terrestrial ecosystems, given their short generation time and environmental hardiness. With thresholds and optimum ranges in bioclimatic conditions (temperature, humidity and wind) determining their maturation, extrinsic parasite incubation and biting behavior; and control of their abundance a function of predator/prey and competition relationships, insect populations rapidly reflect ecosystem health. Paleological records support a strong link between past climatic transitions and increases in insect fauna. *Rodent* populations in arid rural—and urban—settings are another group of rapid responders to environmental change (*e.g.*, food supplies and wastes) and altered biodiversity (loss of predators). In coastal marine systems *algae* are key indicators of ecosystem integrity, and the incidence and abundance of new and old toxic algal species may reflect adaptive responses to enhanced environmental stress and altered biodiversity.

Moreover, insects and rodents are carriers of many plant and animal (including human) viral, bacterial, rickettsial and parasitic diseases, and some are avid consumers of vegetation. Algae transport *Vibrio cholerae* and other human enteric pathogens, and harmful species emit biotoxins that affect finfish, shellfish, marine mammals, sea birds and humans.

---

[a] E-mail:PEPSTEIN@igc.org.

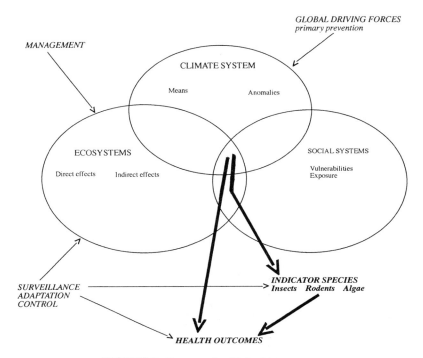

FIGURE 1. Framework with health outcomes.

Combining the monitoring of **biological indicators** and relevant **health outcomes** (to include food security and nutrition) with ecological and meteorological data sets can 1) improve surveillance for emerging diseases, 2) provide a basis for calculating the impacts and **costs** of climate change, 3) contribute to the detection of climate change ("fingerprints"), and 4) support a systems-based approach to the design of adaptative and preventive responses to ecosystem management and environmental change that reduce the emergence of opportunistic pathogens and pests.

AN INTEGRATED ASSESSMENT: DEFINITION OF TERMS

Many diseases of plants, birds, fish and mammals serve as indicators of environmental distress: the direct effects of toxins or indirect effects on species composition and selective pressures. The factors regulating the abundance of species, including parasites and pests, are: 1) Nutrients (chemical), 2) Competition, predation and disease (biological), and 3) Meteorological conditions and habitat (physical). A disturbance in one factor can be destabilizing; multiple perturbations can affect a system's resilience (recovery time) and resistance to invasion of pests.

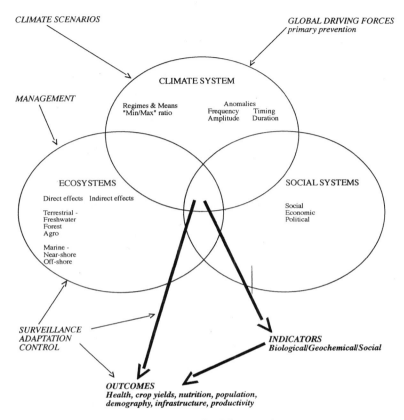

FIGURE 2. Generalized framework.

Stressors and responses occur in biogeochemical and social/economic/political terms. Inputs (*e.g.*, chemicals) or resource depletion have direct and indirect local impacts. Widespread perturbations (*e.g.*, fossil fuel pollutants, deforestation) affect ecosystems. When changes involve biotic feedbacks and occur on a global scale, they can affect the climate system.

FIGURES 1 and 2 show an overlapping of the three systems as each contains forces that affect *and* are impacted by the other systems.

The **climate system** can be characterized by a set of means (of temperatures, pressures and precipitation) and variance or oscillations about the means. A change in means implies a change in regimes. Anomalies or extreme events (*e.g.*, in storm patterns) vary with respect to intensity, frequency, duration, timing and scale. As Greenland ice core records demonstrate, an increase in climate variability may be dynamic over corrections and herald rapid (3–7 years) "jumps" in the non-linear climate system to other stable states. We live in an "unusual" stable period, known as the Holocene, that began about 10,000 years ago with the ending of the last ice age.

The El Niño/Southern Oscillation (ENSO) phenomenon, characterized by anomalous warming of the Pacific Ocean, is considered by meteorologists to be the major climate signal. Coming every 3–5 years, ENSOs alter the Jet stream and are strongly associated with recurrent droughts in some locales (*e.g.*, Northeast Brazil) and heavy rains in others (*e.g.*, Southeast Brazil).

Terrestrial and marine **ecosystems** have biotic and abiotic components, structures and functions, and are characterized by dynamic stability, resilience, vulnerability and sensitivity (see below). **Social systems** have behavioral, cultural, social, economic, military and political components. The latter affect the climate and ecosystems as *driving forces*, and underlie differential *exposures* and *vulnerabilities* to stresses, toxins and pests. Population influences are determined by abundance, composition, density, distribution, movements and migrations.

Indicators may be biological, chemical or physical, as well as behavioral, social, economic or political. **Outcomes** include diseases, disasters, lost food supplies and damaged infrastructures. **Responses** include monitoring, "treatment" (*e.g.*, medical) and compensation for outcomes, withdrawal, anticipatory adjustments, adaptations, technological changes and substitutions, control of indicator species, management on an ecosystem-scale, and energy and forestry policies.

The monetary **costs** of disease events can be measured in terms of health, health services, inspection and surveillance; productivity; nutrition, food exports and commerce; recreation and tourism.

This paper focuses on biological indicators and health outcomes, but presents a general framework for risk assessment. It is implicit that socio/economic and political factors, such as development policies and adaptative strategies, are the primary determinants of global change (*i.e.*, widespread ecological and climate change). Conversely, it is within the social arena that crucial decisions will be made concerning the management of human activities and nurturing of ecosystems, and the mitigation of climate-altering forces.

Bioindicators have thus far been used to monitor environmental accumulations of chemicals. But biotic responses of organisms, populations and communities integrate multiple aspects of ecosystem vulnerability and stresses endured. Monitoring key species that respond rapidly to environmental change (*e.g.*, insects, rodents—urban and rural—and algae) can facilitate impact monitoring, detection of climate changes (*e.g.*, prolonged shifts in the range of species) and can aid the design of adaptations, mitigations and preventive interventions that improve generalized resistance (to the invasion of exotic species and emergence of disease).

A network of regional centers with support from the World Climate Program (Global Climate Observing System or GCOS) is being planned to monitor meteorological data. Other programs are planned to monitor ecosystem integrity and biodiversity (Global Terrestrial and Ocean Observing Systems or GTOS and GOOS), augmented by remote sensing assimilated into geographic information systems. The Global Change System for Analysis, Research and Training (START) program of the International Geosphere-Biosphere Program (IGBP) will involve 13 Regional Research Networks, numerous Regional Research Centers and affiliated Sites. The NOAA Office of Global Programs is initiating regional centers in the Americas to apply climate forecasting to the agriculture, energy and health sectors (water distribution being the pivotable variable). At the same time the Centers for Disease Control and Prevention (CDC) and the World Health Organization (communicating through the PROMED network) are planning an international Consortium of regional centers to monitor health from a clinical, laboratory and epidemiological perspective.

This paper concludes with a proposal for the merging of bioindicators and health outcome surveillance into the monitoring of climate and ecosystems in order to 1) improve emerging disease surveillance, 2) operationalize an integrated assessment of climate change, 3) enhance climate change detection (through the monitoring of species' movements), and 4) improve planning and evaluation of systems-based interventions to confront global change (see FIG. 3).

ECOSYSTEM HEALTH AND INTEGRITY

Living systems begin with "auto-catalytic" reactions (when the waste of one component nourishes another) and are sustained with partnerships and culled with predation and parasitism. Some living communities are intimately symbiotic (coral being algae and animal polyps, lichen being algae and fungi). Within and among systems, feedback fluxes of energy and elements are occurring on individual, population, community and landscape levels.

Ecosystems have **structure** and perform multiple **functions** (*e.g.,* wetlands buffer coasts, filter effluents and nurture marine and seabird species), and their states vary and oscillate around means on daily, seasonal and decadal scales. Temperate and boreal ecosystems depend heavily on temperature for the seasonal succession of species; in the tropics, rainfall patterns (wet and dry season) drive transformations.

Perturbations or **stresses** include human activities and population movements, the introduction of exotic species or elimination of predators, pollutants, habitat fragmentation and loss, and climatic factors. Stresses over time may be strengthening; higher latitude ecosystems, having adapted to seasonal changes, are more resilient than tropical ecosystems. But there are thresholds (*e.g.,* excess habitat fragmentation may reduce more predators than pests, cause excessive extinctions and lead to collapse). **Subsidies** are defined as helpful inputs.

The chief characteristics of **ecosystem health** or **integrity** are stability, resilience, biodiversity, productivity, yields and vigor (see FIG. 4).

Indicators of Vulnerability to Disease

Measures of **vulnerability, exposure,** and pathological **responses** are: *invasability* to exotic species, *resistance* to pathogen/pest emergence, and

CLIMATE	
Means & Regimes	Amplitude/ Frequency of Variance

ECOSYSTEMS	
DIRECT	INDIRECT
Function of: Exposures • Single • Double Vulnerability of hosts and regions Anomalies Means and relative changes in minimums and maximums	Function of: Ecosystems health • sensitivity • resilience Vulnerable regions and populations Means (e.g., isotherms) Anomalies
Agent Dispersion • Direct extension • Hierarchical	

INDICATORS				
Terrestrial	Biological	Chemical	Physical	Social
Agro Forest	Insect pests **Insects**	Soil fertility Soil & leaf nutrients	Plant biomass	Crop prices
Freshwater Arid Marine	Quality **Rodents**	Quality Soils	Quantity Soils	Conflicts Famine
Coastal Ocean	**Algae** Fish	Nutrients Nutrients	Coastal integrity Temperatures, pressures	Tourism Seafood industry, Mariculture

OUTCOMES				
Health	Crop Yields	Human Settlements	Infrastructure	Productive Capacity
Cardiovascular Pulmonary Skin cancer Cataracts Vector-borne diseases— of animals and plants Water-based diseases Person-to-person communicable diseases	Nutrition	Population Displacement & Density	Industrial Agricultural Transport Services	

FIGURE 3. Details of framework.

RESPONSES

Adaptations
("Downstream")
Altered behaviors and technology to change outcomes
(*e.g.,* sunblock and air-conditioning)

Surveillance
Ecosystem and critical region-based

Control
Vector control, sea walls, for example

Ecosystem Integrity
("Midstream")
Coastal management, water filtration systems, for example

Primary Prevention
("Upstream")
Energy and forestry policies

FIGURE 3. (*Continued*)

promoters of vectors/pathogens. Diverse and resilient systems offer the best generalized defense against disease emergence. **Key species** or key elements are those that rapidly respond to and integrate environmental parameters, thus reflecting system integrity. Bioindicators that are disease vectors or reservoirs (*e.g.,* algae in marine systems, rodents and mosquitoes in terrestrial) can provide a crucial link between surveillance for *health outcomes* and the monitoring of global change.

Examples: Ecological Change and Disease Emergence

Several papers in these proceedings provide examples of the interaction of local ecological changes and climate signals in the emergence and redistribution of algal-based diseases (biotoxins and *Vibrio cholerae*). Rodents, involved

- **Stability**: populations in dynamic or cyclical (*e.g.,* seasonal) equilibrium—a fluid, ever shifting, as state of adjustment
- **Resilience**: return-time to equilibrium after a perturbation
- **Biodiversity**: species composition, abundance, redundance and diversity (redundancy in functions provides insurance and enhances resilience in the face of weather changes or disease)
- **Productivity**: primary production is photosynthesis and the level must exceed the limit needed to compensate for constraints imposed by susceptibility to perturbations
- **Yields**: must be at levels to sustain stocks of species
- **Vigor** and metabolism: energy fluxes and metabolic rates

FIGURE 4. The "vital signs" of ecosystem health.

in hantavirus, five emerging arenaviruses in Latin America and agricultural pests, respond rapidly to environmental change. For hantavirus and rodent pests in Africa, prolonged drought affects rodent predators (raptors, snakes), while intermittant rains provide the rodents with nourishment. The *arenaviruses* have emerged in areas of landscape alteration, specifically forest clearing, with subsequent change in rodent species and introduction of vulnerable humans. Mosquitos (Anophelines and Aedes species) have clear seasonalities related to temperature and humidity; once introduced, their abundance rapidly reflects climatic signals and ecological changes (*e.g.*, edge effects in forests).

Underlying Principles

The following are the guidelines used in this framework for modeling and monitoring complex ecological systems.

1. Aggregate changes in locally released aerosolized pollutants (greenhouse gases, tropospheric ozone, "trace" chemicals and total suspended particulates) and widespread landscape alterations are the **anthropogenic** factors cumulatively affecting radiative transfers (heat fluxes), thus the *rate* of climate change.

2. The interaction of stressors and responses within the climate system and ecosystems are **non-linear,** and system dynamics include bimodalities, hystereses (return pathways different from primary), discontinuities and divergences that can help explain "jumps" in system states.

3. Small inputs may lead to large changes in fragile ecosystems where conditions are near **threshold** levels (*e.g.*, depleted fish stocks or those with altered ratio of young to old).

4. Changes in **climate** will affect all parameters. Changes expected include alterations in temperatures, precipitation, humidity, ice cover and sea level. Changes in the **minimum-to-maximum temperatures** (minimum being night-time and winter), with greatest increases over land in higher latitudes, may have the greatest impact on insect generation and maturation times. Changes in means, *i.e.*, a change in regimes, and alterations in the pattern of variability around the means will impact all factors, including breeding grounds. The latter includes changes in storm frequency, amplitude and onset (greater frequency decreasing resilience, *e.g.*, loss of barrier beaches and dunes reducing time for repair).

5. Some responses are "side-effects" of **biotic feedbacks.** While some biotic feedbacks may be negative ("damping climate change"), the impact on species (*e.g.*, increased algae with increased warmth and CO_2 drawdown from the troposphere) may have the side-effect of impacting human societies and human health.

6. **Disease emergence** (new variants or strains), resurgence and redistribution can reflect poor ecosystem health integrated with external stresses.

7. **Dispersion of disease agents** can occur contiguously or hierarchically

(*e.g.*, through air transport or ship ballast water), with amplification and persistence of organisms dependent on the presence of the "right" bioclimatographic factors.

8. **Critical and vulnerable regions** (see below) must be monitored for biological, chemical, physical, socio/economic and political indicators and disease outcomes.

9. **Outcomes, adaptations** and **mitigations** are all associated with variable efficacies, and with social and economic costs and benefits. The best responses are based on ecological principles that foresee (as best one can) untoward responses and those that serve to strengthen generalized defenses.

10. Changes in the distribution of bioindicators and health outcomes will be caused by the interaction of factors within the three systems, to varying degrees according to place and time.

    For example, diseases transmitted person-to-person (*e.g.*, polio, diphtheria, measles, tuberculosis) may more directly reflect population density and dislocations (though the latter may also reflect environmental changes). New outbreaks of illnesses involving vectors (*e.g.*, insects) and animal reservoirs (*e.g.*, birds and deer)—such as dengue and yellow fever, Lyme disease and viral encephalitis—may more immediately reflect environmental changes.

The **sensitivity** of a system to stresses depends on the current state and upon other concurrent factors (*e.g.*, the effects of temperature depend on moisture and nutrient availability). The timing of inputs affects the impact, for **synchronies** in maturation and spawning and varying *degree-days* (days that temperature exceeds threshold for maturation) among biological components, will affect predation pressure and food availability, thus survival and transfers of pathogens. Inputs (*e.g.*, nutrients) at the bottom of food chains will reverberate throughout trophic levels differently than impacts at the middle (*e.g.*, copepod damage from excess uv-bs) or those at the top (*e.g.*, overfishing).

Factors must be evaluated as they *indirectly* cascade through ecosystem dynamics. For example, warm sea surface temperatures not only encourage Northward migration of Northeast U.S. salmon (which may be inocuous); they move mackeral further up the California coast, increasing their predation on salmon larvae, reducing salmon stocks three years later.

Vulnerability is compounded when multiple perturbations occur over a short period, and injured ecosystems are vulnerable to opportunistic species. The ecological niche, whether organisms are specialists (*e.g.*, eat only one plant) or generalists, and the length of the food chain (number of trophic levels) all affect stability and resilience in the face of extreme events. **Ecosystem management** must aim at supporting **generalized defenses** (*e.g.*, preserving mosquito predators). Finally, **indirect effects** of interventions may overwhelm the direction of the response intended. Disease outbreaks may be symptoms of ecosystem dysfunction and are often the first impacts of environmental stress on plant and animal populations.

ECOSYSTEM MONITORING ON A REGIONAL SCALE

The principles of examining marine, terrestrial, and ice-covered systems may be extended to carry out monitoring on regional scales. In 1994, for example, Large Marine Ecosystem (LME) monitoring, funded by the Global Environment Facility, is scheduled for the Gulf of Guinea. Proposals are being submitted for the Chinese Yellow Sea and the Black Sea, with the intention of extension to the world's 49 LMEs. The relative value of the driving forces in each system (*e.g.,* overfishing, pollution, habitat loss and climate) will be evaluated in order to inform policies for mitigation and prevention. Monitoring plankton, bivalves and finfish for biotoxins and vibrios, and surveillance of coastal nations for relevant health outcomes, will form an integral part of these projects.

With respect to life-support systems, terrestrial **regions** (*e.g.,* watersheds, highlands) may be categorized as *sustainable, impoverished, endangered,* or *critical* (see Kasperson *et al.*, in press). **Indicators** to facilitate these characterizations include *environmental degradation* (water availability and quality, soil and air quality, biomass and productivity), *human well-being* (life expectancy, infant and under-fives mortality, nutritional levels and disease burden), and *capacity to respond* (through avoidance, substitutions and mitigation). Other indicators used for monitoring populations are *wealth* (gross domestic product [GDP] or income per capita, savings), *population* growth, movements and density (*urbanization*) and *economic and technological substitutability* (monocultures and cash-crop dependency vs. diversification and technological innovation).

Additional indices are: I. The Human Development Index (UNDP 1992/93) that includes a) Life expectancy (LE), b) education, and c) GDP per capita; II. The International Human Suffering Index (Population Crises Committee 1987/92) that includes a) LE, b) daily caloric intake, c) clean drinking water, d) childhood immunization, e) secondary school enrollment, f) GNP/capita, g) rate of inflation, h) communications technology, i) political freedoms, and j) civil rights.

Monitoring by ecosystem involves a number of strategies, including: 1) Status monitoring (extent, distribution and rates of loss [or gain]), fragmentation and edge effects by remote sensing and fractal dimensions analysis of landscapes; 2) Capacity (storage), 3) Intensity (processes and functions), and 4) Population-community (biodiversity) indices. Stresses and perturbations may be site-specific or generalized and time series are needed to detect shifts and identify early warning signs. Analytical methods utilized are canonical, cluster, discriminant and principal compartment (see Keffers, 1978).

For each region, primary, secondary and tertiary **driving forces** of environmental change will differ. Among the principal forces are: 1) extraction of non-renewable resources (biotic as well as abiotic), 2) exploitation of renewable resources, and 3) generation of wastes beyond the capacity of biogeochemical cycles to assimilate them. These forces are sometimes "exported" to other regions, through the import of contaminated goods or export of aerosolized, liquids and solid wastes. These driving forces are all influenced by population growth, by affluence and development practices, poverty, culture and beliefs, behavioral and technological changes, economic policies, and by political will.

INDICES OF GLOBAL CHANGE

Global indices or "fingerprints" of climate change include: 1) Northern ranges of pelagics and sea mammals, tree populations and land animals; 2) Altitude ranges of plants and insects (carrying malaria, yellow fever and dengue); 3) Fish, submerged vegetation (*e.g.,* eelgrass), sea mammal and forest die-offs; 4) Toxic algal blooms, extent and duration; 5) Coral reef bleaching; 6) "Red snow"—algae, a "litmus" test for warming and uv-bs; 7) Sea levels, sea surface temperatures and total heat retained in the oceans. Increased climate variability may itself be an indicator of instability in the climate system, heralding a change in the climate regime.

CONCLUSIONS

Just as we strive to extract simple principles underlying complex systems, deriving indicators integrating the functions of complex systems becomes a goal simplifying our understanding and surveillance of natural phenomena. Data sets on biological indicators and health outcomes must be "fused" with data sets of meteorology and the quality and distribution of resources and development activities. Certainly human population abundance and distributions figures are essential for projecting inputs and demands on ecosystems.

This integration can be achieved on national levels through coordination at ministry levels to include weather stations, resource managers, agricultural and health authorities. In the US, for example, the Climate Analysis Center (NOAA) defines four regions for weather surveillance; coordinating ecological (EPA), agricultural (FDA) and health data (CDC) through these centers could provide the basis for integrated assessment and monitoring.

Internationally, regional centers could form a network under the rubric of the World Climate Program and its major components: the Global Climate, Terrestrial and Ocean Observing Systems (GCOS, GTOS and GOOS), and be integrated into the planned 13 regional START centers under the direction of the IGBP and the International Council of Scientific Unions. In the Americas, the Inter-American Institute under the NOAA Office of Global Programs is developing multidisciplinary centers with multisectoral applications, including water, agriculture, and health.

This integration of systems through collaborative scientific work, drawing on remote sensing, field and laboratory observations that include key indicator species abundance, composition and distribution, and health outcomes, can comprise an efficient methodology for achieving a dynamic, integrated assessment of climate and ecosystem change and enhance the detection, surveillance and control of emerging infectious diseases.

ACKNOWLEDGMENT

The author would like to acknowledge the advice provided by Dr. Richard Levins, mathematician, botanist, farmer, ecologist and social scientist, in development of this multidisciplinary, multisectoral scheme.

BIBLIOGRAPHY

BARNES, R. S. K. & R. N. HUGHES
  1988   An Introduction to Marine Ecology. Oxford: Blackwell Scientific Publications.
CHAPMAN, V. J.
  1977   Ecosystems of the World 1, Coastal Ecosystems. Amsterdam: Elsevier.
DIMN, S. O.
  1982   Food Webs. UK: Chapman and Hall.
GOLLEY, F. B., Ed.
  1983   Ecosystems of the World 14A, Tropical Rain Forest Ecosystems, Structure and Function. Amsterdam: Elsevier Scientific Publishing Company.
HIRSCH, A.
  1980   Monitoring cause and effects, ecosystem changes. In: D. L. Worf, Ed. op cit., pp. 137–142.
HUNSAKER, C. T. & D. E. CARPENTER, Eds.
  1990   Ecological Indicators for the Environmental Monitoring and Assessment Program (EMAP). EPA 600/3-90/060 U.S. Environmental Protection Agency, Office of Research and Development, Research Triangle Park, NC.
INDIAN NATIONAL SCIENCE ACADEMY INTERNATIONAL UNION OF BIOLOGICAL SCIENTISTS
  1984   International Symposium on Biological Monitoring of the state of Environment, Indian National Science Academy 1984, India. [symposium report], New Delhi 11–13, 1984.
JEFFERS, J. N. R.
  1978   An Introduction to Systems Analysis: With Ecological Applications. London: Edward Arnold.
  1982   Outline Series in Ecology: Modelling. United Kingdom: Chapman and Hall.
KAISER, H. M. & T. E. DRENNEN, Eds.
  1993   Agricultural Dimensions of Global Climate Change. Delray Beach, FL: St. Lucie Press.
KASPERSON, J. X. & R. E. KASPERSON, Eds.
         Global Environmental Risk. Tokyo: United Nations University Press. In press.
KASPERSON, J. X., R. E. KASPERSON & B. L. TURNER II, Eds.
         Regions at Risk: Comparisons of Threatened Systems. Tokyo: United Nations University Press. In press.
KOVACS, M., Ed.
  1992   Biological Indicators and Environmental Protection. United Kingdom: Ellis Horwood.
LIKENS, G. E.
  1992   The Ecosystem Approach: Its Use and Abuse. Germany: Ecology Institute.
MCKENZIE, D. H., D. E. HYATT & V. J. MCDONALD, Eds.
  1992   Ecological Indicators, Volumes I and II. United Kingdom: Elsevier Applied Science.
NAIMAN, R. J. & H. DECAMPES, Eds.
  1990   Man and Biosphere Series: The Ecology and Management of Aquatic-Terrestrial Ecotones. Unesco, France: Parthenon Publishing Group.
PALMER, T. N.
  1993   A nonlinear dynamical perspective on climate change. Weather **48**: 314–326.

RAMADE, F.
  1981   Ecology of Natural Resources. Chichester, UK: John Wiley and Sons.
RICKLEFS, R. E.
  1990   Ecology, 3rd Edition. New York: W. H. Freeman and Company.
ROSENFIELD, A. & R. MANN, Eds.
  1992   Dispersal of Living Organisms into Aquatic Ecosystems. Maryland Sea Grant
          College.
SHERMAN, K., L. M. ALEXANDER & B. D. GOLD, Eds.
  1993   Large Marine Ecosystems: Stress, Mitigation and Sustainability. Washington, DC:
          AAAS Press.
SHUBERT, L. E., Ed.
  n.d.   Algae as Ecological Indicators. London: Academic Press.
SOUTHWICK, C. H.
  1985   Global Ecology. Sunderland, MA: Sinauer Associates Inc.
TEAKALL, D.
  1992   Biomarkers as Pollution Indicators. London, New York: Chapman and Hall.
TELLUS INSTITUTE AND STOCKHOLM ENVIRONMENTAL INSTITUTE
  1994   WEAP: Water Evaluation and Planning Systems. Boston, MA: WEAP User Guide.
          (unpublished guide, Tellus, 617-266-5400)
TUDGE, C.
  1991   Global Ecology. New York: Oxford University Press.
WORF, D. L., Ed.
  1980   Biological Monitoring for Environmental Effects. Lexington, MA: Lexington Books.
WORLD BANK
  1993   World Development Report 1993: Investing in Health. New York: Oxford Univer-
          sity Press.
WHO COMMISSION ON HEALTH AND ENVIRONMENT
  1992   Our Planet, Our Earth. WHO 1992. Geneva.

Prediction and Biological Evolution

Concept Paper

(Summarized by Stephen S. Morse)

SUMMARY

The major issue addressed was how to introduce evolutionary thinking into epidemiology, and the appropriate approach to "evolutionary epidemiology." There was general agreement that disease emergence is not a static but a dynamic process, and that dynamic approaches should therefore be emphasized.

After discussion, the following objectives were reached by consensus:

ASSUMPTIONS

1. Disease emergence includes evolutionary events at several levels, including at the level of genotype, phenotypic expression, and ecologic interactions.
2. Microbial evolutionary events are dynamic and may occur rapidly, but rates are likely to be affected by environmental conditions and different time-scales apply to different levels of evolutionary events.
3. Evolutionary events and other factors in disease emergence may interact in a complex manner.
4. Ecological and demographic changes can drive evolutionary events.

HYPOTHESES

1. Evolutionary processes that affect disease emergence exist on two levels which must be considered: Historical (macroevolutionary events that give rise to new taxonomic categories) and microevolutionary (rapid and reversible appearance and disappearance of variants that affect the course of disease without reaching formal taxonomic states) levels.
2. Human actions can drive evolutionary changes (Assumption 4 above), by creating new habitats, challenging pathogens with strong selection pressures such as antibiotics, changing the communities with which the pathogens interact, altering host vulnerability and promoting unusual genetic recombination or mutation.

The evolution of virulence, which merits serious consideration as an important area of inquiry,[1] may have at least some anthropogenic causes.[1,2] The host defenses are also likely to be an important factor in the evolution of infectious diseases.
3. Ecological events may lead to emergence by altering co-evolutionary (de-

fined for the purposes of this paper as inter-organism) relationships,[2] as well as relationships of organisms to their physical environment and displacement of existing organisms (such as the displacement of a circulating *Salmonella* variety by a newly introduced serovar).

Appropriate methodologies for studying these hypotheses need to be developed; methodologies for analyzing each level, and for understanding the system as a whole, will require different approaches. These include methods for modeling complex dynamical systems, and methods for ecological and population genetics.

PREDICTION

Despite the probabilistic nature of many evolutionary events, and the role of chance, there are also patterns (originating, for example, from evolutionary history as well as from other causes), including stabilizing factors (thus, influenza is static in its usual avian reservoir hosts but undergoes rapid evolution upon introduction into mammals[3]). Better models for understanding these patterns and their underlying causal relationships would allow better prediction of likely evolutionary directions.

In addition, we can begin developing a more systematic understanding of these coevolutionary patterns, and strengthen predictive capabilities by effectively using geographic methods and modeling systems to track disease and better anticipate its spread.[4–6]

This is also an opportune time to better understand the role of genetic variation in a broader context.[7] Although it is still not generally possible to predict biological characteristics from genotype, increased understanding is gradually emerging. Methods for studying these evolutionary events *in vivo* are just beginning to develop,[8,9] including comparative approaches using molecular phylogenetic analysis,[10,11] and one can hope for increasing depth in understanding ecological interactions and coevolution involving viruses and their hosts. Molecular epidemiologic analysis,[12] comparing strains over time or from different geographic regions, and which often also incorporates phylogenetic analysis, can also provide valuable information,[3,13,14] and can also help to track their spread. Combining these phylogenetic and geographic approaches with our understanding of population dynamics of zoonotic agents in their natural hosts would help to resolve questions about extent and timing of various interspecies transfers and to predict where the greatest risk of human exposure might be. Population modeling might also help to identify when ecological conditions are unstable, with increased possibility for emergence.

REFERENCES

1. EWALD, P. W. 1993. The evolution of virulence. Sci. Am. **268**: 86–93.
2. MORSE, S. S. Examining the origins of emerging viruses. *In* Emerging Viruses. S. S. Morse, Ed.: 10–28. New York: Oxford University Press.

3. GAMMELIN, M., A. ALTMÜLLER, U. REINHARDT, J. MANDLER, V. R. HARLEY, P. J. HUDSON, W. M. FITCH & C. SCHOLTISSEK. 1990. Molec. Biol. Evol. **7**: 194–200.
4. GOULD, P., J. KABEL, W. GORR & A. GOLUB. 1991. Interfaces **21**: 80–92.
5. CLIFF, A. D. & P. HAGGETT. 1988. Atlas of Disease Distributions. Analytic Approaches to Epidemiological Data. Oxford, UK: Blackwell.
6. EPSTEIN, P. R., D. J. ROGERS & R. SLOOFF. 1993. Lancet **341**: 1404–1406.
7. MORSE, S. S. 1993. Toward an evolutionary biology of viruses. *In* Evolutionary Biology of Viruses. S. S. Morse, Ed.: 1–28. New York: Raven Press.
8. BERRY, R. J., T. J. CRAWFORD & G. M. HEWITT, Eds. 1992. Genes in Ecology. Oxford, UK: Blackwell Scientific.
9. DOVER, G. A. 1993. Nature **362**: 672–673.
10. BROOKS, D. R. & D. A. McLENNAN. 1991. Phylogeny, Ecology, and Behavior. A Research Program in Comparative Biology. Chicago, IL: University of Chicago Press.
11. HARVEY, P. H. & M. D. PAGEL. 1991. The Comparative Method in Evolutionary Biology. Oxford, UK: Oxford University Press.
12. OU, C.-Y., *et al.* 1992. Science **256**: 1165–1171.
13. BUONAGURIO, D. A., S. NAKADA, J. D. PARVIN, M. KRYSTAL, P. PALESE & W. M. FITCH. 1986. Science **232**: 980–982.
14. SELANDER, R. K. & J. M. MUSSER. 1990. *In* The Molecular Basis of Pathogenesis. B. Iglewski & V. L. Clark, Eds. New York: Academic Press.

Conceptual Framework: Discussion

Part A: A Conceptual Framework of Integrated Epidemiology for Application to Emerging Diseases

(Summarized by P. K. Anderson)

Epidemiology is the science of disease in populations[1] and can be qualified according to the host population of primary interest, *i.e.,* medical epidemiology, veterinary epidemiology or botanical epidemiology.[2]

Science operates and advances through paradigms.[3] A paradigm is a conceptual framework that guides thinking and action within an area of scientific endeavor. Epidemiology, as a science, must have an underlying paradigm. That paradigm, or conceptual framework, may be well-defined, articulated and overt, or empirical and covert. However, the former is more useful.

George Macdonald introduced his book, *Epidemiology and Control of Malaria,*[4] by presenting his overview of epidemiology. Macdonald considered that the science of epidemiology deals with the reasons for the prevalence of disease and the nature and causes of variations in it. He outlined four branches of epidemiological work: circumstantial, etiological, biological and mathematical epidemiology. Circumstantial epidemiology describes the disease and the circumstances in which the disease occurs. Etiological epidemiology deals with identification of the causal agent of the disease, alternative hosts and modes of transmission of the pathogen. Biological epidemiology generates basic knowledge on the organisms involved in the pathosystem: pathogens, hosts and vectors. Even a large body of detailed knowledge on the organisms involved will not, necessarily, lead to a full understanding of disease. Macdonald argued that it is necessary to integrate the circumstantial, etiological and biological data into a coherent whole through mathematical epidemiology. The science of epidemiology, as conceptualized by Macdonald, includes study within all branches: circumstantial, etiological, biological, and mathematical epidemiology.

Macdonald's conceptual framework has been borrowed and, with minor modification, applied to botanical epidemiology to guide research and intervention for insect-transmitted plant pathogens.[5] The branch of epidemiology that Macdonald defined as biological was re-defined as ecological epidemiology. Ecological epidemiology includes not only the biological study of organisms in the pathosystem, but also the study of relationships between them.

439

MODIFICATIONS OF THE EXISTING CONCEPTUAL FRAMEWORK

While Macdonald's conceptual framework is a useful starting point, this framework is fairly static with a short-term (ecological) perspective and biological-biomedical focus. To be useful as a framework to guide continuing work zon vector-borne diseases and incipient work on emerging diseases of varied natures, the framework needs to be further modified.

Circumstantial Epidemiology

In Macdonald's conceptualization this branch of epidemiology describes patterns of disease, as if the patterns were static. Work in the area of emerging diseases illustrates the fact that disease patterns are dynamic; they expand, retract and shift in time and space. Consequently, disease patterns must be continually monitored in order to determine the rate and direction of change for new and reoccurring diseases.

The focus of circumstantial epidemiology must also expand to include the description of spatial and temporal patterns for other parameters of epidemiological significance, such as: a) the organisms in the pathosystem, *i.e.* pathogen, hosts, vectors, pathogen reservoirs, vector hosts; b) climate; c) population structure; d) trade; e) migration; f) ecological change and g) cultural traditions. By tracking and analyzing other parameters, it may be possible to correlate co-varying patterns and generate testable hypotheses to explain the emergence and spread of new and resurgent diseases.

In order to map multiple parameters, it will be necessary to identify and network with the other groups of researchers and practitioners, *e.g.* marine and rodent biologists; ecologists; social scientists; specialists in environmental change, migration, population, commerce; national and international weather services.

Data banks must be created, established and maintained. These data banks will provide the data base for mapping and analysis. The data banks should have both a biological nature (*e.g.*, they should consist of biological specimens—pathogens, vectors, pathogen reservoirs, plant hosts) and an informational nature (*e.g.*, population, migration, trade data). With data permanently stored and maintained it will be possible to develop historical records for disease evolution. These data can be re-analyzed as historical data. The development of new tools (*e.g.*, for the characterization, taxonomy and diagnosis of biological organisms or the analysis of climatic data and environmental change) is a prerequisite.

Most hosts, be they human, animal or plant, are subject to multiple simultaneous infections, not single infections. Thus, there must also be a shift in focus in circumstantial epidemiology from the mapping and analyzing of one pathosystem to the mapping and analyzing of multiple pathosystems that occur simultaneously in time or space.

It may not be possible to predict the future, but it is certainly possible

Pathogen, vector and hosts are present	If pathogen is present, then: host is contacted	If host is contacted, then: transmission occurs	If transmission occurs, then: host is infected
If host is infected, then: what factors lead to disease	If disease results, then: death, chronic infection, or recovery occurs		

FIGURE 1. Etiological pathways of disease emergence.

to plan for it.[a] The study of past and present epidemics and the search of common patterns and principles, will provide powerful insights into vulnerable areas or populations which should be monitored and would enable us to plan for emerging or re-emerging diseases in these vulnerable areas and populations.

Etiological Epidemiology

As conceptualized by Macdonald[4] etiological epidemiology defines the pathogen causing the disease and the principal modes of transmission. This is a strictly biological conceptualization. The presence of a pathogen is necessary but not sufficient to cause disease. There must be a shift in focus from the definition of etiological agent to the definition of etiological pathways. (Fig. 1).

The shift in focus from etiological agent to etiological pathways will require that the study and understanding of human activity, social customs, knowledge and beliefs, *i.e.*, the social determination of diseases, be incorporated into this branch of epidemiology. Etiological epidemiology must become a bio-social construct. This is the branch of epidemiology that must raise the questions of vulnerability. It is expected that vulnerability research will make a significant contribution to etiological epidemiology.

To be applicable to work on emerging diseases, etiological epidemiology must also expand its focus to include the so-called anomalies, *i.e.*, those diseases that do not fall into well-defined and recognized disease syndromes. Active survey work, as in the case of the orphan arboviruses, should be recognized as a valuable activity and funded accordingly.

---

[a] The issue of prediction was discussed very controversially during the workshop. Different opinions regarding this point were expressed by the participants. Pamela Anderson discussed her position in the paper "The emergence of new plant diseases: the case of insect-transmitted plant viruses" in this volume (Anderson and Morales, pp. 181–194).

Ecological Epidemiology

As part of the new conceptual framework, ecological epidemiology must expand its focus to emphasize variation as an epidemiologically important area of study. How much variation exists in pathogens (strains, pathovars), vectors (biotypes), reservoirs, *etc.* and what is the role of this variation?

The basic biological and ecological data which exist on the organisms in defined pathosystems have been generated for purposes other than epidemiological analysis. The data are incomplete and often completely lacking for quantifying many biological and ecological parameters in mathematical models of disease spread. As the efforts to model pathosystems increase and epidemiologically relevant parameters become better defined, networking with biologists and ecologists will become critical in order to stimulate interest in epidemiology within those sciences. The adoption of already existing methodologies or the development of new protocols and methodologies in order to generate data for epidemiologically relevant parameters will result from that networking.

Evolutionary Epidemiology

It is proposed that an additional branch of epidemiology be added to the conceptual framework. Ecological epidemiology deals with the pathosystems as they are currently observed. Evolutionary epidemiology would study the evolutionary processes and the comparative outcome of these processes. Evolutionary epidemiology would, for example, study such questions as: How have hosts and their pathogens co-evolved? What are the evolutionary constraints in nature? Are zoonotic introductions due entirely to opportunities for human exposure, or is there a threshold effect? What are the molecular bases of host range, virulence, pathogenesis and host interactions? How can the potential of a given pathogen for infection and disease be predicted?[6]

Mathematical Epidemiology

As pointed out by Gary Smith,[b] mathematical epidemiology refers to the methodology used in this branch of research while all other branches of epidemiology refer to an area of study. This is probably explained by the fact that Macdonald was a mathematician and, as most scientists, biased towards his profession. Thus, the suggestion that this branch be renamed was accepted. It will be referred to it as *synoptic epidemiology,* although this term is still not completely satisfactory. Synoptic epidemiology analyzes and integrates the knowledge generated in the other branches of epidemiological research into a coherent theory which can guide action and inform interventions and practice.

To date, the bulk of the models that have been developed and utilized,

---

[b] See discussion Part B in this section.

i.e. the analytical tools available for synoptic epidemiology, have been quantitative, biological models. It is necessary that this branch expand in, at least, four directions:

a) Analyses must shift from purely biological to bio-social analyses. It is necessary to develop the capacity to model human activity and behavior;
b) Modeling must shift focus from models of single infections to models of multiple infections;
c) Modeling efforts must expand from quantitative modeling to include qualitative modeling and analytical methodologies; and
d) Synoptic epidemiology must expand from explanatory modeling to include predictive modeling.

CONCLUSIONS

Macdonald's conceptual framework is a reasonable starting point from which to begin the development of a conceptual framework for an integrated epidemiology, but it must be modified and expanded in, at least three dimensions:

1) **Across fields.** The conceptual framework that is created must be applicable to human, animal and plant diseases. Within each of these three fields the framework must be useful for study and intervention in not only vector-borne or contagious diseases but also "environmental" diseases. The conceptual framework must be robust.
2) **Across branches.** Here, it is proposed that Macdonald's framework be expanded to include an additional branch of research, evolutionary epidemiology. Continued analysis of this framework may result in the recommendation of additional branches of epidemiology. However, caution must be taken that unnecessary or counterproductive compartmentalization does not occur.
3) **Across disciplines within each branch.** The social component of integrated epidemiology was consciously not proposed as a separate branch of epidemiology (*i.e.,* social epidemiology); this would have perpetuated the compartmentalization. Work within each branch must be redefined from biological to bio-social.

The proposed framework must incorporate an epistemological dimension.[c] Philosophers of science can promote and strengthen an integrated epidemiology by aiding in the definition, re-definition and clarification of concepts and operational definitions in a way that breaks beyond the boundaries of the discipline where the concepts arose or are proposed.

The understanding generated through epidemiological research will lead to recommendations for continued research and for interventions. But, the conceptual framework for epidemiological research must be linked to a parallel

---

[c] See discussion Part C in this section.

framework for prediction, intervention and population protection. This process of adapting or creating such an intervention framework should begin by reviewing the existing literature on intervention.

Finally, it must be understood that any proposal for a conceptual framework must be viewed as part of an on-going, dynamic dialogue. As the need for these guides to thinking and taking action becomes more widely recognized, accepted and utilized, they will and should continue to be refined and further modified. The principal objective is to promote and develop models, in this case conceptual models, to guide our thinking and actions when working with complex systems, such as emerging diseases.

REFERENCES

1. ZADOKS, J. C. 1974. The role of epidemiology in modern phytopathology. Phytopathology 64: 918–923.
2. VANDERPLANK, J. E. 1963. Plant Diseases: Epidemics and Control. New York: Academic Press.
3. KUHN, T. S. 1970. The Structure of Scientific Revolutions, 2nd edition. Chicago, IL: The University of Chicago Press.
4. MACDONALD, G. 1957. Epidemiology and control of malaria. London: Oxford University Press.
5. ANDERSON, P. K. 1991. Epidemiology of Insect-transmitted Plant Pathogens. D.Sc. Thesis. Harvard School of Public Health, Harvard University, Boston, MA. 304 pp.
6. MORSE, S. S. 1994. The viruses of the future? Emerging viruses and evolution. In Evolutionary Biology of Viruses. S. S. Morse, Ed.: 325–335. New York: Raven Press.

Part B: The Possibilities of an Integrated Epidemiology

RUDI SLOOFF: First, I would like to add one factual comment on the concept of an integrated epidemiology. In addition to pathogen contacts, transmissions, and infections you should explore toxin exposure, absorption, and system damage caused by toxins. Including the possibility of toxin exposure into a survey sometimes makes it easier to understand concurrent physiological phenomena and co-morbidity.

The other comment I would like to make is that we have been restricting ourselves during this workshop to water-related and vector-borne diseases. I come from the environmental health division in WHO which is very much concerned with pollution. Within the current epistemological approach to epidemiology, I think the research on pollution and pollutants is still deficient. We have only the toxicological model. In the framework of this model we make dose-response-relationships and we extract from our calculations acceptable levels of pollution. We are not looking at the behavior of pollutants in an ecosystem.

I would propose shifting the focus from the linear "agent-disease" approach to a more holistic approach. The more holistic approach should take into consideration the various modifications that can take place within the environment due to the behavior of the pollutant and the components of the ecosystems acting on it in that process. I think, we are missing that important aspect completely in this workshop.

Anyway, I appreciate this philosophy you presented with the model of an integrated epidemiology very much. I think this is the way to go.

MICHEL GARENNE: I think we would agree that we need a comprehensive framework if we want to understand the processes that we are looking at. However, in all the discussions that we have had in the last three days it seems that we have forgotten to address a very important parameter of disease: the immunological parameter. The immune system of the host largely determines how the disease evolves.

As an example, look at a disease like chickenpox. About 100 years ago in Europe it was considered a very important and dangerous disease, a major cause of death. In our days it is a very mild disease, although the pathogen and the mode of transmission did not change. What has changed is probably the way our immune system copes with the disease. Going back to your framework of an integrated epidemiology I would like to propose adding immunological epidemiology.

PAMELA ANDERSON: Would you add that as another branch, Michel, or could you assign it to, let's say, ecological epidemiology. Could the study of the genetic variation in the host, which in this case is the human being, incorporate immunology?

GARENNE: Well, I would prefer a separate branch. I don't think that the gene pool in Europe has changed that much over the last 100 years. Nor has the pathogen changed. Maybe you can call this phenomenon an ecological balance between the host and the parasite. I think more research is needed on immunological problems and processes. Immunology works nowadays at the microbiological level, the level of the cell, especially. Those responsible for research design should not forget to explore the effects of changes in the immunological system at the level of populations.

GARY SMITH: I would like to propose a modification to the name "mathematical epidemiology." There are three reasons. Epistemological, circumstantial, etiological, biological or ecological epidemiology all contain some indication of the objective of research in that discipline of science. The word "mathematical" does not refer, in my opinion, to an objective. It describes a technique. Second, in etiological epidemiology, case-control and cohort studies are extremely important. For such studies a very sophisticated mathematical body is usually needed. I think my colleagues in the medical school might find it offensive if we deny etiological epidemiology access to mathematics. Finally, the analyses carried out in the framework of circumstantial, etiological, and biological epidemiology are not solely the domain of mathematical models. I would like to suggest that we change the word "mathematical" to "synoptic," synoptic epidemiology.

STEPHEN MORSE: I want to add that all the suggestions you wrote on the board call for a comparative approach to epidemiology. I don't know to what extent the comparative method or methodologies have really been integrated in epidemiology as legitimate approaches. Maybe we can explore this a little bit further.

ANDERSON: To respond, Stephen, comparative is often defined in a very narrow sense. For example, in regard to fungal epidemiology it means that people are using the same limited paradigm to compare different fungal systems.

In our proposal we thought it is time to start that kind of comparison across fields and across pathosystems within fields. This enterprise is very, very difficult because we do not even talk the same language in the different fields and sub-fields of epidemiology.

MORSE: I agree with you. Much more needs to be done to break down those walls between disciplines and fields that separate us. Very important, in my understanding, are comparisons across humans, animals, and plants. We might find important connections beyond the known zoonotic diseases. We might identify many similar patterns across different (human, animal, and even plant) populations and in different areas which have been exposed to similar ecological conditions, changes or disasters. I also agree with you that the language needs to be developed. In addition, I think a special consciousness needs to be developed. I have some hope because the comparative method has long been a traditional method in evolutionary biology. It apparently has found various applications. Perhaps in epidemiology we are a little bit behind that development.

ANDERSON: I want to add another comment. What we have proposed as a conceptual framework is very restricted attempt at epidemiology in terms of understanding. The whole partner component—action or practical proposals—was not included. Actually, the reason for this is very simple. Dick (Levins) and I did not have enough time to work out a practical proposal for the realization of an integrated epidemiology and could not come up with an example. I am sure that there are more projects on conceptual frameworks for an integrated epidemiology.

The task of transforming our ideas into better decisions remains. The decisions we have to make should be focused on the possible and necessary interventions. Further, we have to be able to actually implement the interventions. To make decisions about interventions we have first to evaluate our interventions in terms of how did the process work, what was the product, what were the consequences, and what were the economic implications? On the basis of the evaluation we could develop a broader range of intervention strategies. Unfortunately, in preparation of this plenary session we could not accomplish this task. We could only make this list. And that was our limitation.

In my opinion, even the task of establishing intervention strategies goes back to epistemology. We have not only to ask the question how do we understand but also the question, how do we act and why do we act?

CRISTINA POSSAS: A comment about epistemological epidemiology. In the beginning of your presentation you mentioned that we would not need to incorporate anything substantially new. We would have to shift our focus and incorporate only new elements into epidemiology. This was your conclusion drawn from our written contributions. I would partly agree with your position. I would suggest that we should also incorporate social epidemiology into our list as a separate branch. We should make clear that we are not suggesting anything new, but that we are focusing on things that have already been done or written and combine them with another perspective. We have notable research on social and epistemological epidemiology in Europe and South America.

I don't understand very well what epistemological epidemiology means. In my understanding, theoretical epidemiology works on the basis of a broad theoretical framework. In the framework of theoretical epidemiology different perspectives in approaching methodologies and policies are identified and discussed. I would not call this epistemological epidemiology because epistemology refers more to a cross-disciplinary, broad perspective. Theoretical epidemiology focuses on a specific issue of epidemiology.

ANDERSON: Which is exactly the point why we need professionals in that area instead of people doing it as a hobby.

NAJWA MAKHOUL: I want to say something similar to Cristina's point. In my research I explore precisely the questions how and why did we move away from the very advanced, social epistemology and how and why medicine took the route of development that it did take? We will find answers to these questions in the history of medicine.

LAURIE GARRETT: I must confess that I also did not understand the concept of epistemological epidemiology. It needs to be explained to me.

ANDERSON: Let's try to explain it with an analogy. We have to have a kind of road map in order to understand and to model complex systems. For me, a conceptual framework is an intellectual road map. I have an intellectual or factual complex problem. To solve the problem I have to "come in," to start somewhere and to proceed from this starting point. The possible roads, highways or dirt roads, I could take are quite numerous and not easy to grasp. Sometimes I will get lost and I need some kind of road map to find my way back. To look at the road map is to ask the question: "what is known about this problem, and what are the existing approaches?" I can locate myself someplace within an existing framework by using a road map. I can then make decisions about where to move and how to approach the problem. Maybe somebody else who actually deals with epistemology wants to answer this. Would you like to answer this, Irina?

GARRETT: I still think that to have a category called "epistemological epidemiology" is not necessary. We have already established that we want the social factors, the cultural factors, and others incorporated into our approach to new diseases. It seems redundant.

RICHARD LEVINS: Part of our problem is turning an experience into an intellectual construct that can then be studied as the direct object of our investigation. For instance, if we talk about "new diseases" immediately the question comes up: Are two genotypes, different in some of their DNA, the prerequisite to identify a new disease?

We have to work that out and establish a common language. A scientific enterprise does not work directly with nature but with our own constructs derived from nature which will not be identical for all participants in research. We are creating artificial entities that we then study and have to relate back to nature. To establish a common language to relate our artificial objects back to nature has to be a self-conscious process. It can not be derived from the history of the special field.

GARRETT: The concern in the social and theoretical workshop was that the social factors, whatever those are, and the cultural factors were thought of only tangentially and separately rather than integrated fundamentally into the entire approach to the emergence of diseases. To identify a separate branch called epistemological epidemiology would be again a segregation. I think all these issues can be included into "etiological epidemiology."

PAUL EPSTEIN: I think a way of resolving this is to think of an epistemological framework as one that integrates the various branches of epidemiology. We can talk about direct and indirect effects of stresses within this framework. PCBs and other chemicals have direct effects on the cellular and genetic level while the indirect impact on the immune system (the vulnerability) is determined by emotional stress, malnutrition, alcoholism, HIV, and depression—the leading reasons for diminished T-cell immunity.

Conversely, people have a direct effect on the environment, removing forests creating "edge effects" through road building, increasing disease vectors directly, or through indirect effects like increased atmosphere CO_2.

We then turn to the question of where we intervene. That's where I suggest a third unifying concept: the integration of research and management. We have interventions, like vaccines, and others concerned with malnutrition, immunity, and equity (inequity/poverty and over-abundance being one of the major driving forces of environmental change). I suggest we examine this emerging framework further, look at some of the research proposals developed here, discuss how we can all contribute to their design based on the emerging framework; developing a more systematic approach to surveillance and primary, secondary, and tertiary level interventions.

IRINA ECKARDT: I would not agree with the term "epistemological epidemiology." Epistemological research in epidemiology or in an approach to new diseases is somehow background work. In my understanding it forms an epistemological dimension of our research. I am not happy with the word dimension, but I can not define it in a better way at the moment. To work on an "epistemological dimension" includes first the development of a certain sensitivity to the terms we are used to. Second, the introduction of new terms and the critical revision of the known terms follows. And third, the construction or design of a conceptual framework—our special "road map"—is an important part within the work on an "epistemological dimension." The conceptual framework does not have to be consistent. We are dealing with a very complex phenomenon which is by itself contradictory. In our theoretical constructs about this part of nature we don't have to eliminate the contradictions. Within the conceptual framework it should be possible to develop a system of terms and definitions. Again, to relate our theoretical construct back to nature, the system of terms can not be static, but dynamic. It can evolve in the process of the research. The meaning and the importance of definitions, like "new disease" or "surveillance" becomes also static. They are moments in the research process. Understanding should be the goal of this enterprise not the definition of certain terms!

People working on and thinking about epistemological questions can introduce concepts and theories originated in different disciplines, for example in evolutionary theory. We can test these concepts if they are additions to our "road map" and we could alter them in relation to the special object of research, the emergence of infectious disease.

I think, in the New Disease Group we worked with the concept of co-evolution, which originated in ecology and evolutionary biology. It is a powerful concept for modeling the emergence of water-borne diseases.

MAKHOUL: I support the discontent with epistemological epidemiology, but not only with epistemological epidemiology. I want to emphasize the point that epistemology deals with the question of the construction and the truth of objectivity and subjectivity of knowledge.

This is not only a philosophical question but a basically political question. It includes that we have to think about the instruments we create and use to make one mode of knowledge possible and other modes of knowledge not possible. I have been trying to make the point during the conference that we need an alternative basis for knowledge. We should not only look at what appears, but why it appears in that way. What are the instruments for creating a special theoretical construct? In my understanding, our scientific methods have strongly focused on the appearance of things. To go further is especially important in relation to the emergence of disease. We have learned from the biologist and virologist that sometimes it is more important to ask about the things that are not detectable at the moment.

To capture the appearance of things and the not detectable it is necessary to develop a comprehensive epistemology or a comprehensive research strategy. In my opinion, circumstantial epistemology, etiological and biological and mathematical epistemology are all the same thing. At the moment they are not dealing with the problem. We are still caught being reactive instead of being proactive.

ANDERSON: One of the values of a conceptual framework is that you get more and more people working within it. They may experience that in some cases the framework or concepts and principles of it just don't work. We can learn something by analyzing why the concept couldn't be applied successfully.

Part C: Cause and Effect in the Evolution of New Diseases

LAURIE GARRETT: A common feature in the reports from the four work-shops is that everybody seems to have some difficulties with the concept of cause and effect. In various ways the four working groups were looking at the cause and effect issue. They had problems marking cause and effect in emergence of a special disease that was discussed as a case example.

I wonder if it is possible to understand cause and effect relationships for primary emergence, because primary emergence may in fact be an isolated, transient event. In addition to that problem, we have to look at what social groups perceive as disease.

PAUL EPSTEIN: In response to Laurie Garrett's point about causality, I think terrestrial systems are more complex than marine ecosystems in considering bio-climatographic conditions (rainfall, temperature and vegetation) that permit persistence of a pathogen or pest. Whether predators of the mosquitoes, frogs, and lace wings are absent, and whether all factors (hosts, reservoirs, agents) are present in a particular place is a very complex equation. One can draw bio-climatographs (where a vector or parasite could persist) and see if that changes if isotherms, for instance, move north or south or ascend mountains.

There are some studies in Argentina and in Rwanda indicating that there may be movement of *Plasmodium vivax* to higher altitudes. It's a very complex equation, however. I appreciate that. In marine systems, causality appears to be much more linear in the sense that eutrophication, nutrients, over-fishing, loss of wetlands (which clean effluents) and perhaps warming sea surface temperature all push in the same direction, to increase algal populations. I think we have a more linear situation with respect to causality.

TAMARA AWERBUCH: I would like to answer Laurie's question about causality. In the working group on mathematical modeling we tried to explore the answers to some of the questions about the design of mathematical models. The very simple model we started with consisted of the input, the mathematics, and the output. We did not explore further the input. We just listed biological inputs, social inputs, environmental inputs, and so forth. It was clear for us that there is no linear relationship. None of the factors, listed as input, contribute the same way to the emergence or reemergence of disease. In the next session of the workshop we want to deal with causality and to see how all these components will effect the emergence of a disease.

IRINA ECKARDT: Personally, I have some difficulties with a linear concept of causality. I think, that linear causality forms the exceptional (aberrant) way in which nature evolves. Anyway, I want to ask Paul if it would be possible to predict, for instance, the influences and changes in the marine ecosystem related to the emergence of a disease on the basis of his more linear model of the relationships between vectors, pathogens and disease. Does your model allow you to predict an outbreak of this disease in that area? Are the differences between terrestrial and marine ecosystems really those of more and less linearity in the relationships of vectors, pathogens and disease?

EPSTEIN: I think it is not a question of predicting one place with certainty, but we can talk about patterns and places, critical regions, that are particularly vulnerable for monitoring.

ECKARDT: Do you think patterns are the same then as cause and effect?

EPSTEIN: I'm talking about how global forces become superimposed on local environmental susceptibilities. We can't say there is going to be a brown tide on Long Island and demoic acid poisoning on Prince Edward Island, but we may say that because of changes in the sea temperature this year, we can expect some events along the east coast in vulnerable areas. Direct effects of warming may have increased cardiovascular disease in heat waves, while indirect effects may occur in terms of vector abundance of communicable disease transmission. With a change in means (in temperature, pressures and prescription) we arrive at a new "regime." Climate values are oscillating around a certain mean, and they can jump and oscillate around another set of means. That is what happened 9,500 years ago at the end of the ice age according to Greenland ice-core records, when the climate system jumped for reasons we don't know and went into the current period (called the Holocene). Whether we will jump into another regime now is uncertain. Secondly, just measuring means may hide other changes which occur. There is evidence that minimum temperatures may go up more than maximum temperatures, so that with an average rise of 2.5 degrees, for instance, the minimum may rise 2.1 and the maximum 2.7 degrees. The rate of change of minimum to maximum may fluctuate. This could affect vectors and parasite cycles much more than just changes in the mean. Thirdly, we have variations and anomalies within the climate system. Abnormal events, abnormal oscillations, in frequency, amplitude, and duration are associated with anomalies in precipitation, storms, *etc.*

Turning to impacts, there is evidence that warming changes species composition among the plankton to favor dinoflagellates and cyanobacteria, which contain more toxic species. Toxic species are less palatable to predators, a factor that may further enhance algal blooms (a positive feedback in the system).

If we are getting a greater number and amplitude of oscillations, with greater perturbations and more chaotic factors impacting ecosystems, the impacts will increase. Global circulation models (GCMS) that couple ocean and atmospheric behavior predict more El Niño events with more warming events and increased atmospheric carbon dioxide. El Niño events have occurred about twice a decade for the past century; since 1983 we have had four El Niño events. In fact, climatologists are reporting we are in a period of stagnation and have been locked into an El Niño for four years. Warming sea surfaces are reflected in lower pressures between Tahiti and Darwin, Australia, and they have been in a "blocked pattern" for the past four years. It is not clear which way it is going to go because there could be a big upwelling (La Niña) that cools the oceans and atmosphere. Prediction of the system is unusually uncertain right now. But we do know that the Western Pacific Warming Center determines global and regional patterns of weather (rain and floods and droughts) that will impact vector distribution, disease transmission and emergence.

RITA COLWELL: I think, I would rather use the analogy of us being in the descriptive stage of an "ecological epidemiology" rather than in the "synoptic," in which we would actually deal with differentiations in cause and effect. In my understanding, what we are really seeking are correlations and patterns from which we may be able to derive the causations. We are still in the earliest stage. This is not a negative statement. I simply want to re-define our position and step back. To jump to the conclusion that there is a direct cause and effect relationship in marine ecosystems we would miss exactly this necessary re-definition which is so important for a conceptual framework. Right now, it would be sufficient to seek out, which has never been done before, a global approach to epidemiology. Within such a global approach to epidemiology we can take into account ecological perspectives and parameters to give a kaleidoscopic instead of a uni-dimensional view.

Development of a Research Agenda

Introduction

The development of a research agenda has to be more than simply listing projects that people would like to see carried out. We begin with the recognition that we are living in a period of abrupt and profound social, demographic, climatic, vegetational, and technical change which is producing new epidemiological challenges. Our goal has to be to minimize epidemiological suprises by assuring that the research program as a whole is broad, imaginative and flexible enough to prepare for the unexpected appearance of new diseases and the resurgence or spread of old ones.

The many specific suggestions made in the discussion groups and plenaries emphasized several general themes:

1. Since parasitism is a general phenomenon affecting all groups of organisms, our understanding would be enhanced by integrating the studies of diseases of plants, domestic and wild animals and of people. The special contributions of plant research include:

a) The large number of species that are studied allows for examining the relation between taxonomic distance between hosts and differences in disease expression.

b) The passage of a pathogen through hosts of different species and the monitoring of attenuation and increased virulence can inform our study of natural selection and adaptation of microorganisms.

c) The immobility of plants allows for precise observation of spatial patterns in an outbreak.

d) Populations of annual crop plants are cohorts of uniform age. The relationship of disease manifestation to development becomes a major consideration in protection.

e) Populations may be made genetically uniform or heterogeneous in desired ways in order to examine the role of genetic diversity in epidemics.

f) Populations have discrete boundaries so that we can distinguish the dynamics of separate epidemics from that of invasion, with population size not only known but also predetermined.

Animal epidemiology is intermediate between plant and human studies in some ways. The number of species we have information about is much smaller than for plants though still allows for taxonomic diversity and the examination of characteristics such as differential immune responses. Special contributions of veterinary epidemiology would include:

a) Controlled nutrition and to some extent environmental conditions among domestic animals allows for the study of the relation of these factors to vulnerability.

b) Discrete populations, with known and to some extent controllable population sizes and age distributions.

c) Comparison of diseases in similar species (*e.g.* domestic and wild swine and cattle).

d) For smaller animals, short generations and large populations amplify the interaction of demography and epidemiology, the co-evolution of host adaptation to disease and the evolution of the parasite, and the role of infection in species interactions.

e) The effect of infection on fertility can be examined with high precision.

The study of human disease contributes to general epidemiology:

a) Long-term historical records of disease;
b) More detailed physiological knowledge than of any other species;
c) Rich descriptions of morbidity since people can tell what they feel.

2. The research agenda has to be multi-leveled, including:

a) The longest range work in evolutionary and systematic epidemiology;
b) The ecology of actual and potential pathogens, vectors and reservoirs;
c) The monitoring of global and local environmental change and changes in disease range;
d) Experimental and modeling work on natural selection in all members of the pathosystems;
e) The analysis of population vulnerability;
f) Surveillance of all members of the relevant pathosystems; and
g) The study of interactions among diseases.

3. Preparation for the unexpected includes prediction, detection with rapid response, reduction of vulnerability and prevention. All are needed. There was some disagreement in the workshop about the possibility of prediction, but this abated when it was clarified that prediction means the reduction of uncertainty, not the announcement of the precise time place and symptoms of new outbreaks.

At present there is much more breadth in the analysis of disease than there is in the proposals for response, which seems to be limited to antibiotics, immunization, and traditional public health measures. Special attention should be given to new approaches to reducing the vulnerability of individuals and populations.

4. There is a need for a diversity of research methods including:

a) Compiling of a database for new and resurgent diseases;
b) Expanded monitoring of ecological change including climate change and also the ecology of agricultural development, deforestation, and urbanization, and of new special habitats such as cooling towers (just as there are population thresholds for the maintenance of diseases such as smallpox—a few hundred thousand—there may be diseases which require populations in the millions and may appear in the new megalopolises of the third world);
c) Ecological studies of relevant species with special emphasis on mosquitoes, rodents and plankton;

   d) Social/ecological study of the vulnerability of populations;
   e) Genetic analysis of variation in pathogens;
   f) Mathematical modeling of epidemics and disease evolution; and
   g) Experimental study of microevolution of pathogens.

   5. To the extent that we are trying to do something new, it becomes important to examine our own processes. This entails:

   a) Conceptual clarification and the development of a common transdisciplinary language;
   b) History and sociology of research in epidemiology;
   c) Identification of the obstacles to disease recognition; and
   d) Invention of new ways of combining the work of health professionals and the general public. On a number of occasions disease problems have been placed on the agenda of public health through the initiatives of neighbors or advocacy groups. This process should be examined and made part of any strategy.

Research Proposals

PAUL R. EPSTEIN

Harvard Medical School
The Cambridge Hospital
1493 Cambridge Avenue
Cambridge, Massachusetts 02139

Benefitting from our Woods Hole setting, a proposal has emerged that integrates research and management in the area of marine biology. Ken Sherman kicked off, with a description of a comprehensive program for monitoring marine ecosystems based on measuring nutrients exiting from watersheds and coasts; the plankton, shellfish and fish communities; currents, winds and sea surface temperatures (SSTs). As initially proposed, the program did not include a health component. We have now developed a plan to carry out such integrated monitoring that includes health indices, along the Gulf of Guinea off West Africa, in a project funded by the Global Environmental Facility (GEF).

The plan calls for an examination of plankton, mussels and fish for biotoxins and for *Vibrio cholerae,* including speciation of vibrios (*e.g.*, for *Vibrio cholerae* O139 Bengal). In addition, we will establish a surveillance tool and a coordinated system for monitoring relevant health outcomes in the five nations involved. Preliminary discussion with WHO representatives of the food and water safety divisions have taken place. Training in laboratory techniques ("building local capacity") for identification of algal biotoxins (Harmful Algal Bloom program of UNESCO) and bacterial pathogens (Maryland Biotechnology Institute) would occur in the initial phase.

It is hoped that this system can serve as a model for integrating data across climatological, ecological, social and health fields. In marine ecosystems we will be looking for early indicators of change, and establishing an early warning system for biotoxins and *Vibrio cholerae* O139 Bengal before they enter nations by way of the marine food chain. Remote sensing of SSTs and algal blooms (with SeaWiFS, a satellite scheduled for launch in 1994) will be used to guide sampling of marine species. Monitoring for O139 Bengal in ballast water has begun elsewhere (Australia), and the International Maritime Organization (IMO) is developing plans to monitor and regulate the transport of ballast water for vibrios and other "nuisance" species.

A Commentary on Research Needs for Monitoring and Containing Emergent Vector-borne Infections

ANDREW SPIELMAN

Department of Tropical Public Health
Harvard School of Public Health
665 Huntington Avenue
Boston, Massachusetts 02115

Outbreaks of vector-borne pathogens tend to increase explosively because such infections generally are exceedingly communicable. Their containment, therefore, depends on timely detection and the rapid transfer of information to a central authority having the means to intervene. Monitoring might seek to detect changes in the vector, non-human reservoir or the human population, itself. Rainfall, or another environmental event, may serve as a surrogate for direct observations on the vector. Sustainable interventions must be parsimonious.

MONITORING VECTOR HOSTS

The recent (1984) invasion of Asian *Aedes albopictus* into North America, for example, seemed to signal an impending outbreak of dengue. The aquatic larval stages of this exotic mosquito were detected during the routine course of a mosquito abatement program in Texas, and quite soon after the species became established. Its distribution subsequently spread to include much of the eastern United States. CDC and university surveys, based on sampling eggs and larvae, traced this rapidly evolving distribution. The cognizant authorities became alert, but no adverse effect on human health has yet been documented.

Introduction of a member of the African *Anopheles gambiae* complex into Natal Province of Brazil, however, produced an exceptionally lethal outbreak of malaria early in the 1930s. The presence of this exotic vector is said to have been detected accidentally by an off-duty Rockefeller Institute entomologist enjoying a Sunday stroll. Action was taken, however, only after many lives were lost. This Brazilian introduction was soon eliminated.

Less dramatic than the discovery of an exotic vector is a more gradual increase in the abundance of a vector or its incremental loss of insecticide susceptibility. These events are commonplace, but are more difficult to detect. No Sunday stroll would document its occurrence, and few pest-abatement efforts would maintain records that can detect such changes.

Observations on the prevalence of arboviral infection in vector arthropods have served as an important basis for public health interventions. Light-trap or resting-box collections of vector mosquitoes are regularly subjected to virological study by health authorities. Sentinel chicken flocks constitute a variant on this monitoring strategy. The results provide a direct transmission index.

A program of research designed to detect threatening changes in vector populations should establish "transmission indices" that quantify levels of risk for particular sites. Such indices have been well developed in the case of peridomestic *Ae. aegypti* and express vector abundance in terms of the occurrence or density of larvae per human residence. Other dengue indices are based on the collection of mosquito eggs in special sampling devices. "Landing" or human-biting collections provide such information in the case of malaria or African sleeping sickness. The immediate need is for locally adapted traps or other collecting systems that produce reliable estimates of vector density that can be compared to some locally derived baseline that predicts outbreaks.

Special attention should be devoted to blood-feeding insects that are locally abundant and that focus their bites on certain potential reservoir hosts. Particular mosquitoes may, therefore, threaten human health precisely because they rarely feed on people.

MONITORING NONHUMAN RESERVOIR HOSTS

The emergence of Lyme disease as a public health threat in parts of North America and Eurasia derives from the recent proliferation of deer. The "chain of causation," however, contains so many links that no threat could have been expected based on observed changes in deer density. Similar complexity surrounds the arboviral encephalitides. Birds that serve as reservoir hosts tend to be particularly dynamic, with such introduced species as house sparrows and starlings replacing native birds. Here too, the link between observed changes in reservoir density and any interpreted threat to the public health is too remote to be used to persuade the health authorities to act.

Observations on the prevalence of particular pathogens in wildlife may help predict outbreaks. Although not vector-borne, rabies is a classical example of this approach. The risk of visceral leishmaniasis appears to relate to the frequency of infection in domestic dogs, and the Brazilian health authorities have acted on this information by destroying infected dogs to reduce risk of human infection.

Research efforts should be directed toward development of improved methods for monitoring the distribution and abundance of selected vertebrate animals, including species composition, their density and prevalence of infections that are relevant to human health. Particular attention should be devoted to abundant animals that establish intense local foci in sites that otherwise contain few hosts on which some indigenous vector feeds. The challenge is to translate these observations into a form that is persuasive to the regional health authorities.

MONITORING HUMAN POPULATIONS

The density of non-immune people resident in a site profoundly affects risk of human infection. Malaria, for example, emerges explosively among non-immune people immigrating from arid or upland regions who seek refuge in an endemic site. Scrub typhus and tick-borne relapsing fever behave similarly. Epidemic typhus is the traditional destroyer of such refugees while in transit. People who have resettled in regions that have been cleared of onchocerciasis would be peculiarly vulnerable to resumed transmission of this filarial worm. Displaced people, then, are peculiarly vulnerable to sweeping outbreaks of vector-borne disease because they are concentrated, non-immune to certain pathogens, and culturally or otherwise unable to protect themselves against vector arthropods.

Drug-resistant malaria pathogens are most likely to develop in sites that are subject to migration. Here, pathogen strains from geographically remote sites would combine through superinfection. Reassortment as well as recombination events would provide the natural variation that would be selected as a function of profligate drug use. For this reason, gem mining and other kinds of economic activity in the tropics would tend to promote emergence of novel drug-resistant malaria parasites.

The health status of moving groups of people is peculiarly difficult to monitor. Rapid and simple diagnostic methodologies would be essential. These include developments such as malaria dip-stick and specific PCR technologies. Potentially more useful would be physical paradigms for population-based diagnoses. Because these efforts would diagnose disease in a group of people as a whole rather than as the sum of individual diagnoses, non-specific signs could be used that would be useless in clinical practice. Moving human populations are "the best targets" for vector-borne infection. Local research efforts should be mounted to devise monitoring strategies for people who recently have moved.

MONITORING ENVIRONMENTAL CHANGE

Although vector arthropods generally derive from the environment rather than from the body of the affected person, host-specificity is a main determinant of their capacity as vectors. Thus, all life-cycle stages will be associated with the vertebrate reservoir host. Mosquito vectors of malaria, dengue and lymphatic filariasis, for example, generally breed in the kinds of water created by human activity. Disturbed environments are the hallmark of human existence, and the many variations on that theme provide the niche exploited by the diverse vectors of human disease. The research challenge is to identify the particular kinds of disturbance that promote vector abundance and to establish appropriate monitoring systems.

INTERVENTION TECHNOLOGY

Powerful intervention technologies for attacking vector populations are already at hand. Fabrics impregnated with the recently developed synthetic pyrethroid insecticides, in particular, permit environmentally non-intrusive and relatively safe attacks on the most vulnerable part of the transmission cycle of vector-borne pathogens. By making life dangerous for vectors that come in contact with people, the longevity of the anthropophagous portion of the vector population is reduced. The present vogue for genetically engineered vectors, however, visualizes an attack on a far less crucial facet of vectorial capacity, seeking merely to modify their competence as hosts for particular pathogens. The technological research challenge is to devise methods for the parsimonious use of methods that attack vulnerable points in the transmission cycle.

To be sustainable, interventions should be used occasionally in place and time. Intensive use, on the other hand, induces resistance, expends resources, reduces herd immunity, causes donor fatigue, and induces unrealistic expectations of health. Iatrogenic outbreaks result. The research need is for the development of interventions that can promptly be launched in response to data that has been transmitted from affected sites.

MODIFIED RESEARCH SUPPORT SYSTEM

Our ability to monitor emergent vector-borne infections worldwide, presently, suffers from a series of fundamental weaknesses. Specialists in vector ecology are increasingly in short supply, as are academic institutions capable of relevant training. Opportunity for research experience in vector ecology similarly is waning, and research on the ecology of vector-borne diseases is becoming increasingly difficult to fund. Although a pervasive shortage of research funds is partly to blame for this weakness, competition from highly reductionist molecular approaches in public health contributes to our progressive inability to cope with substantive problems.

In spite of these trends, the entrepreneurial research spirit of the academic community can effectively be used in an effort to monitor for emerging infections. A novel definition of scientific merit should be developed by granting agencies. Merit is conventionally assigned on the basis of the worth of some stated biological objective and the quality of the reasoning behind the methodology proposed to resolve the issue. Instead, investigators might be encouraged to compete on the basis of the properties of "emergence." The stated objective would be to determine whether risk of human disease is increasing. Priority would be assigned to a proposal describing the likelihood of an outbreak with a steeply sloping epidemic curve and great amplitude as well as a severely debilitating illness. No new funding would be required. Emergent vector-borne diseases should rate well on such an alternative scale of merit.

SUMMARY

Most critical in an approach toward suppressing or containing any vector-borne infection is the ability to select research directions on the basis of substantive rather than technological or opportunistic objectives. Any public health campaign should pursue attainable objectives that are worthwhile, sustainable and quantifiable. Failure to satisfy all of these criteria may result in the worst public health harm, an ultimate increase in prevalence of disease.

The rapidly changing human environment assures us of a continuing series of newly emergent vector-borne diseases. Elements in our ability to monitor, analyze and prevent such events, however, seem to be deteriorating. To strengthen this capacity, granting agencies might permit a modified definition of merit for extramural research support that would harness the entrepreneurial capacities of the academic community.

Research Agenda

General Discussion

RICHARD CASH: Let me comment on a number of points that you have raised here. I agree with your definition of prediction. Though you can not absolutely predict an event, you can reduce your level of uncertainty by gathering information, particularly with regard to interventions during the preplanning phase.

Concerning horizontal and vertical approaches, within the human health field, the approach to malnutrition is certainly a horizontal and not a vertical approach. Severe malnutrition is not caused, in most cases, except during times of famine, simply by the lack of food. Further, I want to support Bob's notion about infection versus disease. There are many more people infected with tuberculosis than develop disease. If we ignore infection and focus only on disease, we would not have predicted many of the outbreaks that we are having now.

Lastly, I think that some of the earlier discussion has attempted to set up a construct that would lead us in a logical stepwise approach to answering specific questions. Unfortunately, scientific discovery does not always develop in linear fashion. There are starts and stops, dead-end paths, and often a lot of serendipity. We should be cautious in trying to reach some sort of model which whould logically lead us to the answer. It just doesn't work that way.

RICHARD LEVINS: But it often leads to answers to other questions.

PAMELA ANDERSON: I have a response to Richard's comments. In my understanding, there was no implication that this stepwise approach is a linear logical sequence. In fact, most of the time the approach to solving a problem is a back and forth process of attempts and decisions between different possible paths to the solution. That is the beauty of this scientific enterprise.

You might decide that you need a specific model. The model tells you what type of circumstantial data you would have to collect. Once you have the data analyzed you might go back and evaluate the model in order to introduce some changes. It is also possible that the data prove your model wrong. It really is a flow between different branches, not a linear process.

LAURIE GARRETT: I have a political question for the scientists in the room. How would you answer the criticism that was raised in relation to the Institute of Medicine (IOM) report[1] that the underlying goal behind all these warnings about new and emerging infections is to get more research money at a time when the budgets are very low in the United States. We are living in a recession in which generally all funds have been cut back to a minimum. How can you demand to get more funds for research? How are you going to create a research proposal to get these funds despite the budgetary constraints?

STEPHEN MORSE: I would agree with the point that the publication of urgent warnings, including the IOM report, are, in one regard, attempts to get more money. We do need more money. I think there are important issues to discuss and to explore. There are diseases that do threaten the world. AIDS had threatened people's health for over 10 years before it became a research problem for health professionals. There is a need to improve health worldwide as well as in our own country, especially in inner cities.

Looking at these necessities, I don't think we should deny the fact that we need more money for research and the improvement of the health systems. I think there has to be a mobilization for action at the political level.

LEVINS: I would like to respond to Laurie's question. The resource base for research on emerging infections and the improvement of the health systems has to be much broader then the resource base for medical research. It is an association of resources, material, and intellectual capacities, from agriculture, veterinary science, ecology, climatology, and so forth, which is needed. Part of it is the process of educating.

The real problem in science is that as budgets get tight, horizons narrow. We know already from our experiences that short horizon planning does not solve any problems, except in case the future will be exactly like the past. The more different the problems might be, the broader the perspective that is needed.

When I was a child, I saw an exhibit on animal behavior at the American Museum of Natural History. The first diorama showed a squid trying to get some food. But there was a transparent screen between this squid and the food. The squid was sort of pushing around. It was incapable of going around the screen. The second diorama showed a chicken. It was blocked by a 3-sided transparent screen. The chicken was able to walk around the edge because it didn't have to turn its back on the food. As long as it could keep its eye on its goal, it reached the food. The third diorama was that of a dog who was able to turn its back completely on the food and go around an obstacle because it could keep an image of where it was headed. The question remains: Is the research funding policy from different agencies more the result of a behavior similar to the squid or the chicken?

PATRICIA TESTER: As someone who has always faced very tight budgets for ecological research, even within the federal government, I could say that the charge Laurie mentioned has always been aimed at people in research. Whatever is proposed in terms of research is misunderstood as an excuse to generate more research dollars. You have to get adapted to that charge. In times of contracted funding you will find that research proposals become a lot more applied—and that is the same as narrowing our horizons. But, I have confidence in the system that the very best research does manage to survive at times like that.

There will be less research in the future and the research that is possible will be very applied for most of the people in this room. But, it will continue. Somehow we will manage to do what we have to do on the slim budget. With one hand we will do our best to fulfill the conditions of the contract for which we got the funding. With the other hand we will do our best to contribute to science and the progress of research, even if this research is not applied research. This is the current pattern.

REFERENCE

1. LEDERBERG, J., R. E. SHOPE & S. C. OAKS, JR., Eds. 1992. Emerging Infections. Microbial Threats to Health in the United States. Institute of Medicine. Washington, DC: National Academy Press.

Summary of Proposals for a Transdisciplinary Research Agenda on New and Emerging Infectious Diseases

The following summary represents a collection of written proposals made by participants of the Workshop on Emerging Diseases. All participants were asked to develop a list of research priorities and to share ideas for a conceptual framework. The proposals served as background materials for the final plenary session. The wide differences in the approaches and recommendations reflect the heterogeneity of the participants and the far-ranging scope of the issues. Many of the ideas expressed in this outline are discussed in other sections of this volume.

The list of proposals is included in this book to stimulate critical thinking about existing research agendas in the field of public health and epidemiology. This list outlines an initial working proposal for a research agenda to understand, model, and predict the evolution of infectious diseases. Questions and priorities are organized by area: ecology and policy, evolution, complexity, prediction, and surveillance.

I. PROPOSALS FOR A RESEARCH AGENDA

Ecology and Policy

- How will a shrinking globe result in spreading of endemic disease?
- Will infectious disease continue to follow the "epidemiological transition" outlined in the World Development Report?
- What are the expected and potential health effects of major environmental changes? How can these be examined? How can future health effects (humans, other animals, plants) be integrated at the planning stage of industrial, marine, and agricultural processes (*e.g.*, change in land use, building factories, other) that will change the environment?
- Preparation of geographic analyses of disease emergence and spread; analyze relationship to areas of ecological change and with routes of migration and trade.

Evolution

- Design an evolutionary framework:
  - study how infections can become severe or lethal,

- study easily transmitted diseases versus diseases with low transmission,
- model population dynamics of co-evolutionary relationships in complex ecological systems,
- study genetic structures of pathogens,
- study parameters of the immune system that cope with the disease,
- study the modes of adaptation between host and pathogen for human diseases versus diseases in mice, rabbits and other animals,
- search for and characterize orphan as well as pathogenic organisms,
- expand research on what allows a pathogen to cross species barriers and ecological niches.
- Develop methods for studying ecological interactions of infectious organisms and hosts:
  - develop other methods for prediction,
  - refine methods for assessing anthropogenic effects on emergence.
- Develop an ecological genetics.

Complexity

- Research the construction and use of mathematical models for dealing with complexity related to new disease:
  - construct data bases to support the model
- Develop methodologies that will link multiple factors, *e.g.,* biological, behavioral, and socio-economic, into structures that make qualitative and quantitative analyses possible.
- Define various levels of reality: molecular, biological, physicochemical, social, bio-social, cultural, economic, political.
- Define various levels of analyses:
  micro level: individual, networks, populations, communities
  macro level: societies, nations, global community:
  - investigate interactions between social events and vulnerability (impact of political/economic crises on emergence),
  - do prospective bio-social and bio-cultural studies on impact of ecological degradation on human health,
  - study social and cultural repercussions of disease emergence and their impact on the biological course of epidemics.

Prediction

Research questions/priorities:

- How can we predict the emergence of a new disease?
- How can we predict the emergence of a known disease?
- How can we increase our chances of noticing a new disease when it occurs?
- What steps should be taken after a new disease has been observed?

Once the research questions have been selected, determine what information is needed to answer the questions. This information will encompass many areas: history, biology, medicine, epidemiology and social, political and economic domains.

- Define the conditions that promote the emergence of new and the reemergence of old diseases:
  - explore, examine, and record previous instances of emergent diseases to identify general principles and factors that promote emergence,
  - examine how previous diseases were recognized and examine methods for facilitating recognition (*i.e.*, development of a responsive infrastructure to notice and report the unusual),
  - broaden our outlook on responses by considering disease rather than merely infection—this change of focus would allow the control of morbidity and mortality,
  - focus on ecological aspects of vulnerability,
  - focus on the consequences of whatever action we might decide to take.

Surveillance

Research questions/priorities:

- Develop a global surveillance and response system:
  - recognition of new diseases requires access to acutely ill patients,
  - this clinical capability must be accompanied by laboratory capacity to provide a specific etiologic diagnosis,
  - an epidemiological capacity has to be developed—to define the population at greatest risk, the mode of transmission, and the target for intervention,
  - recognition of new diseases must take on a global dimension; it can not be limited to a single geographic area or ethnic group,
  - central facilities must serve as a coordinator where requests for assistance are answered, reports of suspicious outbreaks are analyzed, and appropriate responses are organized,
  - a specific target disease should be used to develop the system, for example dengue fever.
- Develop an integrated epidemiology; this demands redefining concepts of surveillance on several levels:
  - vulnerability
  - surveillance/detection
  - response and collateral effects, evaluation of response
  - prediction
- Develop improved surveillance methods:
  - target ecosystems and vulnerable human populations (groups),
  - use remote sensing technologies,
  - establish a truly global data access system, including feed-back mechanisms to disseminate information,

- develop data networks that include water-borne, vector-borne, plant, animal, and human diseases.
- Develop an infrastructure for monitoring:
  - this infrastructure might include a scientific society or organization to help coordinate, integrate and support the required multi-disciplinary research,
  - such umbrella group could help to identify funding sources for the unique multi-disciplinary programs,
  - focused research projects should be designed to identify cost-effective, efficient and productive methodologies that allow us to monitor ecological and other changes that may lead to disease emergence.
- Specific studies might include:
  - infectious causes of "chronic diseases,"
  - development of rapid tests to identify drug resistance,
  - comparative evaluations of various inferences from strategies for emerging infections,
  - development of rapid techniques for the identification of infectious agents in food and water.
- Seafood monitoring
  - set up toxic algal monitoring as well as monitoring for fecal pollution by microorganisms,
  - combine epidemiologic studies with laboratory analyses to determine the role of seafood in transmitting diseases,
  - monitor specific algal blooms and determine trends over time,
  - determine the origins of toxic algal blooms by identifying the toxic species, studying their ecology, and identifying their toxins,
  - determine the role of bacteria in increasing toxic production in plankton,
  - increase surveillance of food- and water-borne diseases in developing as well as industrialized countries,
  - determine more sensitive and specific methods to detect pathogens in food, water, environmental and clinical specimens,
  - establish health hazard evaluation for specific pathogens and their vectors based on the infectious/toxigenic dose, the exposed population, the estimated numbers of annual cases, the severity of the illness, and the social and economic impact.

General Research Priorities

- Develop community grounded systems to provide local surveillance
- Extend social science research to develop better understanding of behavioral factors that increase vulnerability
- Involve evolutionary biologists in helping define range of possibilities
- Compile a list of emergent diseases over last 10–20 years:
  - give ecological characteristics,
  - describe pathogen, vectors and hosts,

- describe social conditions,
- identify the first reported cases (who, how, why),
- contrast the diseases across plants, animals, and humans.
• Replace the concept of "epidemiological transition" with the concept of the present as a period of massive ecological and social change that will give rise to new epidemiological problems.
• Integrate medical, veterinary and plant epidemiology.
• Develop an opportunistic system of awarding contracts or grants based on evidence of increasing risk of human disease

List of Workshop Participants

Name/Address	Phone/Fax/E-mail
1. Pamela Anderson Universidad Nacional Agraria ApartadoOR-8 Managua, Nicaragua	p.: (Sanidad Vegetal) 011-505-2-31505/ (private) 011-505-41-22115 f.: 011-505-2-31619 pamela@nicarao.apc.org
2. Tamara E. Awerbuch* Harvard School of Public Health Department of Population and International Health Building I-11th floor 665 Huntington Avenue Boston, MA 02115	p.: 617-432-0361 TAMAR@HSPH. HARVARD.EDU
3. Ruth L. Berkelman Deputy Director National Center for Infectious Diseases, CDC 1600 Clifton Road NE (C12) Atlanta, GA 30333	p.: 404-639-3945 f.: 404-639-3039 rlbl@cidodl.em.cdc.gov.
4. Agnes Brinkmann* c/o Lau Loskill Bunantstrasse 23 67549 Worms, Germany	p.: 011-06241 76482
5. Ralph T. Bryan National Center for Infectious Diseases, CDC c/o IHS-HQW, Epidemiology Branch 5300 Homestead Drive NE Albuquerque, NM 87110	p.: 505-837-4226 f.: 505-837-4181 rrb2@iddpd2.em.cdc.gov
6. Richard A. Cash* Harvard School of Public Health Department of Population and International Health Building I-11th floor 665 Huntington Avenue Boston, MA 02115	p.: 617-495-9791 f.: 617-566-0365

* Members of the Harvard Working Group on New Diseases.

Name/Address	Phone/Fax/E-mail

7. Lincoln Chen
Harvard School of Public Health
Department of Population and
International Health
Director, Building I-11th floor
665 Huntington Avenue
Boston, MA 02115

p.: 617-432-4615
f.: 617-566-0365

8. Rita R. Colwell
Maryland Biotechnology Institute
Office of the President
4321 Hartwick Road
Room 550
College Park, MD 20740

p.: 301-403-0501
f.: 301-454 8123
colwellr@mbi3.umd.edu

9. Madeline Drexler
74 A Russell Ave.
Watertown, MA 02172

p.: 617-924-4379
f.: 617-923-4956

10. Irina Eckardt*
Falkenberger Ch. 132 (0502)
Berlin D.13057 Germany

p.: 011-49-30-92-10077

11. Paul R. Epstein*
Harvard Medical School
The Cambridge Hospital
1493 Cambridge St.
Cambridge, MA 02139

p.: 617-498-1032
f.: 617-498-1671
PEPSTEIN@Igc.org

12. Harvey V. Fineberg
Harvard School of Public Health
Dean, SPH-3 1005
665 Huntington Avenue
Boston, MA 02115

p.: 617-432-1025
f.: 617-277-5320

13. Timothy E. Ford*
Harvard School of Public Health
Department of Environmental Health
Building I
665 Huntington Avenue
Boston, MA 02115

p.: 617-495-8351
f.: 617-495-5672
FORD@ENDOR.
HARVARD.EDU

14. Michel Garenne
Harvard School of Public Health
Department of Population and
International Health
Building I-11th floor
665 Huntington Avenue
Boston, MA 02115

p.: 617-432-0418
f.: 617-432-2181
mgarenne@HSPH.
Harvard.edu

* Members of the Harvard Working Group on New Diseases.

Name/Address	Phone/Fax/E-mail
15. Laurie Garrett *Newsday*/Science Section 235 Pinelawn Road Melville, NY 11747	p.: 1-800-Newsday x2954 f.: 516-843-2873
16. John W. Glasser National Immunization Program, CDC Mail-Stop E-61 1600 Clifton Road, NE Atlanta, Georgia 30333	p.: 404-639-8256 f.: 404-639-8615 JWG3@NIP.CDC.GOV
17. Anthony E. Kiszewski Harvard School of Public Health Tropical Public Health Room 508, Building I 665 Huntington Avenue Boston, MA 02115	p.: 617-432-2064 AKISZ@HSPH.Harvard.edu
18. Nicholas Komar Harvard School of Public Health Tropical Public Health Room 510, Building I 665 Huntington Avenue Boston, MA 02115	p.: 617-432-2064
19. James W. LeDuc World Health Organization CH 1211 Geneva 27 Switzerland	p.: 011-41-22-791-2111 f.: 011-41-22-788-2937
20. Richard Levins* Harvard School of Public Health Department of Population and International Health Building I-11th floor 665 Huntington Avenue Boston, MA 02115	p.: 617-432-1484
21. Stephen Lichtensteiger New York Academy of Sciences 2 East 63rd Street New York, NY 10021	

* Members of the Harvard Working Group on New Diseases.

Name/Address	Phone/Fax/E-mail

22. Najwa Makhoul*
Harvard University, OEB
26 Oxford Street MCZ
Cambridge MA 02138

p.: 617-432-1484
f.: 617-547-2441

23. Marilia Bernardes Marques
Oswaldo Cruz Foundation
Avenida Brasil 4036 Sala 715
Manguinhos 21040-361
Rio de Janeiro, Brazil

p.: 011-55-21-2605979
f.: 011-55-21-2609944

24. Leonardo Mata
Institute for Health Research
University of Costa Rica
Box 212
2100 Guadalupe, Costa Rica

p.: 011-506-257-1781
f.: 506-224-8167

25. Thomas P. Monath
ORAVAX Inc.
230 Albany Street
Cambridge, MA 02139

p.: 617-494-1339
f.: 617-494-1741

26. Stephen S. Morse
The Rockefeller University
1230 York Avenue
New York, NY 10021-6399

p.: 212-327-7722
f.: 212-327-7172
morse@rockvax.
rockefellr.edu

27. Cristina de A. Possas*
Escola Nacional de Saúde Pública
Fundação Oswaldo Cruz
Avenida Leopoldo Bulhões
1480 Manguinhos
CEP 21041-210
Rio de Janeiro, Brazil

f.: 011-55-21-2702116

28. Charles J. Puccia*
Union of Concerned Scientists
Two Brattle Square
Cambridge, MA 02238

p.: 617-547-5552
f.: 617-864-9405
c.puccia@igc.apc.org

29. Donald R. Roberts
PMB Department
USUHS
4301 Johns Bridge Road
Bethesda, MD 20814

p.: 301-295-3734
f.: 301-295-3860
ROBERTS@USUHSB.
USUHS.MIL

* Members of the Harvard Working Group on New Diseases.

Name/Address	Phone/Fax/E-mail

30. James Robins
Department of Epidemiology
Harvard School of Public Health
Kresge-8th floor
665 Huntington Avenue
Boston, MA 02115

p.: 617-432-0206
f.: 617-566-7805

31. Sonja Sandberg
Mathematics Department
Framingham State College
100 State Street
Framingham, MA 01701

p.: 508-626-4728
ssandberg@rcn.mass.
edu

32. Kenneth Sherman
US Department of Commerce
National Oceanic and Atmospheric
Administration
Northeast Fisheries Science Center
Narragansett Laboratory
28 Tarzwell Drive
Narragansett, RI 02882-1199

p.: 401-782-3210
f.: 401-782-3201

33. Robert E. Shope
Yale Arbovirus Research Unit
Box 3333
New Haven, CT 06510

p.: 203-785-4821
f.: 203-785-4782

34. Rudi Slooff
Division of Environmental Health
World Health Organization CH
1211 Geneva, Switzerland

p.: 011-41-22-7912111
f.: 011-41-22-7910746

35. Gary Smith
University of Pennsylvania
School of Veterinary Medicine
New Bolton Center
382 West Street Road
Kennett Square, PA 19348

p.: 215-444-5800
f.: 215-444-0126
GSMITH@nbc.upenn.edu

36. Johannes Sommerfeld
Applied Diarrheal Disease Research
Project, HIID
1 Eliot Street
Cambridge, MA 02138

p.: 617-495 9791
f.: 617-495 9706
ADDR@HUSC.Harvard.
edu

Name/Address	Phone/Fax/E-mail

37. Andrew Spielman*
Harvard School of Public Health
Tropical Public Health
Building I-5th floor
665 Huntington Avenue
Boston, MA 02115

p.: 617-432-2058
f.: 617-432-4914

38. Robert B. Tesh
Department of Epidemiology and
Public Health
School of Medicine
Yale University
P.O. Box 208034
New Haven, CT 06520-8034

p.: 203-785-2908
f.: 203-785-4782

39. Patricia A. Tester
National Marine Fisheries Service,
NOAA
Southeast Fisheries Science Center
110 Pivers Island Road
Beaufort, NC 28516

p.: 919-728-8792
f.: 919-728-8784

40. Ewen C. D. Todd
Health Protection Branch,
Department of Health
Sir Frederick G. Banting Research
Centre
Ross Avenue
Ottawa ON Canada K1A OL2

p.: 613-957-0887
f.: 613-952-6400

41. Mark L. Wilson
Department of Epidemiology and
Public Health
Yale University
School of Medicine
60 College Street
New Haven, CT 06520

p.: 203-785-2904
f.: 203-785-4782
mlwilson@Biomed.med.
Yale.edu

42. Mary E. Wilson*
Harvard Medical School and
Harvard School of Public Health
Division of Infectious Diseases
Mount Auburn Hospital
330 Mount Auburn Street
Cambridge, MA 02238

p.: 617-499-5026
f.: 617-499-5495

* Members of the Harvard Working Group on New Diseases.

43. Paul H. Wise*
Harvard Institute for Reproductive
& Child Health
221 Longwood Avenue
Boston, MA 02115

p.: 617-278-0098
f.: 617-732-4151
wise@jpnepil.bwh.
harvard.edu

44. George Woodwell
Woods Hole Research Center
13 Church St.
Woods Hole, MA 02543

45. John B. Wyon
143 Fairway Road
Chestnut Hill, MA 02167

* Members of the Harvard Working Group on New Diseases.

Glossary

Advanced Very High Resolution Radiometer (AVHRR): Multispectral sensor (*e.g.*, red and infrared radiation) aboard NOAA satellite

Agenda 21: Document on environmental policies for the 21st century derived from UNCED

Algae (blue green, other): Plankton containing chlorophyll; the primary producers of organic compounds and energy in the marine food web

Allele: One of a pair or series of genes, occupying a particular chromosomal site

Amnesic shellfish poisoning (ASP): Gastroenteritis and central nervous system damage, sometimes permanent or leading to death, from domoic acid, an amino acid produced by a diatom

Anthropogenesis/anthropogenic: Caused by humans

Anthroponosis/anthroponotic: Humans are only natural host for pathogen

Anthropophilic: Preference of insect to feed on humans rather than nonhuman hosts

Aquaculture: The cultivation of plants and animals in water

Arboviruses: Arthropod-borne viruses

Arthropod: Invertebrate animals with chitinous exoskeleton and segmented body; includes insects, crustaceans (including copepods), arachnids, and myripods

Autochthonous: Native to place; indigenous

Axenic: Free of contaminants

Bathymetry: Measurement of depth of large bodies of water

Benthos/benthic: Organisms living on, near or in the bottom sediments of bodies of water

Bight: A bay with a headland at each end; usually fairly shallow

Bioaccumulate: Accumulation of chemicals (*e.g.*, toxins) in organisms with increasing concentration along a food chain

Biological transmission by an arthropod: Transmission of a pathogen by an arthropod in which the pathogen develops or multiplies. *See also mechanical transmission.*

Biomass flips: When a dominant species or group of species rapidly drops to a low level and is succeeded by another species or groups of species, *e.g.*, from over-harvesting

Biomass yield: Amount of living matter produced in milligrams of carbon per unit volume per unit of time

Biotic factor: Produced or caused by living organisms; as opposed to geological (physical) or chemical

Biotic potential: Likelihood of survival of a specific organism in a specific environment

Biotoxin: Toxic substance produced by a living organism

Biovar: Biological variant

Blooms: Excessive planktonic growth in a body of water

Blue-green algae: Cyanobacteria, thought (on the basis of 3.456 billion year old Australian fossil records) to be the first chlorophyllic organism to have evolved

Brevetoxin: Toxin from *Gymnodinum breve* causing neurological shellfish poisoning (NSP)

Bridge vector: An arthropod that carries a pathogen to human or veterinary hosts but that does not contribute to the perpetuation of the pathogen in nature.

CCAMLR: Convention for the Conservation of Antarctic Marine Living Resources; 21 nation membership

477

Chitinaceous and mucilaginous macrobiota: Multi-celled organisms with chitinous or mucilaginous exteriors

Chitinase: Enzyme that breaks down chitin

CIAT: Centro International de Agricultural Tropical

Coastal Zone Color Scanner (CZCS): Remote sensor aboard Nimbus-7 NOAA satellite; collected data worldwide 1979–1986

Copepod: The most numerous marine and fresh water crustaceans (arthropods) >6000 species; filter feeders; some herbivores, others carnivores

Cosmology: Branch of philosophy dealing with the origin, processes, and structure of the universe

CPR: Continuous plankton recorder, begun by Hardy in 1936; dragged behind ships

CULPAD: CUltivated Plant ADapted

Cyanobacteria: Formerly blue-green algae

Diarrheic shellfish poisoning (DSP): Diarrhea from shellfish contaminated with okadaic acid, produced by several dinoflagellates

Diatom: Unicellular algae with yellow-brown pigments, chlorophyll and a siliceous cell wall or "test," associated with nitrogen-fixing bacteria

Digraphs: A branch of mathematics that represents matrix relationships with vertices connected by lines, called graph theory, becomes digraph theory when the lines have a direction, usually indicated with an arrow. Signed digraphs are digraphs with either a positive or negative sign associated with the arrow.

Dinoflagellate: Unicellular plankton (<1 mm), most containing chlorophyll; flagella provide locomotion; "armored" dinoflagellates are found near shore, "naked" occur in open seas; primary producers in marine ecosystems

Dinophysis **toxin:** Dinoflagellate-derived toxin causing diarrheic shellfish poisoning

Diploid: A condition in which the nuclear genetic alleles of an organism are present in pairs

Domoic acid: Excito-toxic amino acid produced by a diatom; causes gastroenteritis and central nervous system damage, including amnesia

Ecosystem: Organization of organisms and their natural environment; a community of organisms and their abiotic environment

Ecosystem health: Defined by stability, resilience, biodiversity, productivity and yields of an ecosystem

EEZ: Exclusive economic zone

Elasmobranchs: Fish with plate-like gills, including sharks, rays, skates, dogfish; hunted for oil

El Niño: An irregularly occurring outward current in the equatorial Pacific Ocean, associated with weather changes and ecological damage

Environmental Management of Enclosed Coastal Seas (EMECS)

Enzootic: Affecting animals of a specific area

Epifluorescence microscopy: The final step in a serological technique for diagnosing pathogens that uses ultraviolet illumination directed through a prism located in the objective of a microscope

Epistemology: Division of philosophy that investigates the nature and origin of knowledge; a theory of the nature of knowledge

Epizootic: Involving large number of animals simultaneously

Eutrophication: Process involving increase in mineral and organic nutrients leading to reduced dissolved oxygen, producing an environment that favors plant over animal life

Exclusive Economic Zone (EEZ)

Extrinsic incubation: The phase of development of a vector-borne pathogen of vertebrate animals that takes place in the vector

Filter-feeding: Filtering and ingestion by an organism of nutrient matter suspended in water

Geographic information system (GIS): A computerized relational database in which information is recorded and displayed on digitized maps

Germ plasm: 1. cytoplasm of germ cell; 2. hereditary material; genes

Gyre systems: A circular pattern of surface currents round an ocean basin.

Global Environment Facility (GEF)

GLOBal ocean ECosystems dynamics (GLOBEC)

Global Ocean Observing System (GOOS)

GLOBEC: Global ocean ecosystems dynamics

GOOS: Global ocean observing system

Ha: *See hectare.*

Haploid: Containing a single set of unpaired chromosomes

Hectare: Equivalent to 10,000 sq meters; 2.477 acres

Hemagglutination-inhibition test: A serological technique for diagnosing infection that depends upon the tendency of red blood cells to attach to common particles

Herd immunity: Resistance of a group to invasion and spread of an infectious agent based on the resistance to infection of a high proportion of the individuals in the group.

Heterotrophic: Obtaining nourishment from organic substances

Heterozygote: An individual having different alleles at one or more genetic loci

Horizontal transmission: Transmission between organisms (vertical transmission refers to transmission between generations)

HPLC: High pressure liquid chromatography

Hydrography: The description and study of bodies of water; the measurement of flow and the investigation of streams

Iatrogenic: Induced unintentionally by a physician's treatment or examination

Ichthyoplankton: Fish eggs and larvae

ICES: International Council for the Exploration of the Sea

ICSEM: International Council for the Scientific Exploration of the Mediterranean Sea

Infection (in contrast to disease): The entry and development or multiplication of an infectious agent in the body of humans, other animals, or plants

Infestation: For persons and animals, the lodgment, development and reproduction of arthropods on the surface of the body or in the clothing.

Intergovernmental Oceanographic Commission: IOC

International Council for the Scientific Exploration of the Mediterranean Sea (ICSEM)

International Union for Conservation of Nature and Natural Resources (UUCN): Old definition. See IUCN.

Intrinsic incubation: The phase of development of a vector-borne pathogen that takes place in the vertebrate host

Introgression: The transfer of genetic information from one species to another following the elimination of reproductive barriers between partially or fully interfertile populations of sexual organisms or, in plants, as the result of hybridization between them and repeated back crossing

IUCN: The World Conservation Union

JGOFS: Joint Global Flux Study, oceanographic component of the International Geosphere-Biosphere Program to study carbon flux in the oceans. Field studies began in 1989.

Large marine ecosystems (LME): Extensive areas of ocean space of approximately 200,000 km² or greater, characterized by distinct bathymetry, hydrography, productivity, and trophically dependent populations.

Limnology: Scientific study of the life and phenomena of lakes, ponds, and streams

Macroalgae: Multi-cellular algae >500 μm.

Marine food web: Organisms of various trophic levels and nutrients and energy utilized by them

Mechanical transmission by arthropod: Transmission of a pathogen by an arthropod that carries the pathogen transiently on its surface or in its gut (no development or multiplication of the pathogen). *See also biological transmission.*

Menhaden: An abundant, herring-like, inedible fish; primarily gets processed as fish meal and oil for animal feed

Microalgae: Algae 50–500 μm size range

Microcosm cultures: Cultures developed in a scaled-down community, representative of a larger community

MT: metric ton

Multispectral satellite data: Remote sensing data from many channels taking data over different wave lengths of emitted or reflected radiation

Multistable ecosystems: Dynamic states of ecosystems; conditions within an ecosystem in which the distribution and abundance of organisms can have more than one equilibrium.

National Oceanic and Atmospheric Administration (NOAA)

Natural Environment Research Council (NERC)

Neap tides: Weak tides produced when the sun and moon positions partially oppose each other's gravitational pull, resulting in the least difference between high and low tides.

Neurotoxic shellfish poisoning (NSP): Result of a toxin in contaminated shellfish that affects the nerves or nervous system

NOAA/NMFS: National Marine Fishery Service

Normalized difference vegetation index (NDVI): Measure of vegetation calculated by a ratio and red and infrared wave lengths as taken by remote sensors, such as AVHRR

Nosocomial: Arising while a patient is in a hospital or as a result of being in a hospital

Nosology: Classification of diseases

Nutrient loading: Enrichment of waters with inorganic material, including nitrogen and phosphorous, and organic material

Ocean Studies Related to Living Resources (OSLR)

Okadaic acid: A newly identified toxin produced by species of the dinoflagellate genus *Dinophysis*; causes diarrheic shellfish poisoning (DSP)

Ornithophilic: Person or other organism that loves birds; among vectors, the tendency to feed most frequently on birds

Palustrine: Of or relating to wetlands

Pathogenicity: The capacity to cause disease

Pelagic current systems: Open seas or oceanic current systems

Petrogenic hydrocarbons: Hydrocarbons isolated or derived from petroleum and natural gas

Phenotypes: Visible properties of an organism produced by the interaction of the genotype and the environment

Photosynthetically active radiation (PAR): Spectrum of ultraviolet radiation used in photosynthesis; 400 to 700 nm

Phycotoxin: Toxin produced by algae

Phytoplankton: Passively floating or weakly swimming minute plant life in a body of water

Planktivores: Organisms that use plankton for primary food source

Plankton (*also zooplankton, phytoplankton*): Passively floating or weakly swimming minute animal or plant life in a body of water

Psychrophilic: Thriving at low temperatures

Red tides: Sea water discolored by the presence of large numbers of dinoflagellates (especially in *Goynaulax* and *Gymnodinium*) that produce toxins poisonous to many forms of marine life and to humans who consume contaminated shellfish

Remote sensing: The gathering of information at a distance from the subject studied; often the observation of the earth's land and water bodies by means of reflected or emitted electromagnetic radiation; the resulting data generally are stored in a computerized relational database displayed on digitized maps

Reservoir host: Hosts in which viable infectious agents remain and from which infection of individuals may occur

River runoff plumes: Nutrient or contaminated plumes of rivers running into estuarine and marine waters

Sand lance: Small marine fish with slender body and forked tail fin; often burrows in sand of tidelands

Saxitoxin: A toxic alkaloid which is synthesized by the dinoflagellates responsible for red tides. Accumulates in mollusks which feed on these dinoflagellates.

Sea-Viewing Wide Field Sensor (Sea-WiFS)

Serologic diagnosis: Identifying current or past infection by testing serum for immune responses induced by pathogens and other antigens

South Atlantic Bight: Large estuarine area

Stochastic: Events that occur with irregular patterns

Toroidal: Ring-shaped with a circular cross-section

Transmission by vector. See biological and mechanical transmission

Transovarial transmission: Passage of a pathogen from a maternal host to the offspring via the egg. *See also horizontal and vertical transmission.*

Trophic levels: A feeding stratum in a food chain of an ecosystem characterized by organisms that occupy a similar functional position in the ecosystem

Ungulate: A hoofed animal

United Nations Convention for the Law of the Sea (UNCLOS)

United Nations Environment Program (UNEP)

Upwelling intensity: Movement of water mass depends on 1) deep currents that meet a mid-ocean ridge and deflect water upward; 2) separation of two contiguous water masses, as along the equator; 3) wind action that drives water masses away from the coastline. When this occurs along a coast with a small continental shelf, the deep ocean waters are sucked to the surface. The last factor is the most significant in many cases of upwelling of bottom waters.

Upwelling of nutrients: The transport of water from deep ocean to the photic zone, which are areas where photosynthesis can occur.

Vector: An organism, such as a mosquito or tick, that carries a pathogen from one host to another. *See also bridge vector.*

Vector competence: The ability of a vector to serve as a biological host for a pathogen. Includes parameters representing the proportion of vectors becoming infected after contact with an infectious reservoir host as well as the quantity of pathogens later transferred to another reservoir host.

Vector reproductive host: The animal on which a vector must feed in order to reproduce.

Vectorial capacity: The ability of a vector to carry a pathogen in nature between reservoir hosts. Described mathematically by an equation that includes entomological variables that contribute to the basic reproduction number of the infection.

Vertical transmission: Passage of an infection from a parental host, usually the mother, to the offspring. *See also horizontal transmission and transovarial transmission.*

Viremia: The presence of a virus in the blood

Virulence: The relative capacity of a microbe to cause to disease; degree of pathogenicity

Virus sink: A host that is frequently bitten by a vector but that is noncompetent for an arbovirus transmitted by that vector. The presence of such hosts powerfully inhibits the force of transmission. *See also zooprophylaxis.*

WILPAD: WILd Plant ADapted
Woods Hole Oceanographic Institute (WHOI)

Zoonosis: Disease that can be transmitted from animals to humans. Natural host is an animal, usually vertebrate.

Zooprophylaxis: A host that is frequently bitten by a vector but that is noncompetent for a pathogen transmitted by that vector. The presence of such hosts, powerfully inhibits the force of transmission. *See virus sink.*

Zooplankton: Animals or heterotrophs inhabiting the water columns, whose large-scale dispersement depends on the currents, with only small, local movements under their own locomotion. Typical organisms include copepods, euphausids, jellyfish, and amphipods.

Subject Index

Index of Contributors[a]

[a] Numbers in italics indicate comments made in discussions.